C000295396

H...

This

WITHDRAWN

DATE:

CANCELLED 2 9 AUG 2007

With the unlimited educational grant of 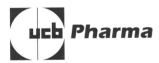 **ucb Pharma**

UCB S.A. Pharma Sector – Allée de la Recherche 60, B-1070 Brussels, Belgium

Springer

Berlin
Heidelberg
New York
Barcelona
Hong Kong
London
Milan
Paris
Singapore
Tokyo

J.-Y. REGINSTER · J.-P. PELLETIER
J. MARTEL-PELLETIER · Y. HENROTIN

Osteoarthritis

Clinical and Experimental Aspects

With editorial assistance by L. CRASBORN

With 92 Figures

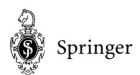 Springer

PROF. J.-Y. REGINSTER, MD, PhD
Department of Epidemiology
and Public Health
University of Liège
CHU Sart-Tilman B23
B-4000 Liège
Belgium

PROF. J.-P. PELLETIER, MD, PhD
PROF. J. MARTEL-PELLETIER, PhD
Osteoarthritis Research Unit
Centre de Recherche L.C. Simard
Centre Hospitalier de l'Université
de Montréal
Campus Notre-Dame
1560 Sherbrooke St. East
Montréal
Québec H2L 4M1
Canada

Y. HENROTIN, PhD
Bone and Cartilage Metabolim
Research Unit
Department of Physical Medicine
Institute of Pathology (+5)
University of Liège
CHU Sart-Tilman B23
B-4000 Liège
Belgium

L. CRASBORN, MD
UCB s.a. Global Marketing
Allée de la Recherche 60
B-1070 Brussels
Belgium

ISBN 3-540-65127-6 Springer-Verlag Berlin Heidelberg New York

Library of Congress Cataloging-in-Publication Data
Osteoarthritis. Clinical and Experimental Aspects / [edited by]
J.-Y. Reginster ... [et al.] ; with editorial assistance by L.
Crasborn.
  p. cm.
Includes bibliographical references and index.
ISBN 3540651276 (softcover)
1. Osteoarthritis. I. Reginster, Jean-Yves.
RC931.O67 E96 1999
616.7'.223-dc21   98-33430

© Springer-Verlag Berlin Heidelberg 1999
Printed in Italy

The use of general descriptive names, registered names, trademarks, etc. in this publication does not imply, even in the absence of a specific statement, that such names are exempt from the relevant protective laws and regulations and free for general use.
Product liability: The publishers cannot guarentee the accuracy of any information about dosage and application contained in this book. In every individual case the user must check such information by consulting the relevant literature.

Coverdesign: Design & Production GmbH, Heidelberg
Typesetting: Fotosatz-Service Köhler GmbH, Würzburg
SPIN: 10668389   22/3134-5 4 3 2 1 0 – Printed on acid-free paper

Preface

Musculoskeletal diseases are rapidly becoming a major health concern. The incidence of osteoarthritis, the most common arthritic disorder, is increasing steadily due to the graying of the world population. This disease is responsible for significant morbidity, particularly in the second half of human life, a time in which the quality of life is of primary importance. The aim of this publication is to bring to physicians and scientists a comprehensive overview of the field, from molecules to men.

The direct costs related to osteoarthritis have been increasing steadily over the years and will soon be comparable to those of other major illnesses, such as cardiovascular diseases. This, of course, does not take into account all of the other costs related to the disease which often cannot be simply calculated in dollars and cents.

There has been a great deal of renewed interest in osteoarthritis in the last few decades. This has been brought on by the need to improve our knowledge of all aspects of the disease, especially with regard to its etiopathogenesis and treatment. The most recent findings and developments on the structural, biochemical, biomechanical and molecular changes observed in clinical and experimental osteoarthritis are presented in this book.

Each chapter highlights the most recent progress made with respect to the understanding of the different mechanisms involved in inducing the structural changes characteristic of the disease. The relevance of experimental models to explore with great detail and precision the very early stages of osteoarthritis and to study cartilage response damage and repair is also reviewed. Several interesting developments have recently occurred with regard to the exploration of the different clinical aspects of the disease. Dimensions of the disease which were long ignored, such as its economic aspects and its impact on the daily life style of the patient, are now receiving much more attention, in part because of the practical implications for the administration of health care programs in industrialized countries around the world.

This review also focuses on recent developments of the imaging techniques used to evaluate osteoarthritic structural changes. Several advances have brought forth new technologies that enable not only the evaluation of the progression of the disease over time, but also allow evaluation of the effectiveness of treatment on the structural changes of osteoarthritis.

The development of new treatments for osteoarthritis has experienced a broad expansion in many ways. The advent of several new drugs has forced the improvement of protocols to accurately evaluate their efficacy. Many of these advances have been made possible through the collaboration of multidisciplinary groups, which has allowed a comprehensive approach. Substantial progress has been made, for instance, in the development of accurate and sensitive tools to evaluate the impact of the disease and its treatment on the quality of life of patients. Recent advances in the understanding of the pathophysiological mechanisms of osteoarthritis have allowed for the development of new agents and drugs, some of which we hope will be found to have structurally protective effects vis-à-vis the disease process. Some very challenging and exciting years lie ahead of us in this field.

Progress in the field of osteoarthritis has been the result of fruitful collaborations among physicians, scientists, epidemiologists and people from many other areas of expertise. We wish to sincerely thank them for their excellent contributions and their dedication. The future looks brighter than ever now that a cure for osteoarthritis may be within reach.

J.-Y. REGINSTER
J.-P. PELLETIER
J. MARTEL-PELLETIER
Y. HENROTIN

Contents

1 Structure and Function of Normal Human Adult Articular Cartilage ... 1
E. J-M. A. THONAR, K. MASUDA, D.H MANICOURT,
and K. E. KUETTNER

2 Epidemiology and Economic Consequences of Osteoarthritis 20

2.1 The American Viewpoint 20
J. C. SCOTT, M. LETHBRIDGE-CEJKU, and M.C. HOCHBERG

2.2 The European Viewpoint 38
X. BADIA LLACH

3 Experimental Models of Osteoarthritis 53

3.1 *In Vitro* Models for the Study of Cartilage Damage and Repair 53
Y. HENROTIN and J.-Y. REGINSTER

3.2 Animal Models of Osteoarthritis 81
K. D. BRANDT

4 Pathophysiology of Osteoarthritis 101

4.1 Role of Mechanical Factors in the Aetiology, Pathogenesis
and Progression of Osteoarthritis 101
G. NUKI

4.2 Role of Biomechanical Factors 115
P. GHOSH

4.3 Genetic and Metabolic Aspects 134
C. J. WILLIAMS and S. A. JIMENEZ

4.4 Biochemical Factors in Joint Articular Tissue Degradation
in Osteoarthritis 156
J. MARTEL-PELLETIER, J. DI BATTISTA, and D. LAJEUNESSE

4.5   Role of Growth Factors and Cartilage Repair 188
      W. B. VAN DEN BERG, P. M. VAN DER KRAAN,
      and H. M. VAN BEUNINGEN

4.6   Role of Crystal Deposition in the Osteoarthritic Joint 210
      G. M. McCARTHY

5   Diagnosis and Monitoring of Osteoarthritis 228

5.1   Direct Visualization of the Cartilage 228
      X. AYRAL and M. DOUGADOS

5.2   Radiographic Imaging of Osteoarthritis 246
      C. BUCKLAND-WRIGHT

5.3   Magnetic Resonance Imaging in Osteoarthritis 268
      Y. JIANG, C. G. PETERFY, J. J. ZHAO, D. L. WHITE, J. A. LYNCH,
      and H. K. GENANT

5.4   The Role of Molecular Markers to Monitor Breakdown and Repair   296
      L. S. LOHMANDER

6   Evolution and Prognosis of Osteoarthritis 312
      E. VEYS and G. VERBRUGGEN

7   Impact of Osteoarthritis on Quality of Life 331
      J. POUCHOT, J. COSTE, and F. GUILLEMIN

8   Medical Management of Osteoarthritis 356

8.1   Medical Aspects 356
8.1.1 Basic Principles in Osteoarthritis Treatment 356
      D. CHOQUETTE, J.-P. RAYNAULD, and E. RICH

8.1.2 Non-steroidal Anti-inflammatory Drug Administration
      in the Treatment of Osteoarthritis 370
      J. T. DINGLE

8.1.3 New and Future Therapies for Osteoarthritis 387
      J.-P. PELLETIER, B. HARAOUI, and J. C. FERNANDES

8.2   Regulatory Requirements 408
8.2.1 Preclinical Studies in Osteoarthritis 408
      M. SISAY and R. D. ALTMAN

8.2.2 Clinical Evaluation of Drug Therapy 421
      J.-Y. REGINSTER, B. AVOUAC, and C. GOSSET

9   **Surgical Treatment of the Cartilage Injuries** 431
M. BRITTBERG

10 **Scientific Basis of Physical Therapy and Rehabilitation
in the Management of Patients with Osteoarthritis** 453
J-M. CRIELAARD and Y. HENROTIN

11 **Conclusion and Perspectives** 480
M. LEQUESNE and L. PUNZI

Subject Index 511

Contributors

R. D. Altman
Rheumatology and Immunology,
Department of Medicine,
University of Miami School of Medicine,
and Geriatric Research, Education
and Clinical Center (GRECC),
Miami Veterans Affairs Medical Center,
Miami VAMC (NH207G),
Miami, FL 33125, USA
(e-mail: raltman@mednet.med.miami.edu)

B. Avouac
Department of Rheumatology,
Hôpital Henri Mondor, Creteil, France

X. Ayral
Department of Rheumatology,
Cochin Hospital, René Descartes University,
Service de Rhumatologie B,
27 rue du Faubourg Saint Jacques,
75679 Paris Cedex 14, France

X. Badia Llach
Catalan Institute of Public Health,
University of Barcelona, Campus de
Bellvitge, Ctra. de la Feixa Llarga s/n 08907
L'Hospitalet de Llobregat, Spain
(e-mail: xbadia@bell.ub.es)

K. D. Brandt
Rheumatology Division, Indiana University
School of Medicine and Indiana University
Multipurpose Arthritis and Musculoskeletal
Diseases Center, 541 Clinical Drive, Room
492, Indianapolis, IN 46202-5103, USA

M. Brittberg
Cartilage Research Unit,
Göteborg University, Department
of Orthopaedics, Kunsgsbacka Hospital,
S-43440 Kungsbacka, Sweden (e-mail:
mats.brittberg@varberg.mail.telia.com)

C. Buckland-Wright
Division of Anatomy and Cell Biology,
United Medical and Dental Schools of Guy's
and St. Thomas's Hospitals, London Bridge,
London SE1 9 RT, UK
(e-mail: c.bucklandw@umds.ac.uk)

D. Choquette
Rheumatic Disease Unit, Centre Hospitalier
de l'Université de Montréal,
Campus Notre-Dame, 1560 Sherbrooke
St. East, Montréal, Québec, H2L 4M1
Canada

J. Coste
Département de Biostatistique,
Hôpital Cochin, Paris, France

J-M. Crielaard
Bone and Cartilage Metabolim Research
Unit, Department of Physical Medicine,
Institute of Pathology, University
of Liège, CHU Sart-Tilman, 4000 Liège,
Belgium

J. Di Battista
Osteoarthritis Research Unit, Centre de
Recherche L.C. Simard, Centre Hospitalier
de l'Université de Montréal,
Campus Notre-Dame, 1560 Sherbrooke
St. East, Montréal, Québec, H2L 4M1
Canada

J. T. Dingle
Cambridge Research Laboratories, 13 Adam
Road, Cambridge CB3 9AD, UK

M. Dougados
Department of Rheumatology,
Cochin Hospital, René Descartes University,
Paris, France

J. C. FERNANDES
Osteoarthritis Research Unit, Centre de
Recherche L.C. Simard, Centre Hospitalier
de l'Université de Montréal, Campus
Notre-Dame, Montréal, Québec, Canada

H. K. GENANT
Osteoporosis and Arthritis Research Group
and Muskuloskeletal Section, Department
of Radiology, University of California,
San Francisco, CA, USA
(e-mail : Harry.Genant@oarg.ucsf.edu)

P. GHOSH
Raymond Purves Bone and Joint Research
Laboratories, Department of Surgery,
University of Sydney, Royal North Shore
Hospital, St. Leonards, NSW 2065, Australia
(e-mail : pghosh@mail.usyd.edu.au)

C. GOSSET
Department of Epidemiology and Public
Health, University of Liège, Liège, Belgium

F. GUILLEMIN
Ecole de Santé Publique, Faculté de
Médecine, 9, avenue de la Forêt de Haye,
BP 184, 54505 Vandoeuvre Cedex, France
(e-mail : guillemi@sante-pub.u-nancy.fr)

B. HARAOUI
Osteoarthritis Research Unit, Centre de
Recherche L.C. Simard, Centre Hospitalier
de l'Université de Montréal,
Campus Notre-Dame, Montréal, Québec,
Canada

Y. HENROTIN
Bone and Cartilage Metabolism Research
Unit, Department of Physical Medicine,
Institute of Pathology (+5), University of
Liège, CHU Sart-Tilman B23, 4000 Liège,
Belgium

M. C. HOCHBERG
Division of Rheumatology and Clinical
Immunology, Department of Medicine,
and Department of Epidemiology
and Preventive Medicine, University of
Maryland School of Medicine, Gerontology
Research Center, National Institute on
Aging, Geriatric Research Education and
Clinical Center, Veterans Affairs Medical
Center, 10 South Pine St., MSTF 8-34,
Baltimore, MD 21201, USA

Y. JIANG
Osteoporosis and Arthritis Research Group
and Muskuloskeletal Section, Department
of Radiology, University of California, 513
Parnassus Avenue, Suite HSW207A,
San Francisco, CA 94143-0628, USA
(e-mail : Yebin.Jiang@oarg.ucsf.edu)

S. A. JIMENEZ
Department of Medicine, Division of
Rheumatology, Thomas Jefferson Univer-
sity, 233 South Tenth Street, Philadelphia,
PA 19107, USA
(e-mail : Sergio.Jimenez@mail.tju.edu)

K. E. KUETTNER
Departments of Biochemistry
and Orthopedic Surgery, Rush Medical
College at Rush-Presbyterian-St. Luke's
Medical Center, Chicago, USA

D. LAJEUNESSE
Osteoarthritis Research Unit,
Centre de Recherche L.C. Simard, Centre
Hospitalier de l'Université de Montréal,
Campus Notre-Dame, 1560 Sherbrooke
St. East, Montréal, Québec, H2L 4M1
Canada

M. LEQUESNE
Department of Rheumatology, Hôpital
Léopold Bellan, 19 rue Vercingétorix,
75014 Paris, France
(e-mail : mlequesne@aol.com)

M. LETHBRIDGE-CEJKU
Division of Rheumatology and Clinical
Immunology, Department of Medicine,
and Department of Epidemiology
and Preventive Medicine, University of
Maryland School of Medicine,
Gerontology Research Center,
National Institute on Aging, Baltimore,
MD, USA

L. S. LOHMANDER
Department of Orthopedics, University
Hospital, SE-22185 Lund, Sweden
(e-mail : Stefan.Lohmander@ort.lu.se)

J. A. LYNCH
Osteoporosis and Arthritis Research Group
and Muskuloskeletal Section,
Department of Radiology, University of
California, San Francisco, CA, USA

D. H. MANICOURT
Service de Rhumatologie, Université Catholique de Louvain, Cliniques Universitaires St Luc, Brussels, Belgium

J. MARTEL-PELLETIER
Osteoarthritis Research Unit, Centre de Recherche L.C. Simard, Centre Hospitalier de l'Université de Montréal, Campus Notre-Dame, 1560 Sherbrooke St. East, Montréal, Québec, H2L 4M1 Canada

K. MASUDA
Departments of Biochemistry and Orthopedic Surgery, Rush Medical College at Rush-Presbyterian-St. Luke's Medical Center, Chicago, USA

G. MCCARTHY
Department of Clinical Pharmacology, Royal College of Surgeons in Ireland, 123 St. Stephen's Green, Dublin 2, Ireland (e-mail : gmccarthy@rcsi.ie)

G. NUKI
University of Edinburgh Rheumatic Diseases Unit, Department of Medicine, Western General Hospital, Crewe Road South, Edinburgh EH4 2XU, Scotland, UK (e-mail : gn@srvO.med.ed.ac.uk)

J.-P. PELLETIER
Rheumatic Disease Unit and Osteoarthritis Research Unit, Centre de Recherche L.C. Simard, Centre Hospitalier de l'Université de Montréal, Campus Notre-Dame, 1560 Sherbrooke St. East, Montréal, Québec, H2L 4M1 Canada

C. G. PETERFY
Osteoporosis and Arthritis Research Group and Muskuloskeletal Section, Department of Radiology, University of California, San Francisco, CA, USA

J. POUCHOT
Service de Médecine Interne, Hôpital Louis Mourier, 178 rue des Renouillers, 92700 Colombes, and Inserm U.292, Hôpital de Bicêtre, 82, rue du Général Leclercq, 94275 Le Kremlin Bicêtre Cedex, France (e-mail : pouchot@ext.jussieu.fr)

L. PUNZI
Division of Rheumatology, University of Padova, via Giustiniani 2, 35128 Padova, Italy

J-P. RAYNAULD
Rheumatic Disease Unit, Centre Hospitalier de l'Université de Montréal, Campus Notre-Dame, Montréal, Québec, Canada

J.-Y. REGINSTER
Bone and Cartilage Metabolism Research Unit, and Department of Epidemiology and Public Health, University of Liège, CHU Sart-Tilman B23, 4000 Liège, Belgium, and Georgetown University Medical Center, Washington DC, USA.

J. RICH
Rheumatic Disease Unit, Centre Hospitalier de l'Université de Montréal, Campus Notre-Dame, Montréal, Québec, Canada

M. SISAY
Rheumatology and Immunology, Department of Medicine, University of Miami School of Medecine, Miami, FL, USA

J. C. SCOTT
Division of Rheumatology and Clinical Immunology, Department of Medicine, and Department of Epidemiology and Preventive Medicine, University of Maryland School of Medicine, Baltimore, MD, USA

E. J-M. A. THONAR
Departments of Biochemistry, Internal Medicine (Section Rheumatology) and Orthopedic Surgery, Rush Medical College at Rush-Presbyterian-St. Luke's Medical Center, 1653 West Congress Parkway, Chicago IL 60612, USA (e-mail : ethonar@rush.edu)

H. M. VAN BEUNINGEN
Department of Rheumatology, University Hospital St Radboud, 6500 HB Nijmegen, The Netherlands

W. B. VAN DEN BERG
Department of Rheumatology, University Hospital St Radboud, Geert Groteplein Zuid 8, PO Box 9101, 6500 HB Nijmegen, The Netherlands (e-mail : w.vandenberg@reuma.azn.nl)

P. M. van der Kraan
Department of Rheumatology,
University Hospital St Radboud,
6500 HB Nijmegen, The Netherlands

G. Verbruggen
Department of Rheumatology,
University of Ghent, University Hospital
of Ghent, De Pintelaan 185, B-9000 Ghent,
Belgium

E. M. Veys
Department of Rheumatology,
University of Ghent, University Hospital
of Ghent, De Pintelaan 185, B-9000 Ghent,
Belgium

D. L. White
Osteoporosis and Arthritis Research Group
and Muskuloskeletal Section, Department
of Radiology, University of California, San
Francisco, CA, USA

C. J. Williams
Department of Medicine, Division of
Rheumatology, Thomas Jefferson
University, 233 South Tenth Street,
Philadelphia, PA 19107, USA
(e-mail : Charlene.Williams@mail.tju.edu)

J. J. Zhao
Osteoporosis and Arthritis Research
Group and Muskuloskeletal Section,
Department of Radiology, University of
California, San Francisco, CA, USA

CHAPTER 1

Structure and Function of Normal Human Adult Articular Cartilage

E. J-M. A. THONAR, K. MASUDA, D. H. MANICOURT and K. E. KUETTNER

1.1
Introduction

Synovial (diarthrodial) joints facilitate mobility by allowing bones to articulate with one another. In synovial joints, the bones are covered by hyaline articular cartilage: a viscoelastic tissue that cushions and thus minimizes the forces that the non-deformable bones are subjected to during load bearing. Each synovial joint contains a vascularized synovium and is enclosed by a tough fibrous capsule [1].

1.2
Structure and Composition of Normal Human Adult Articular Cartilage

1.2.1
Structure

Adult human normal articular cartilage can be divided into several layers or zones (Fig. 1). From the surface inward, these zones are: the superficial or tangential zone (I), the transitional or middle zone (II), the radial or deep zone (III) and the calcified zone (IV). The transitions between zones I and II, but especially between zones II and III, are not sharp boundaries, but rather gradual changes in composition and structure [2]. The junction between uncalcified and calcified articular cartilage is called the "tidemark", a line distinguishable in stained sections of decalcified tissue. It provides a well-defined boundary for the uncalcified tissue [3]. It is also worth noting that the zone of calcified cartilage makes up a relatively constant proportion (6% to 8%) of the total articular cartilage height. In contrast, the total thickness of the articular cartilage, including the zone of calcified cartilage, varies with the magnitude of the forces applied at a specific site and from joint to joint [4]. Intermittent hydrostatic pressure, acting on the ends of the bones, may play a vital role in maintaining the articular cartilage by retarding the ossification front [5].

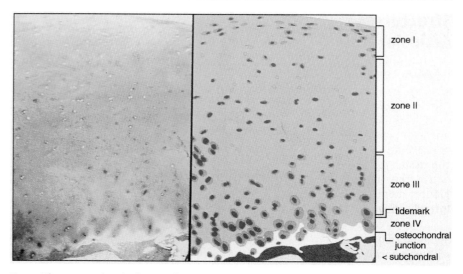

Fig. 1. The zones of articular cartilage. Light micrograph of human articular cartilage from the medial tibial plateau of a 66-year old woman. Weigert's acid iron chloride hematoxylin, Safranin–O and fast green stain (proteoglycans: *red*; collagen: *green*; calcified cartilage: *yellow*). Cartilage thickness: 1.8 mm. The corresponding computer-enhanced schematic illustration of the different layers of articular cartilage from the surface to the subchondral bone is shown on the right. *Zone I*: tangential zone; *zone II*: transitional zone; *zone III*: radial zone, followed by the tidemark which separates the non-calcified cartilage from the calcified zone (*zone IV*). The osteochondral junction links the subchondral bone with the cartilage. Reproduced with permission from Kuettner and Thonar 1998

1.2.2
Cellular Elements

The cells, termed chondrocytes, also exhibit marked variations in density with tissue depth – cell density is highest in zone I and decreases progressively through zones II to IV (Fig. 1). Cartilage is also more cellular in some joints than in others. Further, within each joint, cellularity is inversely related to the thickness of the cartilage and the degree of load bearing at a particular site.

The most superficial chondrocytes are disc-shaped and form a several cell-thick layer (zone I) very close to the surface but beneath a thin layer of matrix; their long axes are parallel to the articular surface. The deepest cells in this layer show a gradual change to a less flattened shape. In zone II, the chondrocytes are more spherical, sometimes arranged in small groups, and appear to be dispersed randomly throughout the matrix [6, 7]. The chondrocytes of zone III are predominantly ellipsoid with their long axes perpendicular to the articular surface and grouped in radially-arranged columns of 2 – 6 cells. In calcified zone IV, the chondrocytes are more sparsely distributed; while some may appear necrotic, most apparently are viable. The cells remain surrounded by non-calcified matrix, since mineralization is restricted to the interterritorial compartment of the matrix.

1.2.3
Extracellular Matrix

Adult human articular cartilage is composed of a hydrated extensive extracellular matrix (ECM) in which a small number of chondrocytes ($\cong 2\% - 3\%$ of the total tissue volume) are embedded. The cells lack cell-cell contact and, consequently, communication between them must involve the ECM. As the tissue has no blood vessels or lymphatics, the delivery of nutrients to, and the removal of waste products from, the cells occurs via diffusion through the ECM. There also are no nerve fibers; neural signals are thus not directly transmitted from the tissue. Although the chondrocytes within the tissue are metabolically very active, they normally do not divide after adolescence. They live in an anoxic environment and are believed to carry out their metabolism mainly through anaerobic pathways [8].

Each chondrocyte can be thought of as a metabolically functional unit of cartilage, isolated from neighboring cells but ultimately responsible for the elaboration and maintenance of the ECM in its immediate vicinity [9]. The ECM in adult cartilage is composed of several compartments (Fig. 2), each with a unique morphological appearance [7] and distinct biochemical composition [10, 11]. The ECM immediately adjacent to the chondrocyte membrane is called the pericellular or lacunar matrix. It is characterized by a high content of large proteoglycan aggregates, bound to the cell via the interaction of hyaluronate (HA) with CD44-like receptors [12], and by the relative absence of organized fibrillar collagens. Contiguous to this pericellular matrix lies the territorial or capsular matrix which is composed of a basket-like network of crosslinked fibrillar collagen that encapsulates individual cells or sometimes groups of

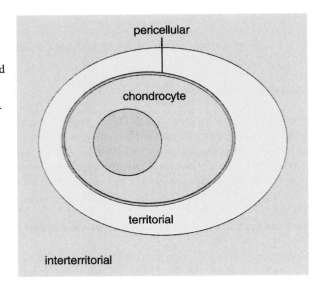

Fig. 2.
Compartmentalization of the articular cartilage matrix. The thin rim of pericellular matrix (*red*) and the territorial matrix (*light blue*) form the cell-associated matrix, the meta-bolically active compart-ment. The metabolically "inert" interterritorial matrix compartment (*dark blue*) makes up more than 90% of the total volume of the matrix in human articular cartilage. Re-produced with permission from [1]

chondrocytes (chondrons) and probably provides a special mechanical support for the cells [1]. The chondrocytes establish contact with the capsular matrix through numerous cytoplasmic processes rich in microfilaments as well as through specific matrix molecules (e.g. anchorin and CD44-like receptors, see below). The largest compartment of the ECM, and the furthest removed from the chondrocyte membrane, is the interterritorial matrix containing most of the collagen fibrils and proteoglycans [7].

The division of the ECM into matrix compartments is more clearly delineated in adult articular cartilage than in immature cartilage [1]. The relative size of each compartment may vary from joint to joint and even within the same cartilage. The resident chondrocytes initially produce, and continuously maintain, their surrounding matrix. Recent studies suggest that in adult tissue chondrocytes exert active metabolic control over their pericellular and territorial matrix compartments but less active control over the interterritorial matrix which may be metabolically "inert" [7, 10].

As mentioned above, articular cartilage is composed primarily of an extensive ECM synthesized, assembled and regulated by the chondrocytes. The tissue macromolecules and their concentrations change during the different phases of development and aging in order to meet altered functional needs. However, it is not known if the cells synthesize all matrix components simultaneously or in regulated phases according to physiological requirements [1]. The concentration and metabolic balance among the various ECM macromolecules and their structural relationships and interactions determine the biochemical properties, and hence the function, of articular cartilage within different joints. The major component of the ECM of human adult articular cartilage is water (65–70% of the total weight). This water is tightly bound within the ECM due to the physical properties of the macromolecular components of the tissue which are composed of collagens, proteoglycans and non-collagenous glycoproteins.

1.3
Biochemical Composition of Normal Human Adult Articular Cartilage

1.3.1
Fibrillar Network

Collagen molecules form the fibrous elements found in the extracellular spaces of most connective tissues. Within this insoluble three-dimensional network of crosslinked fibers, other more soluble components such as proteoglycans, glycoproteins and tissue-specific proteins are enmeshed and, in some cases, non-covalently bound to the collagenous elements.

1.3.1.1
Collagen Type II: The Major Component of the Fibrillar Network

Collagen molecules organized into fibrils make up about 50% of the organic dry weight (or 10–20% of the wet weight). In adult cartilage, approximately

90% of the collagens are of the type II variety, a form found only in a few other tissues (e.g. vitreous body, notochord). Type II belongs to class 1 (fibril forming) collagen molecules. In addition, types IX, XI and small amounts of type VI collagen have been found in adult articular cartilage. The relative amount of type IX in the collagen fibrils decreases from about 15% in fetal cartilage to about 1% in mature (bovine) articular cartilage [13–15].

The type II collagen molecule is composed of three identical polypeptide chains, α_1(II), synthesized and secreted as procollagen precursors whose non-helical extensions are removed by enzymes before the molecule is incorporated into the ECM. Once the trimmed collagen molecules are released extracellularly, they form fibrils within the ECM [1]. In adult articular cartilage, type II collagen forms fibrillar arcades with thicker fibrils in the deeper layers of the tissue and fine fibrils horizontally arranged and enriched at the surface of the tissue [9, 16]. Molecular biological approaches recently have shown that differential splicing of exons occurs. In the type II procollagen gene, a new exon (exon 2) coding for a cysteine-rich domain in the amino-terminal propeptide was recently discovered. This exon is not expressed in mature cartilage but is abundant in early stages of development (early or pre-chondrogenesis) and results in a type II procollagen which is larger in size (type II A) [17]. The expression of this type II A procollagen may be inhibitory to matrix accumulation; the role (if any) it plays during development and cartilage pathology (e.g. inadequate repair, osteophyte formation) remains to be elucidated [18]).

The network of type II collagen fibrils provides the tensile strength and is essential for maintaining the tissue's volume and shape [7, 15]. The tensile strength is increased by covalent, intermolecular crosslinks formed between type II collagen molecules [19]. Extracellularly, the enzyme lysyloxidase produces aldehydes from hydroxylysine which then form the multivalent crosslinking amino acid, hydroxylysyl pyridinoline. The concentration of this mature hydroxypyridinium crosslink in cartilage rises with age but changes little during adult life [20]. On the other hand, articular cartilage shows a marked age-related enrichment in a different type of crosslink produced by non-enzymatic means (browning) [21].

1.3.1.2
Minor Collagens: Essential Players in Fibril Organization and Function

Up to 10% of the total collagen content in adult articular cartilage is made up of other genetically distinct types, the so-called "minor" collagens that contribute to the unique functional properties of the tissue. Type IX collagen belongs to the class 3 short-helix molecules and to the unique group of FACIT-collagens (Fibril-Associated Collagens with Interrupted Triple-helices) [22]. It is assembled from three genetically distinct chains. One of these [the α_2(IX) chain] becomes glycosylated with a chondroitin sulfate (CS) chain, making this collagen molecule a proteoglycan as well. Both mature and immature hydroxypyridinium crosslinks have been identified between helical segments of type IX and the telopeptides of type II collagen (Fig. 3) [23, 24]. Type IX may

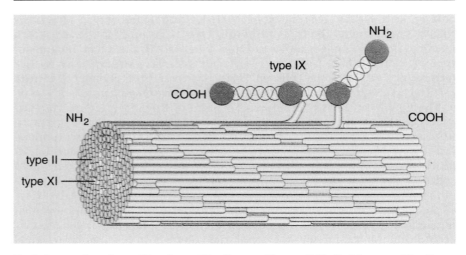

Fig. 3. Interaction of type IX and type XI collagen with type II fibrils. Most type IX collagen molecules in the extracellular cartilage matrix are covalently linked antiparallel onto the surface of type II collagen fibrils that contain in their interior type XI collagen. Adapted from [14, 15]

therefore function as an intermolecular-interfibrillar "connector" (or bridging) molecule between adjacent collagen fibers [25, 26]. Since type IX collagen molecules can also form crosslinks with each other, various homotypic and heterotypic peptides have been identified. The crosslinks between fibers enhance the mechanical stability of the fibrillar three-dimensional network and make it less susceptible to enzymatic attack. They also promote resistance to deformation by restricting swelling of the entrapped proteoglycans. It is also worth noting that in addition to the anionic CS chain, the type IX collagen molecule contains a cationic domain. This makes the surface of the fibrils highly charged and prone to interactions with other matrix macromolecules [27].

Type XI collagen makes up only 2–3% of the total collagen. It belongs to class 1 (fiber forming) collagens and is composed of three distinct α chains. Together with types II and IX, it is co-assembled in the heterotypic fibrils of articular cartilage [15]. Type XI collagen molecules have been located by immunoelectronmicroscopy within the interior of the type II collagen fibrils. Their role may be to organize type II collagen molecules by controlling lateral fibril growth and by determining the diameter of the final heterotypic collagen fibrils [28]. Type XI collagen also is involved in crosslinking but, even in adult cartilage, the crosslinks remain as immature divalent keto-amines [15].

Small amounts of type VI collagen, another representative of class 3 short-helix molecules, have been found in articular cartilage [14, 29]. This collagen forms distinct microfibrils and seems to be concentrated selectively in the capsular matrix of chondrons [30].

1.3.2
Proteoglycans

Proteoglycans are proteins to which are covalently attached at least one glycosaminoglycan chain. They are among the most complicated biological macromolecules. They are ubiquitous in the body and most abundant in the ECM of cartilage. In articular cartilage, these highly hydrophilic proteoglycans are the major space-filling matrix macromolecules. Entrapped in an underhydrated (compressed) form within the fibrillar collagen network, their primary function is to give articular cartilage its ability to undergo reversible deformation [1]. However, they are believed to play other roles that as yet are incompletely understood (for reviews see [31–34]).

1.3.2.1
Aggrecan

Aggrecan is the predominant proteoglycan in articular cartilage: it makes up approximately 90% of the mass of proteoglycans in the tissue. Its protein core (M_r = 230 kilodaltons [kDa]) is glycosylated with numerous covalently-attached glycosaminoglycan chains, as well as N-linked and O-linked oligosaccharides [33] (Fig. 4). The glycosaminoglycan chains, which comprise approximately 90% of the total mass of the macromolecule, are keratan sulfate (KS, containing the repeating sulfated disaccharide ⟨N-acetylglucosamine – galactose⟩, with multiple sulfation sites and other monosaccharide residues such as sialic acid) and CS (containing the repeating disaccharide ⟨N-acetylgalactosamine – glucuronic acid⟩, with a sulfate ester on either the fourth or sixth carbon atom of N-acetylgalactosamine).

The core protein of aggrecan contains three globular (G_1, G_2 and G_3) and two extended interglobular (E_1, E_2) domains. The amino-terminal region contains the G_1 and G_2 domains separated by the 21 nm extended E_1 segment. G_3, present at the carboxy-terminal end, is separated from G_2 by the major (about 260 nm-long) extended E_2 region that carries over 100 CS chains and many of the KS chains (about 15–25) in addition to O-linked oligosaccharides. N-linked oligosaccharides are found mostly within the G_1-E_1-G_2 domains and near the G_3 region. The glycosaminoglycans are clustered in two regions: the largest, termed the CS-rich region, contains all the CS and up to 50% of the KS chains [36]. A KS-rich region is located in the E_2 domain near the G_2 domain and before the CS-rich region [33]. The aggrecan molecules also contain some phosphate esters located primarily on the xylose residues that link CS chains to the core protein, but also are found on some serine residues in the core protein.

A segment of the carboxy-terminal G_3 domain is highly homologous with a hepatic cell-surface lectin specific for galactose and fucose and thus may help anchor proteoglycan molecules within the ECM by binding to select carbohydrate structures [33, 37]. Recent analyses have revealed an alternatively spliced exon encoding an EGF-like sub-domain and a complement B-like sequence within the G_3 domain. Using anti-EGF polyclonal antibodies, the EGF-like epitope has been localized within a peptide of 68 kDa in human aggrecan. Its

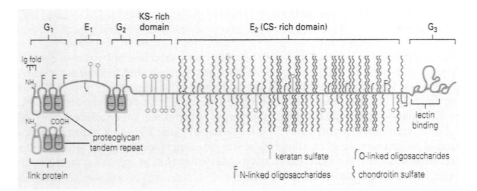

Fig. 4. The structure of cartilage aggrecan and link protein molecules. In aggrecan the three globular domains (G_1, G_2 and G_3) are separated by two extended segments (E_1 and E_2) which carry the glycosaminoglycans chondroitin sulfate (CS, in the CS-rich domain) and keratan sulfate (KS, in the KS-rich domain, but some also in the E_1 segment and within the CS-rich domain). Furthermore, the core protein is substituted with N- and O-linked oligosaccharides. The G_1 and G_2 domains as well as the link protein (LP) contain a double loop structure (proteoglycan tandem repeat, PTR). In addition both G_1 and LP show an additional loop structure (immunoglobulin fold, Ig-fold) which can selectively interact with hyaluronate to form aggregates. The G_3 domain contains a lectin-binding region. Adapted from [35]

function remains to be elucidated [1]. These sub-domains also have been found in adhesion molecules controlling lymphocyte migration [33]. Only about one-third of the aggrecan molecules isolated from adult cartilage actually contain an intact G_3 domain suggesting that within the matrix the aggrecan molecules may be proteolytically reduced in size. The fate and possible function of the released fragments are still unknown [1].

The glycosaminoglycan-bearing E_2 domain is the major "functional" segment of the aggrecan molecule. The KS-rich region closest to G_2 is enriched in the amino acids proline, serine and threonine. Most of the serine and threonine residues are O-glycosylated with an N-acetylgalactosamine residue, which serves as a primer for the synthesis of characteristic oligosaccharides which can become extended as KS chains. The remainder of the E_2 domain contains over 100 serine-glycine sequences in which the serine provides the attachment for the xylosyl residues that initiate the CS chains. Usually both chondroitin 4-sulfate and 6-sulfate exist within the same proteoglycan molecule with the ratio of each molecule varying with tissue source, age and from species to species.

The structure of aggrecan molecules in the cartilage matrix undergoes many changes with development and aging [36, 38–40]. Some of these reflect age-related changes at the level of synthesis; they include a decrease in hydrodynamic size, the result mostly of a change in the average length of the CS chains, and an increase in the number as well as length of KS chains [36]. Aggrecan molecules also undergo changes in the matrix, reflecting the action of proteolytic enzymes (e. g. by aggrecanase and stromelysin) upon their core protein [41]. This results in a progressive decrease in the average length of the core protein of aggrecan molecules in aggregates and in the accumulation, with time spent in the matrix, of G_1-containing fragments relatively deficient in glycosaminoglycan chains.

1.3.2.2
Proteoglycan Aggregates

Aggrecan molecules synthesized by the chondrocytes are secreted into the ECM where they form aggregates stabilized by link protein (LP) molecules. This aggregation involves highly specific non-covalent and cooperative interactions between a strand of HA and up to 200 molecules of both aggrecan and LP. HA is an extracellular, unsulfated, linear, high molecular weight glycosaminoglycan consisting of many repeating units of N-acetylglucosamine and glucuronic acid [12]. The double loop structure of the G_1 domain of aggrecan interacts reversibly with five consecutive HA disaccharide repeat units. LP, which contains a similar (highly homologous) double loop structure [42], interacts with both the G_1 region and the HA molecule and stabilizes the aggregate structure. The ternary complex G_1-HA-LP forms a highly stable interaction that protects the G_1 domain and LP from proteolytic digestion. Two LP molecules with molecular weights between 40 and 50 kDa have been identified; they differ from each other by the degree of glycosylation. Only one LP molecule is present at each HA-aggrecan linkage site. A third smaller LP appears to be derived from the larger species by limited proteolytic cleavage [43].

As many as 200 aggrecan molecules can bind to one single HA molecule to form an aggregate of 5×10^7 to 5×10^8 molecular weight that by electronmicroscopy is more than 8-μm long [31]. In the cell-associated matrix, made up of the pericellular plus territorial matrix compartments, the aggregates retain their association with the cell by binding, via their HA strand, to CD44-like receptors on the cell membrane [12].

The formation of aggregates within the ECM is complex. Newly-synthesized aggrecan molecules exhibit a delay in ability to bind to HA with high affinity [44]. This may act as a regulatory mechanism, allowing newly-synthesized molecules to reach the interterritorial areas of the matrix before becoming immobilized into large-size aggregates [10]. The proportion of newly-synthesized aggrecan and LP molecules able to form aggregates by interacting with HA decreases markedly as a function of age [45]. With age, the size of the aggregates isolated from human articular cartilage also decreases significantly. This is due in part to a reduction in the average length of the HA molecules and in part to the decrease in the average size of the aggrecan molecules, as mentioned above.

Two populations of aggregates have been identified [46]. Most aggregates have an average size of approximately 60 S. A second population of fast sedimenting "superaggregates", with an average S-value of about 120, is enriched in LP molecules [46, 47]. The presence of this superaggregate may play a major role in tissue function; it is more concentrated in the middle layer of the articular cartilage, regains its prominence during tissue recovery after immobilization of the limb, and undergoes a significant decrease in size in osteoarthritic tissues during the early onset of the disease [47].

1.3.2.3
Small Non-Aggregating Proteoglycans

Aside from aggrecan, articular cartilage contains several smaller proteoglycans. Biglycan and decorin, dermatan sulfate-bearing molecules, have molecular weights of approximately 100 kDa and 70 kDa, respectively, and core proteins of about 30 kDa [48]. Biglycan in human articular cartilage contains two dermatan sulfate chains, whereas decorin, the most abundant of the two, contains only one. These molecules make up only a small fraction of the mass of proteoglycans in articular cartilage although they may be as numerous as the larger aggregating proteoglycans. The small proteoglycans interact with other macromolecules within the ECM including collagens, fibronectin and growth factors (and with other macromolecules such as heparin cofactor II) [1]. Decorin is located primarily on the surface of collagen fibrils and inhibits collagen fibrillogenesis [49, 50]. The core proteins bind avidly to the cell-binding domain of fibronectin and probably sterically hinder fibronectin from binding to cell-surface receptors (integrins). Since both decorin and biglycan bind to fibronectin and restrain both cell adhesion and migration as well as clot formation, they may well inhibit processes involved in tissue repair [51].

Fibromodulin in articular cartilage is a proteoglycan (Mr = 50–65 kDa) apparently associated primarily with collagen fibrils [52]. Its core protein, homologous to those of decorin and biglycan, is substituted with a significant number of tyrosine sulfate residues. This glycosylated form of fibromodulin (previously called 59 kDa matrix protein) may help regulate the assembly and maintenance of collagen fibrils [53]. It is noteworthy that both fibromodulin and decorin are located on the surface of the collagen fibrils. Thus, as mentioned previously, any growth in diameter of the fibrils must be preceded by selective removal of these proteoglycans (as well as the type IX collagen molecules bound along the fibrils) [1].

1.3.3
Non-Collagenous Matrix Proteins

Articular cartilage also contains a number of ECM proteins that are neither collagens nor proteoglycans (Fig. 5). They participate in interactions with other matrix molecules to form a network in which most molecules of the ECM are involved (for reviews see [54, 55]. Some of these non-collagenous proteins have been studied in detail and briefly are summarized below.

Anchorin, a 34 kDa protein present on the surface of chondrocytes and within the cell membrane, may mediate interactions between the cell and the matrix. Through its high affinity for type II collagen fibrils, it may act as a mechano-receptor transmitting altered stress on the fibers to the chondrocytes [56].

Fibronectin is a minor component in most cartilaginous tissues and differs slightly from plasma fibronectin [1]. It is thought to contribute to matrix assembly through interactions with the cell membrane and other matrix constituents such as type II collagen and thrombospondin [55]. Fibronectin fragments with deleterious effects upon the metabolism of chondrocytes, i.e.

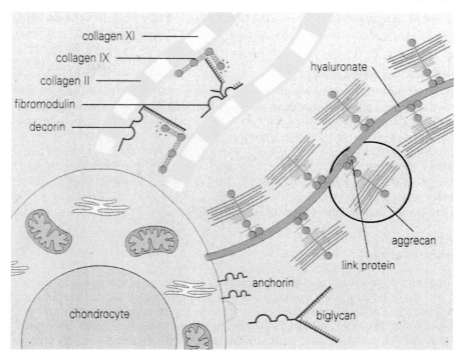

Fig. 5. Some of the major macromolecules in the extracellular matrix of articular cartilage and their possible multiple interactions. Type XI collagen is located within the collagen type II fibers which carry attached to it type IX collagen molecules. Decorin and fibromodulin may bind to the fibers, possibly via the interaction of their negatively charged glycosamino-glycans with the cationic segment of type IX collagen. A proteoglycan aggregate composed of aggrecan, link protein and hyaluronate is shown; it is bound to the cell membrane via the interaction of HA with a cell surface receptor. Some of the aggrecan molecules may lack the G_3 domain. The circle depicts the hydration radius of a compressed aggrecan molecule. Neither the specific location of biglycan, the interaction of anchorin with the collagen fiber, nor the presence of crosslinks between collagen types II and IX are shown. Adapted from [54]

shutdown of aggrecan synthesis and upregulation of catabolic processes, are found in elevated amounts in the joint fluid of patients with osteoarthritis and thus may contribute to the pathogenetic changes that occur in the late stages of this degenerative disease [57]. It is likely that fragments of other matrix molecules that bind in a receptor-mediated fashion to chondrocytes may also produce such effects [58].

Cartilage oligomeric matrix protein (COMP), a member of the thrombospondin superfamily, is a pentamer with five apparently identical subunits with $Mr \cong 83$ kDa. It is found in abundance in articular cartilage, especially in the proliferative cell layer in growth cartilage and may thus be involved in regulating cell growth [55]. This protein is very homologous to thrombospondin, also found in the articular cartilage matrix although in much smaller amounts [55].

Other matrix proteins include the following. A 36 kDa slightly basic cartilage matrix protein expresses high binding affinity for chondrocytes and may mediate interactions of cells with the matrix, e.g. during tissue remodeling. A 39 kDa protein, termed GP-39, is expressed in the superficial layer of articular cartilage and in synovium but its function is not known [55]. A 21 kDa protein synthesized by hypertrophic chondrocytes interacts with type X collagen and may have a function in the tidemark zone [55]. Finally, it is becoming increasingly evident that unglycosylated forms of the small non-aggregating proteoglycans are expressed by the chondrocytes, sometimes in distinct developmental stages and in disease, but their specific functions are still unknown and under investigation.

1.4
Functional Properties of Articular Cartilage

1.4.1
Biochemical Basis

Aggrecan molecules give cartilage its ability to undergo reversible deformation [59]. They show specific interactions within the extracellular milieu and undoubtedly play additional prominent roles in the organization, structure and function of the ECM. Within the tissue, aggrecan molecules reach concentrations as high as 100 mg/ml. They are compressed to about 20% of the volume they occupy when maximally extended in solution and are not freely mobile within the ECM. Collagen fibers form a three-dimensional network that bestows correct tissue shape by preventing these space-filling proteoglycans from further expanding. The proteoglycans entrapped within this collagen network are molecules with high concentrations of negatively charged anionic groups. These charges are fully-ionized under physiological conditions enabling these molecules to provide high local concentrations of negative charges which interact with the mobile cations in the tissue water (interstitial fluid) [1]. Since proteoglycans as highly charged polyelectrolytes occupy only a fraction of their possible hydrodynamic domain, they attract water and thus provide a swelling pressure that is restrained by the stiffness and tensile forces of the collagen fibers [60].

The water content of the ECM is very important. Water defines the volume of the tissue and, entrapped by the proteoglycans of the ECM, offers compressive resistance. It is essentially incompressible and provides for the molecular transport and diffusion within the ECM. The high density of negative charges on the large-size proteoglycans "fixed" in the tissue creates an "excluded volume effect" [1]. The effective pore size within the concentrated proteoglycan solutions is very small and, consequently, the rate of diffusion of large globular proteins into the tissue is very low [61]. Large-size proteins (such as albumin or immunoglobulins) and small negatively-charged proteins tend to be excluded from the ECM.

In the ECM of cartilage some of the water is present within the collagen fibrils, the remainder in the extrafibrillar component. Because of their large size, the proteoglycans are excluded from the intrafibrillar space. It is the extrafibrillar space, therefore, that determines the physiochemical and biomechanical characteristics of cartilage [59]. The water content of the intrafibrillar compartment is dependent upon the concentration of proteoglycans in the extrafibrillar space and increases when the proteoglycan concentration decreases.

The fixed negative (anionic) charges on the proteoglycans determine the ionic composition of the extracellular milieu that contains free cations at high concentrations and free anions at low concentrations [61]. Since the concentration of aggrecan shows a tendency to increase from the surface to the deep zone, the immediate ionic environment of the chondrocytes differs accordingly. In general, the concentration of inorganic ions within the matrix creates a high osmotic pressure.

1.4.2
Effect of Loading on Cartilage

The material properties of articular cartilage depend upon the interplay among its collagen fibers, the entrapped proteoglycans and the fluid phase of the tissue. Structural or compositional changes resulting from an imbalance between synthesis and catabolism, degradation of macromolecules or physical trauma seriously affect the material properties of the tissue and impair its function. Since the concentration, distribution and macromolecular organization of collagens and proteoglycans change with depth from the articular surface, the biomechanical properties of individual zones also vary, with each zone contributing in its own way. For example, the superficial zone with its high concentration of collagen, its tangentially oriented fibers and its relatively low content of proteoglycans shows the highest tensile stiffness and distributes the load evenly over the entire surface of the tissue [1]. In the transitional and radial zones, the high concentration of proteoglycans enables the tissue to bear compressive loads. The material properties change abruptly at the tidemark, from the compliant non-mineralized tissue to the stiffer mineralized cartilage [62]. The continuity of collagen fibers throughout the tidemark provides strength but, at the underlying chondro-osseous junction not crossed by collagen fibers, the highly irregular interdigitating contours between mineralized cartilage and bone serve to lock together the two layers to prevent separation. The calcified cartilage is less stiff than the subchondral bone; thus, it acts as an intermediate layer. At the undulating interface, shear stresses are converted into less damaging compressive forces transmitted to the subchondral bone [63].

Upon loading, a complex distribution of tensile, shear and compressive stresses comes into play. The cartilage matrix is deformed by the expulsion of fluid (together with the metabolic products of the cells) from the loaded region, effectively increasing the ionic concentration within the interstitial fluid [64] (Fig. 6). Movement of water is related directly to the magnitude and duration of the load applied and is retarded by the negative charges (forces) of the proteoglycans. Thus, energy is absorbed by the tissue as water is displaced [65, 66]. Concomitantly, as the tissue is deformed, the proteoglycans are forced closer together, effectively increasing the negative charge density and the inter-

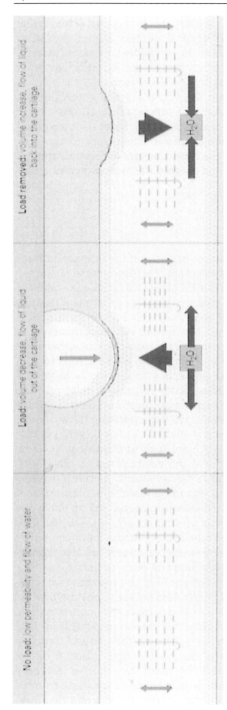

Fig. 6. Water flow within healthy articular cartilage with applied and removed load. Under unloaded conditions, most of the water within the tissue is bound to the underhydrated proteoglycans. If load is applied, water flows toward the load (synovial cavity), carrying with it cellular waste products. (Little water "escapes" downwards and laterally towards the areas rich in proteoglycans.). Once the load is removed, the water returns from the synovial cavity, carrying with it nutrients for the cells. In osteoarthritic cartilage (not shown), the concentration of proteoglycans is diminished and, consequently, during loading water flows not only vertically into the synovial cavity but in other directions as well, thus diminishing the supply of nutrients returning with the water after the load has been released. Reproduced with permission from [1]

molecular charge-charge repulsive forces that in turn increase the resistance of the tissue to further deformation. Ultimately, the deformation reaches an equilibrium in which the external loading force is balanced by the internal forces based upon the swelling pressure (proteoglycan-ionic interactions) and the mechanical stress (proteoglycan-collagen interaction). As the load is removed, the tissue regains its original form by imbibing water (together with nutrients from the surrounding tissue fluids). The unloaded form of the tissue is reached when the swelling pressure of the proteoglycans again is balanced by the resistance of the collagen network to further expansion.

The biomechanical properties of articular cartilage to withstand applied load are based upon the structural integrity of the tissue which in turn is a consequence of the collagen-proteoglycan composition as a "solid" phase, the hydration of the tissue and ion composition of the "solute" phase [67]. The hydrostatic pressure of unloaded articular cartilage, and thus of its embedded chondrocytes, is around one to two atmospheres. This hydrostatic pressure can increase *in vivo* to 100 to 200 atmospheres within milliseconds upon standing and may cycle between 40 to 50 atmospheres when walking. *In vitro* studies have suggested that a hydrostatic pressure of 50 to 150 atmospheres, which is physiological, leads to a moderate increase in cartilage anabolism (increased amino acid and sulfate incorporation) if applied for short periods of time. If applied for two hours, causing fluid loss, no effect is induced, suggesting that this effect is dependent directly upon tissue hydration [68]. It remains to be seen, however, whether the chondrocytes respond as rapidly *in vivo* to these kinds of changes.

An induced decrease in hydration with its concomitant increase in proteoglycan concentration results in the attraction of positive counterions such as H^+ and Na^+ [69]. This leads to a change in the overall ionic composition and the pH of the ECM and thus of the chondrocyte. Prolonged application of load induces a drop in pH with an accompanying decrease in rate of proteoglycan synthesis by cartilage. It is likely that the effect of the extracellular ionic environment on the rate of synthesis also is directly related in part to its effect on intercellular composition. As newly-synthesized aggrecan molecules maintained under mildly acidic conditions exhibit a longer than normal delay before they mature into aggregating forms [70], it is possible that a drop in pH around the chondrocyte, such as occurs during loading, may allow more newly-synthesized aggrecan molecules to reach the interterritorial areas of the matrix [10].

Immobilization or reduced loading leads to a marked decrease in synthesis and tissue content of proteoglycans, whereas increased dynamic loading leads to a moderate increase in synthesis and content of proteoglycans [71]. Strenuous training (20 km/day, 15 weeks) of dogs causes some change in total tissue proteoglycans and specifically depletes the proteoglycans in the superficial zone [72]. Some reversible softening of the cartilage occurs combined with a stimulated remodeling of the subchondral bone. Severe static or impact loading, however, causes cartilage damage and subsequent degeneration. In addition, abnormal changes in the physical-mechanical environment, as occur in osteoarthritis, are initiated by a loss of aggrecan from the ECM [72]. This loss results in water attraction (swelling) by the remaining proteoglycans that are now present in lower concentration with more space available. This dilution leads to a decrease in local fixed-charge density and ultimately in a change in osmolarity with altered feedback to the chondrocytes.

1.5
Concluding Remarks

While we have described the functional properties of normal human adult articular cartilage as the result of the interactions among its three most abundant molecules (collagen type II, aggrecan and water), it is likely that other constituents of the matrix also play important roles. Recent studies have led, for example, to the identification of several matrix proteins found at higher concentrations in cartilage than in any other tissue. At this time, however, their functional roles remain unclear. Future studies should help clarify the roles such minor components of the matrix play in the maintenance of matrix integrity, an absolute requirement for sustaining the normal functions of articular cartilage over the long term.

Acknowledgments. The review was prepared with partial support from grants AR-39239 and AG-04736 from the National Institutes of Health.

References

1. Kuettner KE, Thonar EJ-MA (1998) Cartilage integrity and homeostasis. In: Dieppe P, Klippel J (eds) Rheumatology, 2nd Edition. Mosby-Wolfe, London, pp 8.6.1 – 8.6.13
2. Clark JM (1991) Variation of collagen fiber alignment in a joint surface: a scanning electron microscopy study of the tibial plateau in dog, rabbit and man. J Orthop Res 9:246–257
3. Oegema TR, Thompson RC (1990) Cartilage bone-interface (tidemark). In: Brandt KD (ed) Cartilage changes in osteoarthritis. Indiana University School of Medicine, Indianapolis, pp 43 – 52
4. Oegema TR, Thompson RC (1992) The zone of calcified cartilage. Its role in osteoarthritis. In: Kuettner KE, Schleyerbach R, Peyron J, Hascall VC (eds) Articular cartilage and osteoarthritis. Raven Press, New York, pp 319 – 331
5. Carter DR, Wong M (1990) Mechanical stresses in joint morphogenesis and maintenance. In: Mow VC, Ratcliffe A, Woo SL-Y (eds) Biomechanics of diarthrodial joints, vol II. Springer-Verlag, New York, pp 155 – 174
6. Aydelotte MB, Kuettner KE (1992) Heterogeneity of articular chondrocytes and cartilage matrix. In: Woessner JF, Howell DS (eds) Cartilage degradation: Basic and clinical aspects. Marcel Dekker, New York, pp 37 – 65
7. Hunziker EB (1992) Articular cartilage structure in humans and experimental animals. In: Kuettner KE, Schleyerbach R, Peyron J, Hascall VC (eds) Articular cartilage and osteoarthritis. Raven Press, New York, pp 183 – 199
8. Shapiro IM, Tokuoka T, Silverton SF (1991) Energy metabolism in cartilage. In: Hall B, Newman S (eds) Cartilage: Molecular aspects. CRC Press, Boca Raton, pp 97 – 130
9. Aydelotte MB, Kuettner KE (1988) Differences between subpopulations of cultured bovine articular chondrocytes. I. Morphology and cartilage matrix production. Connect Tiss Res 18:205–222
10. Mok SS, Masuda K, Häuselmann HJ, Aydelotte MB, Thonar EJ-MA (1994) Aggrecan synthesized by mature bovine chondrocytes suspended in alginate: identification of two distinct matrix pools. J Biol Chem 269:33021 – 33027

11. Häuselmann HJ, Masuda K, Hunziker EB, Neidhart M, Mok SS, Michel BA, Thonar EJ-MA (1996) Adult human chondrocytes cultured in alginate form a matrix similar to native human articular cartilage. Am J Physiol 271 (Cell Physiol 40): C742–C752

12. Knudson CB, Knudson W (1993) Hyaluronan-binding proteins in development, tissue homeostasis, and disease. FASEB J 7: 1233–1241

13. Mayne R (1989) Cartilage collagens. What is their function, and are they involved in articular disease? Arthritis Rheum 32: 241–246

14. Eyre DR (1991) The collagens of articular cartilage. Semin Arthritis Rheum 21 (Suppl 2): 2–11

15. Eyre DR, Wu JJ, Woods P (1992) The cartilage-specific collagens: Structural studies. In: Kuettner KE, Schleyerbach R, Peyron J, Hascall VC (eds) Articular cartilage and osteoarthritis. Raven Press, New York, pp 119–131

16. Schenk RK, Eggli PS, Hunziker EB (1986) Articular cartilage morphology. In: Kuettner KE, Schleyerbach R, Peyron J, Hascall VC (eds) Articular cartilage and biochemistry. Raven Press, New York, pp 3–22

17. Ryan MC, Sandell LJ (1990) Differential expression of a cysteine-rich domain in the amino-terminal propeptide of type II (cartilage) procollagen by alternative splicing of mRNA. J Biol Chem 265: 10334–10339

18. Sandell LJ, Goldring MB, Zamparo O, Wu J, Yamin R (1992) Molecular biology of type II collagen: New information in the gene. In: Kuettner KE, Schleyerbach R, Peyron J, Hascall VC (eds) Articular cartilage and osteoarthritis. Raven Press, New York, pp 81–94

19. Eyre DR, Wu J, Niyibizi C, Chun L (1990) The cartilage collagens: Analysis of their cross-linking interactions and matrix organization. In: Maroudas A, Kuettner K (eds) Methods in cartilage research. Academic Press, London, pp 28–33

20. Eyre DR, Dickson IR, Van Ness KP (1988) Collagen cross-linking in human bone and articular cartilage. Age-related changes in the content of mature hydroxypyridinium residues. Biochem J 252: 495–500

21. Monnier VM, Cerami A (1981) Nonenzymatic browning *in vivo*: Possible process for aging of long-lived proteins. Science 211: 491–493

22. Olsen BR (1992) Molecular biology of cartilage collagens In: Kuettner KE, Schleyerbach R, Peyron J, Hascall VC (eds) Articular cartilage and osteoarthritis. Raven Press, New York, pp 151–165

23. Eyre DR, Apon S, Wu JJ, Erickson LH, Walsh KA (1987) Collagen type IX: Evidence for covalent linkage to type II collagen in cartilage. FEBS Lett 220: 337–341

24. van der Rest M, Mayne R (1988) Type IX collagen proteoglycan from cartilage is covalently cross-linked to type II collagen. J Biol Chem 263: 1615–1618

25. Wu JJ, Eyre DR (1989) Covalent interactions of type IX collagen in cartilage. Connect Tiss Res 20: 241–245

26. Muller-Glauser W, Humbel B, Glatt M, Strauli P, Winterhalter KH, Bruckner P (1986) On the role of type IX collagen in the extracellular matrix of cartilage. Type IX collagen is localized to intersections of collagen fibrils. J Cell Biol 102: 1931–1939

27. Vasios G, Nishimura I, Konomi H, van der Rest M, Ninomiya Y, Olsen BR (1988) Cartilage type IX collagen proteoglycan contains a large amino-terminal globular domain encoded by multiple exons. J Biol Chem 263: 2324–2329

28. Eikenberry EF, Mendler M, Bürgin R, Winterhalter KH, Bruckner P (1992) Fibrillar organization in cartilage. In: Kuettner KE, Schleyerbach R, Peyron J, Hascall VC (eds) Articular cartilage and osteoarthritis. Raven Press, New York, pp 133–149

29. Thomas JT, Ayad S, Grant ME (1994) Cartilage collagens: strategies for the study of their organisation and expression in the extracellular matrix. Ann Rheum Dis 53: 488–496

30. Poole CA, Ayad S, Schofield JR (1988) Chondrons from articular cartilage. 1. Immuno-localization of type VI collagen in the pericellular capsule of isolated canine tibial chondrons. J Cell Sci 90: 635–643

31. Rosenberg LC, Buckwalter JA (1986) Cartilage proteoglycans. In: Kuettner KE, Schleyerbach R, Peyron J, Hascall VC (eds) Articular cartilage and biochemistry. Raven Press, New York, pp 39–58

32. Wight T, Mecham R (1987) Biology of proteoglycans (Biology of extracellular matrix). Academic Press, New York
33. Hardingham TE, Fosang AJ, Dudhia J (1992) Aggrecan: the chondroitin sulphate/keratan sulphate proteoglycan from cartilage. In: Kuettner KE, Schleyerbach R, Peyron J, Hascall VC (eds) Articular cartilage and biochemistry. Raven Press, New York, pp 5–20
34. Sandy JD (1992) Extracellular metabolism of aggrecan. In: Kuettner KE, Schleyerbach R, Peyron J, Hascall VC (eds) Articular cartilage and biochemistry. Raven Press, New York, pp 21–33
35. Hardingham T, Bayliss M (1990) Proteoglycans of articular cartilage: Changes in aging and in joint disease. Semin Arthritis Rheum 20 (Suppl 1):12–33
36. Thonar EJ-MA, Kuettner KE (1987) Biochemical basis of age-related changes in proteoglycans. In: Wight TN, Mecham RP (eds) Biology of proteoglycans. Academic Press, Orlando, pp 211–246
37. Halberg DF, Pronix G, Doege K, Yamada Y, Drickamer K (1986) A segment of the cartilage proteoglycan core protein has lectin-like activity. J Biol Chem 261:8108–8111
38. Roughley PJ, Mort JS (1986) Aging and the aggregating proteoglycans of human articular cartilage. Clin Sci 71:337–344
39. Thonar EJ-MA, Buckwalter JA, Kuettner KE (1986) Maturation-related differences in the structure and composition of proteoglycans synthesized by chondrocytes from bovine articular cartilage. J Biol Chem 261:2467–2474
40. Bayliss MT (1990) Proteoglycan structure and metabolism during maturation and ageing of human articular cartilage. Biochem Soc Trans 18:799–802
41. Plaas AHK, Sandy JD (1995) Proteoglycan anabolism and catabolism in articular cartilage. In: Kuettner KE, Goldberg VM (eds) Osteoarthritic Disorders. American Academy of Orthopedic Surgeons, Rosemont, pp 103–116
42. Neame PJ, Christner JE, Baker JR (1987) Cartilage proteoglycan aggregates. The link protein and proteoglycan amino-terminal globular domains have similar structure. J Biol Chem 262:17768–17778
43. Roughley PJ, Nguyen Q, Mort JS (1992) The role of proteinases and oxygen radicals in the degradation of human articular cartilage, In: Kuettner KE, Schleyerbach R, Peyron J, Hascall VC (eds) Articular cartilage and osteoarthritis. Raven Press, New York, pp 305–317
44. Sandy JD, Plaas AHK (1989) Studies on the hyaluronate binding affinity of newly synthesized proteoglycans in chondrocyte cultures. Arch Biochem Biophys 271:300–314
45. Bayliss MT (1992) Metabolism of animal and human osteoarthritic cartilage. In: Kuettner KE, Schleyerbach R, Peyron J, Hascall VC (eds) Articular cartilage and osteoarthritis. Raven Press, New York, pp 487–500
46. Manicourt DH, Pita JC, McDevitt CA, Howell DS (1988) Superficial and deep layers of dog normal articular cartilage. Role of hyaluronate and link protein in determining the sedimentation coefficients distribution of the nondissociatively extracted proteoglycans. J Biol Chem 263:13121–13129
47. Pita JC, Müller FJ, Manicourt DH, Buckwalter JA, Ratcliffe A (1992) Early matrix changes in experimental osteoarthritis and joint disuse atrophy. In: Kuettner KE, Schleyerbach R, Peyron J, Hascall VC (eds) Articular cartilage and osteoarthritis. Raven Press, New York, pp 455–469
48. Fisher LW, Termine JD, Young MF (1989) Deduced protein sequence of bone small proteoglycan I (biglycan) shows homology with proteoglycan II (decorin) and several non-connective tissue proteins in a variety of species. J Biol Chem 264:4571–4576
49. Vogel KG, Paulsson M, Heinegård D (1984) Specific inhibition of type I and type II collagen fibrillogenesis by the small proteoglycan of tendon. Biochem J 223:587–597
50. Scott JE (1990) Proteoglycan-collagen interactions and subfibrillar structure in collagen fibrils. Implications in the development and ageing of connective tissues. J Anat 169:23–35
51. Rosenberg L (1992) Structure and function of dermatan sulfate proteoglycans in articular cartilage. In: Kuettner KE, Schleyerbach R, Peyron J, Hascall VC (eds) Articular cartilage and osteoarthritis. Raven Press, New York, pp 45–63

52. Oldberg Å, Antonsson P, Lindblom K, Heinegård D (1989) A collagen-binding 59-kd protein (fibromodulin) is structurally related to the small interstitial proteoglycans PB-S1 and PG-S2 (decorin). EMBO J 8:2602–2604
53. Plaas AHK, Barry FP, Wong-Palms S (1992) Keratan sulfate on cartilage matrix molecules. In: Kuettner KE, Schleyerbach R, Peyron J, Hascall VC (eds) Articular cartilage and osteoarthritis. Raven Press, New York, pp 69–79
54. Heinegård D, Oldberg A (1989) Structure and biology of cartilage and bone matrix non-collagenous macromolecules. FASEB J 3:2042–2051
55. Heinegård D, Lorenzo P, Sommarin Y (1995) Articular cartilage matrix proteins. In: Kuettner KE, Goldberg VM (eds) Osteoarthritic Disorders. American Academy of Orthopedic Surgeons, Rosemont, pp 229–237
56. von der Mark K, Mollenhauer J, Pfäffle M, van Menxel M, Mueller PK (1986) Role of anchorin CII in the interaction of chondrocytes with extracellular collagen. In: Kuettner KE, Schleyerbach R, Peyron J, Hascall VC (eds) Articular cartilage and biochemistry. Raven Press, New York, pp 125–141
57. Homandberg GA, Meyers R, Xie D-L (1992) Fibronectin fragments cause chondrolysis of bovine articular cartilage slices in culture. J Biol Chem 267:3597–3604
58. Poole AR (1995) Imbalances of anabolism and catabolism of cartilage matrix components in osteoarthritis. In: Kuettner KE, Goldberg VM (eds) Osteoarthritic Disorders. American Academy of Orthopedic Surgeons, Rosemont; pp 247–260
59. Maroudas A, Schneiderman R, Popper O (1992) The role of water, proteoglycan and collagen in solute transport in cartilage. In: Kuettner KE, Schleyerbach R, Peyron, J, Hascall VC (eds) Articular cartilage and osteoarthritis. Raven Press, New York, pp 355–371
60. Maroudas A (1975) Biophysical properties of collagenous tissues. Biorheology 12:233–248
61. Urban JPG (1990) Solute transport between tissue and environment. In: Maroudas A, Kuettner K (eds) Methods in cartilage research. Academic Press, London, pp 241–273
62. Donohue JM, Buss D, Oegema TR, Thompson RC (1983) The effects of indirect blunt trauma on adult canine articular cartilage. J Bone Joint Surg 65A:948–957
63. Radin EL, Martin RB, Burr DB, Caterson B, Boyd RD, Goodwin C (1984) Effects of mechanical loading on the tissues of the rabbit knee. J Orthop Res 2:221–234
64. Urban JPG (1994) The chondrocyte: A cell under pressure. Br J Rheumatol 33:901–908
65. Torzilli PA (1988) Water content and equilibrium partition in immature cartilage. J Orthop Res 6:766–769
66. Maroudas A, Grushko G (1990) Measurement of swelling pressure of cartilage. In: Maroudas A, Kuettner KE (eds) Methods in cartilage research. Academic Press, London, pp 298–301
67. Myers ER, Armstrong CG, Mow VC (1984) Swelling pressure and collagen tension. In: Hukins DWL (ed) Connective tissue matrix. MacMillan, New York, pp 161–168
68. Sah RL, Kim YJ, Grodzinsky AJ, Plaas AHK, Sandy JD (1992) Effects of static and dynamic compression on matrix metabolism in cartilage explants. In: Kuettner KE, Schleyerbach R, Peyron J, Hascall VC (eds) Articular cartilage and osteoarthritis. Raven Press, New York, pp 373–392
69. Urban J, Hall A (1992) Physical modifiers of cartilage metabolism. In: Kuettner KE, Schleyerbach R, Peyron J, Hascall VC (eds) Articular cartilage and osteoarthritis. Raven Press, New York, pp 393–406
70. Plaas AHK, Sandy JD (1986) The affinity of newly synthesized proteoglycan for hyaluronic acid can be enhanced by exposure to mild alkali. Biochem J 234:221–223
71. Palmoski MJ, Brandt KD (1981) Running inhibits the reversal of atrophic changes in canine knee cartilage after removal of a leg cast. Arthritis Rheum 24:1329–1337
72. Helminen HJ, Kiviranta I, Säämänen A-M, Jurvelin JS, Arokoski J, Oettmeier R, Abendroth K, Roth AJ, Tammi MI (1992) Effect of motion and load on articular cartilage in animal models. In: Kuettner KE, Schleyerbach R, Peyron J, Hascall VC (eds) Articular cartilage and osteoarthritis. Raven Press, New York, pp 501–510

Chapter 2

Epidemiology and Economic Consequences of Osteoarthritis

2.1
The American Viewpoint

J. C. Scott, M. Lethbridge-Cejku and M. C. Hochberg

2.1.1
Overview

Arthritis and musculoskeletal diseases are the most common chronic diseases and causes of physical disability in the United States [1]. Based on data from the 1989–1991 National Health Interview Survey (NHIS), 15.1 percent of the civilian, noninstitutionalized population of the United States reported the presence of a musculoskeletal condition that was classified as arthritis by the National Arthritis Data Work Group [2]. The prevalence of arthritis increased with increasing age; the majority of persons aged 65 and above reported the presence of an arthritis diagnosis (Fig. 1). Age-adjusted prevalence was higher in women than men, and in persons of non-Hispanic than of Hispanic ethnicity; there was no difference in age-adjusted prevalence between whites and blacks, but the ratio was lower in Asians [2, 3]. Other factors associated with the presence of arthritis, analyzed in a subset of this cohort aged 18 and above, included being overweight, defined as having a body mass index (BMI) of 25 kg/m^2 of greater, and having low levels of formal education, defined as not being a high school graduate [4].

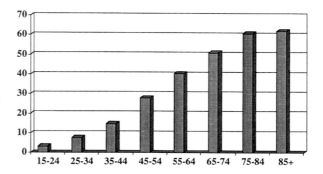

Fig. 1.
Age-specific average annual prevalence of self-reported arthritis. Data derived from the National Health Interview Survey – United States, 1989–1991 [2]

Applying the overall prevalence ratio to 1990 population census figures, an estimated 38 million persons in the United States are affected by arthritis [2].

The impact of arthritis in the United States can be estimated by examining its relationship with disability and its associated economic costs. In the NHIS, disability was defined as some difficulty in performing one or more activities of daily living or instrumental activities of daily living. Overall, almost 3 percent of persons reported that they had an activity limitation attributable to arthritis [2]. Disability attributed to arthritis increased with increasing age, and was higher in women than men, blacks than whites, as well as in people with lower levels of formal education, and people with lower incomes [2]. In an examination of baseline data from the NHIS Longitudinal Supplement on Aging, Verbrugge and colleagues noted that people with other chronic diseases or illnesses in addition to arthritis, and people who were either underweight (BMI < 20 kg/m^2) or severely overweight (BMI > 30 kg/m^2) were also more likely to have arthritis resulting in disability [5].

Musculoskeletal diseases such as arthritis exact a heavy economic burden in the United States [6-9]. The total cost to the U.S. economy (including inpatient and out-patient care, nursing home care, medications, and lost productivity) in 1988 of arthritis was estimated at $54.6 billion [8]; in 1992 dollars, this figure was $64.8 billion [9]. Less than a quarter of these costs are due to direct medical care, including inpatient and outpatient hospital and physician charges, and costs of pharmaceuticals. The vast majority of costs are attributable to indirect costs, predominantly due to lost wages.

More than 100 diseases make up the spectrum of arthritis and musculoskeletal disorders. Most of these diseases are uncommon, are of unknown cause, and allow little opportunity for primary or secondary prevention in the general population [10]. One disorder, osteoarthritis, makes up the vast majority of the disability and economic costs of arthritis, and is subject to primary and secondary prevention initiatives. The remainder of this chapter reviews the epidemiology of osteoarthritis, highlighting studies conducted in the U.S., and notes recent data on economic costs of osteoarthritis.

2.1.2
Definitions of Osteoathritis

Prior to 1986, no standard definition of osteoarthritis, formerly known as degenerative joint disease, existed; most authors described osteoarthritis as a disorder of unknown etiology(ies) in which articular cartilage was primarily affected in contrast to rheumatoid arthritis which primarily affects the synovial membrane. In 1986, the Subcommittee on Osteoarthritis of the American College of Rheumatology Diagnostic and Therapeutic Criteria Committee, proposed the following definition of osteoarthritis: "A heterogeneous group of conditions that lead to joint symptoms and signs which are associated with defective integrity of articular cartilage, in addition to related changes in the underlying bone at the joint margins." [11].

A more comprehensive definition of osteoarthritis was developed at a conference on the Etiopathogenesis of Osteoarthritis sponsored by the National

Institute of Arthritis, Diabetes, Digestive and Kidney Diseases, National Institute on Aging, American Academy of Orthopaedic Surgeons, National Arthritis Advisory Board and Arthritis Foundation [12]. This definition summarizes the clinical, pathophysiologic, biochemical and biomechanical changes that characterize osteoarthritis: "Clinically, the disease is characterized by joint pain, tenderness, limitation of movement, crepitus, occasional effusion, and variable degrees of local inflammation, but without systemic effects. Pathologically, the disease is characterized by irregularly distributed loss of cartilage more frequently in areas of increased load, sclerosis of subchondral bone, subchondral cysts, marginal osteophytes, increased metaphyseal blood flow, and variable synovial inflammation. Histologically, the disease is characterized early by fragmentation of the cartilage surface, cloning of chondrocytes, vertical clefts in the cartilage, variable crystal deposition, remodeling, and eventual violation of the tidemark by blood vessels. It is also characterized by evidence of repair, particularly in osteophytes, and later by total loss of cartilage, sclerosis, and focal osteonecrosis of the subchondral bone. Biomechanically, the disease is characterized by alteration of the tensile, compressive, and shear properties and hydraulic permeability of the cartilage, increased water, and excessive swelling. These cartilage changes are accompanied by increased stiffness of the subchondral bone. Biochemically, the disease is characterized by reduction in the proteoglycan concentration, possible alterations in the size and aggregation of proteoglycans, alteration in collagen fibril size and weave, and increased synthesis and degradation of matrix macromolecules."

A more recent definition of osteoarthritis was developed in 1994 at a workshop entitled "New Horizons in Osteoarthritis" sponsored by the American Academy of Orthopaedic Surgeons, National Institute of Arthritis, Musculoskeletal and Skin Diseases, National Institute on Aging, Arthritis Foundation and Orthopaedic Research and Education Foundation [13]. This definition underscores the concept that osteoarthritis may not represent a single disease entity: "Osteoarthritis is a group of overlapping distinct diseases, which may have different etiologies but with similar biologic, morphologic, and clinical outcomes. The disease processes not only affect the articular cartilage, but involve the entire joint, including the subchondral bone, ligaments, capsule, synovial membrane, and periarticular muscles. Ultimately, the articular cartilage degenerates with fibrillation, fissures, ulceration, and full thickness loss of the joint surface."

2.1.3
Classification of Osteoarthritis

Osteoarthritis, as noted above, is a disorder of diverse etiologies. A classification schema for osteoarthritis developed at the "Workshop on Etiopathogenesis of Osteoarthritis" is shown in Table 1 [12]. Idiopathic osteoarthritis is divided into two forms: localized or generalized; the latter represents the form of osteoarthritis described by Kellgren and Moore involving three or more joint groups. Patients with an underlying disease that appears to have caused their osteoarthritis are classified as having secondary osteoarthritis. Some forms of secondary osteoarthritis [e. g., that due to chronic trauma from leisure and/or

Table 1. Classification of osteoarthritis[a]

I. Idiopathic
  A. Localized
    1. Hands
    2. Feet
    3. Knee
    4. Hip
    5. Spine
    6. Other single sites
  B. Generalized

II. Secondary
  A. Traumatic
  B. Congenital or developmental diseases
  C. Metabolic diseases
    1. Ochronosis
    2. Hemochromatosis
    3. Wilson's disease
    4. Gaucher's disease
  D. Endocrine diseases
    1. Acromegaly
    2. Hyperparathyroidism
    3. Diabetes mellitus
    4. Hypothyroidism
  E. Calcium deposition disease
    1. Calcium pyrophosphate dihydrate deposition disease
    2. Apatite arthropathy
  F. Other bone and joint diseases
  G. Neuropathic (Charcot) arthropathy
  H. Endemic disorders
  I. Miscellaneous conditions

[a] Modified from [11].

occupation activities] may be considered as risk factors for idiopathic osteoarthritis; conversely, risk factors for idiopathic osteoarthritis [e. g., overweight] may be considered as causes of secondary osteoarthritis.

2.1.3.1
Radiographic Criteria

Classically, the diagnosis of osteoarthritis in epidemiologic studies has relied on the characteristic radiographic changes described by Kellgren and Lawrence in 1957 [14], and illustrated in the Atlas of Standard Radiographs [15]. These features include 1) formation of osteophytes on the joint margins or in ligamentous attachments; 2) periarticular ossicles, chiefly in relation to distal and proximal interphalangeal joints; 3) narrowing of joint space associated with sclerosis of subchondral bone; 4) cystic areas with sclerotic walls situated in the subchondral bone; and 5) altered shape of the bone ends, particularly the head of the femur. Combinations of these changes considered together led to the development of an ordinal grading scheme for severity of radiographic features of osteoarthritis: 0 = normal, 1 = doubtful, 2 = minimal, 3 = moderate, and 4 = severe.

Potential limitations of the use of the Kellgren-Lawrence grading scales, as illustrated in the Atlas on Standard Radiographs, have been noted [16]. Radiographic grading scales which focus on individual radiographic features of osteoarthritis at specific joint groups have now been published for the hand [17], hip [18, 19], knee [20, 21], as well as all three peripheral joint groups [22].

2.1.3.2
Clinical Criteria

As noted above, the are potential limitations to the use of purely radiographic criteria for case definition, especially in clinical studies of osteoarthritis. At the Third International Symposium on Population Studies of the Rheumatic Diseases in 1966, the Subcommittee on Diagnostic Criteria for Osteoarthrosis recommended that future population–based studies should investigate the predictive value of certain historical, physical and laboratory findings for the typical radiographic features of osteoarthritis on a joint–by–joint basis [23]. Such historical features included pain on motion, pain at rest, nocturnal joint pain, and morning stiffness. Features on physical examination included bony

Table 2. Algorithm for classification of osteoarthritis of the knee, Subcommittee on Osteoarthritis, American College of Rheumatology Diagnostic and Therapeutic Criteria Committee

---

Clinical[a]
1. Knee pain for most days of prior month
2. Crepitus on active joint motion
3. Morning stiffness ≤30 minutes in duration
4. Age ≥38 years
5. Bony enlargement of the knee on examination

Clinical, Laboratory and Radiographic[b]
1. Knee pain for most days of prior month
2. Osteophytes at joint margins (Xray spurs)
3. Synovial fluid typical of osteoarthritis (laboratory)
4. Age ≥40 years
5. Morning stiffness ≤30 minutes
6. Crepitus on active joint motion

Modified from [11, 27]. Reproduced from Silman AJ, Hochberg MC (1993) Epidemiology of the rheumatic diseases. Oxford University Press, Oxford.
[a] Osteoarthritis present if items 1, 2, 3, 4 or items 1, 2, 5 or items 1, 4, 5 are present. Sensitivity is 89% and specificity is 88%.
[b] Osteoarthritis present if items 1, 2 or items 1, 3, 5, 6 or items 1, 4, 5, 6 are present. Sensitivity is 94% and specificity is 88%.

enlargement, limitation of motion, and crepitus. Laboratory features included erythrocyte sedimentation rate, tests for rheumatoid factor, serum uric acid and appropriate analyses of synovial fluid.

The Subcommittee on Osteoarthritis of the American College of Rheumatology's Diagnostic and Therapeutic Criteria Committee has proposed sets of clinical criteria for the classification of osteoarthritis of the knee [11, 24], hand [25], and hip [26]; these criteria sets have been amplified into algorithms by Altman for ease of use in clinical research and population–based studies (Tables 2 – 4) [27]. These criteria sets identify patients with clinical osteoarthritis, as the major inclusion parameter is joint pain for most days of the prior month. This contrasts with the use of radiographic features alone wherein many, if not most, subjects do not report joint pain. Thus, prevalence estimates using different case definitions will likely be systematically lower when based

Table 3. Algorithm for classification of osteoarthritis of the hand, Subcommittee on Osteoarthritis, American College of Rheumatology Diagnostic and Therapeutic Criteria Committee

Clinical[a]
1. Hand pain, aching, or stiffness for most days of prior month
2. Hard tissue enlargement of ≥ 2 of 10 selected hand joints[b]
3. Fewer than 3 swollen MCP joints
4. Hard tissue enlargement of 2 or more DIP joints
5. Deformity of 2 or more of 10 selected hand joints

Modified from [25, 27]. Reproduced from Silman AJ, Hochberg MC (1993) Epidemiology of the rheumatic diseases. Oxford University Press, Oxford.
DIP = distal interphalangeal, PIP = proximal interphalangeal, MCP = metacarpophalangeal, CMC = carpo–metacarpal.
[a] Osteoarthritis present if items 1, 2, 3, 4 *or* items 1, 2, 3, 5 are present. Sensitivity is 92% and specificity is 98%.
[b] Ten selected hand joints include bilateral 2nd and 3rd DIP joints, 2nd and 3rd PIP joints and 1st CMC joints.

Table 4. Algorithm for classification of osteoarthritis of the hip, Subcommittee on Osteoarthritis, American College of Rheumatology Diagnostic and Therapeutic Criteria Committee

Clinical, Laboratory and Radiographic[a]
1. Hip pain for most days of the prior month
2. Femoral and/or acetabular osteophytes on radiograph
3. Erythrocyte sedimentation rate ≤ 20 mm/hr
4. Axial joint space narrowing on radiograph

Modified from references 26 and 27. Reproduced from Silman AJ, Hochberg MC (1993) Epidemiology of the rheumatic diseases. Oxford University Press, Oxford.
[a] Osteoarthritis present if items 1, 2 *or* items 1, 3, 4 are present. Sensitivity is 91% and specificity is 89%.

on the American College of Rheumatology classification criteria as opposed to traditional radiographic criteria [28]; readers need to be aware of this when reviewing published studies.

2.1.4
Descriptive Epidemiology of Osteoarthritis

2.1.4.1
Prevalence

The prevalence of osteoarthritis has been estimated in two national studies: the National Health Examination Survey (NHES), conducted from 1960 to 1962, [29], and the First National Health and Nutrition Examination Survey (NHANES-I), conducted from 1971 to 1975 [30]. The case definition of osteoarthritis was based on radiographic changes in the hands and feet in the NHES and on radiographic changes in knees and hips in NHANES-I. In addition, a physician's clinical diagnosis of osteoarthritis was also available in NHANES-I. These data were summarized by the National Arthritis Data Work Group in 1989 and again in 1998 [31, 32].

Overall, about one third of adults aged 25 to 74 years have radiographic evidence of osteoarthritis involving at least one site. Specifically, 33 percent had changes of definite osteoarthritis of the hands, 22 percent of the feet, and 4 percent of the knee [31]. Among persons aged 55 to 74, corresponding prevalence ratios were 70 percent for the hands, 40 percent for the feet, 10 percent for the knees, and 3 percent for the hips [32]. Overall, a clinical diagnosis of osteoarthritis, based on symptoms and physical findings, was made by the examining physician in 12 percent of 6,913 examinees aged 25 to 74 years in NHANES-I [30]; using estimates for the 1990 U.S. Population, the National Arthritis Data Work Group estimated that over 20 million adults have physician-diagnosed osteoarthritis [32].

Radiographs of the knees obtained in the NHANES-I were not weight-bearing; hence, joint space narrowing may not have been present in subjects with cartilage loss, leading to an underestimate of the prevalence of radiographic knee osteoarthritis. Population-based data from the Framingham Osteoarthritis Study, a prevalence survey of radiographic knee osteoarthritis in white elders aged 63 to 93 years, suggest that one-third of persons in this age group have evidence of definite radiographic osteoarthritis of the knees [33]. These results are similar to those from the Baltimore Longitudinal Study on Aging [34].

The prevalence of symptomatic knee osteoarthritis can also be estimated from NHANES-I and the Framingham Osteoarthritis Study. Subjects are considered to be symptomatic if they report pain in or around their knees on most days of at least one month. The prevalence of symptomatic knee osteoarthritis was 1.6 percent in adults aged 25 to 74 years using data from NHANES-I [30], and 9.5 percent among adults aged 63 to 93 years in the Framingham Osteoarthritis Study [33].

2.1.4.2
Demographic Factors

Prevalence of osteoarthritis, as well as the proportion of cases with moderate or severe disease, increases with increasing age at least through age 65 to 74 years. Osteoarthritis is more common among men than women under age 45 and more common among women than men over age 54. Clinically, patterns of joint involvement also demonstrate sex differences, with women having on average more joints involved and more frequent complaints of morning stiffness and joint swelling. Among adults in the United States who participated in NHANES-I, radiographic knee osteoarthritis was more common among black women than white women [35]. No racial differences have been noted for hip osteoarthritis [36].

2.1.4.3
Geographic Distribution

Data from national surveys suggest that arthritis and associated disability are more prevalent in the South and least prevalent in the Northeast [2]. Possible explanations for these patterns include lower socioeconomic status and greater proportion of the population employed in manual labor in the South. No specific studies, however, have been conducted to determine reasons for these regional variations.

2.1.4.4
Time Trends

No data are available on time trends in the prevalence of osteoarthritis in the United States. The National Center for Health Statistics recently released the clinical data from NHANES–III, conducted from 1988 to 1993; this study also included radiographs of the hands and knees in elders. When these radiographic data become available, they will be useful for comparing the prevalence of osteoarthritis with the prevalence based on earlier national surveys.

2.1.5
Modifiable Risk Factors for the Development of Osteoarthritis

Risk factors for the development of osteoarthritis have been the subject of many studies. These factors include genetic and nongenetic host factors, and environmental factors (Table 5). Results have been reviewed elsewhere [37–40]; this section will focus on three potentially modifiable factors associated with osteoarthritis of the knee and hip: overweight, occupation and physical activity, and joint injury/trauma. The reader is referred to the above cited reviews for a detailed discussion of the role of other factors in the development of osteoarthritis at these joint groups as well as at other sites, including the hand and spine.

Table 5. Factors associated with the presence of osteoarthritis

Genetic factors
  Gender
  Inherited disorders of type II collagen gene [e.g., Stickler's syndrome]
  Other inherited disorders of bones and joints
  Race/ethnicity
Nongenetic host factors
  Increasing age
  Overweight
  Depletion of female sex hormones [e.g., postmenopausal state] (?)
  Developmental and acquired bone and joint diseases
  Previous joint surgery [e.g., meniscectomy]
Environmental factors
  Occupations and physical demands of work
  Major trauma to joints
  Leisure and/or sports activities

2.1.5.1
Overweight

Overweight is clearly the most important modifiable risk factor for the development of knee osteoarthritis in both sexes; however, its role as a risk factor for the development of osteoarthritis of the hip remains controversial. Many epidemiologic studies have found a cross-sectional association between obesity and radiographically-defined knee osteoarthritis [35, 41–46].

Anderson and Felson studied the association between overweight and radiographic osteoarthritis of the knee in 5,193 subjects aged 35 to 74 years who participated in NHANES-I of whom 315 had definite osteoarthritis of one or both knees [35]. In age-adjusted multiple logistic regression models, there was a significant direct association between BMI and osteoarthritis of the knee in both sexes: for each 5 unit increase in BMI the odds ratio (95% confidence intervals) for the association with osteoarthritis of the knee was 2.10 (1.70, 2.58) in men and 2.20 (1.95, 2.50) in women. After adjustment for potential confounders, the odds ratio increased in men to 2.53 (1.75, 3.68) but remained constant in women at 2.17 (1.74, 2.77). Finally, these authors demonstrated a dose-response relationship between overweight and osteoarthritis in both sexes: in models adjusted for age and race, subjects who were obese and very obese, defined as BMI between 30 kg/m² and 35 kg/m², and over 35 kg/m², respectively, had higher odds of knee osteoarthritis than subjects who were only overweight, defined as body mass index between 25 kg/m² and 30 kg/m², compared to those of normal weight.

Davis and colleagues studied the association between overweight and unilateral and bilateral radiographic osteoarthritis of the knee in 3,885 subjects aged 45 to 74 years who participated in NHANES-I of whom 226 (4.9%) had bilateral osteoarthritis and 75 (1.8%) had unilateral osteoarthritis [44]. Overall, 65.0 percent of subjects with bilateral knee osteoarthritis had a BMI above 30 kg/m², compared to 37.4 percent of 37 subjects with right knee osteoarthritis, 43.3 percent of 38 subjects with left knee osteoarthritis, and 17.7 percent of 3,584 with normal radiographs. In multiple polychotomous logistic regression analysis adjusting for age, sex, and history of knee injury, the odds ratio (95% confidence intervals) for the association of overweight with bilateral knee osteoarthritis was 6.58 (4.71, 9.18) as compared with right knee osteoarthritis and left knee osteoarthritis of 3.26 (1.55, 7.29) and 2.35 (0.96, 5.75), respectively.

Is the association of overweight with osteoarthritis of the knee related to the distribution of body weight and/or the amount of body fat? Davis and colleagues examined the relationship between body fat distribution and osteoarthritis of the knees in subjects aged 45 to 74 years in NHANES-I [45]. Central fat distribution was measured as subscapular skinfold thickness, while peripheral fat distribution was measured as triceps skinfold thickness. There was no association of either subscapular skinfold thickness or triceps skinfold thickness with either unilateral or bilateral osteoarthritis of the knees in men or women after adjustment for age, race and body mass index. BMI remained significantly associated with bilateral knee osteoarthritis in both sexes and unilateral knee osteoarthritis in men only.

Hochberg and colleagues examined the relationship between body fat distribution and percent body fat in 465 Caucasian men and 275 Caucasian women participants in the Baltimore Longitudinal Study of Aging; 169 men and 99 women had radiographic features of definite knee osteoarthritis [46]. Body fat distribution was measured using the ratio of waist and hip girth, while percent body fat was estimated from standard equations using the subscapular, triceps and abdominal skinfold thicknesses. As expected, BMI was significantly associated with the presence of knee osteoarthritis in both sexes. A central body fat distribution, defined as a higher waist-hip ratio, was weakly associated with bilateral knee osteoarthritis in both sexes; however, after adjustment for BMI, body fat distribution was no longer significantly related to the presence of knee osteoarthritis. A higher percent body fat was significantly related to knee osteoarthritis in women but not men; similarly, however, after adjustment for BMI, percent body fat was no longer significantly related to the presence of knee osteoarthritis. Thus, based on these two studies, it appears that being overweight is the important factor related to the presence of knee osteoarthritis, not whether the weight is predominantly fat vs. lean body weight or where the weight is distributed.

Is the relationship of overweight with knee osteoarthritis mediated by biomechanical factors or metabolic factors related to obesity? Davis and colleagues examined the role of metabolic factors in subjects participating in NHANES-I [42]. They found that the strength of the association between overweight and the presence of knee osteoarthritis was not diminished by adjustment for potential confounding variables including blood pressure, serum cholesterol, serum uric acid, body fat distribution and history of diabetes. Similar results have been found in analyses from the Baltimore Longitudinal Study of Aging which failed to demonstrate significant confounding or effect modification of the association of BMI with definite knee osteoarthritis by blood pressure, fasting and 2-hour serum glucose and insulin levels, and fasting serum lipid levels, including cholesterol, triglycerides and HDL-cholesterol [47].

These cross-sectional data demonstrating an association between overweight and osteoarthritis of the knee were confirmed in an analysis of longitudinal data from the Framingham study [48]. These authors examined the relationship between weight measured at examination 1, between 1948–1952, and the presence of radiographic knee osteoarthritis measured 36 years later at the 18th biennial examination in 1983–1985. When subjects were grouped into quintiles based on their sex- and height-adjusted weight at baseline, both men and women in the highest quintiles were significantly more likely to have developed knee osteoarthritis; the relative risks (95 percent confidence intervals) were 1.51 (1.14, 1.98) and 2.07 (1.67, 2.55) in men and women, respectively. Furthermore, women in the fourth quintile also had an elevated relative risk of developing knee osteoarthritis: 1.44 (1.11, 1.86).

Does prevention of weight gain or weight loss among those overweight result in a decreased risk of developing knee osteoarthritis? Felson and colleagues analyzed data from the Framingham study to examine the effect of weight change from the baseline examination on the incidence of symptomatic knee osteoarthritis in women [49]. The outcome in this analysis was the recalled year of onset of knee symptoms in those with radiographic knee osteoarthritis at the 18th biennial examination who also had current knee symptoms. After adjusting for baseline BMI, they showed a relationship between weight change from 6 to 12 years prior to the radiographic examination; women whose weight increased by 2 kg/m^2 had between a 25 and 35 percent increased risk of having current symptomatic knee osteoarthritis compared to women without weight change, while those whose weight decreased by the same magnitude had a reduced risk of developing current symptomatic knee osteoarthritis. Focusing on the 10-year interval prior to the radiographic examination, the authors showed that the odds of having current symptomatic knee osteoarthritis were reduced by 50 percent for a loss of every 2 kg/m^2. Thus, these data suggest that weight loss during adulthood can reduce the risk of developing symptomatic knee osteoarthritis.

The results of cross-sectional studies examining the association of obesity with hip osteoarthritis are inconsistent, suggesting that the relationship is of lower strength than that with osteoarthritis of the knee [36, 41].

Tepper and Hochberg studied the association between overweight and radiographic osteoarthritis of the hip in 2,358 subjects aged 55 to 74 years who participated in NHANES-I of whom only 73 (3.1%) had definite osteoarthritis of one or both hips [36]. In multiple logistic regression models adjusted for age, race and education, there was not a significant association between overweight, defined as a BMI exceeding 27.3 kg/m^2 and 27.8 kg/m^2 in women and men, respectively, and osteoarthritis of the hip in either sex. When the analysis was performed examining the relationship between overweight and either unilateral or bilateral hip osteoarthritis, however, the odds ratio (95% confidence intervals) for the association of overweight with bilateral hip osteoarthritis was 2.00 (0.97, 4.15) as compared with unilateral hip osteoarthritis of 0.54 (0.26, 1.16).

2.1.5.2
Occupation and Physical Activity

Certain occupations which require repetitive use of particular joints over long periods of time have been associated with the development of site-specific osteoarthritis. Specific occupational groups with increased risks of osteoarthritis include miners, who have an excess of knee and lumbar spine disease; dockers and shipyard workers, who have an excess of hand and knee osteoarthritis; cotton and mill workers, who have an excess of hand osteoarthritis involving specific finger joints; pneumatic tool operators, who have an excess of elbow and wrist osteoarthritis; concrete workers and painters, who have an excess of knee osteoarthritis; and farmers, who have an excess of hip osteoarthritis. The relationship between occupation and osteoarthritis has been the subject of several reviews [50, 51]. In addition, Buckwalter has reviewed the biomechanical mechanisms underlying the relationship between abuse of joints and development of osteoarthritis [52].

Anderson and Felson examined data from NHANES-I to study the relationship between occupation and knee osteoarthritis in the general population [35]. Occupation was coded into one of seven broad categories and the physical demand and knee-bending requirement for each code were categorized into 3-level variables: low/moderate/high or none/some/much, respectively. Occupations associated with high strength demands included laborers and service workers, while those associated with much knee-bending included laborers and service workers and craftsmen. In multiple logistic regression models adjusted for race, BMI and education levels, subjects in both sexes aged 55 to 64 years who worked in jobs with either increasing strength demands or higher knee-bending demands had greater odds of radiographic knee osteoarthritis.

The association between occupational physical demands and knee osteoarthritis was confirmed in men in the longitudinal Framingham study [53]. Occupational status was assessed between examinations 1 and 6, i.e., 1948–51 through 1958–61, and presence of radiographic knee osteoarthritis was determined at examination 18 in 1983–85. Occupations which involved at least a medium level of physical demand and knee-bending included craftsmen, operators/transporters, and laborers/service workers. Men who were employed in jobs requiring knee-bending and medium, heavy or very heavy physical demands had a 2-fold greater risk of developing radiographic knee osteoarthritis than men employed in jobs not requiring knee-bending and with only sedentary or light physical demands. Furthermore, these authors estimated that the proportion of radiographic knee osteoarthritis in men attributable to these occupational factors was 15 percent. Thus, certain occupations which repetitively stress apparently normal knee joints through repeated use appear to predispose to the development of knee osteoarthritis.

Occupational physical activity has also shown to be associated with hip osteoarthritis in several studies conducted in Europe; these are reviewed elsewhere [40, 50]. In the only U.S. Study which examined the relationship between occupation and hip osteoarthritis, Roach and colleagues compared occupational work load, defined based on estimated joint compression forces produced by an occupational activity, in 99 men with primary hip osteoarthritis and 233 male controls known to be free of radiographic hip osteoarthritis [54]. Work load was categorized as light, intermediate or heavy based on the type and duration of exposure to different levels of sitting, standing, walking or lifting in their jobs. In multiple logistic regression models, adjusting for obesity and history of sports actitivies, men with hip osteoarthritis had a 2.5-fold greater odds of having performed heavy workloads than controls. Furthermore, duration of performing heavy workloads also appeared to be significantly related to increasing odds of hip osteoarthritis.

2.1.5.3
Sports and Exercise

Many studies have been conducted to examine the relationship between regular physical activity and osteoarthritis; most of the recent European studies have included elite athletes, particularly football players, runners, and soccer players. Panush and Lane [55], and Lane and Buckwalter, [56], reviewed these and older studies, and concluded that individuals who participate in sports at a highly competitive level [i.e., elite athletes] or who have abnormal or injured joints appear to be at increased risk of developing osteoarthritis as compared to persons with normal joints who participate in low impact activites.

Running as a recreational activity does not appear to be a risk factor for the development of osteoarthritis of the knee in the absence of knee injury [57–59].

2.1.5.4
Joint Injury/Trauma

As noted above, leisure physical activity does not appear to be associated with an increased risk of either knee or hip osteoarthritis in the absence of joint injury. Furthermore, knee injury, especially rupture of the anterior cruciate ligament, is associated with an increased risk of knee osteoarthritis in elite soccer players. Is joint injury associated with knee and hip osteoarthritis in the general population?

Davis and colleagues studied the association between knee injury and unilateral and bilateral radiographic osteoarthritis of the knee in 3,885 subjects aged 45 to 74 years who participated in NHANES-I of whom 226 (4.9%) had bilateral osteoarthritis and 75 (1.8%) had unilateral osteoarthritis [44]. Overall, a history of right knee injury was present in 5.8 percent of subjects with bilateral knee osteoarthritis, 15.8 percent of 37 subjects with right knee osteoarthritis and 1.5 percent of controls, while a history of left knee injury was present in 4.6 percent of those with bilateral knee osteoarthritis, 27.0 percent of subjects with left knee osteoarthritis and 1.8 percent of controls. In multiple polychotomous logistic regression analysis adjusting for age, sex, and BMI, the odds ratio (95% confidence intervals) for the association of knee injury with bilateral knee osteoarthritis was 3.51 (1.80, 6.83) as compared with right knee osteoarthritis and left knee osteoarthritis of 16.30 (6.50, 40.9) and 10.90 (3.72, 31.93), respectively.

Tepper and Hochberg studied the association between hip injury and radiographic osteoarthritis of the hip in 2,358 subjects aged 55 to 74 years who participated in NHANES-I of whom only 73 (3.1%) had definite osteoarthritis of one or both hips [36]. In multiple logistic regression models adjusted for age, race and education, a history of hip injury was significantly associated with higher odds of hip osteoarthritis: odds ratio (95% confidence intervals) 7.84 (2.11, 29.10). When the analysis was performed examining the relationship between hip injury and either unilateral or bilateral hip osteoarthritis, however, the odds ratio (95% confidence intervals) for the association of hip injury with unilateral hip osteoarthritis was 24.2 (3.84, 153) as compared with bilateral hip osteoarthritis of 4.17 (0.50, 34.7). Thus, these data suggest that hip and knee injury are an important risk factor for hip and knee osteoarthritis, respectively, especially unilateral hip and knee osteoarthritis.

2.1.5.5
Population – Attributable Risk

Several studies provide data on the estimated proportion of knee osteoarthritis attributable to individual risk factors. For overweight, based on data from the Baltimore Longitudinal Study of Aging, Hochberg and colleagues estimated that the proportion of knee osteoarthritis attributed to overweight, defined as being in the highest tertile of BMI, was 31.6 percent in men and 52.4 percent in women [46]. For occupational activity, Felson and colleagues estimated that the proportion of cases of radiographic knee osteoarthritis attributable to jobs with both physical demands and knee bending was 15 percent [51]. The amount of knee osteoarthritis attributable to sports and joint injury/trauma would be expected to be lower because of the low prevalence of these exposures in the general population. Thus, for knee osteoarthritis, overweight is the most important modifiable risk factor followed by occupational activity.

Data on which to base estimates for osteoarthritis of the hip are limited to studies from Scandinavia, and are discussed elsewhere [40].

2.1.6
Prevention of Osteoarthritis

2.1.6.1
Primary Prevention

Epidemiologic considerations in the primary prevention of osteoarthritis have been reviewed elsewhere [38, 40]. Primary prevention strategies directed towards preventing overweight through dietary instruction and regular low intensity physical exercise, workplace modification to reduce the physical stress on lower extremity joints, and preventing major joint injury would be expected to reduce the incidence of hip and knee osteoarthritis in the population. National recommendations include reducing obesity (BMI > 27.8 for men and > 27.3 for women) to a prevalence of no more than 20% among adults and 15% among

Table 6. Factors associated with progression of osteoarthritis of the knee

Older age

Female sex

Overweight

Generalized osteoarthritis
  Heberden's nodes

Low dietary intake of antioxidants

Low dietary intake (serum levels) of vitamin D

adolescents and reducing the number of nonfatal unintentional injuries, especially those that are work-related.

2.1.6.2
Secondary Prevention

Factors associated with the progression of osteoarthritis have been reviewed elsewhere and are listed in Table 6 [60, 61]. Secondary prevention strategies directed towards weight loss through dietary instruction and regular low intensity aerobic physical exercise have been shown to decrease symptoms and functional limitation in patients with knee osteoarthritis [62]; it is possible that this intervention may slow progression of knee osteoarthritis and reduce the need for total joint replacement. In addition, recent data from the Framingham Osteoarthritis Study suggest that elders with a low dietary intake of antioxidants, especially vitamin C and vitamin E, as well as those with low serum levels of vitamin D, have higher rates of progression of radiographic changes of knee osteoarthritis [63–65]. Hence, dietary supplementation with vitamin C 1000 mg/day, vitamin D 400 IU/day, and vitamin E 400 IU/day, may be indicated in elders with knee osteoarthritis.

2.1.7
Economic Impact of Osteoarthritis

As noted above, arthritis and related musculoskeletal diseases exact a tremendous economic burden in the United States. Gabriel and colleagues estimated the economic burden attributable to osteoarthritis using data from the Rochester Epidemiology Project [66, 67]. They identified all prevalent cases of osteoarthritis among Olmsted County residents as off January 1, 1987, and examined billing data for all health services, including pharmacy charges for prescription medications, using the Olmsted County Health Care Utilization and Expenditures Database [66]. The prevalence cohort included 6,742 individuals aged 35 and above with osteoarthritis who had a mean age of 69 years; these cases represented 17 percent of the Olmsted County population aged 35 and above. Eighty-five percent of the osteoarthritis cases received medical care in the index year and had average direct medical charges of $2,654 per person; the age-, and sex-adjusted median charge per person was $664. These charges were significantly greater that those for patients without arthritis, but were significantly lower that for patients with rheumatoid arthritis.

Indirect medical costs and nonmedical costs were examined in a sample of 200 patients with osteoarthritis drawn from this prevalent cohort [67]. One hundred sixteen (58%) completed a self-administered questionnaire detailing their use of and expenditures for nonmedical practitioners, total number of days missed from work due to illness, use of home health care services due to illness, and other factors which may contribute to indirect costs for the calendar year 1992. Forty percent of respondents with osteoarthritis incurred indirect or nonmedical expenditures in 1992; the average indirect and nonmedical expenditures, excluding wage losses, were $726 per person. These costs were significantly greater than persons without arthritis, but were significantly lower than those among patients with rheumatoid arthritis.

References

1. Kelsey JL, Hochberg MC (1988) Epidemiology of chronic musculoskeletal disorders. Ann Rev Public Health 9:379–401
2. Centers for Disease Control (1994) Arthritis prevalence and activity limitations – United States, 1990. MMWR 43:433–438
3. Centers for Disease Control (1996) Prevalence and impact of arthritis by race and ethnicity – United States, 1989–1991. MMWR 45:373–378
4. Centers for Disease Control (1996) Factors associated with prevalent self-reported arthritis and other rheumatic conditions – United States, 1989–1991. MMWR 45:487–491
5. Verbrugge LM, Gates DM, Ike RW (1991) Risk factors for disability among US adults with arthritis. J Clin Epidemiol 44:167–182
6. Felts W, Yelin E (1989) The economic impact of the rheumatic diseases in the United States. J Rheumatol 16:867–884
7. Yelin EH, Felts WR (1990) A summary of the impact of musculoskeletal conditions in the United States. Arthritis Rheum 33:750–755
8. Praemer A, Furner S, Rice DP (eds) (1992) Musculoskeletal Conditions in the United States. Park Ridge, American Academy of Orthopaedic Surgeons
9. Yelin E, Callahan LF, for the National Arthritis Data Work Group (1995) The economic cost and social and psychological impact of musculoskeletal conditions. Arthritis Rheum 38:1351–62
10. Hochberg MC, Flores RH (1995) Arthritis and connective tissue diseases. In: Thoene J (ed) Physician's Guide to Rare Diseases. Second edition. Montvale, Dowden Publishing Co. Inc. 745–86
11. Altman R, Asch E, Bloch D, Bole G, Borenstein D, Brandt K et al. (1986) Development of criteria for the classification and reporting of osteoarthritis: classification of osteoarthritis of the knee. Arthritis Rheum 29:1039–1049
12. Brandt KD, Mankin HJ, Shulman LE (1986) Workshop on etiopathogenesis of osteoarthritis. J Rheumatol 13:1126–1160
13. Kuttner K, Goldberg VM (eds) (1995) Osteoarthritic Disorders. American Academy of Orthopaedic Surgeons, Rosemont xxi–v
14. Kellgren JH, Lawrence JS (1957) Radiologic assessment of osteoarthrosis. Ann Rheum Dis 16:494–501
15. The Department of Rheumatology and Medical Illustration, University of Manchester (1973) The Epidemiology of Chronic Rheumatism, Vol 2, Atlas of Standard Radiographs of Arthritis. F. A. Davis Company, Philadelphia 1–15

16. Spector TD, Hochberg MC (1994) Methodological problems in the epidemiological study of osteoarthritis. Ann Rheum Dis 53:143–146
17. Kallman DA, Wigley FM, Scott WW Jr, Hochberg MC, Tobin JD (1989) New radiographic grading scales for osteoarthritis of the hand. Arthritis Rheum 32:1584–1591
18. Croft P, Cooper C, Wickham C, Coggon D (1990) Defining osteoarthritis of the hip for epidemiologic studies. Amer J Epidemiol 132:514–522
19. Lane NE, Nevitt MC, Genant HK, Hochberg MC (1993) Reliability of new indices of radiographic osteoarthritis of the hand and hip and lumbar disc degeneration. J Rheumatol 20:1911–1918
20. Spector TD, Cooper C, Cushnaghan J, Hart DJ, Dieppe PA (1992) A Radiographic Atlas of Knee Osteoarthritis. Springer-Verlag, London
21. Scott WW Jr, Lethbridge–Cejku M, Reichle R, Wigley FM, Tobin JD, Hochberg MC (1993) Reliability of grading scales for individual radiographic features of osteoarthritis of the knee: the Baltimore Longitudinal Study of Aging atlas of knee osteoarthritis. Invest Radiol 28:497–501
22. Altman RD, Hochberg MC, Murphy WA Jr, Wolfe F, Lequesne M (1995) Atlas of individual radiographic features in osteoarthritis. Osteoarthritis Cart 3 (Suppl A): 3–70
23. Bennett PH, Wood PHN (eds) (1968) Population Studies of the Rheumatic Diseases, International Congress Series No. 148. Excerpta Medica Foundation, Amsterdam 417–419
24. Altman RD, Meenan RF, Hochberg MC, Bole GG Jr, Brandt K, Cooke TDV, et al. (1983) An approach to developing criteria for the clinical diagnosis and classification of osteoarthritis: a status report of the American Rheumatism Association Diagnostic Subcommittee on Osteoarthritis. J Rheumatol 10:180–183
25. Altman R, Alarcon G, Appelrough D, Bloch D, Borenstein D, Brandt K et al. (1990) The American College of Rheumatology criteria for the classification and reporting of osteoarthritis of the hand. Arthritis Rheum 33:1601–1610
26. Altman R, Alarcon G, Appelrough D, Bloch D, Borenstein D, Brandt K, et al. (1991) The American College of Rheumatology criteria for the classification and reporting of osteoarthritis of the hip. Arthritis Rheum 34:505–514
27. Altman R (1991) Classification of disease: osteoarthritis. Semin Arthritis Rheum 20 (6, Suppl 2): 40–47
28. Hart DJ, Leedham-Green M, Spector TD (1991) The prevalence of knee osteoarthritis in the general population using different clinical criteria: the Chingford Study. Br J Rheumatol 30 (S 2): 72
29. Engle A (1966) Osteoarthritis in adults by selected demographic characteristics, United States – 1960–1962. Vital Health Stat, Series 11, No. 20, Washington, D.C.
30. Maurer K (1979) Basic data on arthritis knee, hip and sacroiliac joints in adults ages 25–74 years, United States, 1971–1975. Vital Health Stat, Series 11, No. 213, Washington, D.C.
31. Lawrence RC, Hochberg MC, Kelsey JL, et al. (1989) Estimates of the prevalence of selected arthritic and musculoskeletal diseases in the United States. J Rheumatol 16:427–441
32. Lawrence RC, Helmick CG, Arnett FC, et al. (1998) Prevalence estimates of the arthritis and selected musculoskeletal diseases in the United States. Arthritis Rheum 41: in press
33. Felson DT, Naimark A, Anderson J, Kazis L, Castelli W, Meenan RF (1987) The prevalence of knee osteoarthritis in the elderly. Arthritis Rheum 30:914–918
34. Lethbridge-Cejku M, Tobin JD, Scott WW Jr, Reichle R, Plato CC, Hochberg MC (1994) The relationship of age and gender to prevalence and pattern of radiographic changes of osteoarthritis of the knee: data from the Baltimore Longitudinal Study of Aging. Aging Clin Exp Res 6:353–7
35. Anderson JJ, Felson DT (1988) Factors associated with osteoarthritis of the knee in the First National Health and Nutrition Examination Survey (NHANES-I): evidence for an association with overweight, race, and physical demands of work. Am J Epidemiol 128:179–189
36. Tepper S, Hochberg MC (1993) Factors associated with hip osteoarthritis: data from the National Health and Nutrition Examination Survey (NHANES-I). Amer J Epidemiol 137:1081–1088

37. Scott JC, Hochberg MC (1987) Epidemiologic insights into the pathogenesis of hip osteo-arthritis. In Hadler NM (ed) Clinical Concepts in Regional Musculoskeletal Illness. Orlando, Grune & Stratton 89–107
38. Hochberg MC (1991) Epidemiologic considerations in the primary prevention of osteo-arthritis. J Rheumatol 18:1438–1440
39. Silman AJ, Hochberg MC (1993) Epidemiology of the Rheumatic Diseases. Oxford, Oxford University Press 257–88
40. Hochberg MC, Lethbridge-Cejku M (1997) Epidemiologic considerations in the primary prevention of osteoarthritis. In Hamerman D (ed) Osteoarthritis: Public Health Implications for an Aging Population. Johns Hopkins University Press, Baltimore 169–186
41. Hartz AJ, Fischer ME, Brill G et al. (1986) The association of obesity with joint pain and osteoarthritis in the HANES data. J Chron Dis 39:311–319
42. Davis MA, Ettinger WH, Neuhaus JM (1988) The role of metabolic factors and blood pressure in the association of obesity with osteoarthritis of the knee. J Rheumatol 15:1827–1832
43. Davis MA, Ettinger WH, Neuhaus JM, Hauck WW (1998) Sex differences in osteoarthritis of the knee: the role of obesity. Am J Epidemiol 127:1019–1030
44. Davis MA, Ettinger WH, Neuhaus JM, Cho SA, Houck WW (1989) The association of knee injury and obesity with unilateral and bilateral osteoarthritis of the knee. Am J Epidemiol 130:278–288
45. Davis MA, Neuhaus JM, Ettinger WH, Mueller WH (1990) Body fat distribution and osteo-arthritis. Am J Epidemiol 132:701–707
46. Hochberg MC, Lethbridge-Cejku M, Scott WW Jr, Reichle R, Plato CC, Tobin JD (1995) The association of body weight, body fatness and body fat distribution with osteoarthritis of the knee: data from the Baltimore Longitudinal Study of Aging. J Rheumatol 22:488–493
47. Martin K, Lethbridge-Cejku M, Muller D, Elahi D, Andres R, Plato CC, Tobin JD, Hochberg MC (1997) Metabolic correlates of obesity and radiographic features of knee osteoarthri-tis: data from the Baltimore Longitudinal Study of Aging. J Rheumatol 24:702–707
48. Felson DT, Anderson JJ, Naimark AA, Walker AM, Meenan RF (1988) Obesity and knee osteoarthritis: the Framingham study. Ann Intern Med 109:18–24
49. Felson DT, Zhang Y, Anthony JM, Naimark A, Anderson JJ (1992) Weight loss reduces the risk for symptomatic knee osteoarthritis in women: the Framingham Study. Ann Intern Med 116:535–539
50. Cooper C (1995) Occupational activity and the risk of osteoarthritis. J Rheumatol 22 (suppl 43): 10–2
51. Felson DT (1994) Do occupation-related physical factors contribute to arthritis? Balliere's Clin Rheumatol 8:63–77
52. Buckwalter JA (1995) Osteoarthritis and articular cartilage use, disuse, and abuse: ex-perimental studies. J Rheumatol 1995;22(suppl 43):13–5
53. Felson DT, Hannan MT, Naimark A, Berkeley J, Gordon G, Wilson PWF, Anderson J. Occupational physical demands, knee bending, and knee osteoarthritis: results from the Framingham study. J Rheumatol 18:1587–1592
54. Roach KE, Persky V, Miles T, Budiman-Mak E (1994) Biomechanical aspects of occupation and osteoarthritis of the hip: a case-control study. J Rheumatol 21:2334–2340
55. Panush RS, Lane NE (1994) Exercise and the musculoskeletal system. Balliere's Clin Rheumatol 8:79–102
56. Lane NE, Buckwalter JA (1993) Exercise: a cause of osteoarthritis? Rheum Dis Clin N.A. 19:617–633
57. Lane NE, Bloch DA, Jones HH, Marshall W Jr, Wood PD, Fries JF (1986) Long distance run-ning, bone density and osteoarthritis. JAMA 255:1147–1151
58. Lane NE, Bloch DA, Hubert HB, Jones H, Simpson U, Fries JF (1990) Running, osteo-arthritis, and bone density: initial 2-year longitudinal study. Am J Med 88:452–459
59. Lane NE, Michel B, Bjorkengren A, Oehlert J, Shi H, Bloch DA, Fries JF (1993) The risk of osteoarthritis with running and aging: a 5-year longitudinal study. J Rheumatol 20:461–468

60. Felson DT (1993) The course of osteoarthritis and factors that affect it. Rheum Dis Clin N.A. 19:607–615
61. Hochberg MC (1996) Progression of osteoarthritis. Ann Rheum Dis 55:685–688
62. Martin K, Nicklas BJ, Bunyard LB, et al. (1996) Weight loss and walking improve symptoms of knee osteoarthritis. Arthritis Rheum 39 (Suppl 9): S225
63. McAlindon RE, Lacques P, Zhang Y, et al. (1997) Do antioxidant micronutrients protect against the development and progression of knee osteoarthritis? Arthritis Rheum 39:648–656
64. McAlindon RE, Lacques P, Zhang Y, et al. (1996) The relationship between vitamin D status and knee osteoarthritis progression. Ann Intern Med 125:353–359
65. McAlindon T, Felson DT (1997) Nutrition: risk factors for osteoarthritis. Ann Rheum Dis 56:397–402
66. Gabriel SE, Crowson CS, Campion ME, O'Fallon WM (1997) Direct medical costs unique to people with arthritis. J Rheumatol 24:719–725
67. Gabriel SE, Crowson CS, Campion ME, O'Fallon WM (1997) Indirect and nonmedical costs among people with rheumatoid arthritis and osteoarthritis compared with non-arthritic controls. J Rheumatol 24:43–48

2.2
The European Viewpoint

X. BADIA LLACH

2.2.1
Introduction

Data on epidemiological aspects of osteoarthritis (OA) in various European countries has become increasingly available over recent years, to the point where it is beginning to be possible to put together a broad picture of prevalence in different populations, and of the risk factors associated with the disease. Nevertheless, problems still arise in providing an overview of the situation, particularly at a European level, largely for two reasons: firstly, because of a lack of published data in some countries, and, secondly, because very few of the epidemiological studies carried out to date are strictly comparable. In particular, the use of different criteria for classifying individuals with OA, and the use of different methodologies for measuring prevalence, may well account for a considerable amount of the variation in prevalence found in different studies. Though many studies of the prevalence of OA have used Kellgren and Lawrence's system of radiographic changes [1], recent studies have used other measurements, such as self-reports of joint pain, and even where Kellgren and Lawrence's system is used there is still disagreement about how subjects should be classified using that system, for example, whether subjects with Grade II changes should be included in study protocols or dealt with as a separate group [2]. In the case of self-reports of joint pain there is evidence of a lack of reliability [3], and in the case of combined methods there is evidence that they may produce excessively low prevalence rates [2].

Agreement on classification and measurement is essential if data is to be compared across studies and across countries; the use of standardised measures would also provide more accurate information on the prevalence and incidence of OA. The discrepancies between studies and the rather partial information available, as well as the growing importance of OA, not only in terms of its effects on health but also its impact on health care systems, would appear to make studies at a European level essential. Such studies, using standardized classifications and measurement techniques, would not only help to fill in the gaps concerning various epidemiological aspects of the disease, but would also provide important opportunities for co-operation on means of tackling the disease.

That new approaches are necessary seems beyond doubt, especially given the rising costs associated with the disease. Though readily available data on the economic impact of OA is also somewhat lacking in Europe, there can be little doubt that the condition is a major contributor to both direct and indirect (social) costs, and that these costs are likely to increase in the long-term, given the combination of the degenerative nature of the disease and the ageing of populations in Europe, together with the increasing availability and rising costs of health care used to treat patients with the disease. Again, the limited number of cost-based studies to date make it difficult to estimate costs on a European scale, though an approximate idea can be gained from the data that do exist. Further studies are required to make more accurate estimations, to estimate likely trends in future costs, and to find the most cost-effective ways of improving the quality of life of people with the disease.

2.2.2
Prevalence

2.2.2.1
General

In Spain, a study carried out in 1990 which used self-reports to study the prevalence of rheumatic disease in the community, found that 12.7% of all respondents reported some form of rheumatic complaint (25.7% in individuals over 60), of which 43% were reported to be osteoarthritic complaints. Reporting of osteoarthritic complaints differed between the sexes, with 29.4% of men and 52.3% of women reporting osteoarthritic complaints [4]. A survey of the prevalence of chronic conditions in the Scottish highlands showed that symptomatic OA had an overall prevalence of 65 per 1000 but rose from one in 20 of those aged 40–50 years to one quarter of those aged over 70 [5].

2.2.2.2
Small Joints of the Hand

Petersson has provided a very useful review of the occurrence of OA in the peripheral joints in European populations [6], reporting that OA of the finger joints was present in about 10% of individuals aged 40–49, rising to 92% in individuals over 70 (>90% in females; 80% in males). A comparison of Swedish and Dutch elderly populations using a similar methodology found prevalence figures of 92% and 75% respectively. In individuals over 15, prevalence figures were 22% and 29% for males and females.

2.2.2.3
Hip OA

In Britain, Kellgren and Lawrence reported prevalence rates of hip OA in individuals over 55 as 8.4% in women and 3.1% in men for OA grade 3 or 4 on the Kellgren and Lawrence system [7], Jørring reported figures for Denmark in persons over 60 of 5.6% in women and 3.7% for men [8], while a retrospective Swedish study of 12,051 radiographs indicated that prevalence of coxarthrosis rose from less than 1% in the population aged under 55 to 10% in those over 85, with an average prevalence of 3.1% for subjects over age 55, and no differences between sexes [9]. The Swedish figures were identical to figures reported 20 years previously [10]. In Holland, prevalence of hip OA has also been reported to be approximately 3% in the 45 – 49 age group for OA of Kellgren and Lawrence grade 2 or more [11].

2.2.2.4
Knee OA

As Petersson states, prevalence figures for knee OA vary substantially across studies. For example, in 1958 Kellgren and Lawrence reported figures of 40.7% for women and 29.8% for men in subjects aged 55 – 64, whilst more recent figures range between 2.9% in women aged 45 – 65 [12] to 7.7% – 14.3% in individuals aged 45 – 49 years [11]. A Swedish study which made use of self-reports of joint pain to measure prevalence of OA in an elderly population found that 30 – 43% of female subjects and 15 – 25% of male subjects between the ages of 70 and 79 reported joint complaints, and that knee joints were the most common site of complaints in both sexes. It should be noted, however, that reporting did not appear to be consistent, with complaints tending to 'disappear' with repeated measurements. In all, 15% of women and 3% of men reported joint complaints on all three occasions (at baseline and at 4 and 5 year intervals), though an association was found between repeatedly reported complaints and radiographic OA [13].

2.2.2.5
Cervical and Lumbar Spine OA

Surprisingly, given the importance of lower back pain as a prime determinant of lost work days and physician visits, data on the prevalence of lumbar and cervical OA is relatively scarce, although at least one study found that it was one of the most prevalent sites of OA, with peak rates as high as 84% and 70% for cervical and lumbar spine OA, respectively, in older age groups and based on radiological OA [11].

Finally, at least two studies have been carried out which suggest that there may be substantial regional variation in prevalence within countries. An interview survey carried out in Sweden found that reported long-standing illness, complaints, handicap or other debility due to OA were most prevalent in northern and south-eastern areas of Sweden, with these variations being attributed principally to differences in climatic (hot and cold) conditions at work, though also to variations in the amount of physical strain at work [14]. Likewise, in a recent French study of 20,325 individuals aged between 35 and 50, OA was one of the conditions in which statistically significant regional variations were found, with the likelihood of having OA being lower than the national mean in western France (odds ratio 0.6–0.79) and higher in the South (odds ratios 1.24–1.46) [15].

2.2.3
Incidence

Relatively few studies of the incidence of OA have been reported in the literature in Europe. A 12-year follow up study of 258 individuals aged over 45 from the general population showed that approximately 25% of women and 10% of men developed radiographic knee OA during the study period [16], whilst in individuals between 75 and 79 the incidence in small joints of the hand was 13.6% and of knee OA 4.5% over a 5 year period [13]. A 1992 French study found that the mean ages for onset of chronic pain in women with lateral femoro-patellar, medial femora-tibial, and lateral femoro-tibial OA were 56.6 (+/–12), 62.7 (+/–12), and 69.2 (+/–10) years, respectively. Onset of pain was slightly later in men (60.5 +/–10 for lateral femoro-patellar OA, and 64 +/–10 in medial femoral-tibial OA) [15].

2.2.4
Risk Factors

2.2.4.1
Genetic

Few epidemiological studies of the impact of genetic factors on osteoarthritis have been carried out in Europe. However, a recent study carried out in England found significant differences between identical and non-identical twins in terms of prevalence in both twins, with a clear genetic effect of hand or knee OA in women, and genetic influences ranging from 39 to 65% [17]. A further study, also based in England, suggested that the relative risk of undergoing total knee or hip replacement was higher in siblings than in spouses of those who had already undergone such an operation, with relative risks of 1.86 and 4.8 in the sibling group for hip and knee replacements, respectively [18]. Though some progress has been made in identifying hereditary defects, such as those in type II collagen, which appear to predispose to the early development of osteoarthritis in affected family members, considerable further research is necessary to understand the epidemiological role of genetic factors in OA. Again, given the size of combined European populations, and the range of genetic bases, the possibility of co-operation at European level seems to provide an ideal opportunity for the epidemiological study of the role of genetic factors in the development of OA, though to date it is an opportunity which has not been taken advantage of to any great extent.

2.2.4.2
Overweight

The association between increased risk of developing OA and being overweight is increasingly clear, with recent studies showing, for example, close associations between body mass index (BMI) and bilateral coxarthrosis, with adjusted odds ratios of having bilateral coxarthrosis for those with a BMI >35 of 2.8 (1.4–5.7) compared to subjects with a BMI of <25 [19]. A study of middle-aged women in an English sample of the general population also found that obesity was a strong and important risk factor in the development of knee OA with odds ratios of 17.99 for the upper tertile of the sample on BMI of having bilateral knee OA compared to the lowest tertile, though associations between obesity and OA of the small joints of the hand were not so strong [20]. In a study of the association between various risk factors and coxarthrosis, it was found that although being overweight was a risk factor in the development of hip OA, it appeared to be less important than physical work load and sport, with the etiologic fraction related to the three factors being 55% for sports, 40% for physical work load and 15% for obesity. Together, however, these three factors explained 80% of the idiopathic coxarthrosis [21].

2.2.4.3
Occupation

Several studies have shown that occupation can be a significant risk factor in the development of OA, with sites of OA being associated with the type of work performed. For example, it was found that knee OA was more common among carpet and floor layers than among painters [22], and that OA of the acromioclavicular joint was more common among construction workers than among foremen, with odds ratios of 2.62 and 7.67 for right and left sides, respectively [23]. The increased prevalence of coxarthrosis among farmers when compared with controls in mainly sedentary jobs (odds ratios of 9.3 in farmers who had farmed for over 10 years) led to the suggestion that hip OA should be a prescribed industrial disease in farmers [24]. Activities principally identified with the development of OA are regular lifting for OA of the hip, and knee bending for OA of the knee [25].

2.2.4.4
Age

Although it is clear that most forms of OA are very much age-related, with prevalence being very low below the age of 45–50, OA is not an inevitable consequence of ageing, but depends on many interacting factors such as the site of OA, gender, lifestyle, etc., that make it difficult to generalise as to age of onset (though see [15] for further data).

There have also been relatively few studies of the effect of ageing on disease progression, though at least one follow-up study suggested that long term prognosis was good in a large proportion of patients with OA, with no change over an 11 year follow-up period in 60% of knees studied, and mild deterioration in 33%, using the Kellgren and Lawrence system. In the same study, no significant differences were found in terms of self-reported pain using visual analogue scales between the two administrations. The study did suggest, however, that reporting of knee pain might have prognostic significance [26].

2.2.4.5
Gender

It is also becoming increasingly clear that gender plays an important role in the development of OA, with women being more susceptible to OA in many sites, though perhaps not all. A Finnish study of 6,647 farmers aged 40–64 published in 1996 for example found that being female was an independent predictor of having disabling knee OA, with odds ratios in women compared to men of 7 (2.5–19.7), 3.3 (1.1–9.8), and 4.8 (2.4–9.3) of having right unilateral, left unilateral and bilateral knee OA, respectively [27]. Also, a review of 29 epidemiological studies of hip and knee OA from 14 countries, appeared to show that the presence of radiographic OA of the hip was higher in men than in women, though the pattern was reversed for OA of the knee, especially over age 45 [28]. Nevertheless, the majority of studies reviewed for this chapter suggest that hip OA is also more prevalent in women. It has been suggested that the sharp increase in the incidence of knee OA in women over age 50 may be due to changes in hormonal status associated with menopause [28]. Again, although the evidence of gender being a risk factor is fairly conclusive for some OA sites, there is nevertheless conflicting evidence for other sites, and much work needs to be done to on understanding the mechanisms which produce increased levels of risk, particularly in women, and on means of tackling this differential, both at a biological and public health level.

2.2.4.6
Sport

There is an increasing amount of evidence regarding the role of sport as a risk factor for OA. For example, it has been found that incidence of admission to hospital for OA of the hip, knee or ankle is between 1.73 and 2.17 times higher in athletes than in control subjects, with athletes practising mixed and power sports having higher rates of admissions for premature OA, and admissions being at an older age in endurance athletes [29]; that in a comparison of overweight, physical work-load and sport as risk factors for coxarthrosis showed the etiologic fraction related to sport to be 55%, compared to 40% for physical work-load and 15% for overweight [21]; and that weight-bearing sports activity

in runners and tennis players produced a 2- to 3-fold increased risk for radiologic OA of the knees and hips in the study group compared to matched control
groups [30]. Soccer has also been shown to lead to a possible increased risk of
hip OA [31].

2.2.4.7
Others

At least one recent European study has provided evidence that the risk of
developing hip OA leading to total hip replacement (THR) is greater among
smokers than non-smokers (OR 1.5), as well as suggesting that the use of
contraceptive pills appeared to increase the relative risk for THR, this risk
was decreased by oestrogen substitution [32]. Ethnicity is a further risk factor
to be taken into account, with the review of 29 epidemiological studies from
14 countries mentioned above finding that radiographic hip OA was higher
in Caucasian populations than in non-Caucasian populations, though there
appeared to be no differences in prevalence of radiographic knee OA [28].
Other studies have shown that rural populations appear to be at greater risk
of developing coxarthrosis than urban populations, though the increased risk
was attributed primarily to the heavy labour involved in farming in the rural
population [33]. Finally, physical trauma is also positively associated with the
presence of coxarthrosis, one study finding odds ratios of 2.1 of unilateral
coxarthrosis and 1.5 of bilateral coxarthrosis in a sample which had suffered
physical trauma compared to controls [19].

2.2.5
Resource Implications

Given the relatively high prevalence rates of various types of OA and its fairly severe impact on health and functional capacity, it is hardly surprising that the resource implications of treating OA should be enormous. This section reports
some of the data which are available regarding some aspects of treatment for OA,
and is intended to provide an impression of the impact of OA on health care
resources, and by no means is intended to provide a detailed picture. Other
aspects of caring for individuals with OA, such as home help or informal care-
giving, are not covered here, though their importance should not be understated.
   A Finnish study of hip and knee arthroplasties [34] showed that between
1980 and 1988, 25,966 such operations were performed, of which 56% were for
primary OA, 22% for rheumatoid arthritis, and 6.3% for secondary arthrosis. In
1988, the total number of arthoplasties was 4,268 of which about two thirds were
hip arthoplasties and one third knee replacements. Over 40% of patients were
under 65 years of age, and the annual frequency of rearthroplasty increased between 1980 and 1988 from 9.8 to 13.6%, indicating an increasing orthopaedic
work load in the future. Other studies have shown that the while the percentage
of knee arthroplasties performed due to rheumatoid arthritis has declined, the
number of such operations performed for OA have steadily increased [35].
Apart from the need for surgical interventions, another Finnish study found

that OA, especially of the hip, was a strong determinant of both occasional and regular need for assistance and that, together with chronic low back pain and inflammatory arthritis, it was one of the disorders with the highest community impact [36].

In terms of overall impact, a very useful French study which aimed to quantify the social and financial burden imposed by OA estimated that 6 million new diagnoses of OA were reported in France each year, and that it was responsible for 8.7 million physician visits in 1993. The annual number of hospital admissions was 93,000. In a further study to determine the economic and social impact of rheumatic complaints, it was found that 40.5 % of lost work days were due to rheumatic diseases, and that osteoarthritis was the most frequent cause of lost work days within this category. It was also found that OA was the third most frequent cause of visits to a primary care centre [37].

2.2.6
Costs of Osteoarthritis

Again, it is not possible at present to develop a reliable overall picture of the costs associated with OA in Europe, as relatively little data is available on the costs associated with the disease in many countries, and there are still large gaps regarding the cost implications of different types of OA. Likewise, though substantial information may be available on certain aspects of treatment, such as the cost of total hip replacement or expenditure on pharmacological treatments, very little information is available on other aspects of resource implications such as the cost of home care, or physiotherapeutic measures. Nevertheless, it is abundantly clear that OA is an extremely costly disease, not only in terms of direct costs to health care systems, but also in terms of indirect costs attributable to lost work days, reduced production, invalidity payments, etc. Considerable further research is required into both epidemiological aspects and economic aspects of the disease in order to be able to predict future resource implications with any accuracy. Given the huge costs associated with OA, it is imperative to develop means of regulating expenditure on the disease and of finding ways to reduce both direct and indirect costs.

2.2.6.1
Overall Costs

One of the few papers reporting the direct costs of OA to the health care system [37], estimated that total direct costs for OA in France in 1992 amounted to 4 billion French francs (606 million ECUs), of which physician visits accounted for 950 million FF (144 million ECUs), prescribed drugs for 965 million FF (146 million ECUs), laboratory tests, roentgenograms, and rehabilitation therapy for 330 million FF (50 million ECUs), and hospital costs (with average stay ranging from 11 to 16 days) for 1.6 billion FF per year (242 million ECUs). Indirect costs in terms of sick leave benefit were estimated to be 556 million FF (84 million ECUs). The total of direct and indirect costs therefore amounted to 6.2 billion FF (939.4 million ECUs).

2.2.6.2
Cost of Pharmacological Treatment

An increasingly important component of costs associated with OA is represented by expenditure on pharmacological treatment for the condition. Pharmacological treatment is largely directed at the control of pain as the disease proceeds, with surgical options being resorted to in the case of severe symptomatic OA which fails to respond to medical therapy. Pharmacological treatment ranges from non-opioid and opioid analgesics, to nonsteroidal antiinflammatory drugs (NSAIDs), to intraarticular steroid injections in the case of knee OA. Recent guidelines [38] indicated that acetaminophen should be the initial drug of choice in the treatment of knee osteoarthritis, but that in patients who fail to respond to acetaminophen or other oral analgesics, NSAIDs would be indicated.

The cost implications of NSAID use are considerable. For example, in the UK in 1990 prescriptions for NSAIDs accounted for approximately 1 in 20 UK National Health Service prescriptions, while the total cost of antirheumatic prescriptions (mainly NSAIDs) was 219 million pounds sterling (336 million ECUs). As Wynne and Campbell [39] suggest that half of all NSAID prescription use is attributable to the control of degenerative diseases, and especially OA, then the cost of NSAID use associated with OA is easy to appreciate. In Spain, in 1996, NSAIDs were the 8th most costly drug in terms of cost to the National Health Care System, with a total cost for the period of January to September of 22,500 million pesetas (134 million ECUs). Increase in expenditure compared to 1995 was equivalent to 5.9% [40].

One of the major disadvantages of NSAIDs, however, is the likelihood of adverse drug reactions, particularly those affecting the gastrointestinal system. The incidence of adverse drug events related to NSAIDs are well-known and widely covered in the medical literature [41, 42]. The treatment of such adverse events represents a significant part of the total costs associated with treatment with NSAIDs. Since the efficacy of available NSAIDs has been shown to be similar, an economic evaluation of these drugs must place an emphasis on the cost of treating adverse drug reactions, and not simply the cost of the drug itself, in order to give a complete idea of the total medical costs of NSAIDs. De Pouvourville for example calculated what he called the 'shadow price' of an NSAID by adding the direct medical costs of treatment of NSAID-induced gastrointestinal complications to the public price of the drug in the following way [43]:

$$(1 - T/100) \times P + T/100 \times (C + P/2)$$

where P is the price of the drug over a given period, $T\%$ designates the known rate of complications related to the prescription of the NSAID, and C represents the direct medical cost for the treatment of such complications. When the 'shadow price' derived from this formula is related to the cost of NSAID therapy the iatrogenic cost factor, i.e. the ratio of shadow price to treatment cost is derived, as follows:

iatrogenic cost factor = shadow price/cost of NSAID therapy

Thus, as de Pouvourville states, 'if the [iatrogenic] cost factor is 2 this means that each dollar spent for a prescription of this drug will incur an extra dollar for the treatment of its secondary effects.' The iatrogenic cost factor will vary depending on the cost of treatment with different drugs and on assumptions regarding scenarios for treatment of secondary effects, but is nevertheless useful in determining the 'true' cost of different NSAIDs. De Pouvourville reported that the iatrogenic cost factor for the least safe NSAID ranged between 2.16 and 3.6 depending on the scenario chosen for treatment of secondary effects [43], and similar results were obtained in a British context [44].

In a recent unpublished study, the iatrogenic cost factor was calculated for a number of different NSAIDs used in Spain, but took into account not only gastrointestinal adverse events but other adverse events associated with NSAID use such as abdominal pain and nausea, which, though not as serious as the gastrointestinal events included in de Pouvourville's study, are nevertheless more common and also imply the use of health care resources above and beyond the cost of the drug itself. The cost analysis of the NSAID was based on the total medical cost of NSAID treatment, i.e. the total cost for each option is the NSAID drug cost (market price) plus all described ADR-related costs of a particular NSAID. Resource use related to each ADR (Adverse Drug Reaction) was estimated by a panel of rheumatologists who had participated in clinical trials with different NSAIDs. Resource use centred on issues related to the treatment of ADR including specific pharmacological treatment for the ADR (drug, dose and treatment duration), number of medical visits associated with the ADR (phone, home, ambulatory or hospital visits), length of hospital stay (when indicated), diagnostic tests, and the need to discontinue treatment with the given NSAID and the substitution treatment after that point. Cost variables included in the analysis were therefore related to direct medical resources employed in treatment using NSAIDs, i.e. drug costs for the different NSAID options, ADR related costs, and drug replacement treatment for cases where NSAID treatment was discontinued.

Of the 7 NSAIDs included in the analysis, there was a wide range in iatrogenic cost factors (ICF) derived from the analysis, with the lowest ICF being 1.67 and the highest being 6.01, when a three-month time horizon was used. Sensitivity analysis showed that the results were stable when data on key variables such as ADR treatment costs, efficacy, and time of ADR occurrence were manipulated.

The results of this type of study indicate that the 'true' cost of an NSAID will not normally be reflected by its prescription price, and also that the cheapest drug may not be the least expensive in terms of total medical costs. From the point of view of estimating costs associated with OA and its treatment, the first of these is an important factor to take into account, and both will be important from the point of view of cost control and purchasing decisions, though at present the repercussions of such analyses on both cost estimation and purchasing decisions is undoubtedly limited. Nevertheless, they highlight the need for continuing appraisal of safety and effectiveness studies in clinical practice, i.e. in real patients under real conditions.

2.2.6.3
Costs of Surgical Treatment

The costs of surgical interventions related to OA are clearly of considerable importance, given that procedures such as total hip replacement and knee arthroplasties are some of the most costly procedures currently provided in terms of overall expenditure on health care. Again, demographic trends suggest that the demand for this type of procedure can be expected to increase, and that such trends will be coupled with rising costs due to technological advances, which not only involve higher costs *per* se but also mean that such procedures are increasingly performed in patients who would once have been considered too old or too impaired to benefit from them, with a concomitant rise in the cost of such procedures due to factors such as an increased length of hospital stay and higher complication rates [45].

A number of studies are available which calculate the costs of hip and knee arthroplasties in different European countries. A study of costs in Sweden published in 1991 reported that the cost of hip replacement was 34,092 Swedish crowns and for knee replacement 56,200 Swedish crowns (4,010 and 6,611 ECUs, respectively). In a British study to calculate the total cost of primary total hip replacement [46], a primary replacement episode was assumed to cost 3,500 pounds sterling (4,900 ECUs), with revision surgery costing twice that amount. The results of this study highlighted the importance of the recipient's age and the influence of life expectancy on total costs, and also illustrated the influence of quality on costs by using the idea of insurance premiums based on a life-time care package, finding that the use of the best available procedure would result in significantly reduced premiums when compared with the worst available procedure (880 ECUs compared to 4,312 ECUs respectively). For comparison, a French study conducted in 1987 estimated the total cost of a THR to be 2,725 ECUs at 1987 prices, which, assuming an annual rate of inflation of 5% would give a figure in today's prices very similar to that cited above for UK.

In terms of overall costs, a recent Norwegian study found that, for the period 1987 to 1994, the annual costs of THR were $70 million (77 million ECUs), though obviously only a certain proportion of these costs, not specified by the authors, are attributable to OA. The authors also highlight the fact that variations in the procedure used produce additional revision costs of approximately $1.7 million per year compared to the reference procedure (Charnley prothesis fixed with high viscosity cement containing antibiotic and with systemic antibiotic prophylaxis) [47].

2.2.7
Cost Containment Strategies

It is clear from a number of the observations made above that there are various means of implementing strategies which will help to contain if not reduce spending on OA. The development of more sophisticated methods for analysing the true cost of pharmacological treatment and their incorporation into purchasing plans would help to curtail spending on drugs such as NSAIDs, as would the development of prescribing guidelines which took true costs into account. Bloor and Maynard, for example, suggest that reducing the prescribing of NSAIDs, reducing dosage, switching to less toxic NSAIDs and using targeted prophylaxis could lead to a reduction of up to 50% in spending on these drugs, which would represent a saving of 86 million pounds (approximately 120 million ECUs) [48]. Careful cost-based analysis of surgical interventions would also provide useful data on which to base purchasing decisions, especially if the concept of iatrogenic cost factors is employed, and may lead to the purchase of interventions which are initially more expensive but which in fact lead to substantial savings compared to present practices in terms of complications, revision and replacement rates.

Other studies have pointed the way to means of containing costs. For example, it has been suggested that patient management by multidisciplinary teams which involve extensive use of prior screening, better patient education before admission and surgery, improved communication between team members on patient progress and co-ordination of care across the continuum resulted in a reduction in the length of hospital stay to 4 days, a reduction in direct costs per patient of $667 (734 ECUs), no reported cases of readmission for complications in a 2 year follow up period, reductions in length of stay for patients referred to extended care facilities, and a shortened period in home health services [49]. Other initiatives which are perhaps underused in current treatment approaches to OA include patient educational and self-management programs, health professional social support via telephone, weight loss, physical and occupational therapy, and aerobic aquatic exercises, all of which can produce excellent results at relatively low cost in the treatment of hip and knee OA [38]. Other options for cost reduction include the use of transitional home care programmes, though the extent to which such programmes reduce costs to date remains unclear [50].

2.2.8
Conclusions

Currently, the data which is available on both the epidemiological and economic aspects of OA in Europe, though not ideal, does nevertheless allow us to build up a picture of the condition which highlights both its prevalence and its costs. The picture is perhaps a cause for concern, particularly in terms of costs, given current demographic trends and technological advances in health care. However, a number of tools are available to control, to a substantial extent, the economic consequences of the disease. These tools range from public health interventions which target at risk groups, to cost-effectiveness analyses of interventions and treatment associated with the disease, the development of treatment guidelines and protocols which take into account both the health and economic consequences of treatment, and the implementation of co-ordinated disease management programs. It is clear, however, that continuing research on both the epidemiological and economic aspects of the disease are vital, and that increased co-operation between European countries and studies at European level would be of great value in providing much needed information, and in developing common approaches to dealing with what is likely to be one of the major health care challenges of the coming millennium.

References

1. Kellgren JA and Lawrence JS (1963) Atlas of standard radiographs. The epidemiology of chronic rheumatism, Vol 2. Oxford: Blackwell Scientific
2. Spector TD, Hochberg MC (1994) Methodological problems in the epidemiological study of osteoarthritis. Ann Rheum Dis 53:143–146
3. Bagge E, Bjelle A, Eden S, Svanborg A (1992) A longitudinal study of the occurrence of joint complaints in elderly people. Age-Ageing 3:160–7
4. Martín P, Paredes B, Fernández C, Hernández R, Ballina FJ (1992) Los reumatismos en la comunidad. Aten Primaria 10:567–70
5. Steven MM (1992) Prevalence of chronic arthritis in four geographical areas of the Scottish Highlands. Ann Rheum Dis 2:186–194
6. Petersson I (1996) The occurrence of osteoarthrosis of the peripheral joints in European populations. Ann Rheum Dis 55:659–664
7. Kellgren JA and Lawrence JS (1958) Osteoarthrosis and disk degeneration in an urban population. Ann Rheum Dis 17:388–397
8. Jørring K (1980) Osteoarthritis of the hip. Epidemiology and clinical role. Acta Orthop Scand 51:523–30
9. Lindberg H (1985) Epidemiological studies on primary coxarthosis. Malmö: University of Lund
10. Danielsson LG (1966) Incidence of osteoarthritis of the hip. Clin Orthop 45:67–72
11. Van Saase JLCM, van Romunde LKJ, Cats A, Vandenbroucke JP, Valkenburg HA (1989) Epidemiology of osteoarthritis: Zoetermeer study. Comparison of radiological osteoarthritis in a Dutch population with that in 10 other populations. Ann Rheum Dis 48 (4):271–280
12. Spector TD, Hart DJ, Leedham-Green M (1991) The prevalence of knee and hand osteoarthritis (OA) in the general population using different clinical criteria: the Clingford study. Arthritis-Rheum 34:S171
13. Bagge E, Bjelle A, Svanborg A (1992) Radiographic osteoarthritis in the elderly. A cohort comparison and a longitudinal study of the "70-year old people in Göteburg". Clin Rheumatol 11:486–91
14. Bjelle A (1982) Epidemiological aspects of osteoarthritis: an interview survey of the Swedish population and a review of previous studies. Scand J Rheumatol Suppl 43:35–48
15. Masse JP, Glimet T, Kluntz D (1992) Age de debut et frequences des douleurs chroniques dans la gonarthrose. Rev Rhum Mal Osteoartic 1:17–21
17. Spector TD, Cicuttini F, Baker J, Loughlin J, Hart D (1996) Genetic influences on osteoarthritis in women: a twin study. BMJ 7036:940–3
18. Chitnavis J, Sinsheimer JS, Clipsham K, Loughlin J, Sykes B, Burge PD, Carr AJ (1997) Genetic influences in end-stage osteoarthritis. Sibling risks of hip and knee replacement for idiopathic osteoarthritis. J Bone Joint Surg Br 79(4):660–4
19. Heliovaara M, Makela M, Impivaara O, Knekt P, Aromaa A, Sievers K (1993) Association of overweight, trauma and workload with coxarthrosis. A health survey of 7,217 persons. Acta Orthop Scand 5:513–518
20. Hart DJ and Spector TD (1993) The relationship of obesity, fat distribution and osteoarthritis in women in the general population: the Chingford study. J Rheumatol 20(2): 331–5
21. Olsen O, Vingard E, Koster M, Alfredsson L (1994) Etiologic fractions for physical work load, sports and overweight in the occurrence of coxarthrosis. Scand J Work Environ Health 3:184–8

22. Kivimaji J, Riihimaki H, Hanninen K (1992) Knee disorders in carpet and floor layers and painters. Scand J Work Environ Health 5:310–316
23. Stenlund B, Goldie I, Hagberg M, Hogstadt C, Marions O (1992) Radiographic osteoarthrosis in the acromioclavicular joint resulting from manual work or exposure to vibration. Br J Ind Med 8:588–593
24. Croft P, Coggon D, Cruddas M, Cooper C (1992) Osteoarthritis of the hip: an occupational disease in farmers. BMJ 6837:1269–1272
25. Spector TD (1993) Epidemiology of the rheumatic diseases. Curr Opin Rheumatol 2:132–7
26. Spector TD, Dacre JE, Harris PA, Huskisson EC (1992) Radiological progression of osteoarthritis: an 11 year follow up study of the knee. Ann Rheum Dis 51:1107–1110
27. Manninen P, Riihimaki H, Feliovaara M, Makela P (1996) Overweight, gender and knee osteoarthritis. Int J Obes Relat Metab Disord 6:595–7
28. Sun Y, Sturmer T, Gunther KP, Brenner H (1997) Inzidenz una Pravalenz der Cox- und Gonarthrose in der Allgemeinbevolkerung. Z Orthop Ihre Grenzgeb 135(3):184–92
29. Kujala UM, Kaprio J, Sarna S (1994) Osteoarthritis of weight-bearing joints of low limbs in former elite male athletes. BMJ 6923:231–4
30. Spector TD, Harris PA, Hart DJ, Cicuttini FM, Nandra D, Etherington J, Wolman RL, Doyle DV (1996) Risk of osteoarthritis associated with long-term weight-bearing sports: a radiologic survey of the hips and knees in female ex-athletes and population controls. Arthritis-Rheum 39(6):988–95
31. Lindberg H, Roos H, Gardsell P (1993) Prevalence of coxarthrosis in former soccer players: 286 players compared with matched controls. Acta Orthop Scand 2:165–167
32. Vingard E, Alfredsson L, Malchau H (1997) Lifestyle factors and hip arthrosis. A case referent study of body mass index, smoking and hormone therapy in 503 Swedish women. Acta Orthop Scand 3:216–220
33. Forsberg K, Nilsson BE (1992) Coxarthrosis on the island of Gotland: increased prevalence in a rural population. Acta Orthop Scand 1:1–3
34. Paavolainen P, Hamalainen M, Mustonen H, Slatis P (1991) Registration of arthroplasties in Finland. A nationwide prospective project. Acta Orthop Scand Suppl 241:27–30
35. Knutson K, Lewold S, Robertsson O, Lidgren L (1994) The Swedish knee arthroplasty register: a nation-wide study of 30,003 knees 1976–1992. Acta Orthop Scand 4:375–386
36. Makela M, Heliovaara M, Sievers K, Knent P, Maatela J, Arimaa A (1993) Musculoskeletal disorders as determinants of disability in Finns aged 30 years or more. J Clin Epidemiol 6:549–559
37. Levy E, Ferme A, Perocheau D, Bono I (1993) Les couts socio-economiques de l'arthrose en France. Rev Rhum 6(pt 2):63S–67S
38. Hochberg MC, Altman R, Brandt KD, Clark BM, Dieppe PA, Griffin MR, Moskowitz RW, Schnitzer TJ (1995) Guidelines for the medical management of osteoarthritis. Parts I and II. Arthritis-Rheum 11:1535–1540
39. Wynne HA, Campbell M (1994) Pharmacoeconomics of nonsteroidal anti-inflammatory drugs (NSAIDs). PharmacoEconomics 3(2):107–23
40. Insalud (1996) Indicadores de la prestación sanitaria en el SNS. Septiembre
41. Brand KD (1993) Should nonsteroidal anti-inflammatory drugs be used to treat osteoarthritis? Rheumatic Disease Clinics of North America 19:29–44
42. Scholes D, Stergachis A (1995) Nonsteroidal anti-inflammatory discontinuation in patients with osteoarthritis. J Rheum 22:708–712
43. De Pouvourville G (1995) The iatrogenic cost of non-steroidal anti-inflammatory drug therapy. Br J Rheumatol 34(suppl. 1):19–24
44. Knill-Jones RP (1992) The economic consequences of NSAID-induced gastropathy in the United Kingdom and commentary on the article by G. De Pouvourville. Scand J Rheumatol Suppl. 96:59–62
45. Jacobsson SA, Rehnberg C, Djerf K (1991) Risks, benefits and economic consequences of total hip arthroplasty in an aged population. Scand J Soc Med 19(1):72–8
46. Pynsent PB, Carter SR, Bulstrode CJ (1996) The total cost of hip-joint replacement; a model for purchasers. J Public Health Med 2:157–68

47. Furnes A, Lie SA, Havelin LI, Engesaeter LB, Vollset SE (1996) The economic impact of failures in total hip replacement surgery: 28,997 cases from the Norwegian Arthroplasty Register, 1987–1993. Acta Orthop Scand 2:115–21

48. Bloor K, Maynard A (1996) Is there scope for improving the cost-effective prescribing of nonsteroidal anti-inflammatory drugs? PharmacoEconomics 9(6):484–496

49. Lindsrom CC, Laird J, Soscia J (1995) High quality and lower cost: they can coexist! Semin Nurse Manag 3:133–6

50. Rothman NL, Moriarty L, Rothman RH, Silver C, O'Connor PC, Aguas J (1994) Establishing a home care protocol for early discharge of patients with hip and knee arthroplasties. Home Healthc Nurse 1:24–30

CHAPTER 3

Experimental Models of Osteoarthritis

3.1
In Vitro Models for the Study of Cartilage Damage and Repair

Y. HENROTIN and J.-Y. REGINSTER

3.1.1
Introduction

Cartilage is a very specialized tissue containing only one type of cell and characterized by the absence of blood and lymphatic vessels. Nutrition is mainly assumed by synovial fluid imbibition. Chondrocyte metabolism is regulated by soluble factors produced locally by chondrocytes themselves and also by neighboring tissues. Chondrocyte functions are also influenced by the composition of the extracellular environment (O_2 tension, ionic concentration, pH, etc), the extracellular matrix composition, the matrix-cell interactions and the physical signals. The first challenge of *in vitro* research is to reproduce in culture this complex extracellular environment without modifying the specific phenotype of mature chondrocytes. The second goal is to perform culture models to study the precocious, delayed, brief or sustained responses of chondrocyte to chemical and/or physical signals. *In vitro* culture also provides an opportunity to study chondrocytes behaviors during osteoarthritis (OA). The third aim is to develop co-culture systems that would allow investigation of the interactions between different tissues of the joint. The fourth goal is to prepare cartilage implants for further transplantation. Finally, *in vitro* research aims to screen growth factors, cytokines or therapeutic agents that could stimulate cartilage repair and/or reduce cartilage resorption. Over the last decade, different culture models have been developped. Monolayer culture, suspension culture, chondron culture, explant culture, co-culture systems and immortalized cell cultures will be described in this chapter. Each culture system presents advantages and disavantages and each is particularly suitable to explore one particular aspect of chondrocyte metabolism. Cartilage explant culture is an excellent model system for studying matrix turnover or mechanisms requiring original cell surface receptors and normal cell-matrix and matrix-matrix interactions. On the other hand, if the study aims to investigate matrix deposition or the regulatory pathways of chondrocyte metabolism, an isolated cell culture system is recommended to avoid the presence of a pre-existing matrix. Low density monolayer culture is appropriate to investigate cell dedifferentiation processes. Freshly isolated chondrocytes are recommended to investigate active oxygen species production and avoid the scavenging effect of matrix components. Suspended culture in a natural or synthetic matrix is a suitable model to analyze the adaptive responses of chondrocytes to mechanical stress. This chapter aims to review and analyze the culture models described in the literature.

3.1.2
Chondrocytes in Culture

3.1.2.1
Tissue Harvest

Several important considerations must be taken into account in the selection of cartilage tissue used for *in vitro* investigations. Matrix composition and metabolic activity vary within individual joints as well as among different joints. It is well recognized that the metabolic activity of chondrocytes varies through the depth of the tissue. This fact has been reported in several studies where subpopulations of chondrocytes isolated from different depths of the cartilage were cultured. Some morphological and biochemical differences are clearly evident between superficial and deep chondrocytes cultured in agarose gel. Superficial cells synthesize a sparse, proteoglycan-poor fibrillar matrix whereas the deeper cells produce an abundant matrix rich in proteoglycan [1, 2]. Moreover, superficial cells produce relatively more small non-aggregating proteoglycans and hyaluronic acid but less aggrecan and keratan sulfate than deep cells [3–5]. Another important metabolic difference between chondrocytes isolated from different depths of the cartilage is their responsiveness to exogenous stimuli. Based on both their anabolic and catabolic responses, bovine chondrocytes derived from the superficial zone revealed a greater sensitivity to IL-1 than deep zone chondrocytes [6,7].

Cell behavior also differs according to the localization of the tissue. Rib and ear chondrocytes isolated from the same animal respond differently to growth factors such as bFGF and TGFβ. bFGF increases thymidine, proline and leucine incorporation into rib, but not into ear, primary cultured chondrocytes. TGFβ enhances thymidine incorporation into both chondrocytes but does not affect proline or leucine incorporation into the ear cells [8]. Cartilage excised from high-load-bearing areas differs from that of low-load-bearing areas. In adult ovine stiffle joint, chondrocytes from the central region of the tibial plateau not covered by the meniscus, which is subject to high mechanical loads *in vivo*, synthesized less aggrecan but more decorin than cells from regions covered by the meniscus [9]. This study serves to emphasize the importance of using cartilage from identical joint areas when examining chondrocyte synthesis.

Chondrocytes metabolism and responsiveness to regulatory factors vary greatly according the age of the donor, the skeletal development and the pathological status of the joint from which the cartilage is harvested. Human chondrocytes show a continuous age-related decline in the proliferative response to serum. The greatest decrease is noted between cells of 40–50 year old donors and those from donors a decade older. Moreover, the magnitude of the proliferative response to growth factors (i.e. TGFβ or PDGF) decreased with the age of the donor. In addition to the quantitative changes in the proliferatives of chondrocytes, there is a qualitative change in the pattern of growth responsiveness during development. Cells from young donors (10–20 years of age) respond better to platelet derived growth factor (PDGF) than to transforming growth factor (TGFβ), while the inverse pattern is observed in cells from adult donors [10]. Different mechanisms have been suggested to explain age-related change in the synthetic pattern and growth factor responsiveness of chondrocytes. Reductions of cell surface receptor number and affinity, changes in cytokine or growth factor synthesis and bioactivity, or modifications in post-receptor signaling events are possible explanations.

The pathological status of the joint also alters chondrocyte morphology and metabolic activity. Recently, Kouri et al. [11] have identified three distinct chondrocyte subpopulations in osteoarthritic (OA) cartilage. Chondrocytes from the superficial and upper middle of fibrillated cartilage form clusters and synthetize higher levels of proteoglycan and collagen [12, 13]. Moreover, a focal onset of type III collagen expression was observed. TGFβ and IGF are able to stimulate proteoglycan synthesis by chondrocytes and partially reverse adverse effects of IL-1 and TNFα. Interestingly, osteoarthritic cartilage explants and isolated chondrocytes from osteoarthritic cartilage are much more sensitive to stimulation by TGFβ than healthy cartilage. This difference is largely attributed at phenotypically changed chondrocytes present in the damaged upper layer of osteoarthritic chondrocytes [14].

3.1.2.2
Chondrocyte Isolation

Isolation of the individual chondrocyte is generally achieved through sequential proteolytic digestion of the extracellular matrix. After their release from the matrix, isolated cells are ideally suited for the study of *de novo* synthesis of matrix components. Some authors use only clostridial collagenase whereas others previously incubate cartilage dices with trypsin, pronase, DNAse and/or hyaluronidase. In this session, we report personal data on the effects of the enzymatic isolation method on the amount of matrix components contaminating the isolated cells. The residual amounts of protein and aggrecan contained in the cellular pellet after collagenase digestion (24 h; collagenase clostridial, type IA, 1 mg/320 U/ml) and after successive enzymatic digestion with hyaluronidase (30 min.; Type IV S; 0.5 mg/400 U/ml), pronase (1 h; 1 mg/4000 U/ml) and collagenase (24 h; collagenase clostridial, type IA, 1 mg/320 U/ml) are compared. Chondrocyte clusters were obtained after collagenase digestion whereas chondrocytes were well isolated from each other after three successive enzymatic digestions with hyaluronidase, pronase and collagenase (Fig. 1). Cell numbers isolated from 1 g of tissue were also widely varied. When collagenase was used alone, only 1.4×10^6 cells were isolated from 1 g of tissue whereas

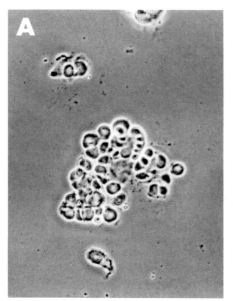 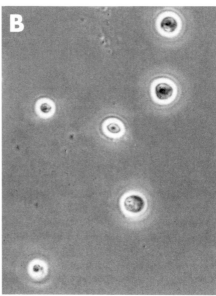

Fig. 1. Microscopic observation (magnification: ×100) of human chondrocytes isolated from cartilage by a single digestion with collagenase (**A**) or by a triple digestion with hyaluronidase, pronase and collagenase (**B**)

4.3×10^6 cells were isolated after pronase, hyaluronidase and collagenase treatments. Aggrecan, total proteins, IL-6 and IL-8 amounts found in the cell pellet obtained after collagenase digestion were significantly more elevated than in the cell pellet obtained after three successive enzymatic digestions (Table 1). Seventy-two hours after isolation, proteoglycan and cytokine synthesis also fully differed according the isolation method used. Mono-digested chondrocytes produced more IL-6, PGE_2 and IL-8 but lower levels of aggrecans than tri-digested chondrocytes (Fig. 2). Some information found in the literature contributes to the explanation of differences observed between the two isolation systems.

- Receptors may be down-regulated or damaged by enzymatic treatment [15]. TGFβ inhibits DNA and proteoglycan synthesis of freshly isolated chondrocytes (first day) while the DNA and proteoglycan synthesis of chondrocytes cultured in monolayer (7 days) was stimulated by TGF-β [16]. Therefore, adequate time for re-expression of such a membrane component is essential before the initiation of experiment.
- The exogenously applied proteases can disrupt cell-matrix interactions mediated by integrins. The integrin family of transmembrane adhesion receptors mediates attachment of chondrocytes to extracellular matrix molecules [17]. Disruption of normal integrin mediated cell-matrix interactions may influence matrix gene expression [18].

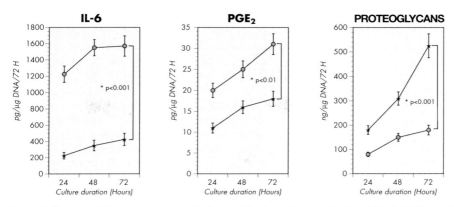

Fig. 2. Influence of the enzymatic isolation method on the synthesis of IL-6, PGE$_2$ and proteoglycans by human articular chondrocytes *in vitro*. Chondrocytes were isolated from the cartilage by a single enzymatic digestion (o) or by triple digestion with hyaluronidase, pronase and collagenase (*). Results are expressed as mean values of three cultures from the same donor. Comparison of mean values was performed using the unpaired Student's t-test

Table 1. Proteins, cytokines and proteoglycans contained in the cell pellets collected after digestion of the cartilage by collagenase alone (mono-digestion) or by three successive enzymatic treatments (tri-digestion) with hyaluronidase, pronase and collagenase. Before assays, cell pellets were homogenized by ultrasonic dissociation. IL-6 and IL-8 were measured by two specific EASIAs (Enzyme Amplified Sensitivity Immunoassays) and proteoglycans by a radioimmunoassay in which the antiserum is directed against the core protein of the aggrecan. The data are expressed as amounts of proteins, cytokines and proteoglycans found in the cell pellet per µg of DNA and presented as the mean and standard deviation of triplicate cultures. Comparison of mean values was performed using the unpaired Student's t-test

Isolation method	Proteins (µg/µg DNA)	IL-8 (pg/µg DNA)	IL-6 (pg/µg DNA)	Proteoglycans (ng/µg DNA)
Mono-digestion	14 ± 0.07	58 ± 0.61	61 ± 5	210 ± 3.15
Tri-digestion	9.7 ± 0.04[a]	3.7 ± 0.93[b]	6.5 ± 0.91[b]	41 ± 3.75[b]

[a] $p < 0.01$.
[b] $p < 0.001$.

- Residual matrix components contaminating isolated cells may regulate chondrocyte synthesis. Integrins can recognize degradation products of the extracellular matrix, suggesting an important role in tissue repair following proteolytic matrix degradation. Larsson et al. [19] reported that the addition of intact or fragmented proteoglycans to cell cultures stimulate the synthesis of protein and proteoglycans. On the other hand, high level of hyaluronic acid (HA) was shown to cause an important reduction of the sulphate incorporation into proteoglycans synthesized by chick embryo chondrocytes, adult pig chondrocytes and Swarm rat chondrosarcoma cells [20–23].

Furthermore, HA is a potent inhibitor of the release of proteoglycans from the cell matrix layer into the medium even in the presence of IL-1β, TNFα, or FGF suggesting that HA can counteract the biological activity of cytokines and growth factors [24]. The precise mechanism underlying the action of HA remains unknown but chondrocytes contain a receptor for hyaluronate which is associated with cytosolic actin filament and thereby influence its organization [25, 26]. Binding of HA to receptors stimulates the tyrosine phosphorylation of proteins [27]. Thus, all together, these findings demonstrate that fragmented or native cartilage matrix molecules may modulate chondrocytes metabolic functions via the activation of cell membrane receptors.

–   The rapid up-regulation of chondrocyte matrix protein synthesis upon enzymatic resuspension of cells could also be a consequence of the change in chondrocyte shape and/or cytoskeletal reorganization.
–   Some cytokines (IL-8) and growth factors (i.e., IGF-1, TGFβ) are trapped in the cartilaginous extracellular matrix [28–30]. The best known example is the binding of TGFβ by decorin. Indeed, it has been reported that the interaction between TGFβ and decorin is partially responsible for the decreased ability of TGFβ to induce cell growth in Chinese hamster ovary cells [31]. There is evidence that the decorin content in the cartilage increases with age suggesting that the bioavailability of TGFβ could decrease with age [32]. Growth factors and cytokines could be released from the residual matrix during the culture period and then directly modulate the chondrocyte functions.

3.1.3
Chondrocyte Culture Models

3.1.3.1
Culture in Monolayer

The differentiated phenotype of articular chondrocytes is primarily characterized by the synthesis of type II collagen and cartilage-specific proteoglycans and by the low level of mitotic activity. Many studies have shown that cultures in monolayer on plastic subtrata for prolonged periods or upon repeated passages lead to the loss of chondrocytes spherical shape and to the acquisition of an elongated fibroblast-like morphology [33]. The synthesis pattern is fully modified by this dedifferentiation process. A progressive reduction in the synthesis of type II, IX and XI collagens and an increase in the synthesis of type I, III and V collagens were observed during fibroblastic metaplasia [34, 35]. Small non-aggregating proteoglycans are synthesized at the expense of functional aggrecan [36–38]. The synthesis of cathepsin B and L are extremely low in differentiated cells, but are soon increased in parallel with the loss of the differentiated state. Inversely, collagenase-1 is strongly expressed by differentiated chondrocytes and declines rapidly with successive subculture [39] while TIMP production progressively increases [35].

Interestingly, dedifferentiated chondrocytes re-express the differentiated collagen phenotype when they are transferred from monolayer to suspension culture [34, 40 – 42]. Differentiation process is not yet clearly identified but seems to be related to the shape of the cells [43]. This characteristic is regularly used by researchers investigating cartilage defect grafting with autologous chondrocytes. A small number of cells obtained from the biopsy specimen may be amplified in monolayer and therefore reinvested in a three-dimensional matrix before transplantation. The re-expression of cartilage specific phenotype by dedifferentiated chondrocytes transferred in agarose culture may be promoted by TGFβ, osteogenin and vitamin C [44].

Chondrocyte responses to growth factors and cytokines are modified during the dedifferentiation process. Cellular responses to cytokines and growth factors differ between primary chondrocytes and dedifferentiated cells. IL-1 stimulates fibroblast proliferation, whereas primary chondrocytes are growth inhibited by IL-1 [45]. DNA synthesis is stimulated by IGF-1 in flattened chondrocytes but not in rounded cells [46]. IL-1β and TNFα stimulating effect on procollagenase production is more pronounced on dedifferentiated chondrocytes than on differentiated cells [47].

3.1.3.2
Culture in Suspension

Maintenance of chondrocytes in suspension in a liquid medium or in a natural or synthetic three-dimensional matrix stabilizes the chondrocyte phenotype. Chondrocytes conserve their spherical shape and continue to produce cartilage-specific proteins. Suspension culture is particularly recommended to study new pericellular matrix formation. Culture of chondrocytes within synthetic or natural absorbable polymers have also been developed for implantation of cells into cartilage defects to promote regeneration of the articular joint surface. Cell scaffolds for cartilage engineering should meet several criteria: (1) Implants should provide a pore structure that allows cell adhesion and growth. (2) Neither the polymer nor its degradation products should provoke inflammation or toxicity when implanted in vivo. (3) Transplantation vehicles should also provide binding capacity to adjacent cartilage or subchondral bone. (4) The scaffold should be absorbable and the degradation should match the rate of tissue regeneration. (5) To facilitate cartilage repair, the chemical structure and pore architecture of the matrix should allow the seeded cells to maintain the chondrocytes phenotype and the synthesis of cartilage-specific proteins. (6) The scaffolds need to be mechanically studied enough at the time of *in vivo* implantation.

Suspension in a Liquid Phase. Cellular attachment to the supporting plastic culture flask may be prevented by maintaining chondrocytes under constant agitation [37, 48] or by coating the plastic dishes with a viscous solution of methyl cellulose, agarose, hydrogel (poly-(2-hydroxyethyl methacrylate) or a composite collagen-agarose [49]. In these conditions, chondrocytes form clusters and synthesize mainly aggrecan and cartilage-specific collagens (II, IX, XI collagens). Nevertheless, two types of cells are usually observed. The cells in the center of the nodules remains spherical and are surrounded by an abundant cartilaginous extracellular matrix, as evidenced by histochemical and ultra-structural examinations. The cells in the periphery have a discoid morphology and are surrounded by a sparse extracellular matrix. Little is known about the synthetic and functional characteristics of the flattened surface cells. On the other hand, plates coated with fibronectin and type I and type II collagens allow chondrocyte attachment and promote direct motility of cells in a haptotatic and chemotatic fashion [50].

Chondrocytes can also be cultured on microcarriers maintained in suspension by constant agitation in a siliconized spinner flask [51, 52]. Different types of microcarriers, including dextran beads (Cytodex), dextran beads collagen coated (Cytodex III) and non-porous type I collagen microspheres (Cellagen), have been tested for chondrocytes suspension culture. In these culture conditions, chondrocytes attach to the microcarrier surface and keep their spherical shape and produce a matrix-like material. Moreover, Cellagen culture promotes chondrocytes proliferation and re-expression of chondrocytic phenotype [52]. Therefore, Cellagen culture could be used for bulk production of chondrocytes that continue to express their original phenotype before transplantation.

Another method consists of culturing chondrocyte as a pellet of high density cells obtained by centrifugation. The high density pellet culture system (0.5 to $1 \cdot 10^6$ cells) has been widely used to study epiphyseal and growth plate chondrocyte differentiation and hypertrophy [53]. Recently, it was also applied to the culture of adult bovine nasal and articular chondrocytes [54]. In this method, chondrocyte suspension is centrifuged and cultured for at least 3 weeks in poly-propylene tubes. This study showed that adult chondrocytes cultured as pellets deposit a cartilage-like matrix that contains abundant proteoglycan and type II collagen but not type I as judged by histological, immunohistochemical and quantitative methods.

Suspension in a Natural Extracellular Matrix. Chondrocytes may also be cultured in suspension within a three-dimensional matrix such as soft agar, agarose, collagen gel and sponge, hyaluronan, fibrin glue or alginate beads.

Chondrocytes cultured in agarose are known to maintain their cartilage phenotype and synthesized type II collagen and tissue-specific aggrecan aggregated [42]. In the agarose culture, most of the proteoglycan remains in the agar but is continuously released into the medium for more than 50 days. In the monolayer culture, by comparison, the cellular phase becomes saturated with GAG after 5–6 days whereas in the culture medium an increase initially occurs and is followed by a time-dependent decrease after the first 8–10 days [55]. Nevertheless, chondrocytes in agarose do not have exactly the same behavior than *in vivo*. In agarose, the majority of the synthesized aggrecan aggregates contain less than 20 aggrecan molecules and are smaller than *in vivo* [56]. TGF-β increased proteoglycan synthesis in explant culture [57, 58] but down-regulates aggrecan by the same cells in agarose [59].

Alginate is a linear polysaccharide isolated from brown algae and composed by two uronic acids, L-guluronic and D-manuronic acid linked by $\beta 1,4$ and $\alpha 1,4$ glucoside binds. In the presence of divalent cations such as Ca^{++}, the polymer undergoes instant ionotrophic gelation [60]. Each chondrocyte entrapped in alginate is surrounded by a negatively charged polysaccharide matrix that has a pore size comparable to that of hyaline articular cartilage. The matrix formed by adult human chondrocytes in alginate beads is composed in two compartments; a thin rim of cell-associated matrix that corresponds to the pericellular and territorial matrix of articular cartilage and a more abundant further removed matrix, the equivalent of the interritorial matrix in the tissue. On day 30 of culture, the relative and absolute volumes occupied by the cells and each of the two compartments in the beads are nearly identical to those in native cartilage [61, 62]. The chondrocytes maintain a spherical appearance for at least 30 days and mainly produce aggrecan of similar hydrodynamic size to aggrecan molecules present in the matrix of articular cartilage as well as cartilage characteristic collagens including type II, IX and XI [62 – 64]. Meanwhile, as observed in other supension culture models, flattened cells are present at the surface of the beads. These flattened cells produce small amounts of type I collagen molecules which are directly released in the culture medium and do not become incorporated in the extracellular matrix [62]. Chondrocytes proliferate moderately in the alginate beads. After 8 months in alginate gel, adult chondrocytes are still metabolically active and continue to synthesize cartilage specific type II collagen and aggrecan [65]. Tanaka et al. [66] investigated the diffusion characteristics of a variety of naturally occurring molecules into alginate and found that the diffusion of molecules larger than 70 Kda was excluded out of the matrix. This culture system is very well suited for the investigation of the regulation of matrix biosynthesis and extracellular matrix organization. Additionally, culture in alginate has the advantage that rapid depolymerization of the matrix can be achieved in the presence of a calcium chelating agent that allows the cells and matrix to be harvested for further analysis. The accessibility of the cells allows further investigation of the mode of action of peptide regulatory factors and pharmacological agents at the transcriptional, post-transcriptional and translational levels.

Chondrocytes are also cultured within type I and type II collagen matrices [67, 68]. Recently, Nehrer et al. [69, 70] compared the behaviors of canine chondrocytes in a porous collagen-glycosaminoglycan copolymer matrix comprising different collagen types. They observed an important difference in the morphology and biosynthetic activities of the cells in the type I and type II collagen matrices. The cells in the type II collagen matrix retain their spherical shape, while in the type I matrix chondrocytes displayed a fibroblastic morphology. Moreover, chondrocytes cultured in type II matrix produce higher amounts of GAG than in type I sponge. In addition, cell numbers increase with culture time in all collagen matrices. Van Susante et al. [71] compared viability, phenotype, proliferation and sulfate incorporation of bovine chondrocytes cultured in alginate or type I collagen gel. The author observed a significant increase in cell numbers in collagen gel, but the chondrocytes dedifferentiated into fibroblast-like cells from day 6. In alginate gels, initial cell loss occurred but the cells maintained their typical chondrocyte phenotype. The total quantity of proteoglycans initially synthesized per cell in collagen gel was significantly higher. However, in collagen gel, matrix production decreased from day 6, whereas in alginate gel it continued to increase. Subsequently, proteoglycan synthesis in alginate gel, expressed per chondrocytes, surpassed that in collagen gel on day 6.

Solid three-dimensional fibrin matrices represent a natural substance which also sustains suspended chondrocytes in a differentiated phenotype. Three-dimensional fibrin matrix was also tested as a vehicle in chondrocyte transplantation [72]. The benefits of fibrin include its absence of cytotoxicity, space-filling capabilities and adhesive capacity [73, 74]. Histology, autoradiography, electron microscopy and biochemical investigations revealed that chondrocytes seeded in fibrin glue kept their morphology, multiplied and produced matrix even after 14 days of culture [74]. Nevertheless, Homminga et al. [72] reported that glue desintegration began after 3 days and cell dedifferentiation progressed.

Suspension in a Synthetic Matrix. Cartilage implants for potential use in reconstructive or orthopedic surgery can be created by growing isolated chondrocytes *in vitro* into a synthetic, biocompatible and biodegradable scaffold.

Chondrocytes cultures in polyglycolic acid (PGA) scaffolds proliferate and keep their morphology and phenotype for 8 weeks. Chondrocyte-PGA constructs consisted of cells, GAG and collagen, and had an outer collagenous capsule. Nevertheless, both type I and type II collagen were present in the cell-PGA implants. Moreover, the authors reported that implants based on dedifferentiated chondrocytes by serial passage had similar cellularities, higher GAG contents and higher collagen contents than those based on primary chondrocytes. These findings indicate that tissue engineering can be amplified by a previous serial passage prior to seeding chondrocytes on PGA scaffolds [75]. Freed and collaborators [76] also compared the behaviors of human and bovine chondrocytes cultured on fibrous polyglycolic acid (PGA) and porous poly(L)-lactil acid (PLLA). Over 6–8 weeks of *in vitro* culture, bovine chondrocytes cultured on PGA or PLLA proliferated and regenerated cartilaginous matrix. On PGA, chondrocytes appeared rounded and within lacunae surrounded by cartilaginous matrix. After 8 weeks of *in vitro* culture, regenerated tissue accounted for 50% of the construct dry weight (4% cell mass, 15% GAG and 31% collagen) [77]. In contrast, on PLLA the cells appeared spindle-shaped and minimal matrix staining for GAG and collagen was observed. Moreover, the cell growth rate was approximately twice as high on PGA as it was on PLLA [51]. *In vivo*, chondrocytes grown on both PGA and PLLA for 1–6 months produced tissue appearing glistening white macroscopically and resembling cartilage histologically. At this time, implants contained GAG, type I and type II collagen as shown by immunostaining [51].

Porous high density hydrophobic or hydrophilic polyethylene (HDPE) substrates have also been tested to culture fetal bovine chondrocytes. After 7 days of incubation, the cells within both subtrates remained spherical and contained mainly type II collagen. After 21 days, the majority of the cells had spread. The hydrophilic matrices contained significantly more type II collagen than the hydrophobic matrice [78].

Bioresorbable co-polymer fleeces of vicryl and polydioxanon (Ethicon) or polylactic acid soaked with poly-L-lysine or type II collagen were tested for cartilage tissue engineering in perfusion culture [79, 80]. The biomaterial containing cells were encapsulated in agarose gel to improve retention and accumulation of extracellular matrix component synthesized by the chondrocyte. The fleece organization offers a maximun of available internal polymer surface and a minimun of solid polymer volume and therefore allows attachment of a great number of cells. Culture perfusion avoids repetitive culture manipulation, decreases the risk of bacterial contamination and achieves a constant supply of nutrient by diffusion. Moreover, perfusion not only stabilizes the components provided by the culture medium, it also stabilizes secreted autocrine factors at a constant level. For example, it was demonstrated that glucose concentrations fluctuate at each culture medium change when chondrocytes are cultured in monolayer in a stagnant medium environment [80]. Using a perfusion culture system, a constant concentration of nutrients like glucose is provided. However, the measured concentrations of lactate are unstable and significantly increase during the perfusion culture of cell-Ethicon system tissue due to the hydrolytic degradation of the poly-hydroxy acids [81]. Furthermore, chondrocytes cultured on bioresorbable polymer of polylactic acid rapidly adhered onto bioresorbable carrier fleece but conserved their rounded morphology. The chondrocytes in cell-polymer cultures continued and maintained synthesis of type II collagen and proteoglycan as analysed by immunohistochemistry.

Cartilaginous tissue may also be obtained by culturing chondrocytes as monolayer on Millicell-CM filters. Precoating the filters with collagen was necessary for attachment of the chondrocytes. Histological examination of the culture showed that the chondrocytes over time accumulated an extracellular matrix which contained proteoglycans and type II collagen and formed a continuous layers of cartilaginous tissue. No type I collagen was detected. Chondrocytes within the tissue were spherical but appeared flattened on the surface. The thickness of the tissue generated increased over time and was dependent on the initial plating density. Under optimal culture conditions, the cartilaginous tissue attains a thickness of 110 µm and shows organization of cells and collagen into superficial and deeper layers similar to that previously described for articular cartilage. The extracellular matrix contains approximately three-fold more collagen than proteoglycan, which is similar to *in vivo* cartilage. After 2 weeks, there was sufficient matrix accumulation that the tissue could be handled and removed easily from the supporting filter and used for transplantation. *In vivo*, engineered tissue did not integrate to the host cartilage and tissue fixation was needed. Moreover, fibrovascular tissue was observed in some transplants [82, 83].

More recently, Sims et al. [84] investigated the utilization of polyethylene oxide gels as encapsulating polymer scaffolds for delivering large numbers of isolated chondrocytes via injection. As early as 6 weeks after injection into the subcutaneous tissue of athymic mice, new cartilage was formed exhibiting a white opalescence similar to that of hyaline cartilage. Histologic and biochemical analysis showed the presence of actively proliferating chondrocytes with production of a well-formed cartilaginous tissue in the transplant.

Culture chondrocytes in a three-dimensional synthetic matrix seems to be suitable for long-term study of cartilage formation. Nevertheless, little information is available concerning the utilization of these systems for cartilage resorption investigation. One major disavantage of suspension cultures utilizing gel matrices is the difficulty of harvesting the cells once they have been encapsulated within the artificial matrix.

3.1.3.3
Explant Culture

Cartilage explant culture has been used by many investigators to study various aspects of the anabolic and catabolic metabolism of articular cartilage [85, 86]. Articular cultures offer a panel of advantages for the *in vitro* study of matrix homeostasis, resorption and repair. The chondrocytes in cartilage explants maintain their phenotype and the extracellular matrix is similar to that observed *in vivo*. After 5 days in culture in the presence of serum, steady-state rates of synthesis and turnover were reached [87, 88]. Resorption may be accelerated in both basal and serum-supplemented culture by several agents including IL-1β, TNFα, bacterial lipopolysaccharides, retinoic acid derivative or active oxygen species flux. Repair capacity of the cartilage may also be investigated. Initial injury to the cartilage is usually induced by soluble mediators of inflammation (H_2O_2, IL-1, TNFα) or by physical disruption of the matrix. Thereafter, healing of the tissue may be easily studied.

Organotypic culture is also an adequate in vitro model to study the effects of isolated environmental factors on chondrocytes and the surrounding matrix. *In vivo*, chondrocytes are sparsely distributed in the extracellular matrix and do not have contact between one another. Cartilage explant cultures conserve these structural organizations and the multiple interactions between chondrocytes and their direct extracellular environment.

This model is also used to test the effect of mechanical stress, pharmacological agents, growth factors, cytokines or hormones on the cartilage metabolism. The system yields some information on the possible interactions of the tested compounds with the matrix and their accessibility to the chondrocytes.

Another advantage is that chondrocytes are not damaged by enzymatic or mechanical stress occurring during cell isolation. Receptors and other menbrane proteins and glycoproteins are protected from damaging stress. Removal and dicing of full-thickness cartilage to randomize the influence of geographic effects are recommended. On the other hand, there are no clear guidelines on the surface and the volume of the dice. Too large an explant may induce central necrosis. The shape of the explant may influence the size of the exchange surface between explant and culture medium. It is well known that the alteration in surface area of the explant cartilage may produce an initial increase in the rate of proteoglycan loss from the tissue.

3.1.3.4
Chondron Culture

Chondron is a morphological entity in articular cartilage composed of chondrocyte, its pericellular matrix and a compacted filamentous capsule [89–92].

They are considered as the primary structural, functional and metabolic unit in hyaline cartilage responsible for matrix homeostasis. Chondrons are mechanically extracted from cartilage and collected by serially low-speed homogenisation. Chondrons isolated from full-deep articular cartilage are classified in four broad categories; single chondrons, double chondrons, multiple linear column (three or more chondrons) and chondron clusters/matrix chips. Single chondron represent the smallest chondron unit identified and is commonly found in the middle layers of intact cartilage. Double chondrons are typically identified in the middle-to-deep layers of intact tissue. Multiple chondron columns consist of three or more chondron units organized in a linear array typical of those seen in the deep layers of intact cartilage. Finally, clusters consist of randomly organized groups of single and double chondrons that remain aggregated during the homogenization procedure. Chips are described as large cartilage fragments usually containing several chondrons aligned and spatially organized in parallel with radial collagen fibres typical of the deep layer matrix [93]. Techniques have now been introduced to immobilize chondrons in transparent agarose allowing a range of structural, molecular and metabolic investigations. This chondron-agarose system is considered as a micro-cartilage explant model and differs from traditional chondrocyte-agarose cultures in that the natural microenvironment is retained and need not be resynthesized and assembled [94]. Microscopy and immunohistochemistry analysis have ushered in a clearer understanding of the composition of the pericellular environment of the chondrocytes as well as the cell matrix interaction [93, 95–100]. Chondrons are presented as a model system to study cell-matrix interaction in articular cartilage health and disease. Nevertheless, little information is available on the maintenance of chondrons in culture.

3.1.3.5
Immortalized Chondrocytes

Recombinant DNA or virus containing oncogene with an "immortalizing" function has been used with various cell types to establish permanent cell lines [101–104]. Immortalization of chondrocytes in culture, displaying both infinite proliferation capacity and stable phenotype, could be of interest because chondrocytes lose their phenotype when grown in monolayer. Mallein-Gerin et al. [104] showed that SV40 large T oncogene is able to induce mouse chondrocyte proliferation without loss of expression of type II, IX and XI collagens, as well as cartilage aggrecan and link protein. Nevertheless, the cell line obtained also synthesized type I collagen when cultured in monolayer or in agarose gel. Horton et al. [101] described an immortalized cell line having a low level of type II collagen mRNA expression. These cells were created by transformation with a murine retrovirus carrying the v-myc and v-raf oncogenes. This cell type represents a unique model to study cartilage matrix interactions in the absence of type II collagen and also the type II collagen synthesis regulatory pathway [103]. Finally, it was shown that rat chondrocytes immortalized by myc express mRNA transcript coding for the proα2 chain of type I collagen when cultured in monolayer, but not in suspension as normal chondrocytes.

Chondrocytes with mutated or knock-out genes important for cartilage physiology can also be maintained in culture. This approach is of particular interest to investigate the role of specific molecules in the organization of cartilage matrix or the effect of regulatory factors on the cartilage metabolism. Chondrocytes knock-out for type IX collagen gene synthesize type II collagen fibrils larger than normal type II collagen fibrils suggesting that type IX collagen acts as a fibril diameter regulator [104]. Recently, molecular and genetic analyses have demonstrated the presence of mutations in COL2A1, the gene coding for type II collagen, in family with primary generalized osteoarthritis. To examine the influence of mutant type II collagen molecules on cartilage matrix, Dharmaravan et al. [105] performed stable transfection of COL2A1 construct containing the Arg^{519} – Cys mutation into human fetal chondrocytes *in vitro*.

3.1.3.6
Co-Culture System

In the joint, the articular cartilage develops a relationship with other cell types contained in synovial membrane, synovial fluid, ligament and subchondral bone. Chondrocytes metabolism may be influenced by soluble factors synthesized by these cells. In arthritis, cartilage is directly degraded by enzymes and free radicals produced by synovial cells. Many reseachers have developed culture models studying the interactions between cartilage and neighboring tissues.

Lacombe-Gleize et al. [106], cultured rabbit chondrocytes and osteoblasts in a co-culture system (COSTAR) in which cells were separated by a microporous membrane (0.4 µm) that permitted exchanges between the two cell types without any direct contact. This study demonstrated that osteoblasts are able to stimulate growth of chondrocytes by way of soluble mediators. This model should be of interest to understand interaction between chondrocytes and osteoblasts.

Another model described by Malfait and collaborators [107], studied the relation between peripheral blood mononuclear cells and chondrocytes. This model was particularly useful to investigate cytokine-mediated events at the cartilage-synovial pannus junction in destructive arthropathies. In this model, agarose cultures were performed in tissue culture inserts consisting of a low-protein binding membrane with 0.4 µm pores. Chondrocytes culture in agarose were then placed in a Petri dish on the top of mononuclear cells. This study showed that mononuclear cells stimulated by LPS produced IL-1 and TNFα which thereby depressed chondrocyte aggrecan synthesis and provoked the breakdown of newly synthesized aggrecan aggregates.

Tada et al. [108] established an *in vitro* model in which vascular endothelial cells on type I collagen in an inner chamber, which featured a 0.4 µm millipore filter, are co-cultured with chondrocytes in an outer chamber. In this model, human endothelial cells formed tubes in the collagen gel in the presence of epidermal growth factor (EGF) or transforming growth factor-α. Interestingly, TGF-dependent tube formation by endothelial cells was inhibited when human chondrocytes were co-cultured in the outer chamber. This chondrocyte-induced inhibition is partly abrogated by anti-TGFβ antibodies suggesting that avascularity of cartilage is partly due to TGFβ produced by chondrocytes themselves.

Groot et al. [109] co-cultured chondrocytes from the hypertrophic and proliferative zones of 16-day-old fetal murine bone with pieces of cerebral tissue. After 4 days of co-culture, some chondrocytes had transdifferentiated into osteoblasts and started to form osteoids. After 11 days, part of the cartilage was replaced by bone and the bone matrix was partially calcified. The nervous system produces neuropeptides and neurotransmitters, of which some are known to affect osteoblast metabolism or have receptors on osteoblastic cells, such as norepinephrine [110], vasoactive intestinal peptide [111, 112], calcitonin gene-related peptide [113, 114], substance P [114] and somatostatin [115]. The co-cultured pieces of cerebral tissue may produce some of these factors capable of inducing transdifferentiation process of chondrocytes into osteoblasts.

3.1.4
Chondrocyte Culture Environment

3.1.4.1
Effects of Oxygen Tension on Chondrocyte Metabolism

Most chondrocyte cultures are developed within an atmospheric oxygen tension. Nevertheless, it is widely assumed that chondrocytes live in a hypoxic environment and that oxygen tension may vary in pathological situations. Morever, during maturational process, there are marked changes in the vascular supply to epiphysis. In concert with the observation that the vascular supply varies from zone to zone in the growth plate, sharp differences in the oxygen tension accross the plate have been noted. Brighton and Heppenstall [116], demonstrated that in the tibial plate of the rabbit, the oxygen tension is lower in the hypertrophic zone than in surrounding cartilage. Measurement of a number of metabolic parameters indicated that chondrocytes are able to rapidly respond to local alterations in the oxygen concentration. Firstly, oxygen consumption by chondrocytes decreases at low oxygen tension [117]. Secondly, glucose utilization, glycolytic enzyme activity and lactate synthesis progressively increase when the oxygen tension is lowered from 21% to 0.04%. Thirdly, the absolute levels of ATP, ADP or AMP remain stable even at very low oxygen tension [118]. These data demonstrate that chondrocytes exhibit metabolic characteristics directed at preserving maximum energy levels for vital processes. Nevertheless, synthetic activity, and thus repair processes, is altered by hypoxic conditions. Low oxygen tension inhibits sulfate incorporation and DNA synthesis [119].

High oxygen tension may also induce adverse effects on chondrocyte metabolism including reduction of the proteoglycan and DNA synthesis [119, 120] or cartilage matrix degradation [121]. These effects may be conducted by active oxygen species production [122, 123].

3.1.4.2
Effects of Ionic and Osmotic Environment on Chondrocyte Function

In cartilage, the extracellular ionic environment is different from that of most cells, extracellular Na^+ being 250–350 mM and extracellular osmolality 350–450 mOsm. When chondrocytes are isolated from the matrix and incubated in a standard culture medium (DMEM; osmolality 250–280 mOsm), their extracellular environment changes sharply. Furthermore, Ca^{++} and K^+ concentrations in the medium are considerably lower than in the tissue, and anion concentration are higher.

Hyperosmotic stimuli produced by addition of sucrose concentration, induces a transient intracellular elevation of proton and calcium anions in the cytosol [124]. This intracellular change may affect several cell processes such as chondrocyte differentiation and metabolic activity. Urban et al. [125] demonstrated that ^{35}S-sulphate and ^3H-proline incorporation rates by isolated cells incubated in DMEM for 2–4 h is only 10% of that in the tissue. Synthesis reached a maximum when the extracellular osmolality is 350–400 mOsm for both freshly isolated and for cartilage explant. Moreover, the cell volume of chondrocytes increased by 30–40% when the cells were removed from their in situ environment into DMEM. If, however, chondrocytes are maintained for 12–16 h in non-physiological osmolalities, they appear to adapt to some extent to their new extracellular environment so that as before, synthesis rates decreased in proportion to any further change in extracellular osmolality. Another study reported the effect of osmolarity on pig chondrocyte growth, synthesis and morphology when cultured at high density. This study showed a similar biochemical and morphological behavior of chondrocytes cultured at 0.28 and 0.38 osM. At 0.48 osM, cell proliferation and protein synthesis are reduced during the first 4–6 h of culture and then progressively recovered their rate and nearly reached the control value. In contrast, cells cultured in 0.58 osM medium are unable to sustain their proliferative rate and after 6-days of exposure cell number drastically decline indicating cell detachment or death. At 0.58 osM, protein synthesis is highly inhibited and protein synthesis does not restore to the control rate level during the subsequent period of observation. Furthermore, while chondrocytes cultured in 0.28–0.38 osM medium maintained phenotypic characteristic in culture, the higher osmolarities (0.48–0.58) caused morphological change resulting in loss of phenotypic stability as demonstrated by their taking on a fibroblast-like shape as well as a lack of ability to assemble matrix proteoglycans [126]. These findings suggest that chondrocytes possess adaptative mechanisms capable of responding quickly at limited osmolarity variation. The change in concentration of other ionic species as the result of cell isolation may also affect matrix synthesis. Incorporation rates of ^{35}S-sulphate increased by 50% as the medium concentration of K^+ was raised from 5 mM (DMEM concentration) to 10 mM (extracellular concentration in cartilage). Extracellular HCO_3^- has no effect on the synthesis rate over the physiological range. In addition, Ca^{++} had no effect on tracer incorporation rates in cells or cartilage slices over 0–10 mM [125, 127]. Nevertheless, $CaCl_2$ concentration below 0.5 mM to the selectively promoted the production of collagen by adult bovine chondrocytes whereas the lowest levels of collagen synthesis were reached at calcium concentrations of 1–2 mM (which corresponded at the amount found in DMEM). A moderate increase occurred at high levels of calcium (2–10 mM) [127]. SO_4^- became rate-limiting at 0.3 mM, but had no significant effect above this concentration. Moreover, cations were required for chondrocytes attachment and provided a mechanism to differentially regulate attachment to ECM protein. Mg^{2+} and Mn^{2+} supported attachment to fibronectin and type II collagen while Ca^{2+} did not support adhesion to collagen [128]. These data indicate that synthesis rates in chondrocytes incubated in DMEM after isolation are affected by changes in extracellular K^+, Na^+, Ca^{++} and osmolality.

3.1.4.3
Effects of Mechanical Stress on Chondrocyte Metabolism

Joint immobilization causes reversible cartilage athrophy suggesting that mechanical stimuli are required for physiologic turnover of the extracellular matrix. The majority of culture models reported in the literature is realised at normal atmospheric pressure and fails to expose chondrocytes at tensile or compressive strength. However, it has been clearly demonstrated that chondrocyte metabolism is influenced by the mechanical environment, with the level of response dependent on both the strain and frequency of the compressive load [129]. Loading experiments using intact articular cartilage explants *in vitro* have indicated that static loading reduces PG and protein synthesis, while dynamic loading may stimulate synthesis in a frequency dependent manner [5, 130, 131]. The exact signaling pathways are complex and believed to involve cell deformation [132], hydrostatic pressure [133], osmotic pressure [125], streaming potentials [134], or cell surface receptor for matrix molecule [135]. To assess the exact influence of each of the parameter, it is necessary to develop systems in which one parameter can be varied independently. For example, explant culture is not adapted to study cell deformation but may be used to investigate the general effect of pressurization on chondrocyte metabolic activity. Indeed, compression of cartilage results in deformation of cells but it is also accompanied by hydrostatic pressure gradients, fluid flow, streaming potentials and currents as well as physiochemical changes such as altered matrix water content, fixed charge density and modifications in osmotic pressure. Cell deformation can be studied using isolated cells embedded in agarose gel or collagen gel [132].

A variety of experimental system have been developped to investigate the effect of mechanical stimulation on cultured chondrocytes. Some groups used an experimental system where pressure is applied to the cultured chondrocytes via a gas phase. Using pressure of 13 kPa above atmospheric at a low frequency of 0.3 Hz for 15 min, Veldhuijzen et al. [136] demonstrated an increase in cytoplasmic cyclic AMP and proteoglycan synthesis and a reduction in DNA synthesis. Complementarily, Smith el al. [137] showed that primary bovine chondrocytes cultured at high density in the presence of fetal bovine serum and exposed to hydrostatic pressure (10 MPA) applied intermittently at 1 Hz for 4 h increased aggrecan and type II collagen mRNA signals whereas constant pressure had no effect on either mRNA. In a similar system, Wright et al. [129] reported that cyclical pressurization is associated with hyperpolarization of chondrocyte cell membranes and activation of Ca^{2+}-dependent K-ion channels. This effect is associated with changes in microstrain applied on the base of the culture plate and subsequent stretching of the attached chondrocytes suggesting that effect observed after intermittent pressurization is mediated by stretch-activated ion channels in chondrocytes plasma membrane. The chondrocyte reaction to hydrostatic pressure depends on culture conditions and testing regimens. Cyclic hydrostatic pressure (5 MPa) decreases sulfate incorporation in chondrocyte monolayers when applied at 0.05, 0.25 and 0.5 Hz but stimulates sulfate incorporation when applied to cartilage explants at 0.5 Hz [133].

Fluid-induced shear can be applied on chondrocytes monolayer culture using a cone viscometer rotating within the cell culture medium at a constant speed. Chondrocytes submitted at fluid-induced shear adapted an elongate shape and align tangentially to the direction of the cone rotation. Fluid induced shear stimulated glycosaminolycan and increased the length of newly synthesized chain in human and bovine chondrocytes [138]. Moreover, the release of prostaglandin E_2 and mRNA signal for tissue inhibitor of metalloproteinase was enhanced by fluid-induced shear. In contrast, mRNA signals for the neutral metalloproteinases did not show major changes.

Recently, Buschmann et al. [139] reported that chondrocytes in agarose gel respond biosynthetically to static and dynamic mechanical load in a manner similar to that of intact organ culture. However after the level of matrix development was more advanced, the response to compression was more pronounced in culture. This method has also demonstrated that mechanical loads generate a hyperosmotic stimulus and subsequent pH decrease at the level of the chondrocytes.

The effect of mechanical tensile may be studied within a gel embedded cell system or on adherent support cells. Tensile strain may be determinated with a system in a computer-controlled vacuum unit and a base plate to hold the culture dishes. When a precise vacuum level is applied to the system, the culture plate bottoms are deformed to a known percentage elongation which is maximal at the edge and decrease at the center. The strain is translated to the cells cultured. By this way, Holmval et al. [135] showed that chondrosarcoma cells cultured on collagen type II-coated dishes increased the mRNA expression of α2- but not α1-integrin. The integrin α2β1 is able to bind type II collagen. Therefore, it is an excellent candidate for mechanoreceptors since it interacts with actin-binding proteins and thereby links the extracellular matrix with the cytoskeleton.

3.1.4.4
Effect of pH on Chondrocyte Metabolism

Chondrocytes exist in an extracellular environment where the pH of the interstitial fluid is more acidic than that of other tissues and which changes with tissue loading. Values of pH 6.9 have been measured for the matrix of articular cartilage [140] and there are reports of values as low as 5.5 for diseased tissue [141]. Chondrocytes live at low pO_2 implicating that metabolism is largely by glycolysis (up to 95% of all glucose metabolism), with consequent production of significant quantities of lactic acid [142]. In addition to this acidification which arises from metabolism, there is also a contribution from the components of the matrix itself. The large numbers of fixed negative charges on proteoglycans modify the extracellular ionic composition. There are high levels of free cations (e.g., H^+, Na^+, K^+) and low concentration of anions (e.g., Cl^-, HCO_3^-) [143]. Furthermore, the water present in the matrix can be expressed during tissue loading, resulting in a higher concentration of fixed negative charges, and so attracting more positive ions into the matrix. This includes a decrease of the extracellular pH, which is known to affect the intracellular pH, thereby modifying intracellular metabolism. Recently, Wilkins and Hall [144] have studied the effect of extracellular and intracellular pH on matrix synthesis by isolated bovine chondrocytes. They have observed that matrix synthesis exhibited a bimodal relation with decreased pH. Slight reductions ($7.4 < pH < 7.1$) increased $^{35}SO_4$ and ^3H-proline incorporation by up to 50% whereas profound acidification of the media ($pH < 7.1$) inhibited syntheses by up to 75% of the control value. On the other hand, direct imposition of a sustained intracellular acidosis ($pH = 6.65$) using ammonium prepulse with amiloride inhibited matrix synthesis by only 20%. These findings suggest that the modification of the matrix synthesis by extracellular pH, could not be entirely explained by changes of the intracellular pH. Moreover, chondrocytes possess a power regulating system of intracellular pH involving a Na^+-H^+ exchanger, a Na^+-dependent Cl^- HCO_3 transporter and H^+-ATPase pump [145].

3.1.4.5
Culture Medium Composition

The culture medium must be adapted according the experimental requirement. Fetal calf serum has often been used in the past decade to optimize culture condition, but several problems with the use of serum should be noted: (1) outgrowth of cells from the periphery of tissue in organ cultures; (2) variability between the composition of different batches of serum [146]; [3] presence of an unknown amount of components; (4) elevated risks of interferences with the results of studies on the influence of various biologic factors on metabolic activities of cells. A example of interference was recently related to the effect of EGF on rat articular chondrocytes. EGF stimulated ^3H-thymidine incorporation and increased DNA content of cultures. The effect was strongest when serum concentration was low ($\leq 1\%$) and was lost at high ($\geq 7.5\%$) concentration [147]. Moreover, it is well known that levels of synthesis and degradation in DMEM supplemented with fetal calf serum are greatly elevated compared with *in vivo*. The differences between metabolism *in vivo* and *vitro* may be caused by differences between the synovial fluid and medium in which cells are batched. Therefore, Lee et al. [148] cultured steer chondrocytes into agarose using a nutrient medium containing Dulbecco's Minimal Essential Medium supplemented with 20% FCS and an increased amount of normal allogenic synovial fluid. Dilution of medium with synovial fluid induced an increase in proteoglycan amounts to levels of 80 % synovial fluid. On the other hand, tritiated thymidine uptake decreased with increasing concentrations of synovial fluid. These results suggest that culture in synovial fluid induces a metabolic state similar to that seen *in vivo*, with high levels of glycosaminoglycan synthesis and low levels of cell division.

Some substitutes of serum with a standardized composition are available commercially. The most currently used are ultroser G and ITS+ (Insulin, transferrin, selenium, BSA and linoleic acid). In order to avoid interferences, a completely defined serum-free culture media can be prepared in a composition adapted at the goals of the *in vitro* study. In a very interesting study, Verbruggen et al. [149] demonstrated that ^{35}S-aggrecan synthesis by human chondrocytes cultured in agarose in serum-free DMEM was between 20 and 30 % of the value observed in DMEM supplemented with 10 % fetal calf serum. They determined the extent to which IGF-1, IGF-2, TGF-β or insulin were able to restore aggrecan production in serum-free medium. The authors conclude that 100 ng/ml of insulin, IGF-1 or IGF-2 partly restored aggrecan synthesis to 39 – 53 % of the control level. No cumulative or synergic activities were observed when these factors were combined. Interestingly, 10 ng/ml of TGF-β, in the presence of 100 ng/ml of insulin, stimulated aggrecan synthesis to more than 90 % of the reference level. Finally, human serum transferrin, alone or in combination with insulin, had no effects on aggrecan synthesis. When FCS was replaced by BSA, the proportion of aggrecan aggregates decreased dramatically. Supplementing the culture media with IGF, insulin or TGF-β partly restored the ability of the cells to produce aggrecan-aggregates. On the other hand, IGF-1 and insulin have been shown to maintain homeostasis in organ cultures. After 40 days of culture, 10 to 20 ng/ml IGF-1 maintained PG synthesis at the same or higher levels than in a medium containing 20 % fetal calf serum. Catabolic rates were slower in IGF-1 medium than in medium with only 0.1 % albumin, but somewhat faster than for culture in medium with 20 % FCS. In long-term cultures, 20 ng/ml IGF-1 maintained a steady-state condition [88].

Lee et al. [46] compared the effect of DMEM + 20 % FCS, DMEM and DMEM + 20 ng of IGF-1 on DNA synthesis in explant culture, monolayer culture or in suspension culture over agarose. When cultured over agarose in the presence of serum, there was a tendency for chondrocytes to clump together, forming large clusters. Cells cultured without serum or with IGF-1 remained rounded over agarose, clumping in small groups, but failed to form large aggregates. In monolayer, DNA synthesis was significantly greater in serum containing cultures than in cultures supplemented with IGF-1, which in turn, was significantly greater than in serum free cultures. In contrast, when chondrocytes were cultured in suspension over agarose, no difference in DNA synthesis was observed between serum-free culture and culture supplemented with IGF-1. However, serum containing cultures incorporated significantly more radionucleotide (^{3}H-TdR) than in the other treatments.

Vitamin C is required for the activity of prolyl hydroxylases, RER enzymes that hydroxylate proline residues in the nascent procollagen chains and allow folding of the chains into a stable triple helix. Scorbutic chondrocytes synthesized underhydroxylated non-helical precursors of collagens that were secreted very slowly and accumulated in the RER. Acute ascorbic acid treatment (50 µg/ml), type II and IX underwent hydroxylation and were secreted at normal high rates. On the other hand, proteoglycans synthesis and secretion were unchanged by acute acorbic acid treatment. These findings suggest that secretion of collagens is regulated independently of proteoglycan secretion and that RER must possess mechanisms able to discriminate between proteoglycans core protein and procollagens [150].

3.1.5
Concluding Remarks

Maintenance of chondrocytes in culture is challenging because chondrocyte phenotype and metabolism are strongly regulated by their close environment. Chondrocyte isolation from the extracellular matrix drastically modifies its extracellular environment and deeply alters its behavior. Chondrocytes are suddenly exposed to abnormal oxygen tension, ionic and osmotic environment and are released from cell-matrix interactions. Moreover, chondrocyte phenotype is not stable. When chondrocytes are seeded in a support plastic they lose their cartilage-specific phenotype and show a fibroblastic-like morphology. Monolayer culture does not allow a long-term study of chondrocyte metabolism but is particularly recommended to study cell dedifferenciation. Since the discovery that chondrocytes re-express the differentiated phenotype when they are transferred from monolayer to suspension, some tri-dimensional culture models have been developped. Chondrocytes were embedded in natural or synthetic matrix or maintained in suspension by constant agitation. In these culture conditions, chondrocytes conserve their phenotype for several weeks and are suitable to study matrix formation. Morever, cultures of chondrocytes in a tridimensional matrix allow tissue engineering for transplantion in cartilage defects. This culture method granted the study of matrix homeostasis, resorption and repair in environmental conditions close to that observed *in vivo*.

We can conclude that *in vitro* studies on cartilage explants or isolated chondrocytes provide important information on normal and pathological chondrocyte metabolic functions and may help to define the mode of action of regulatory factors and drugs. Nevertheless, some discrepancies in the conclusion can appear according the origin of the cartilage, the culture model and the experimental conditions used.

References

1. Aydelottte M, Kuettner K (1988a) Differences between subpopulations of cultured bovine articular chondrocytes. I Morphology and cartilage matrix production. Connect Tiss Res 18:205–222
2. Archer C, McDowell J, Bayliss M, Stephens M, Bentley G (1990) Phenotypic modulation in sub-populations of human articular chondrocytes in vitro. J Cell Sci 97:361–371
3. Manicourt D, Pita J (1988) Quantification and characterization of hyaluronic acid in different topographical areas of normal articular cartilage from dogs. Coll Rel Res 1:39–47

4. Siczkowski M, Watt F (1990) Subpopulations of chondrocytes from different zones of pig articular cartilage-isolation, growth and proteoglycan synthesis in culture. J Cell Sci 97:349–360

5. Korver T, van de Stadt R, Kiljan E, van Kampen G, van der Korst J (1992) Effects of loading on the synthesis of proteoglycans in different layers of anatomically intact articular cartilage in vitro. J Rheumatol 19:905–912

6. Aydelotte M, Raiss R, Schleyerbach R, Kuettner K (1988b) Effects of interleukin-1 on metabolism of proteoglycans by cultured bovine articular chondrocytes. Orthop Trans (J Bone Joint Surg) 12:359

7. Aydelotte M, Schmid T, Greenhill R, Luchene L, Schumacher B, Kuettner K (1991) Synthesis of collagen by cultured bovine chondrocytes derived from different depths of articular cartilage. Trans Orthop Res Soc 16:26

8. Lee J, Hwang O, Who Kim S, Han S (1997) Primary cultured chondrocytes of different origins respond differently to bFGF and TGF-β. Life Sciences 61:293–299

9. Little C, Ghosh P (1997) Variation in proteoglycan metabolism by articular chondrocytes in different joint regions is determined by post-natal mechanical loading. Osteoarthritis and Cartilage 5:49–62

10. Guerne P-A, Blanco F, Kaelin A, Desgeorges A, Lotz M (1995) Growth factor responsiveness of human articular chondrocytes in aging and development. Arthritis Rheum 7:960–968

11. Kouri J, Jimenez S, Quintero M, Chico A (1996) Ultrastructural study of chondrocytes from fribrillated and non-fibrillated human osteoarthritic cartilage. Osteoarthritis and Cartilage 4:111–125

12. Lafeber F, van der Kraan P, Van Roy J, Vitters E, Huber-Brining O, Bijlsma J, van den Berg W (1992a) Local changes in proteoglycan synthesis during culture are different for normal and osteoarthritic cartilage. Am J Pathol 140:1421–1429

13. Aigner T, Gluckert K, von der Mark K (1997) Activation of fibrillar collagen synthesis and phenotypic modulation of chondrocytes in early human osteoarthritic cartilage lesions. Osteoarthritis Cartilage 5:183–189

14. Lafeber F, van Roy H, van der Kraan P, van den Berg W, Bijlsma J (1997) Transforming growth factor-β predominantly stimulates phenotypically changed chondrocytes in osteoarthritic human cartilage. J Rheumatol 24:536–542

15. Loeser R (1993) Integrin-mediated attachment of articular chondrocytes to extracellular matrix proteins. Arthritis Rheum 36:1103–1110

16. van der Kraan P, Vitters E, van den Berg W (1992) Differential effect of transforming growth factor β on freshly isolated and cultured articular chondrocytes. J Rheumatol 19:140–145

17. Shakibaei M, De Souza P, Merker H-J (1997) Integrin expression and collagen type II implicated in maintenance of chondrocyte shape in monolayer culture: an immunomorphological study. Cell Biol Intern 21:115–125

18. Hering T, Kollar J, Huynh T, Varelas J, Sandell L (1994) Modulation of extracellular matrix gene expression in bovine high-density chondrocyte cultures by ascorbic acid and enzymatic resuspension. Arch Biochem Biophys 314:90–98

19. Larsson T, Aspden R, Heinegard D (1989) Large cartilage proteoglycan (PG-LA) influences the biosynthesis of macromolecules by isolated chondrocytes. Matrix 9:343–352

20. Nevo Z, Dorfman A (1972) Stimulation of chondromucoprotein synthesis in chondrocytes by extracellular chondromucoprotein. Proc Natl Acad Sci USA 69:2069–2072

21. Wiebkin O, Muir H (1973) The inhibition of sulphate incorporation in isolated adult chondrocytes by hyaluronic acid. FEBS Lett 37:42–46

22. Solursh M, Vaerewyck S, Reiter S (1974) Depression by hyaluronic acid of glycosaminoglycan synthesis by cultured chick embryo chondrocytes. Dev Biol 41:233–244

23. Bansal M, Ward H, Mason R (1986) Proteoglycan synthesis in suspension cultures of rat chondrosarcoma chondrocytes and inhibition by exogenous hyaluronate. Arch Biochem Biophys 246:602–610

24. Shimazu M, Jikko A, Iwamoto M, Koike T, Yan W, Okada Y, Shimnei M, Nakamura S, Kato Y (1993) Effects of hyaluronic acid on the release of proteoglycans from the cell matrix in rabbit chondrocyte cultures in the presence and absence of cytokines. Arthritis Rheum 36:247–253
25. Lacy B, Underhill C (1987) The hyaluronate receptor is associated with actin filaments. J Cell Biol 105:1395–1404
26. Aruffo A, Stamenkovic I, Melnick M, Underhill C, Seed B (1990) CD44 is the principal cell surface receptor for hyaluronate. Cell 61:1303–1313
27. Turley E (1989) Hyaluronic acid stimulates protein kinase activity in intact cells and isolated protein complex. J Biol Chem 264:8951–8955
28. Luyten F, Hascall v, Nissley S, Morales T, Reddi A (1988) Insulin-like growth factors maintain steady-state metabolism of proteoglycans in bovine articular cartilage explants. Arch Biochem Biophys 267:416–425
29. Morales T, Joyce M, Sobel M, Danielpour D, Roberts A (1991b) Transforming growth factor-b in calf articular cartilage organ cultures: synthesis and distribution. Arch Biochem Biophys 288:397–405
30. Recklies A, Gold E (1992) Induction of synthesis and release of interleukin-8 from human articular chondrocytes and cartilage explants. Arthritis Rheum 35:1510–1519
31. Yamaguchi Y, Mann d, Ruoslahti E (1990) Negative regulation of transforming growth factor-β by the proteoglycan decorin. Nature 346:281–284
32. Roughley P, Melching L, Recklies A (1994) Changes in the expression of decorin and bi-glycan in human articular cartilage with age and regulation by TGF-β. Matrix Biol 14:51–59
33. Von der Mark K, Gauss V, von der Mark H, Muller P (1977) Relationship between cell shape and type of collagen synthesized as chondrocytes lose their cartilage phenotype in culture. Nature 267:531–532
34. Elima K, Vuorio E (1989) Expression of mRNAs for collagens and other matrix components in dedifferentiating and redifferentiating human chondrocytes in culture. FEBS Lett 258:195–197
35. Lefebvre V, Peeters-Joris C, Vaes G (1990a) Production of collagens, collagenase and collagenase inhibitor during the differentiation of articular chondrocytes by serial subculture. Biochem Biophys Acta 1051:266–275
36. Okayama M, Pacifici M, Holtzer H (1976) Differences among sulfated proteoglycans synthesized in nonchondrogenic cells, presumptive chondroblasts, and chondroblasts. Proc Natl Acad Sci 73:3224–3228
37. Kuettner K, Memoli V, Pauli B, Wrobel N, Thonar E, Daniel J (1982) Synthesis of cartilage matrix by mammalian chondrocytes in vitro. II. Maintenance of collagen and proteoglycan phenotype. J Cell Biol 93:751–757
38. Watt F (1988) Effect of seeding density on stability of the differentiated phenotype of pig articular chondrocytes in culture. J Cell Sci 89:373–378
39. Kostoulas G, Lang A, Trueb B, Baici A (1997) Differential expression of mRNAs for endopeptidases in phenotypically modulated ('dedifferentiated') human articular chondrocytes. FEBS Letters 412:453–455
40. Desmukh K, Kline W (1976) Characterization of collagen and its precursors synthesized by rabbit-articular-cartilage cells in various culture systems. Eur J Biochem 69:117–123
41. Norby D, Malemud C, Sokoloff S (1977) Differences in the collagen types synthesized by lapine articular chondrocytes in spinner and monolayer culture. Arthritis Rheum 20:709–716
42. Benya P, Schaffer J (1982) Dedifferentiated chondrocytes reexpress the differentiated collagen phenotype when cultured in agarose gels. Cell 30:215–224
43. Loty S, Forest N, Boulekbache H, Sautier J-M (1995) Cytochalasin D induces changes in cell shape and promotes in vitro chondrogenesis: a morphological study. Biol Cell 83:149–161
44. Harrison E, Luyten F, Reddi A (1992) Transforming growth factor-beta: its effect on phenotype reexpression by dedifferentiated chondrocytes in the presence and absence of osteogenin. In Vitro Cel Dev Biol 28A:445–448

45. Guerne P, Sublet A, Lotz M (1994) Growth factor responsiveness of human articular chondrocytes: distinct profiles in primary chondrocytes, subcultured chondrocytes, and fibroblasts. J Cell Physiol 158:476–484
46. Lee D, Bentley G, Archer C (1993) The control of cell division in articular chondrocytes. Osteoarthritis Cartilage 1:137–146
47. Lefebvre V, Peeters-Joris C, Vaes G (1990b) Modulation by interleukin 1 and tumor necrosis factor α of production of collagenase, tissue inhibitor of metalloproteinases and collagen types in differentiated and dedifferentiated articular chondrocytes. Biochem Biophys Acta 1052:366–378
48. Bujia J, Sittinger M, Pitzke P, Wilmes E, Hammer C (1993) Synthesis of human cartilage using organotypic cell culture. ORL 55:347–351
49. Reginato A, Iozzo R, Jimenez S (1994) Formation of nodular structures resembling mature articular cartilage in long-term primary cultures of human fetal epiphyseal chondrocytes on a hydrogel substrate. Arthritis Rheum 37:1338–1349
50. Shimizu M, Minakuchi K, Kaji S, Koga J (1997) Chondrocyte migration to fibronectin, type I collagen, and type II collagen. Cell Struct Func 22:309–315
51. Freed L, Vunjak-Novakovic G, Langer R (1993a) Cultivation of cell-polymer cartilage implants in bioreactors. J Cell Biochem 51:257–264
52. Fronroza C, Sohrabi A, Hungerford D (1996) Human chondrocytes proliferate and produce matrix components in microcarrier suspension culture. Biomaterials 17:879–888
53. Ronzière M-C, Farjanel J, Freyria A-M, Hartmann D, Herbage D (1997) Analysis of type I, II, III, IX and XI collagens synthesized by fetal bovine chondrocytes in high-density culture. Osteoarthritis Cartilage 5:205–214
54. Xu C, Oyajobi B, Frazer A, Kozaci D, Russel RGG, Hollander A (1996) Effects of growth factors and interleukin-1a on proteoglycan and type II collagen turnover in bovine nasal and articular chondrocyte pellet cultures. Endocrinology 137:3557–3566
55. Spirito S, Goldberg R, Di Pasquale G (1993) A comparison of chondrocyte proteoglycan metabolism in monolayer and agarose cultures. Agents Actions 39:C160–C162
56. Cornelissen M, Verbruggen G, Malfait A-M, Veys E, Dewulf M, Hellebuyck P, DeRidder L (1993) Size distribution of native aggrecan aggregates of human articular chondrocytes in agarose. In Vitro Cell Biol 29:356–358
57. Morales T, Roberts A (1988) Transforming growth factor beta regulates the metabolism of proteoglycans in bovine cartilage organ cultures. J Biol Chem 263:12828–12831
58. Pujol J-P, Galera P, Redini F, Mauviel A, Loyau G (1991) Role of cytokines in osteoarthritis: comparative effects of interleukin 1 and transforming growth factor -beta on cultured rabbit articular chondrocytes. J Rheumatol 18:75–76
59. Skantze K, Brinckerhoff C, Collier J-P (1985) Use of agarose culture to measure effect of transforming growth factor β and epidermal growth factor on rabbit articular chondrocytes. Cancer Res 45:4416–4421
60. Guo J, Jourdian G, MacCallum D (1989) Culture and growth characteristics of chondrocytes encapsulated in alginate beads. Connect Tissue Res 19:277–297
61. Hauselmann H, Masuda K, Hunziker E, Neidhart M, Mok S, Michel B, Thonar E (1996) Adult human chondrocytes cultured in alginate form a matrix similar to native human articular cartilage. Am J Physiol 271:C742–C752
62. Petit B, Masuda K, D'Souza A, Otten L, Pietryla D, Hartmann D, Morris N, Uebelhaert D, Schmid T, Thonar E (1996) Characterization of crosslinked collagen synthesized by mature articular chondrocytes cultured in alginate beads: comparison of two distinct matrix compartments. Exp Cell Res 225:151–161
63. Mok S, Masuda K, Hauselmann H, Aydelotte M, Thonar E (1994) Aggrecan synthesized by mature bovine chondrocytes suspended in alginate. J Biol Chem 269:33021–33027
64. Platt D, Wells T, Bayliss M (1997) Proteoglycan metabolism of equine articular chondrocytes cultured in alginate beads. Res Vet Sci 62:39–47
65. Hauselmann H, Fernandes R, Mok S, Schmid T, Block J, Aydelotte M, Kuettner K, Thonar E (1994) Phenotypic stability of bovine articular chondrocytes after long term culture in alginate beads. J Cell Sci 107:17–27

66. Tanaka H, Matsumara M, Veliky A (1984) Diffusion of peptides through polymerized alginate. Biotechnol Bioeng 26:53–57
67. Schuman L, Buma P, Versleyen D, de Man B, van der Kraan P, van den Berg W, Homminga G (1995) Chondrocyte behaviour within different types of collagen gel *in vitro*. Biomaterials 16:809–814
68. Fujisato T, Sajiki T, Liu Q, Ikada Y (1996) Effect of basic fibroblast growth factor on cartilage regeneration in chondrocyte-seeded collagen sponge scaffold. Biomaterials 17:155–162
69. Nehrer S, Breinan H, Ramappa A, Shortkroff S, Young G, Minas T, Sledge C, Yannas I, Spector M (1997) Canine chondrocytes seeded in type I and II collagen implants investigated *in vitro*. J Biomed Mater Res 38:95–104
70. Nehrer S, Breinan H, Ramappa A, Young G, Shortkroff S, Louie L, Sledge C, Yannas I, Spector M (1997) Matrix collagen type and pore size influence behaviour of seeded canine chondrocytes. Biomaterials 18:769–776
71. Van Susante J, Buma P, van Hosh G, Versleyen D, van der kraan P, van der Berg W, Homminga G (1995) Culture of chondrocytes in alginate and collagen carrier gels. Acta Orthop Scand 66:549–556
72. Homminga G, Buma P, Koot H, van der Kraan P, van den Berg W (1993) Chondrocyte behavior in fibrin glue *in vitro*. Acta Orthop Scand 64:441–445
73. Hendrickson D, Dixon A, Erb H, Lust G (1994) Phenotypic and biological activity of neonatal equine chondrocytes cultured in a three-dimensional fibrin matrix. Am J Vet Res 55:410–414
74. Fortier L, Nixon A, Mahommed H, Lust G (1997) Altered biological activity of equine chondrocytes cultured in three-dimensional fibrin matrix an supplemented with transforming growth factor β-1. Am J Vet Res 58:66–70
75. Freed L, Vunjak-Novakovic G, Biron R, Eagles D, Lesnoy D, Barlow S, Langer R (1994b) Biodegradable polymer scaffolds for tissue engineering. Biotechnology; 12:689–693
76. Freed L, Marquis J, Nohria A, Emmanual J, Mikos A, Langer R (1993b) Neocartilage formation *in vitro* and *in vivo* using cells cultured on synthetic biodegradable polymers. J Biomed Mater Res 27:11–23
77. Freed L, Grande D, Lingbin Z, Emmanual J, Marquis J, Langer R (1994a) Joint resurfacing using allograft chondrocytes and synthetic biodegradable polymer scaffolds. J Biomed Mater Res 28:891–899
78. Livecchi A, Tombes R, Laberge M (1994) *In vitro* chondrocyte collagen deposition within porous HDPE: substrate microstructure and wettability effects. J Biomed Mater Res 28:839–850
79. Sittinger M, Bujia J, Minuth W, Hammer C, Burmester G (1993) Engineering of cartilage tissue using bioresorbable polymer carriers in perfusion culture. Biomaterials 15:451–456
80. Bujia J, Sittinger M, Minuth W, Hammer C, Burmester G, Kastenbauer E (1995) Engineering of cartilage tissue using bioresorbable polymer fleeces and perfusion culture. Acta Otolaryngol 115:307–310
81. Sittinger M, Schultz O, Keyszer G, Minuth W, Burmester G (1997) Artificial tissues in perfusion culture. Int J Artif Organs 20:57–62
82. Kandel R, Chen H, Clark J, Renlund D (1995) Transplantation of cartilaginous tissue generated *in vitro* into articular joint defects. Art Cells, Blood Subs, and Immob Biotech 23:565–577
83. Boyle J, Luan B, Cruz T, Kandel R (1995) Characterization of proteoglycan accumulation during formation of cartilaginous tissue *in vitro*. Osteoarthritis Cartilage 3:117–125
84. Sims C, Butler P, Casanova R, Lee B, Randolph M, Lee A, Vacanti C, Yaremchuk M (1996) Injectable cartilage using polyethylene oxide polymer substrates. Plast Reconstr Surg 98:843–850
85. Campbell M, Handley C, D'Souza S (1989) Turnover of proteoglycans in articular-cartilage cultures. Characterization of proteoglycans released into culture medium. Biochem J 259:21–25

86. Sandy J, Flannery C, Neame P, Boynton R, Flannery C (1991) Catabolism of aggrecan in cartilage explants. J Biol Chem 294:115–122

87. Hascall V, Handley C, McQuillan D, Hascall G, Robinson H, Lowther D (1983) Effect of serum on biosynthesis of proteoglycans by bovine articular cartilage in culture. Arch Biochem Biophys 224:206–223

88. Campbell M, Handley C, Hascall V, Campbell R, Lowther D (1984) Turnover of proteoglycans in cultures of bovine articular cartilage. Arch Biochem Biophys 234:275–289

89. Poole CA, Flint M, Beaumont B (1984) Morphological and functional interrelationships of articular cartilage matrices. J Anat 138:113–138

90. Poole CA, Flint M, Beaumont B (1985) Morphology of pericellular capsule in articular cartilage revealed by hyaluronidase digestion. J Ultrastruct Res 91:13–23

91. Poole CA, Flint M, Beaumont B (1986) Chondrons from articular cartilage. Scand J Rheumatol (Suppl) 60:20

92. Poole CA, Flint M, Beaumont B (1987) Chondrons in cartilage: ultrastructural analysis of the pericellular microenvironment in adult human articular cartilage. J Orthopaed Res 5:509–522

93. Poole CA, Wotton S, Duance V (1988c) Localisation of type IX collagen in chondrons isolated from porcine articular cartilage and rat chondrosarcoma. Histochem J 20: 567–574

94. Poole C (1997) Articular cartilage chondrons: form, function and failure. J Anat 191:1–13

95. Poole CA, Ayad S, Schofield J (1988a) Chondrons from articular cartilage:. I. Immuno-localization of type VI collagen in the pericellular capsule of isolated canine tibial chondrons. J Cell Sci 90:635–643

96. Poole CA, Flint M, Beaumont B (1988b) Chondrons extracted from canine tibial cartilage: preliminary report on their isolation and structure. J Orthopaed Res 6:408–419

97. Poole CA, Honsa T, Skinner S, Schofield J (1990) Chondrons from articular cartilage (II). Analysis of the glycosaminoglycans in the cellular microenvironment of isolated canine chondrons. Connect Tiss Res 24:319–330

98. Poole CA, Glant T, Schofield J (1991) Chondrons from articular cartilage. (IV). Immuno-localization of proteoglycans epitopes in isolated canine tibial chondrons. J Histochem Cytochem 39:1175–1187

99. Poole CA, Ayad S, Gilbert R (1992) Chondrons from articular cartilage. V. Immuno-histochemical evaluation of type VI collagen organisation in isolated chondrons by light, confocal and electron microscopy. J Cell Sci 103:1101–1110

100. Chang J, Nakajima H, Poole CA (1997) Structural colocalisation of type VI collagen and fibronectin in agarose cultured chondrocytes and isolated chondrons extracted from adult canine tibial cartilage. J Anat 190:523–532

101. Horton W, Cleveland J, Rapp U, Nemuth G, Bolander M, Doege K, Yamada Y, Hasssell J (1988) An established rat cell line expressing chondrocytes properties. Exp Cell Res 178:457–468

102. Thenet S, Benya P, Demignot S, Feunteun J, Adolphe M (1992) SV40-Immortalization of rabbit articular chondrocytes: Alteration of differentiated functions. J Cell Physiol 150:158–167

103. Oxford J, Doege K, Horton W, Morris N (1994) Characterization of type II and type IX collagen synthesis by an immortalized rat chondrocyte cell line (IRC) having a low level of type II collagen mRNA expression. Exp Cell Res 213:28–36

104. Mallein-Gerin F, Ruggeiro F, Quinn T, Bard F, Grodzinsky A, Olsen B, van der Rest M (1995) Analysis of collagen synthesis and assembly in cultured by immortalized mouse chondrocytes in the presence or absence of $\alpha 1(IX)$ collagen chain. Exp Cell Res 219: 257–265

105. Dharmavaram R, Liu G, Jimenez S (1997) Stable transfection of human fetal chondrocytes with a mutant Arg^{519}-Cys type II procollagen (COL2A1) gene construct and expression of the mutated protein in vitro. Arthritis Rheum 9 (Suppl):S184

106. Lacombe-Gleize S, Gregoire M, Demignot S, Hecquet C, Adolphe M (1995) Implication of TGFβ1 in co-culture of chondrocytes-osteoblasts. In Vitro Cell Dev Biol 31:649–652

107. Malfait A-M, Verbruggen G, Almqvist K, Broddelz C, Veys E (1994) Co-culture of human articular chondrocytes with peripheral blood mononuclear cells as a model to study cytokine-mediated interactions between inflammatory cells and target cells in the rheumatoid joint. In Vitro Cell Dev Biol 30:747–752

108. Tada K, Fukunaga T, Wakabayashi Y, Masumi S, Sato Y, Izumi H, Kohno K, Kumano M (1994) Inhibition of tubular morphogenesis in human microvascular endothelial cells by co-culture with chondrocytes and involvement of transforming growth factor β: a model for avascularity in human cartilage. Biochem Biophys Acta 1201: 135–142

109. Groot C, Thesingh W, Wassenaar A-M, Scherft J (1994) Osteoblasts develop from isolated fetal mouse chondrocytes when co-cultured in high density with brain tissue. In Vitro Cell Dev Biol 30:547–554

110. Kumagai H, Sakamoto H, Guggino S (1989) Neurotransmitter regulation of cytosolic calcium in osteoblast-like bone cells. Calcif Tissue Int 45:251–254

111. Bjurholm A, Kreicberg A, Brodin E (1988a) Substance P- and CGRP-immunoreactive nerves in bone. Peptides 9:165–171

112. Bjurholm A, Kreicbergs A, Terenius L (1988b) Neuropeptide Y-, tyrosine hydroxylase-, vasoactive intestinal polypeptide-immunoreactive nerves in bone and surrounding tissues. J Autonom Nerv Syst 25:119–125

113. Michelangeli V, Fletcher A, Allan E (1989) Effects of calcitonin gene-related peptide on cyclic AMP formation in chicken, rat, and mouse bone cells. J Bone Min Res 4: 269–272

114. Bjurholm A, Kreicbergs A, Dahlberg L (1990) The occurrence of neuropeptides at different stage of DBM-induced heterotopic bone formation. Bone Miner 10:95–107

115. Mackie E, Trechsel U, Bruns C (1990) Somatostatin receptors are restricted to a subpopulation of osteoblast-like cells during endochondral bone formation. Development 110:1233–1239

116. Brighton C, Heppenstall R (1971) Oxygen tensions in zones of the epiphysial plate, the metaphisis and diaphysis. J Bone Joint Surg 53:712–728

117. Haselgrove J, Shapiro I, Silverton S (1993) Computer modeling of the oxygen supply and demand of cells of the avian growth cartilage. Am J Physiol 265:C497–C506

118. Rajpurohit R, Koch C, Tao Z, Teixeira C, Shapiro I (1996) Adaptation of chondrocytes to low oxygen tension: relationship between hypoxia and cellular metabolism. J Cell Physiol 168:424–432

119. Lane J, Brighton C, Menkowitz B (1977) Anaerobic and aerobic metabolism in articular cartilage. J Rheumatol 4:334–342

120. Lemperg R, Bergenholtz A, Smith T (1975) Calf articular cartilage in organ culture in a chemically define medium. 2. Concentration of glycosaminoglycans and ^{35}S-sulfate incorporation at different oxygen tensions. In vitro 11, 291–301

121. Sledge C, Dinle J (1965) Oxygen-induced resorption of cartilage in organ culture. Nature 205:140–141

122. Henrotin Y, Deby-Dupont G, Deby C, Franchimont P, Emmerit I (1992) Active oxygen species, articular inflammation and cartilage damage. In "Free radicals and Aging". Ed by Emmerit I and Chance B. Birkhauser Verlag, Basel: pp 308–322

123. Henrotin Y, Deby-Dupont G, Deby C, Debruyn M, Lamy M, Franchimont P (1993) Production of active oxygen species by isolated human chondrocytes. Br J Rheumatol 32:562–567

124. Dascalu A, Korestein R, Oron Y, Nevo Z (1996) A hyperosmotic stimulus regulates intracellular pH, calcium, and S-100 protein levels in avian chondrocytes. Biochem Biophys Res Comm 227:368–373

125. Urban J, Hall A, Gehl K (1993) Regulation of matrix synthesis rates by the ionic and osmotic environment of articular chondrocytes. J Cell Physiol 154:262–270

126. Borghetti P, Della Salda L, De Angelis E, Maltarello M, Petronini P, Gabassi E, Marcato P, Maraldi N, Borghetti A (1995) Adaptative cellular response to osmotic stress in pig articular chondrocytes. Tiss Cell 27:173–183

127. Koyano Y, Hejna M, Flechtenmacher J, Schmid T, Thonar E, Mollenhauer J (1996) Collagen and proteoglycan production by bovine fetal and adult chondrocytes under low levels of calcium and zinc ions. Connect Tisssue Research 34:213–225
128. Loeser R (1994) Modulation of integrin-mediated attachment of chondrocytes to extracellular matrix proteins by cations, retinoic acid, and transforming growth factor β. Exper Cell Res 211:17–23
129. Wright M, Jobanputra P, Bavington C, Salter D, Nuki G (1996) Effects of intermittent pressure-induced strain on the electrophysiology of cultured human chondrocytes: evidence for the presence of stretch-activated membrane ion channels. Clin Sci 90: 61–71
130. Saamanen A, Tammi M, Jurvelin J (1990) Proteoglycan alteration following immobilization and remobilization in the articular cartilage of young canine joint. J Orthop Res 8:863–873
131. Parkkinen J, Lammi M, Helminen H, Tammi M (1992) Local stimulation of proteoglycan synthesis in articular cartilage explant by dynamic compression in vitro. J Orthop Res 10:610–620
132. Lee D, Bader D (1995) The development and characterization of an in vitro system to study strain-induced cell deformation in isolated chondrocytes. In Vitro Cell Dev Biol 31:828–835
133. Parkkinen J, Ikonen J, Lammi M, Tammi M (1993) Effects of cyclic hydrostatic pressure on proteoglycan synthesis in cultured articular chondrocytes and explants. Arch Biochem Biophys 300:458–465
134. Frank E, Grodzinsky A (1987) Cartilage electromechanics I: Electrokinetic transduction and the effect of electrolyte pH and ionic strength. J Biomech 20:615–627
135. Holmvall K, Camper L, Johansson S, Kimura J, Lundgren-Akerlund E (1995) Chondrocyte and chondrosarcoma cell integrins with affinity for collagen type II and their response to mechanical stress. Exp Cell Res 221:496–503
136. Veldhuilzen J-P, Bourret L, Rodan G (1979) In vitro studies of the effect of intermittent compressive forces on cartilage cell proliferation. J cell Physiol 98:299–306
137. Smith R, Rusk S, Ellison B, Wessels P, Tsuchiya K, Carter D, Caler W, Sandell L, Schurman D (1996) In vitro stimulation of articular chondrocytes mRNA and extracellular matrix synthesis by hydrostatic pressure. J Bone Joint Surg 14:63–60
138. Smith R, Donlon B, Gupta M, Mohtai M, Das P, Carter D, Cooke J, Gibbons G, Hutchinson N, Shurman D (1995) Effects of fluid-induced shear on articular chondrocyte morphology and metabolism in vitro. J Bone Joint Surg 13:824–831
139. Bushmann M, Gluzband Y, Grodzinsky A, Hunziker E (1992) Mechanical compression modulates matrix biosynthesis in chondrocyte/agarose culture. J Cell Sci 108:1497–1508
140. Maroudas A (1980) Metabolism of cartilaginous tissues: a quantitative approach. In: Studies in joint disease. A Maroudas, E Holborow (eds) Pitman, Tunbridge Wells: pp 59–86
141. Diamant B, Karlsson J, Nachemson A (1968) Correlation between lactic acid levels and pH in discs of patients with lumbar rhizopathies. Experientia 24:1195–1196
142. Stefanovic-Racic M, Stadler J, Georgescu H, Evans C (1994) Nitric oxide and energy production in articular chondrocytes. J Cell Physiol 159:274–280
143. Lesperance L, Gray M, Burstein D (1992) Determination of fixed charge density in cartilage using nuclear magnetic resonance. J Othop Res 10:1–13
144. Wilkin R, Hall A (1995) Control of matrix synthesis in isolated bovine chondrocytes by extracellular and intracellular pH. J Cell Physiol 164:474–481
145. Dascalu A, Nevo Z, Korenstein R (1993) The control of intracellular pH in cultured avian chondrocytes. J Physiol 461:583–599
146. Morales T (1991a) Transforming growth factor-b1 stimulates synthesis of proteoglycan aggregates in calf articular organ cultures. Arch Biochem Biophys 286:99–106
147. Ribault D, Khatib A, Panasyuk A, Barbara A, Bouisar Z, Mitrovic R (1997) Mitogenic and metabolic actions of epidermal growth factor on rat articular chondrocytes: modulation by fetal calf serum, transforming growth factor-β, and thyrosin. Arch Biochem Biphys 337:149–158

148. Lee D, Salih V, Stockton E, Stanton J, Bentley G (1997) Effect of normal synovial fluid on the metabolism of articular chondrocytes *in vitro*. Clin Orthop Rel Res 342:228–238
149. Verbruggen G, Malfait A-M, Dewulf M, Broddelez C, Veys E (1995) Standardization of nutrient media for isolated human articular chondrocytes in gelified agarose suspension culture. Osteoarthritis Cartilage 3:249–259
150. Pacifici M (1990) Independent secretion of proteoglycans and collagens in chick chondrocyte cultures during acute ascorbic acid treatment. Biochem J 272:193–199

3.2
Animal Models of Osteoarthritis

K. D. BRANDT

3.2.1
Introduction

As discussed by Pritzker [1], an animal model can be defined as "a homogenous set of animals which have an inherited, naturally acquired, or experimentally induced biological process, amenable to scientific investigation, that in one or more respects resembles the disease in humans." Animal models of osteoarthritis (OA) are useful in studying the evolution of structural changes in joint tissues, determining how various risk factors may initiate or promote these changes, and evaluating therapeutic interventions. Because it is difficult to obtain joint tissues from humans with OA until the pathological changes are far advanced and to obtain them sequentially, use of animal models provides the only practical way to examine the processes involved with initiation of the disease, the associated morphologic biochemical, metabolic and molecular biological changes in articular cartilage, and how, e.g., the balance of matrix cartilage synthesis and degradation influences disease progression. However, it must be borne in mind that OA is not a disease of only a single tissue – articular cartilage – but that all of the tissues of the joint are affected, i.e., the subchondral bone, synovium, menisci, ligaments, periarticular muscles and the afferent nerves whose terminals lie both within and external to the joint capsule. To date, studies of OA in animal models of pharmacologic agents have focused chiefly on their effects on articular cartilage. The effects, for example, of quadriceps weakness, which is a major cause of disability in humans with knee OA [2] and a risk factor for knee OA in humans [3], have received essentially no attention in animal models of knee OA. Indeed, if such studies were performed in quadripeds, their relevance to the disease in humans would be questionable. Furthermore, because joint pain is the chief clinical feature of OA leading the human subject to seek medical attention, it is worth emphasizing that the effects of a drug on joint pain in humans cannot be studied adequately in any animal model.

A comprehensive, although not exhaustive, list of animal models of OA is provided in Table 1, modified from the excellent recent review of the subject by

Table 1. Examples of Animal Models of OA

Underlying mechanism	Species/strain	Inducing agent	Reference
Spontaneous OA	Guinea pig, Hartley	Age/obesity	5, 6
	Mouse, STR/ORT, STR/INS	Unidentified genetic predisposition	7–9
	Mouse, C57 black	Unidentified genetic predisposition	10–13
	Mouse	Type II collagen mutation	14
	Mouse	Type IX collagen mutation	15
	Rat, Wister, Fischer 344		16
	Dog	Hip dysplasia	17
	Primate	Unidentified genetic predisposition	18–20
Chemically-induced	Chicken	Intra-articular iodoacetate	21
	Rabbit	Intra-articular papain	22–24
	Guinea pig	Intra-articular papain	25
	Dog	Intra-articular chymopapain	26
	Guinea pig	Intra-articular papain	27
	Mouse	Intra-articular papain	28
	Mouse	Intra-articular collagenase	28
	Mouse	Intra-articular TGF-β	29
	Rabbit	Intra-articular hypertonic saline	30
Physically-induced	Dog	Anterior cruciate ligament transection (unilateral)	31, 32
	Dog	Anterior cruciate ligament transection (bilateral)	33
	Rabbit	Anterior cruciate ligament transection	34, 35
	Sheep	Meniscectomy	36
	Rabbit	Meniscectomy	37–39
	Guinea pig	Meniscectomy	5
	Guinea pig	Myectomy	40–42
	Rabbit	Patellar contusion	43, 44
	Rabbit	Immobilization	45, 46
	Dog	Immobilization	47–49
	Dog	Denervation followed by anterior cruciate ligament transection	50

Modified from Doherty N et al. [4].

Doherty et al. [4–50]. In general, the greater the similarity of OA changes in the model to those in humans, the more desirable the model. However, practical issues, such as the availability of the animal species, the rate at which changes of OA develop, the ease of handling and maintenance, and cost all are important considerations.

Great interest currently exists in therapeutic agents which may slow the progression of OA, i.e., disease-modifying OA drugs (DMOADs) [51]. Although several drugs have been shown to slow the progression, or prevent the development, of experimentally-induced or spontaneous OA in animals, none has yet been shown to be effective in humans with OA. Clinical trials of diacerhein and of doxycycline are now in progress and trials of other matrix metalloproteinase (MMP) inhibitors and of an antiresorptive agent (targeting bone rather than articular cartilage) will soon be initiated in patients with knee OA.

Surgical models of OA and models which involve intra-articular injection of a degradative enzyme to destabilize the joint by damaging articular cartilage or other structures are currently popular; whether they are more relevant to post-traumatic OA than to primary (idiopathic) OA in humans, however, at least with regard to their suitability for evaluating therapeutic agents, remains to be seen. The development of spontaneous knee OA in a variety of animal species – bipeds as well as quadripeds – provide alternatives to these surgically or chemically induced models (Table 1). However, because no animal model can mirror fully all of the variables which may modify the disease in humans, use of models for discovery of DMOADs represents, as noted by Billingham [52], "… an expensive gamble that what can be achieved in animals will translate to the OA diseases of man."

Over the past several years, numerous reviews of animal models of OA have been published. This chapter draws extensively on two recent excellent comprehensive reviews: one, by Billingham [52], emphasizes the advantages attached to the use of animal models of OA while the other, by Doherty [4], deals with the limitations associated with the use of models.

3.2.2
Spontaneous OA in Animals

Medial compartment knee OA has been described in mouse strains, the Dunkin Hartley strain of guinea pig, Rhesus and Cynomolgus macaque monkeys and the Wistar and Fischer 344 strains of rats (see Table 1). Whether OA in larger species will prove to be more important to the study of idiopathic knee OA in humans than OA in rodent models and whether mechanisms of initiation and progression of the disease may be elucidated in macaques which are more relevant to human OA than those in small quadripeds remains to be seen.

3.2.2.1
Mice

Nearly all inbred strains of mice develop OA, although the incidence, severity and localization of the disease varies among strains. The highest incidence and most severe joint pathology are seen in STR/ORT and STR/INS strains [53]. In STR/ORT mice, the disease is more prevalent and more severe in males than in females. The initial articular cartilage lesion appears to develop in the medial tibial plateau. It has been suggested that patellar displacement precedes the changes in the cartilage but Evans et al. [54] and Collins et al. [55] found that all mice had cartilage damage by 11 months of age, although not all had patellar displacement.

Chondro-osseous metaplasia in tendinous structures around the knee joint and in ligament insertions is also common in this model [54, 55] and precedes the cartilage changes, suggesting that it may be of primary pathogenetic importance in these strains of mice. It is possible that ligamentous calcification alters the mechanical stress on intra-articular structures, and that the ensuing cartilage changes reflect unsuccessful attempts to maintain normal loading of the joint. In contrast to the guinea pig and macaque models, in which subchondral bone changes precede the development of cartilage degeneration, sclerosis of subchondral bone is a late feature of OA in this model.

Even though several months of treatment are required to evaluate a DMOAD in mice, their small size is advantageous insofar as less compound is required to study a drug in mice than in guinea pig or macaque models of OA. On the other hand, the small quantity of articular cartilage available from mice is a disadvantage for biochemical studies of pathogenetic mechanisms and drug effects. Molecular biology techniques, such as the differential display of genes which are activated or repressed during development of OA, can be used to assess a pharmacologic effect on very small amounts of tissue over a shorter time span than is needed to evaluate the effects of a DMOAD on the pathoanatomy of the joint, but cannot replace morphologic evaluation.

3.2.2.2
The Guinea Pig

The studies of Bendele et al. [56, 57] and Meacock et al. [58] describing the natural history of the disease, have stimulated interest in the guinea pig model of OA. All male guinea pigs of the Dunkin Hartley strain begin to show cartilage degeneration after 13 months of age [57, 62]. Similar changes are seen in females but are somewhat delayed and less severe than in males. By one year of age, full-thickness loss of articular cartilage on the medial femoral condyle and tibial plateau has occurred. Increases in body weight increase the severity of the disease and diet restriction, limiting body weight to less than 900 g, can decrease the severity of joint pathology by 50 % [59].

Magnetic resonance imaging studies [60] have identified a change within the subchondral bone in this model as early as 8 weeks of age, i. e., preceding any apparent change in the articular cartilage. Radiography of 1 mm-thick undecalcified sections revealed extensive thinning of the subchondral trabeculae in the tibia and femur at the sites of insertion of the cruciate ligaments at an even earlier age. As seen with spontaneous OA in mice, cartilage degeneration in this guinea pig model is apparently preceded by a change in the subchondral bone. Although a change within the cruciate ligaments may precipitate the bone remodeling, it is possible that a subtle change in the articular cartilage leads to remodeling of the underlying bone.

Few drug studies have been reported in the guinea pig model of OA. Bendele et al. found that oral administration of diacerhein [61], the acetylated derivative of the anthroquinone, rhein, from 3 months to 12–15 months of age reduced the rate of progression of joint damage by some 50 per cent.

In 1986, Arsever and Bole [40] described changes of osteoarthritis in both the hip and knee of Hartley guinea pigs after unilateral resection of the gluteal muscles and/or transection of the infrapatellar ligament. Abnormalities also developed in joints of the contralateral hind limb. While this model provided an opportunity to examine early OA events unaffected by post-operative synovitis or local joint trauma, factors which may confound other physically-induced models of OA, interpretation of the results is confounded by the changes of OA that develop spontaneously in this species (see above).

3.2.2.3
Rhesus and Cynomolgus Macaques

Although OA develops spontaneously in rhesus monkeys [20, 62–64], the availability of this species for study is limited. However, development of a similar disease in the much more readily available Cynomolgus species has permitted study of naturally occurring medial compartment knee OA in a primate species [22, 65, 68]. The disease occurs in middle-aged to elderly animals which, unlike mice and guinea pigs, are bipedal. The earliest histological change is thickening of the subchondral plate, which is followed by fibrillation of the articular cartilage in the medial plateau [65]. Eventually, the lateral compartment becomes involved. Notably, degeneration of the cartilage does not occur until the subchondral bone undergoes thickening to 400 µm [66]. Both the prevalence and severity of knee OA increase with age in this model but, in contrast to the epidemiology of knee OA in humans [67], these are not affected by either gender or weight. This model has not yet been employed for studies of potential DMOADs.

3.2.3
Surgical Models of OA

Models based on surgically induced laxity of the knee joint, altering the mechanical stresses, have most frequently utilized rabbits and dogs. The most extensively studied surgical model is the cruciate-deficient dog, described by Marshall and Olsson [30] and by Pond and Nuki [31], and characterized in detail by our unit [32]. In the rabbit, a variety of surgical procedures on ligaments and menisci have been described [68], including cruciate ligament transection, with and without medial and collateral ligament section, total and partial meniscectomy, and creation of bucket-handle tears of the meniscus. In the guinea pig, partial meniscectomy and cruciate and collateral ligament transection have been studied [58, 69]. Partial meniscectomy leads to osteophyte formation within 2 weeks and extensive cartilage degeneration within 6 weeks, greatly accelerating the underlying spontaneous disease in this species (see above).

Because the natural history of OA in the canine cruciate-deficiency model has been well elucidated and the pathology, not only in articular cartilage but also in other joint tissues, has been characterized to a greater extent than in other animal models of OA [32], it is described in some detail below.

3.2.3.1
The Natural History of OA in the Canine Cruciate-Deficiency Model

Until recently, because of an apparent absence of progressive changes and lack of full-thickness cartilage ulceration (as seen in human OA), the cruciate-deficient dog was widely viewed with skepticism as a model of OA. Studies by Marshall and Olsson [30] had suggested that the articular cartilage changes 2 years after ligament transection were no more severe than those seen only a few months after surgery. It was presumed that mechanical factors, e. g., capsular fibrosis and buttressing osteophytes, stabilized the cruciate-deficient knee and prevented progressive cartilage breakdown. The apparent lack of progressive cartilage changes led a number of investigators to contend that this was a model of cartilage injury and repair, rather than of OA.

Our studies, however, which documented the findings in the unstable knee after a lengthier period of observation than had been employed previously, clearly validate the cruciate-deficient dog as a model of OA [70]. They emphasize, furthermore, the striking capacity of the chondrocyte for repair in the earlier stages of OA [71], as outlined below:

McDevitt and Muir had noted that an increase in proteoglycan (PG) synthesis by chondrocytes in articular cartilage of the unstable knee occurs within days after ligament transection [72, 73]. We found that cartilage from the OA knee, while showing typical biochemical, metabolic and histological changes of OA, remained thicker than normal for as long as 64 weeks after the onset of knee instability [71], and showed that this thickening was associated with a sustained increase in PG synthesis and increases in both the content and concentration of PGs in the OA cartilage (Fig. 1). By magnetic resonance imaging (MRI) [74], we showed that this hypertrophic cartilage was maintained for as long as 3 years after cruciate transection, but that progressive loss of articular cartilage then occurred, so that 45 months after cruciate ligament transection extensive areas of the joint surface were devoid of articular cartilage. Studies of dogs sacrificed 54 months after cruciate ligament transection provided pathological confirmation of our MRI observations. In summary, given sufficient time, the changes of OA in this model are progressive; this is, indeed, a model of OA.

The phenomenon of hypertrophic repair of articular cartilage in OA is illustrated particularly well by the canine cruciate-deficiency model. It is, however, by no means unique to that model. It was recognized first in human OA cartilage by Bywaters [75] and subsequently by Johnson [76], and evidence exists of its presence in OA cartilage from rabbits subjected to partial meniscectomy [77] and from Rhesus macaques developing OA spontaneously [21, 78].

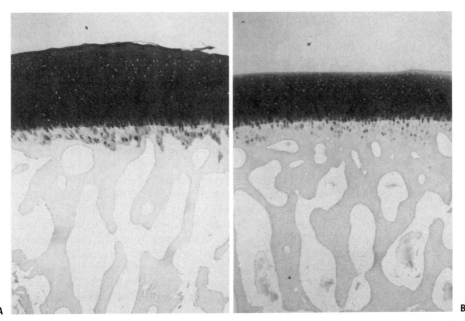

A   B

Fig. 1. Full thickness sections of articular cartilage from a mongrel. The sections were stained with safranin-O and fast green. The right anterior cruciate ligament was transected 12 weeks before sacrifice. The thickness of the articular cartilage from the OA knee and intensity of staining with safranin-O are greater in the OA knee (**A**) than in the contralateral knee (**B**). Original magnification X 40. Taken from [71]

Although contemporary descriptions of the pathology of OA emphasize the progressive loss of articular cartilage, they often fail to take into account the increases in cartilage thickness and PG synthesis in the earlier stages of OA, which are consistent with a homeostatic phase of compensated, stabilized OA. In this phase, repair may keep place with cartilage breakdown and maintain the joint in a reasonably functional state for years. The repair tissue, however, often does not hold up as well to mechanical stress as normal hyaline cartilage and, eventually, at least in some cases, the rate of PG synthesis falls and the cells can no longer successfully maintain the matrix. End-stage OA then develops, with full-thickness loss of the articular cartilage [70]. In marked contrast to this protracted time course, Fernandes et al. [79] described a surprisingly extensive loss of articular cartilage in this model within only a few weeks after cruciate ligament transection.

Recently, Manolopoulos et al. [80] have used mongrel dogs in which the anterior cruciate ligament was transected in both knees, leading to development of bilateral OA, to compare the effects of a pharmacologic agent which was administered by intra-articular injection in one knee with the findings after placebo (saline) injection into the contralateral knee [33]. It is possible that the loading of the unstable hind limbs in that model is quantitatively and qualitatively different from that of the unstable knee in the unilateral canine cruciate-deficiency model; no direct comparisons of pathology in the two models are available. It should be emphasized, however, that the contralateral knee of dogs with unilateral knee instability is not a truly normal control [81].

3.2.3.2
Neurogenic Acceleration of OA

As described above, in the canine cruciate-deficiency model of OA, cartilage degeneration, with fibrillation and thinning of the cartilage, develops gradually and failure of the joint, with loss of cartilage down to bone, may take 3-5 years. However, we have shown that if ligament transection is preceded by dorsal root ganglionectomy [50] or articular nerve neurectomy [82], full-thickness ulceration of the cartilage occurs within only weeks [83].

This observation is relevant to Charcot (neuropathic) arthropathy, a joint disorder characterized by severe, chaotic joint destruction, with osteochondral fractures, loose bodies, effusions, ligament instability and formation of new bone and new cartilage within the joint. The general concept of the pathogenesis of Charcot arthropathy is that interception of sensory input from the extremity by a neurologic disease (e.g., tabes dorsalis, syringomyelia) deprives the central nervous system of information from nociceptive or proprioceptive nerve fibers, leading to recurrent episodes of joint trauma and, ultimately, to joint breakdown.

A problem exists with this proposed mechanism, however: it is impossible to consistently produce Charcot arthropathy experimentally by neurosurgical procedures which interrupts the sensory nerve supply from an extremity. For example, we were unable to induce knee joint pathology in normal dogs subjected to unilateral L4-S1 dorsal root ganglionectomy [83]. On the other hand, if we transected the ipsilateral anterior cruciate ligament in dogs which had previously undergone dorsal root ganglionectomy, cartilage in the ipsilateral knee broke down within weeks. These results stand in sharp contrast to the very slowly progressive changes seen in the neurologically intact dog with a cruciate-deficient knee (see above).

The accelerated canine model of OA has proved very useful for evaluation of pharmacologic agents, the impact of which on progressive joint damage can be observed within only a few weeks (Fig. 2) [84]. However, the pathogenetic processes underlying the initiation of OA, i.e., the homeostatic hypertrophic repair phase (see above) may be different from those associated with the stage of progression of joint damage [85-87]. It is possible that a drug may show efficacy in the slowly progressing (neurologically intact) cruciate deficiency model but not in the accelerated model, as was the case with diacerhein [86-87]; the converse may also be expected.

3.2.3.3
Periarticular Muscle

Several years ago we showed that when the hind limb of a normal dog was immobilized in an orthopedic cast, the articular cartilage soon developed

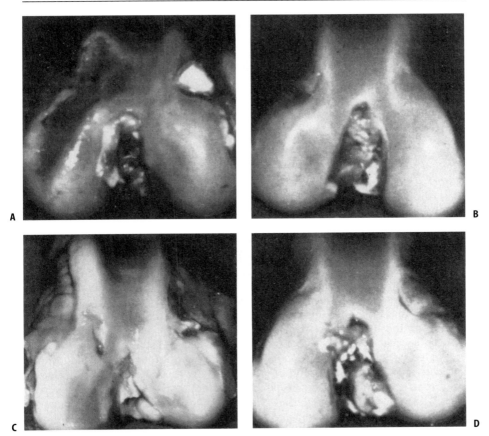

Fig. 2. Gross appearance of femoral condyles from doxycycline-treated and untreated dogs. Distal femur from the osteoarthritic knee of an untreated dog (**A**). Note the extensive full-thickness ulceration of the central, weight-bearing region of the medial femoral condyle. Contralateral, stable knee of the same animal as in **A** (**B**). The cartilage is grossly normal. Unstable knees of dogs treated prophylactically with doxycycline (**C** and **D**). The knee shown in C has only partial thinning of cartilage over the weight-bearing region of the medial condyle (**arrow**); however a linear cartilage ulcer is present on the medial trochlear ridge. The articular cartilage shwon in D, was grossly normal. Taken from [84]

striking atrophic changes, with thinning, a decrease in proteoglycan concentration, reduction in net proteoglycan synthesis and a defect in proteoglycan aggregation [88]. Notably, if the unstable knee is immobilized immediately after cruciate ligament transection, OA does not develop, but changes of cartilage atrophy are seen [89], identical to those noted after immobilization of a dog with normal knee stability, emphasizing the importance of altered joint mechanics in the genesis of OA in this model. Studies aimed at elucidating the pathogenesis of the cartilage changes seen with immobilization indicated that these were not due principally to a decrease in oscillatory motion of the joint, but to reduction in the contraction of the periarticular muscles that span the joint (e. g., hamstrings, quadriceps), and stabilize the limb during stance [90].

In patients with knee OA, quadriceps weakness is common and is generally believed to be due to atrophy of the muscle, secondary to unloading of the painful extremity [91]. Recently, an additional explanation for the quadriceps weakness in subjects with knee OA has been suggested, based on epidemiologic data. In a study of a community cohort of elderly individuals from central Indiana we found that among women with radiographic changes of knee OA, quadriceps weakness was common even among those who have no history of knee pain and hypertrophy (rather than atrophy) of the quadriceps muscle, due to their obesity [91]. Furthermore, longitudinal analysis of women in this cohort strongly suggested that baseline quadriceps weakness was a risk factor for radiographic changes of knee OA (i. e., for structural damage) [92]. The proposed mechanism by which quadriceps weakness in humans may predispose to knee joint damage is as follows: although hamstring activity decelerates the forward swing of the leg, at the end of swing, the leg is pulled toward the ground (toward heel-strike) by gravity, assisted by continuous hamstring action. Quadriceps action at this point retards the rate of descent, acting to brake the fall of the leg. Furthermore, because the quadriceps is important in providing anteroposterior stability to the knee [93], quadriceps weakness may alter sites of mechanical loading of the joint surface, resulting in damage to the articular cartilage. Experimental paralysis of the quadriceps in a normal subject was shown to result in a marked heelstrike transient and an estimated 5-fold increase in forces acting at the knee at touchdown [94]. Among subjects with normal knee radiographs, those with knee pain were found to exhibit a significantly greater heelstrike transient than those without knee pain [95]. The authors suggested that the gait pattern in the former group, the consequence of which was repeated impact loading of the lower extremity, led to a "pre-osteoarthritic" state, although no evidence was provided that those with knee pain developed OA or that the increased heelstrike transient was the cause, rather than the result, of knee pain.

Experimentally, some support exists for the above hypothesis: rabbits subjected to repeated acute (50 msec) impact loading of the knee incurred damage to articular cartilage and subchondral bone [96] while impulsive loads of greater magnitude, if applied more gradually (500 msec), were innocuous (Radin, E., personal communication). Very rapid application of load does not allow sufficient time for the periarticular muscles, the major shock absorbers protecting the joint, to absorb the load through eccentric contraction [97, 98]. Why some normal subjects generate a large heelstrike transient when walking, while others do not, is also unknown, but may reflect individual differences in central program generators, i. e., neurologic mechanisms based in the central nervous system which coordinate complex limb movements during gait [99].

Finally, the importance of muscle spindles (sensory nerve endings within muscle) in modulating muscle tone in response to changes in the position of a limb, thereby protecting the joint from injury, has received attention recently [93]. Joint position sense, measured both as the ability to reproduce passive positioning and to detect the onset of movement (kinesthesia), was significantly impaired in normal subjects after completion of a strenuous exercise protocol [100]. Hence, maintenance of quadriceps strength appears to be important also in preserving the integrity of protective muscular reflexes.

A variety of evidence suggests that the pathogenesis of knee OA in women may be different from that in men. For example, in women, knee OA tends to be more strongly associated with obesity and to be bilateral than in men, in whom it is more likely to be related to prior trauma and to be unilateral [101]. Although the association between knee OA and obesity is well-established, the mechanism by which they are related is unclear. Both biomechanical and metabolic mechanisms have been postulated. Martin et al. [102] found recently that, after adjustment for age and for obesity, metabolic correlates of obesity (measurements of glucose and lipid metabolism) did not exhibit an independent association with knee OA, indirectly favoring a mechanical basis.

Our data suggest that among women with incident OA, the greater their body weight, the poorer their quadriceps function. Regardless of the cause, our findings raise the possibility that the well-recognized association of obesity with knee OA in women is mediated through quadriceps weakness. Clearly, quadriped models of OA are unlikely to prove suitable for study of the relationship between periarticular muscle strength and development of OA; whether primate models will prove suitable in this respect remains to be seen.

3.2.3.4
Subchondral Bone

Some investigators have suggested that stiffening of the subchondral bone may be of primary importance in the etiopathogenesis of OA in man [103]. Radiographic studies of dogs that had undergone cruciate ligament transection revealed typical bony changes of OA, including subchondral sclerosis, by 24 months after surgery [104]. However, direct examination by computerized tomographic microdensitometry of the subchondral plate and the subchondral trabeculae in samples from dogs which were maintained as long as 72 weeks after cruciate ligament transection showed no increase in thickness of the subchondral plate and thinning of the underlying cancellous bone [103]. Only later was a trend noted for thickening of the subchondral plate. The osteopenia in the subchondral trabeculae is presumably due to the decrease in loading of the unstable limb after cruciate ligament transection [105] and to the synovitis which characterizes this model [106].

Our observations make it clear that typical articular cartilage changes of OA can occur in the presence of osteopenia; stiffening of subchondral bone is not a requisite for *initiation* of the early cartilage changes in this OA model. Indeed, the loss of subchondral bone could theoretically increase mechanical strain in the overlying articular cartilage, leading to degeneration [107]. Thickening of the subchondral plate, a relatively late phenomenon in the canine model, could, however, contribute to the failure of intrinsic repair mechanisms and to the *progression* of cartilage breakdown. Recently, we have shown that administration of a bisphosphonate can effectively inhibit resorption and formation of subchondral bone in the canine cruciate-deficiency model of OA [108], although it had no effect on osteophyte formation. Formation of new subchondral bone in the OA knee is presumably coupled to osteoclastic resorption, which can be inhibited pharmacologically [109, 110]; because osteophyte formation involves bony metaplasia of new fibrous connective tissue and bears no relationship to bone resorption, the absence of a pharmacologic effect on osteophytosis, while formation of subchondral bone was blocked by the bisphosphonate, is not surprising. A multi-center clinical trial to evaluate the effectiveness of a bisphosphonate as a DMOAD in patients with knee OA is currently planned.

Despite the costs associated with the model, several drug studies have been undertaken in the canine cruciate-deficiency dog. The NSAID, tiaprofenic acid, was reported to reduce both the severity of OA and protease levels within the cartilage [111], although evidence for a DMOAD effect in humans with this or any other NSAID is lacking. Tenidap, a nonsteroidal anti-inflammatory drug with cytokine-inhibitory properties, has also been reported to prevent cartilage damage in this model [79]. However, the extent of cartilage damage in that study was unusually severe only 8 weeks after cruciate ligament transection and confirmation of the results is needed. Corticosteroid treatment in relatively high doses, either oral or intra-articular, has been shown to prevent osteophyte formation and to reduce levels of stromelysin in extracts of the articular cartilage [111–113] in the canine cruciate-deficiency model. However, when prednisone was given orally in a lower dose (which, on a weight basis, would have been the equivalent of 5 mg/d for a 70 kg human), no effect on OA pathology was noted [114]. This model [115], and the lapine partial medial meniscectomy model [116], have been used to demonstrate the efficacy of glycosaminoglycan polysulfate acid ester. Co-administration of petosan sulfate and IGF-1 protected against cartilage damage and resulted in a reduction in the levels of MMP and increase in the levels of TIMP within the cartilage [117]. Finally, we have shown that oral doxycycline administration strikingly inhibited joint breakdown in the accelerated canine cruciate-deficiency model (i.e., in which sensory input from the ipsilateral limb was interrupted by L4–5 dorsal root ganglionectomy prior to ligament transection, see above) [84]. This treatment prevented the extensive loss of cartilage seen in this model and dramatically reduced the levels of MMP within the cartilage.

3.2.4
Pitfalls Associated with the Use of Animal Models in the Discovery of DMOADs

Because the etiology of OA is poorly understood, it is impossible to measure how well any animal model, although it may display some features of OA in humans, mimics the disease in humans. It is impossible to determine how closely a therapeutic effect in any animal model will predict therapeutic activity in man. In particular, the importance of inflammation in OA is uncertain. Therefore, use of models in which joint damage is mediated by an inflammatory response could give misleading indications of efficacy. Similar uncertainty concerning the importance of other etiologic factors, such as a systemic increase in bone density, ligamentous laxity, inherited defects in the structure of cartilage collagen and, as indicated above, periarticular muscle weakness.

It should also be noted that, as emphasized by Doherty et al. [4], major differences exist among species with respect to the relative contribution to the pathologic changes of OA of various mediators, receptors or enzymes which could lead to inappropriate extrapolation to humans of therapeutic activity seen in animal models. For example, results in rodent models of inflammatory arthritis, in which NSAID treatment profoundly inhibits disease activity [117], led to *over*estimation of the efficacy of NSAIDs in treatment of arthritis in humans, in whom prostaglandins do not play the same fundamental role in the pathogenesis of the disease as they do in rodents and in whom the clinical benefits of NSAIDs are therefore limited to treatment of symptoms rather than modification of joint damage.

On the other hand, *under*estimation of the therapeutic potential of novel agents on the basis of animal data could lead to the abandonment of potentially useful agents. For example, gold, penicillamine, chloroquine and sulfasalazine, all of which have some efficacy in the treatment of rheumatoid arthritis, are not effective in the animal models routinely employed to screen antirheumatic drugs [118]. Discovery of their efficacy in treatment of patients with rheumatoid arthritis was serendipitous and their mechanisms of action in this disease are unknown. The point is this: excessive reliance on animal models of disease in drug screening could lead researchers to discard novel mechanism-based agents with potential utility in the treatment of arthritis in humans.

A species difference particularly relevant to the development of DMOADs relates to cartilage collagenase, an enzyme widely assumed to contribute importantly to cartilage damage in OA. Although inhibitors of interstitial collagenase (collagenase-1, MMP-1) are frequently evaluated in rodent models [116], a rodent homologue of collagenase-1 has not been identified and probably does not exist. Inhibitors specific for human collagenase-1 would, therefore, not exhibit therapeutic activity in a rodent model of arthritis. Fortunately, however, most MMP inhibitors which have been developed to date do not have great selectivity [120] and will inhibit also the collagenase now shown to be involved in cartilage damage in rodents, collagenase-3 (MMP-13). Furthermore, human collagenase-3 [121], recently shown to be expressed in human osteoarthritic cartilage, may play an important role in human OA [122].

Finally, even assuming that a given mediator, receptor or enzyme plays a role in the pathogenesis of OA in a particular animal model, similar to that it plays in human OA, the ability of a drug to interfere with a molecular target may differ among species [4]: for example, although the chemotactic potency of leukotriene B_4 for human, murine and lapine neutrophils is similar, some antagonists show differences in potency as great as 1,000-fold in some of these species. In the evaluation of a mechanism-based agent, such species-specific differences in potency can be detected and methods can be developed to permit *in vivo* pharmacodynamic studies, for example, by evaluating the effects of compounds which inhibit an exogenously administered human enzyme or mediator. This technique has been used to evaluate MMP inhibitors by determining the ability of drugs to inhibit release of proteoglycans from the articular cartilage after injection of human stromelysin into the lapine knee [123].

Despite the fact that results obtained from animal models of OA may be misleading in the evaluation of potential DMOADs, models have an important role to play in basic research. By examining the pathogenetic mechanisms underlying joint damage in animal models, potential roles in human OA of enzymes, mediators or receptors may be identified. However, evidence of the importance a molecular mechanism of joint damage in an animal model provides no assurance that it is important in man. Perhaps the strongest evidence of the pathogenetic importance of a postulated disease mechanism is the demonstration of a therapeutic effect after pharmacologic interference with that mechanism. Therefore, development of mechanism-based drugs and demonstration of their efficacy in animal models of OA may be integral to our understanding of the pathogenesis of the disease; however, validation of a molecular target in human disease will be obtained only after Phase III clinical trials *in humans*.

References

1. Pritzker KPH (1994) Animal models for osteoarthritis: processes, problems and prospects. Ann Rheum Dis 53: 406–420
2. McAlindon TE, Cooper C, Kirwan JR, Dieppe PA (1993) Determinants of disability in osteoarthritis of the knee. Ann Rheum Dis 52: 258–262
3. Slemenda C, Heilman DK, Brandt KD, Katz BP, Mazzuca S, Braunstein EM, Byrd D Reduced quadriceps strength relative to body weight. A risk factor for knee osteoarthritis in women? Arthritis Rheum. In press
4. Doherty NS, Griffiths RJ, Pettipher ER (1998) The role of animal models in the discovery of novel disease-modifying osteoarthritis drugs (DMOADs). In: Brandt KD, Doherty M, Lohmander LS. Osteoarthritis. Oxford: Oxford University Press pp 439–449
5. Bendele AM (1987) Progressive chronic osteoarthritis in femorotibial joints of partial medial meniscectomized guinea pigs. Vet Pathol 24: 444–448
6. Bendele AM, Hulman JF, Bean JS (1989) Spontaneous osteoarthritis in Hartley albino guinea pigs: effects of dietary and surgical manipulations. Arthritis Rheum 32: S106
7. Das-Gupta EP, Lyons TJ, Hoyland JA, Lawton DM, Freemont AJ (1993) New histological observations in spontaneously developing osteoarthritis in the STR/ORT mouse questioning its acceptability as a model of human osteoarthritis. Int J Exp Pathol 74: 627–634
8. Dunham J, Chambers MG, Jasani MK, Bitensky J, Chayen J (1989) Quantitative criteria for evaluating the early development of osteoarthritis and the effect of diclofenac sodium. Agents Actions 28: 1–2
9. Dunham J, Chambers MG, Jasani MK, Bitensky L, Chayen J (1990) Changes in the orientation of proteoglycans during the early development of natural murine osteoarthritis. J Orthop Res 8: 101–104
10. Okabe T (1989) Experimental studies on the spontaneous osteoarthritis in C57 black mice. J Tokyo Med Coll 47: 546–557
11. Stanescu R, Knyszynski A, Muriel MP, Stanescu V (1993) Early lesions of the articular surface in a strain of mice with very high incidence of spontaneous osteoarthritis-like lesions. J Rheumatol 20: 102–110
12. Takahama A (1990) Histological study on spontaneous osteoarthritis of the knee in C57 black mouse. J Jpn Orthop Assoc 64: 271–281
13. van der Kraan PM, Vitters EL, van Beuningen HM, van de Putte LB, van den Berg WB (1990) Degenerative knee joint lesions in mice after a single intra-articular collagenase injection. A new model of osteoarthritis. J Exp Pathol 71: 19–31

14. Garofalo S, Vuorio E, Metsaranta M, Rosati R, Toman D, Vaughan J, et al. (1991) Reduced amounts of cartilage collagen fibrils and growth plate anomalies in transgenic mice harboring a glycine-to-cysteine mutation in the mouse type II procollagen α_1-chain gene. Proc Natl Acad Sci (USA) 88 : 9648 – 9652

15. Nakata K, Ono K, Miyazaki J-I, Olsen B, Muragaki Y, Adachi E, et al. (1993) Osteoarthritis associated with mild chondrodysplasia in transgenic mice expressing α_1(IX) collagen chains with a central deletion. Proc Natl Acad Sci (USA) 90 : 2870–2874

16. Alexander JW (1992) The pathogenesis of canine hip dysplasia. Vet Clin North America: Small Animal Practice 22 : 503–511

17. Smale G, Bendele AM, Horton WE (1995) Comparison of age-associated degeneration of articular cartilage in Wistar and Fischer 344 rats. Lab Anim Sci 45 : 191 – 194

18. Alexander CJ (1994) Utilisation of joint movement range in arboreal primates compared with human subjects: an evolutionary frame for primary osteoarthritis. Ann Rheum Dis 53 : 720 – 725

19. Carlson CS, Loeser RF, Jayo MJ, Weaver DS, Adams MR, Jerome CP (1994) Osteoarthritis in Cynomolgus macaques: a primate model of naturally occurring disease. J Orthop Res 12 : 331 – 339

20. Châteauvert JM, Grynpas MD, Kessler MJ, Pritzker KP (1990) Spontaneous osteoarthritis in rhesus macaques. II. Characterization of disease and morphometric studies. J Rheumatol 17 : 73 – 83

21. Kalbhen DA (1987) Chemical model of osteoarthritis – a pharmacological evaluation. J Rheumatol 130 : 130 – 131

22. Marcelon G, Cros J, Guiraud R (1976) Activity of anti-inflammatory drugs on an experimental model of osteoarthritis. Agents Actions 6 : 191 – 194

23. Coulais Y, Marcelon G, Cros J, Guiraud R (1983) Studies on an experimental model for osteoarthritis. I. Induction and ultrastructural investigation. Pathol Biol 31 : 577 – 582

24. Coulais Y, Marcelon G, Cros J, Guiraud R (1984) An experimental model of osteoarthritis. II. – Biochemical study of collagen and proteoglycans. Pathol Biol 32 : 23 – 28

25. Leipold HR, Goldberg RL, Lust G (1989) Canine serum keratan sulfate and hyaluronate concentrations. Relationship to age and osteoarthritis. Arthritis Rheum 32 : 312 – 321

26. Tanaka H, Kitoh Y, Katsuramaki T, Tanaka M, Kitabayashi N, Fujimori S, et al. (1992) Effects of SL-1010 (sodium hyaluronate with high molecular weight) on experimental osteoarthritis induced by intra-articularly applied papain in guinea pigs. Folia Pharmacol Jpn 100 : 77 – 86

27. van der Kraan PM, Vitters EL, van den Berg WB (1989) Development of osteoarthritis models in mice by "mechanical" and "metabolical" alterations in the knee joints. Arthritis Rheum 32: S107

28. van den Berg WB (1995) Growth factors in experimental osteoarthritis: transforming growth factor beta pathogenic? J Rheumatol 43 (Suppl): 143 – 145

29. Vasilev V, Merker HJ, Vidinov N (1992) Ultrastructural changes in the synovial membrane in experimentally-induced osteoarthritis of rabbit knee joint. Histol Histopathol 7 : 119 – 127

30. Marshall JL, Olsson S-E (1971) Instability of the knee: a long-term experimental study in dogs. J Bone Joint Surg 53 A: 1561 – 1570

31. Pond MJ, Nuki G (1973) Experimentally-induced osteoarthritis in the dog. Ann Rheum Dis 32 : 387 – 388

32. Brandt KD (1994) Insights into the natural history of osteoarthritis provided by the cruciate-deficient dog: An animal model of osteoarthritis. Ann NY Acad Sci 732 : 199 – 205

33. Marshall KW, Chan AD (1996) Bilateral canine model of osteoarthritis. J Rheumatol 23 : 344 – 350

34. Christensen SB (1983) Localization of bone-seeking agents in developing experimentally induced osteoarthritis in the knee joint of the rabbit. Scand J Rheumatol 12 : 343 – 349

35. Vignon E, Mathieu P, Bejui J, Descotes J, Hartmann D, Patricot LM, et al. (1991) Study of an inhibitor of plasminogen activator (tranexamic acid) in the treatment of experimental osteoarthritis. J Rheumatol 27 (Suppl): 131–133

36. Ghosh P, Armstrong S, Read R, Numata Y, Smith S, McNair P, et al. (1993) Animal models of early osteoarthritis: their use for the evaluation of potential chondroprotective agents. Agents Actions 39 (Suppl): 195–206

37. Fam AG, Morava-Protzner I, Purcell C, Young BD, Bunting PS, Lewis AJ (1995) Acceleration of experimental lapine osteoarthritis by calcium pyrophosphate microcrystalline synovitis. Arthritis Rheum 38 : 201–210

38. Moskowitz RW, Goldberg VM (1987) Studies of osteophyte pathogenesis in experimentally induced osteoarthritis. J Rheumatol 14 : 311–320

39. Ehrlich MG, Mankin HJ, Jones H, Grossman A, Crispen C, Ancona D (1975) Biochemical confirmation of an experimental osteoarthritis model. J Bone Joint Surg [Am] 57 : 392–396

40. Arsever CL, Bole GG (1986) Experimental osteoarthritis induced by selective myectomy and tendotomy. Arthritis Rheum 29 : 251–261

41. Layton MW, Arsever C, Bole GG (1987) Use of the guinea pig myectomy osteoarthritis model in the examination of cartilage-synovium interactions. J Rheumatol 125 : 125–126

42. Dedrick DK, Goulet R, Huston L, Goldstein SA, Bole GG (1991) Early bone changes in experimental osteoarthritis using microscopic computed tomography. J Rheumatol 27 (Suppl): 44–45

43. Oegema TRJ, Lewis JLJ, Thompson RCJ (1993) Role of acute trauma in development of osteoarthritis. Agents Actions 40 : 3–4

44. Mazieres B, Maheu E, Thiechart M, Vallieres G (1990) Effects of N-acetyl hydroxyproline (oxaceprol (R)) on an experimental post-contusive model of osteoarthritis. A pathological study. J Drug Dev 3 : 135–142

45. Langenskiold A, Michelsson JE, Videman T (1979) Osteoarthritis of the knee in the rabbit produced by immobilization. Attempts to achieve a reproducible model for studies on pathogenesis and therapy. Acta Orthop Scand 50 : 1–14

46. Videman T (1982) Experimental osteoarthritis in the rabbit: comparison of different periods of repeated immobilization. Acta Orthop Scand 53 : 339–347

47. Howell DS, Muller F, Manicourt DH (1992) A mini review: proteoglycan aggregate profiles in the Pond-Nuki dog model of osteoarthritis and in canine disuse atrophy. Br J Rheumatol 31 : 7–11

48. Ratcliffe A, Beauvais PJ, Saed-Nejad F (1994) Differential levels of synovial fluid aggrecan aggregate components in experimental osteoarthritis and joint disuse. J Orthop Res 12 : 464–473

49. Palmoski M, Brandt K (1981) Running inhibits the reversal of atrophic changes in canine knee cartilage after removal of a leg cast. Arthritis Rheum 24 : 1329–1337

50. Vilensky JA, O'Connor BL, Brandt KD, Dunn EA, Rogers PI (1994) Serial kinematic analysis of the canine knee after L4-S1 dorsal root ganglionectomy: implications for the cruciate deficiency model of osteoarthritis. J Rheumatol 21 : 2113–2117

51. Lequesne M, Brandt K, Bellamy N, Moskowitz R, Menkes CJ, Pelletier JP, Altman RD (1994) Guidelines for testing slow-acting and disease-modifying drugs in osteoarthritis. J Rheumatol 21 (Suppl 41): 65–71

52. Billingham MEJ (1998) Advantages afforded by the use of animal models for evaluation of potential disease-modifying osteoarthritis drugs (DMOADs). In: Brandt KD, Doherty M, Lohmander LS, editors. Osteoarthritis. Oxford: Oxford University Press pp 429–438

53. Sokoloff L (1956) Natural history of degenerative joint disease in small laboratory animals. 1. Pathological anatomy of degenerative joint disease in mice. Arch Pathol 62 : 118–128

54. Evans RG, Collins C, Miller P, Ponsford PM, Elson CJ (1994) Radiological scoring of osteoarthritis progression in STR/ORT mice. Osteoarthritis Cart 2 : 103–109

55. Collins C, Evans RG, Ponsford F, Miller P, Elson CJ (1994) Chondro-osseous metaplasia, bone density and patella cartilage proteoglycan content in the osteoarthritis of STR/ORT mice. Osteoarthritis Cart 2 : 111 – 118

56. Bendele AM, Hulman JF (1988) Spontaneous cartilage degeneration in guinea pigs. Arthritis Rheum 31 : 561 – 565

57. Bendele AM, White SL, Hulman JF (1989) Osteoarthritis in guinea pigs: histopathologic and scanning electron microscopic features. Lab Anim Sci 39 : 115 – 121

58. Meacock SCR, Bodmer JL, Billingham MEJ (1990) Experimental osteoarthritis in guinea pigs. J Exp Path 71 : 279 – 293

59. Bendele AM, Hulman JF (1991) Effects of body weight restriction on the development and progression of spontaneous osteoarthritis in guinea pigs. Arthritis Rheum 34 : 1180 – 1184

60. Watson PJ, Carpenter TA, Hall LD, Tyler JA (1994) Spontaneous joint degeneration in the guinea pig studied by magnetic resonance imaging. Br J Rheumatol 33 (Suppl 1): 105

61. Bendele AM, Bendele RA, Hulman JF, Swann BP (1996) Effets bénéfiques d'un traitement à la diacérhéine chez des cobayes atteints d'arthrose. Revue du Praticien 46 : 35 – 39

62. DeRousseau CJ (1985) Aging in the musculoskeletal system of rhesus monkeys. II. Degenerative joint disease. Am J Phys Anthropol 67 : 177 – 184

63. Kessler MJ, Turnquist JE, Pritzker KPH, London WT (1986) Reduction of passive extension and radiographic evidence of degenerative knee joint disease in cage-raised and free-ranging aged rhesus monkeys (Maccaca mulatta). J Med Primato 15 : 1 – 9

64. Pritzker KPH, Chateauvert J, Grynpas MD, Renlund RC, Turnquist J, Kessler MJ (1989) Rhesus macaques as an experimental model for degenerative arthritis. PR Health Sci J 8 : 99 – 102

65. Carlson CS, Loeser RF, Johnstone B, Tulli HM, Dodson DB, Caterson B (1995) Osteoarthritis in Cynomolgus macaques. II. Detection of modulated proteoglycan epitopes in cartilage and synovial fluid. J Orthop Res 13 : 399 – 409

66. Carlson CS, Loeser RF, Purser CB, Gardin JF, Jerome CP (1996) Osteoarthritis in Cynomolgus macaques. III. Effects of age, gender, and subchondral bone thickness on the severity of disease. J Bone Miner Res 11 : 1209 – 1217

67. Felson DT (1998) Epidemiology of osteoarthritis. In: Brandt KD, Doherty M, Lohmander LS (eds) Osteoarthritis. Oxford: Oxford University Press pp 13 – 22

68. Moskowitz RW (1992) Experimental models of osteoarthritis. In: Moskowitz RW, Howell DS, Goldberg VM. Osteoarthritis: Diagnosis and Medical/Surgical Management. Philadelphia, PA: W.B. Saunders pp 213 – 232

69. Bendele AM, White SL (1987) Early histopathologic and ultrastructural alterations in femorotibial joints of partial medial meniscectomised guinea pigs. Vet Pathol 24 : 436 – 443

70. Brandt KD, Braunstein EM, Visco DM, O'Connor B, Heck D, Albrecht M (1991) Anterior (cranial) cruciate ligament transection in the dog: a bona fide model of canine osteoarthritis, not merely of cartilage injury and repair. J Rheumatol 18 : 436 – 446

71. Adams ME, Brandt KD (1991) Hypertrophic repair of canine articular cartilage in osteoarthritis after anterior cruciate ligament transection. J Rheumatol 18 : 428 – 435

72. McDevitt C, Gilbertson E, Muir H (1977) An experimental model of osteoarthritis: early morphological and biochemical changes. J Bone Joint Surg 59 B : 24 – 35

73. McDevitt CA, Muir H, Pond MJ (1973) Canine articular cartilage in natural and experimentally induced osteoarthrosis. Biochem Soc Trans 1 : 287 – 289

74. Braunstein EM, Brandt KD, Albrecht M (1990) MRI demonstration of hypertrophic articular cartilage repair in osteoarthritis. Skeletal Radiol 19 : 335 – 339

75. Bywaters EGL (1937) Metabolism of joint tissues. J Pathol Bacteriol 44 : 247 – 268

76. Johnson LC (1959) Kinetics of osteoarthritis. Lab Invest 8 : 1223 – 1241

77. Vignon E, Arlot M, Hartmann D, Moyen B, Ville G (1983) Hypertrophic repair of articular cartilage in experimental osteoarthrosis. Ann Rheum Dis 42 : 82 – 88

78. Châteauvert J, Pritzker KP, Kessler MJ, Grynpas MD (1989) Spontaneous osteoarthritis in rhesus macaques: I. Chemical and biochemical studies. J Rheumatol 16 : 1098 – 1104

79. Fernandes JC, Martel-Pelletier J, Otterness LG, Lopez Anaya A, Mineau F, Tardiff G et al. (1995) Effects of tenidap on canine experimental osteoarthritis. I. Morphologic and metalloprotease analysis. Arthritis Rheum 38 : 1290 – 1303

80. Manolopoulos V, Mancer K, Marshall KW (1998) Amelioration of disease severity by intra-articular hyalan therapy in bilateral canine osteoarthritis. Trans Orthop Res Soc 23 : 291

81. Brandt KD, Schauwecker DS, Dansereau S, Meyer J, O'Connor BL (1997) Bone scintigraphy in the canine cruciate-deficiency model of osteoarthritis. Comparison of the unstable and contralateral knee. J Rheumatol 24 : 140 – 145

82. O'Connor BL, Visco DM, Brandt KD, Myers SL, Kalasinski L (1992) Neurogenic acceleration of osteoarthritis: The effects of prior articular nerve neurectomy on the development of osteoarthritis after anterior cruciate ligament transection in the dog. J Bone Jt Surg 74 A: 367 – 376

83. O'Connor BL, Palmoski MJ, Brandt KD (1985) Neurogenic acceleration of degenerative joint lesions. J Bone Joint Surg 67 A: 562 – 572

84. Yu LP, Smith Jr GN, Brandt KD, Myers SL, O'Connor BL, Brandt DA (1992) Reduction of the severity of canine osteoarthritis by prophylactic treatment with oral doxycycline. Arthritis Rheum 35 : 1150 – 1159

85. Dedrick DK, Goldstein SA, Brandt KD, O'Connor BL, Goulet RW, Albrecht M (1993) A longitudinal study of subchondral plate and trabecular bone in cruciate-deficient dogs with osteoarthritis followed for up to 54 months. Arthritis Rheum 36 : 1460 – 1467

86. Brandt KD, Smith G, Kang SY, Myers S, O'Connor B, Albrecht M (1997) Effects of diacerhein in an accelerated canine model of osteoarthritis. Osteoarthritis Cart 5 : 438 – 449

87. Smith GN Jr, Myers SL, Brandt KD, Mickler EA, Albrecht ME Diacerhein treatment reduces the severity of osteoarthritis in the canine cruciate-deficiency model of osteoarthritis. Arthritis Rheum. In press

88. Palmoski M, Perricone E, Brandt KD (1979) Development and reversal of a proteoglycan aggregation defect in normal canine knee cartilage after immobilization. Arthritis Rheum 22 : 508 – 517

89. Palmoski MJ, Brandt KD (1982) Immobilization of the knee prevents osteoarthritis after anterior cruciate ligament transection. Arthritis Rheum 25 : 1201 – 1208

90. Palmoski MJ, Colyer RA, Brandt KD (1980) Joint motion in the absence of normal loading does not maintain normal articular cartilage. Arthritis Rheum 123 : 325 – 334

91. Slemenda C, Brandt KD, Heilman DK, Mazzuca S, Braunstein EM, Katz BP, Wilinsky FD (1997) Quadriceps weakness and osteoarthritis of the knee. Ann Int Med 127 : 97 – 104

92. Slemenda C, Heilman DK, Brandt KD, Katz BP, Mazzuca S, Braunstein EM, Byrd D (1998) Reduced quadriceps strength relative to body weight. A risk factor for knee osteoarthritis in women? Arthritis Rheum. In press

93. Johansson H, Sjölander P, Sojka P (1991) A sensory role for the cruciate ligaments. Clin Orthop 268 : 161 – 178

94. Jefferson RJ, Collins JJ, Whittle MW, Radin EL, O'Connor JJ (1990) The role of the quadriceps in controlling impulsive forces around heel strike. Proc Inst Mech Eng [H] 204 : 21 – 28

95. Radin EL, Yang KH, Riegger C, Kish VL, O'Connor JJ (1991) Relationship between lower limb dynamics and knee joint pain. J Orthop Res 9 : 398 – 405

96. Radin EL, Boyd RD, Martin RB, Burr DB, Caterson B, Goodwin C (1985) Mechanical factors influencing cartilage damage. In: Peyron JG (ed) Osteoarthritis: Current Clinical and Fundamental Problems. Paris: Geigy pp 90 – 99

97. Hill AV (1960) Production and absorption of work by muscle. Science 131 : 897

98. Radin EL, Paul IL (1970) Does cartilage compliance reduce skeletal impact loads? The relative force attenuating properties of articular cartilage, synovial fluid, periarticular soft-tissue and bone. Arthritis Rheum 13 : 139

99. O'Connor B, Brandt KD (1993) Neurogenic factors in the etiopathogenesis of osteoarthritis. In: Moskowitz RW (ed) Rheumatic Disease Clinics of North America. Philadelphia: WB Saunders Co. pp 450 – 468

100. Skinner HB, Wyatt MP, Hodgdon JA, Conard DW, Barrack RL (1986) Effect of fatigue on joint position sense of the knee. J Orthop Res 4:112–118
101. Davis MA, Ettinger WH, Neuhaus JM, Cho SA, Hauck WW (1989) The association of knee injury and obesity with unilateral and bilateral osteoarthritis of the knee. Am J Epidemiol 130:278–288
102. Martin K, Lethbridge-Cejku, Muller DC, Elahi D, Andres R, Tobin JD et al. (1995) Metabolic correlates of obesity and radiographic features of knee osteoarthritis: data from the Baltimore longitudinal study of aging. J Rheumatol 24:702–707
103. Dedrick DK, Goldstein SA, Brandt KD, O'Connor BL, Goulet RW, Albrecht M (1993) A longitudinal study of subchondral plate and trabecular bone in cruciate-deficient dogs with osteoarthritis followed up for 54 months. Arthritis Rheum 36:1460–1467
104. Visco DM, Hill MA, Widmer WR, Johnstone B, Myers SL (1996) Experimental osteoarthritis in dogs: a comparison of the Pond-Nuki and medial arthrotomy methods. Osteoarthritis Cart 4:9–22
105. O'Connor BL, Visco DM, Heck DA, Myers SL, Brandt KD (1989) Gait alterations in dogs after transection of the anterior cruciate ligament. Arthritis Rheum 32:1142–1147
106. Myers SL, Brandt KD, O'Connor BL, Visco DM, Albrecht ME (1990) Synovitis and osteoarthritic changes in canine articular cartilage after cruciate ligament transection. Effect of surgical hemostasis. Arthritis Rheum 33:1406–1415
107. Brown TD, Radin EL, Martin RB, Burr DB (1984) Finite element studies of some juxtaarticular stress changes due to localized subchondral stiffening. J Biomech 17:11–24
108. Myers SL, Brandt KD, Schauwecker DS, Burr DB, O'Connor BL, Albrecht M Effects of a bisphosphonate on bone histomorphometry and dynamics in the canine cruciate-deficiency model of osteoarthritis. Submitted for publication
109. Rodan GA, Fleisch HA (1996) Bisphosphonates: mechanisms of action. J Clin Invest 97:2692–2696
110. Lin JH (1996) Bisphosphonates: a review of their pharmacokinetic properties. Bone 18:75–85
111. Pelletier JP, Martel-Pelletier J (1991) In vivo protective effects of prophylactic treatment with tiaprofenic acid or intraarticular corticosteroids on osteoarthritic lesions in the experimental dog model. J Rheumatol 27 (Suppl): 127–130
112. Pelletier JP, Martel-Pelletier J (1989) Protective effects of corticosteroids on cartilage lesions and osteophyte formation in the Pond-Nuki dog model of osteoarthritis. Arthritis Rheum 32:181–193
113. Pelletier JP, Mineau F, Raynauld JP (1994) Intraarticular injections with methylprednisolone acetate reduce osteoarthritic lesions in parallel with chondrocyte stromelysin synthesis in experimental osteoarthritis. Arthritis Rheum 37:414–423
114. Myers SL, Brandt KD, O'Connor BL (1991) "Low-dose" prednisone treatment does not reduce the severity of osteoarthritis in dogs after anterior cruciate ligament transection. J Rheumatol 18:1856–1862
115. Altman RD, Dean DD, Muniz OE, Howell DS (1989) Therapeutic treatment of canine osteoarthritis with glycosaminoglycan polysulfuric acid ester. Arthritis Rheum 32:1300–1307
116. Howell DS, Carreno MR, Pelletier JP, Muniz OE (1986) Articular cartilage breakdown in a lapine model of osteoarthritis: action of glycosaminoglycan polysulfate ester (GAGPS) on proteoglycan degrading enzyme activity, hexuronate and cell counts. Clin Orthop 21:69–76
117. Rogachevsky RA, Dean DD, Howell DS, Altman RD (1994) Treatment of canine osteoarthritis with insulin-like growth factor (IGF1) and sodium pentosan polysulfate. Ann N Y Acad Sci 732:392–394
118. Zhang J, Weichman BM, Lewis AJ (1995) Role of animal models in the study of rheumatoid arthritis: An overview. In: Henderson B, Edwards JCW, Pettipher ERP (eds) Mechanisms and models in rheumatoid arthritis. New York: Academic Press pp 363–372
119. Karran EH, Young TJ, Markwell RE, Harper GP (1995) In vivo model of cartilage degradation – effects of a matrix metalloproteinase inhibitor. Ann Rheum Dis 54:662–669

120. Beeley NRA, Ansell PRJ, Docherty AJP (1994) Inhibitors of matrix metalloproteinases (MMPs). Curr Opin Ther Patents 4:7–16
121. Freije JMP, Diez-Itza I, Balbib M, Snachez LM, Blasco R, Tolivia J et al. (1994) Molecular cloning and expression of collagenase-3, a novel human matrix metalloproteinase produced by breast carcinomas. J Biol Chem 269:16766–16773
122. Mitchell PG, Magna HA, Reeves LM, Lopresti-Morrow LL, Yocum SA, Rosner PJ et al. (1996) Cloning of matrix metalloproteinase-13 (MMP-1, collagenase-3) from human chondrocytes, expression of MMP-13 by osteoarthritic cartilage and activity of the enzyme on type II collagen. J Clin Invest 97:761–768
123. Ganu V, Parker D, MacPherson L, Hu S-I, Goldberg R, Raychaudhuri A et al. (1994) Biochemical and pharmacological profile of a non-peptidic orally active inhibitor of matrix metalloproteinases. Osteoarthritis Cart 2 (Suppl 1): 34

CHAPTER 4

Pathophysiology of Osteoarthritis

4.1
Role of Mechanical Factors in the Aetiology, Pathogenesis and Progression of Osteoarthritis

G. NUKI

Motion and mechanical stimulation play a critical role in the development of the skeleton and normal joints [1, 2]. Movement, loading and intermittent mechanical strain are also crucial for the maintenance of healthy articular cartilage, [3], bone mineral [4] and muscle [5]. Paradoxically mechanical factors also play an important role in the development and progression of osteoarthritis.

4.1.1
Definition and Classification

Osteoarthritis (OA) is currently defined as *"a group of overlapping distinct diseases, which have different aetiologies but with similar biological, morphologic and clinical outcomes. The disease processes not only affect the articular cartilage, but involve the entire joint, including the subchondral bone, ligaments, capsule, synovial membrane and periarticular muscles. Ultimately, the articular cartilage degenerates with fibrillation, fissures, ulceration and full thickness loss of the joint surface"* [6]. This long, clumsy and rather wide ranging definition does at least emphasise that OA is not a single disease, or process, but rather the clinical and pathological outcome of a variety of disorders that lead to structural and functional failure of one or more synovial joints [7, 8].

Current concepts [9] emphasise the dynamic nature of the OA process which is characterized by new bone formation, increased turnover of cartilage matrix components and joint remodelling as well as by degeneration of articular tissues.

Osteoarthritis is usually classified as *primary* (*idiopathic*) or *secondary* when it follows some clearly defined predisposing disorder [10]. An abbreviated classification, [11], based on recommendations of an osteoarthritis sub-committee of the American College of Rheumatology is shown in Table 1. Although distinct from the more common type of idiopathic OA, many of the rarer subsets of secondary osteoarthritis are good examples of *accidents of nature* which can

Table 1. Classification: subsets of osteoarthritis [11]

Primary (idiopathic)	Secondary

Localized
  Hands and feet
  Knee
  Hip
  Spine
  Other
	Post traumatic
	Congenital/developmental
	  Localised
	    Hip diseases, e.g., Perthes
	    Mechanical and local factors, e.g., obesity,
	    hypermobility, valgus/varus

Generalized
3 or more joint areas
	Generalised
	  Bone dysplasias
	  Metabolic diseases
	Calcium deposition diseases
	  Calcium pyrophosphate deposition disease
	  Hydroxyapatite arthropathy
	  Destructive arthropathies

	Other bone and joint disorders
	  Avascular necrosis
	  Rheumatoid arthritis
	  Paget's disease

	Miscellaneous other diseases Endocrine, e.g., acromegaly, neuropathic

serve as models for understanding some of the pathological mechanisms that can lead to joint failure. Mechanical factors play a role in all types of primary, as well as secondary, OA. Joint failure results from an imbalance between the combination of mechanical stresses and catabolic processes acting on the joint and the capacity of its tissues to withstand the strains and repair the damage. In broad terms structural failure of articular cartilage and bone either result from abnormal mechanical stresses causing damage to normal tissues, or failure of pathologically impaired articular cartilage and bone under the influence of physiologically normal mechanical strains (Fig. 1).

Post traumatic OA, the OA that complicates Paget's disease, Perthes disease, congenital dislocation of the hip, slipped capital epiphyses or any one of a number of skeletal dysplasias are examples of secondary OA that can result from the generation of abnormal mechanical stresses which cause injury to initially normal articular cartilage. In contrast, the premature osteoarthritis that is associated with acromegaly, crystal deposition diseases and metabolic disorders such as haemochromatosis or ochronosis are examples of secondary OA in which the articular cartilage is impaired by the primary pathological process and cartilage degeneration and joint failure then progress even under the influence of physiologically normal mechanical stresses.

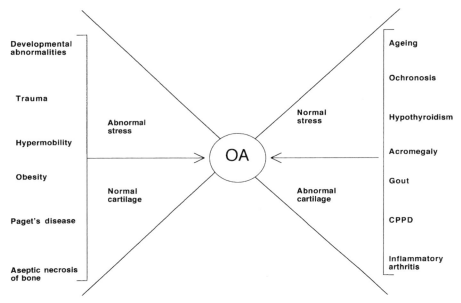

Fig. 1. Pathways leading to secondary osteoarthritis

4.1.2
Risk Factors

It is likely that in the majority of patients with *primary, idiopathic* and *secondary* OA, multiple genetic and environmental factors are contributing to the pathogenesis and progression of joint failure. The importance of ageing and as yet undefined genetic factors, as contributory *risk factors* is well illustrated in patients who develop osteoarthritis of the knee after meniscectomy – an apparently straightforward example of mechanically determined secondary OA. Although overall about 70% of patients develop radiological evidence of knee OA 20 years after meniscectomy there is evidence that post-meniscectomy OA may occur more frequently in patients with primary hand OA [12] and more rapidly in older patients [13].

4.1.2.1
Ageing

The prevalence and incidence of osteoarthritis of the hands, hip and knee increase dramatically in men and women between the ages of 50 and 80 years [14] but the basis for this is far from clear. Age-related changes in articular cartilage matrix chemistry and structure are distinct from those that are seen in osteoarthritis and mechanically induced experimental osteoarthritis [15] (Table 2). Ageing cartilage is characterised by a progressive increase in keratan sulphate and a decrease in chondroitin sulphate without significant change in the total

Table 2. Structural and biochemical changes in ageing articular cartilage, osteoarthritis and mechanically induced experimental osteoarthritis compared

	Ageing	OA/Experimental OA
Cartilage thickness	Decreased	Initially increased, later decreased
Tensile modulus	Slighty decreased	Greatly decreased
Collagen fibre network	Largely intact	Grossly disrupted
Collagen fibrillogenesis	Decreased	Decreased
Collagen synthesis	Unchanged	Increased
Total sulphated glycosaminoglycans	Unchanged	Initially increased, later decreased
Proteoglycan synthesis	Decreased	Increased
Keratan sulphate	Increased	Decreased
Chondroitin sulphate	Decreased	Initally increased, later decreased
Low molecular weight proteoglycans	Increased	Increased
Aggrecan size	Decreased	Decreased
Water content	Decreased	Increased
Hyaluronan content	Increased	Increased
Hyaluronan size	Decreased	Unchanged
Chondroitin sulphate neoepitopes	Not expressed	Re-expressed
Cartilage oligomeric protein	Unchanged	Increased

tissue content of sulphated glycosaminoglycans [15] The average size of the proteoglycan aggregates decreases in older cartilage, as does the water content, and there are increased amounts of proteolytically cleaved link protein, biglycan [16] and hyaluronan of shorter chain length [17]. The decreases in tensile stiffness and fracture stress of articular cartilage that occur with ageing [18, 19] are, however, more likely to be related to thinning, loss of packing and increased cross-linking of collagen fibrils [20, 21].

Age-related decreases in the capacity of chondrocytes to synthesize normal matrix proteins and age-related decline in muscle strength, capsular collagen and joint proprioception may also have an influence on mechanical stresses in ageing joints.

4.1.2.2
Hypermobility

Evidence that constitutional hypermobility might be an important risk factor for the development of generalised osteoarthritis remains sparse [22–24] and unconvincing as premature osteoarthritis is not a feature of many inherited disorders of connective tissue which are associated with striking hypermobility [25]. Recent studies have however suggested that prominent osteoarthritis of the carpometacarpal joints of the thumbs constitutes a localised clinical and radiological subset of hand OA which is associated with constitutional hyper-mobility [26].

4.1.2.3
Direct Trauma and Sporting Injury

In addition to meniscus injuries and other intra-articular derangements, osteochondral injuries, post-traumatic incongruities of articular surfaces and malaligned fractures are important causes of premature, localised osteoarthritis [27]. The relative risk of developing knee OA is increased more than threefold following major knee injuries [28] and the average time to develop secondary OA of the hip, severe enough to warrant arthoplasty, following fracture-dislocation is seven years [29]. Cruciate ligament deficiency leads to premature knee OA in orthopaedic practice [30] as well as in canine veterinary practice [31] and in experimentally induced OA in the stifle joints of dogs [32]. The high prevalence of knee OA in former soccer players [33, 34] and American football players [35] has been largely attributed to the high incidence of meniscectomy and cruciate ligament injuries in these professional athletes. Although there is some data to suggest that long-distance running may be associated with an increase in radiographic OA of the knee [36] and hip [37] other controlled studies found no increase in hip OA in marathon runners after 20 years [38] and little increase in knee OA in top level long-distance runners [39]. A retrospective cohort study of former elite women runners and tennis players showed a two- to threefold increase in radiographic OA, but this was predominantly the development of osteophytes [40]. A recent review of sports related osteoarthritis has analysed the methodological problems that beset many of the reported clinical studies and emphasized that radiographic osteophyte formation in former athletes may not correlate with articular cartilage loss [41]. These authors also suggest that joint dysplasia, muscle weakness, neurological deficits and increased weight may be additional risk factors for the development of OA in athletes.

4.1.2.4
Occupational Risks

Repetitive mechanical stress, particularly in occupations that involve regular knee bending and the lifting of heavy loads is associated with the development of knee OA [42]. Industrial surveys in Scotland in the 1960's showed that osteoarthritis of the elbows, knees and spine were significant clinical problems in miners working at the coal face [43] and subsequent studies in dockyard workers [44] confirmed that the risk of knee OA was increased in occupations involving heavy manual labour. More recent epidemiological studies have identified occupational risks for the development of OA in the hips and knees in farmers, firefighters and construction workers [45].

Farming is associated with a particularly high risk of developing OA of the hip. Croft's case-control studies suggested that farmers were ten times more likely to develop radiographic signs of hip OA after farming for ten years than controls employed in sedentary occupations [46].

Data from the US national health and nutritional examination survey (NHANES-1) showed a threefold increase in radiographic OA of the knee in people undertaking heavy work that involved bending of the knees [47] and the role of occupations involving knee bending was confirmed by data from the Framingham Study [48].

Lawrence's classical studies [49] showing an increase in hand OA in cotton mill workers in Lancashire, were followed by a detailed study of job related activities in 3 groups of workers in a Virginia textile mill [50]. Hadler demonstrated that women whose jobs involved using a pinch grip which was associated with increased stress through the distal interphalangeal joints had more OA in the DIP joints than women whose jobs involved using a power grip which did not stress the DIP joints [50].

4.1.2.5
Body Weight

After many years of uncertainty, conflicting data and opinion, evidence is now accumulating to show that obesity is definitely associated with a significant increase in risk of developing knee OA; and possibly with an increase in risk for hip and hand OA as well [51].

Cross sectional data from the US health and nutrition examination survey showed that men and women with a body mass index of 30–35 had an approximately fourfold increase in knee OA compared with normal weight controls [47]. Excess weight is associated with OA in both the patellofemoral and tibiofemoral compartments of the knee [52, 53], and twin studies from St Thomas' Hospital in London also showed a small but statistically significant increase in risk for the development of hand OA in the CMC joints of the thumbs [53].

The data from the Framingham study shows that obesity precedes the development of knee OA with a 40% increase in risk (odds ratio 1.4; CI 1.1–1.8) for every 10 lb (5 kg) gain in weight [54]. In this study, where changes in weight and radiographic status were recorded over an eight year period, there were also commensurate decreases in incident knee OA for every 10 lb (5 Kg) weight lost, suggesting that obesity is a *modifiable* risk factor, and that even modest reductions in weight, in overweight individuals might slow the progression of disease.

Although the relationships between weight and knee OA are likely to be attributable to mechanical strains the associations with hand OA require some alternative explanation. The fact that the relationship between obesity and OA is stronger in women than in men has suggested the possibility of an unidentified endocrine factor. Alternatively the increase in bone mineral density which occurs in obese people could itself be a risk factor for OA [55].

4.1.3
Subchondral Bone and Bone Mineral Density

The biomechanical properties of the cortical and subchondral bone are key to the protection of articular cartilage from damage following impact loading.

Table 3.
Force attenuation in joints
[56]

Tissue	Attenuation (%)
Subchondral bone	30
Cortical bone	30–35
Articular cartilage	1–3
Joint capsule/synovium	35
Synovial fluid	0

Cortical and subchondral bone are far more effective than articular cartilage in attenuating force through joints and synovial fluid plays no significant role [56] (Table 3). The presence of subchondral bone limits the radial deformation of articular cartilage under load [57] and the undulating structure of the tidemark and osteochondral junction help to transform shear stresses into potentially less damaging tensile and compressive stresses in the articular cartilage [58]. Radin [59] has suggested that the process of OA is initiated by an increase in stiffness and density in subchondral bone following microfractures caused by impulsive loading of joints. It is suggested that loss of viscoelasticity of the bone results in steep stiffness gradients, stretching of the overlying articular cartilage and induction of cartilage fibrillation [59]. Progression to full thickness cartilage loss would depend on continued impulsive loading of the stiffened subchondral bone plate, but finite element mathematical models [60] suggest that such a mechanism could not generate sufficient mechanical strains in the articular cartilage to cause progressive cartilage loss. There is no doubt however that the development of subchondral bone sclerosis in osteoarthritic joints is associated with loss of shock absorbing capacity of the bone. OA knees only absorb half the load absorbed by normal joints [61].

Indirect support for Radin's hypothesis that OA is initiated by changes in bone stiffness comes from studies of the relationship between osteoporosis and osteoarthritis. Following the observation that severe OA changes were seldom observed on femoral heads removed after femoral neck fractures Byers showed that bone mineral density was increased in patients with hip OA [62]. There is some evidence to suggest that reduced bone mineral density may protect women from developing severe osteoarthritis [63], and that the presence of OA may retard the development of osteoporosis [64]. Dequeker's suggestion that OA and osteoporosis tend to be mutually exclusive [63] was supported to some extent by an epidemiological study which showed that less than 1% of a population had coexistent osteoporosis and OA of the hip [65].

4.1.4
Developmental Abnormalities

Abnormal joint loading secondary to alterations in the geometry of joints leads to secondary OA in patients with a wide range of developmental abnormalities and gene mutations.

Slipped capital femoral epiphyses, congenital dislocations of the hip and Perthe's disease are three examples of *localised* developmental abnormalities which commonly lead to premature *secondary* OA of the hip. In many cases the nature of the preceding abnormality can be easily recognised but in others presenting with advanced disease it can be very difficult to discern what was the underlying abnormality. Two studies have suggested that about a quarter of patients with "primary" osteoarthritis of the hip presenting for orthopaedic surgery have evidence of an underlying acetabular dysplasia [66, 67]. Although there is little doubt that acetabular dysplasia can progress to OA of the hip in a high proportion of patients [68], a large study of pelvic radiographs taken for non-skeletal indications suggested that acetabular dysplasia was unlikely to be an important pre-disposing cause of the common form of hip OA in men [69]. The possibility of a more *generalized* multiple epiphyseal or spondyloepiphyseal dysplasia must always be considered in patients presenting with bilateral premature hip OA. Short stature and clinical evidence of spinal deformity may be useful pointers, but a family history suggesting dominant inheritance of premature OA may be the only clinical clue in some cases.

Following the identification of mutations in the type II procollagen gene (COL2A1) in families with chondrodysplasia and premature OA 10 years ago [70, 71] numerous collagen gene mutations have been associated with structural abnormalities of articular cartilage, bone and other connective tissues in mouse and man [72, 73]. The rapid advance in detecting mutations responsible for familial OA has been greatest in identifying mutations in COL2A1, the gene that codes for the most abundant type of collagen in articular cartilage. Recently, however, a number of mutations in genes for type X collagen (COL101A) have been found in patients with the Schmid type of metaphyseal osteochondrodysplasia [74] where growth plate cartilage is affected. It will be interesting to see if mutations in the genes coding for collagen type VI, IX and XI, which are also found in articular cartilage, will be associated with familial forms of OA in the future. At the present time mutations responsible for the development of most cases of multiple epiphyseal dysplasia, a relatively frequently recognised familial disorder associated with the development of premature OA, cannot be identified, but this situation may change rapidly following the identification of mutations in the cartilage oligomeric matrix protein (COMP) in three patients with MED/pseudoachondroplasia [75].

4.1.5
Neuropathic Joint Disease

Neuropathic (Charcot) arthritis is a complication of neurological disorders associated with prominent loss of proprioception. Classically it occurs in the knees in about 5% of patients with Tabes dorsalis and in the elbows and other upper limb joints of up to 25% of patients with syringomyelia. Neuropathic arthritis is, however, most commonly encountered in the mid and hindfoot joints of diabetics, and up to 5% of patients with a diabetic neuropathy may be affected. Charcot joints are among the most hypertrophic forms of OA. The dramatic outgrowths of new bone and cartilage in this form of OA emphasizes the point that osteoarthritis is associated with *regeneration*, as well as *degeneration* of cartilage and bone. O'Connoll and Brandt [76] have shown that the speed with which experimental osteoarthritis develops in the stifle joints of dogs following anterior cruciate ligament transection is greatly accelerated by ipsilateral deafferentation: emphasizing the protective role of muscular reflexes triggered by joint receptors. Abnormalities of proprioception have also been detected in patients with OA knees [77] and this may play a part in pathogenesis by facilitating inappropriate joint loading. Radin [78] has suggested that minor neuromuscular incoordination may also contribute to the development of knee OA, but clearly we need to know a great deal more about the influence of afferent nerves on the metabolism of joints.

4.1.6
Articular Cartilage Loading

When external loads are applied to joints during movement and weight bearing shear, tensile and compressive stresses are generated in the articular cartilage as it changes in shape and the congruence and contact areas of opposing cartilage surfaces are increased. In addition to mechanical deformation, joint-loading leads to changes in hydrostatic pressure, fluid flow, loss of water and alterations in pH and osmolality within the cartilage matrix [79]. The articular cartilage behaves as a viscoelastic material so that deformation and recovery of shape are time-dependent and accompanied by creep and energy dissipation [80]. The mechanical functions of articular cartilage and its ability to withstand loading are critically dependent on the structural integrity of its extracellular matrix proteins. In general the collagen network imparts tensile strength and the negatively charged proteoglycan aggregates within it resist compression [81]. A few measurements with implanted pressure transducers have shown that peak contact pressures of 10 – 20 MPa can be generated in the hip on standing [82] and articular cartilage may be compressed in volume by as much as 13 % [83]. Static loading is associated with depression of matrix synthesis while dynamic, high frequency, cyclical loading is associated with increases of up to 50 % in proteoglycan synthesis [84, 85]. Cyclical compression of articular cartilage can have variable effects on proteoglycan synthesis depending on the nature of the loading and whether measurements of synthesis are made during or following compression [85]. In general, loads which raise hydrostatic pressure and cause fluid movement without significant fluid loss lead to an increase in matrix synthesis rates whilst loading regimes that cause fluid loss decrease synthesis. Overloading [86] and unloading [87] of articular cartilage are both associated with proteoglycan depletion while proteoglycan synthesis and articular cartilage thickness are increased by the mechanical stresses associated with physiological exercise [88]. Articular chondrocytes are the cells responsible for the synthesis of matrix proteoglycans and collagen. Compression of articular cartilage results in deformation of chondrocytes which strain at contact points between the cells and the pericellular matrix but compression is also accompanied by hydrostatic pressure gradients, fluid flow, streaming potentials and currents and physico-chemical changes such as alterations in matrix water content, fixed charge density, fluxes in ion concentrations and changes in osmotic pressure [85, 86].

Cyclical pressurisation of cultured chondrocytes results in increases in cyclic AMP and proteoglycan synthesis and decreases in DNA synthesis [89] but the signal transduction mechanisms that lead to these metabolic changes have still to be elucidated.

In Edinburgh we have developed experimental techniques that allow us to measure membrane potentials and proteoglycan metabolism in human articular chondrocytes in monolayer cell culture following cyclical pressure-induced microstrain. Early results showed that chondrocytes, unlike fibroblasts, hyperpolarise following cyclical pressurisation [90] as a consequence of activation of apamin sensitive, charybdotoxin and iberiotoxin resistant low conductance Ca^{2+}-activated K^+ ion channels [91]. Cyclical pressure induced strain also led to increased expression of the immediate early response gene c-fos [92] and increases in proteoglycan synthesis [93]. Membrane hyperpolarisation and accelerated proteoglycan synthesis could be blocked with 10μm gadolinium, a blocker of stretch-activated ion channels [93]. Subsequent experiments showed that the membrane hyperpolarisation response following cyclical pressure-induced strain was inhibited by RGD containing oligopeptides and antibodies to β1 and α5 integrins, but not by antibodies to other integrins expressed by human articular chondrocytes [94]. This suggests that α5β1, the classical fibronectin receptor, which is strongly expressed in human articular cartilage may be a mechanoreceptor which could function as a regulator of chondrocyte responses to strain. More recently we have demonstrated that neutralizing antibodies to IL-4 and IL-4 receptor α will block mechanically induced membrane hyperpolarisation [95] suggesting a novel regulatory function for this cytokine in articular cartilage. Most recently we have obtained preliminary evidence that the p38 MAP Kinase pathway is involved in the upregulation of proteoglycan synthesis that follows cyclical pressure-induced strain [96].

Further studies are clearly necessary to clarify the intracellular pathways involved in mechanical signalling in chondrocytes and also to clarify whether IL-4 does have an important role as an autocrine/paracrine regulator of mechanically induced responses in cartilage. Better understanding of these basic mechanisms may lead to new targets for therapeutic intervention in patients with osteoarthritis where progression of disease is so dependent on mechanical factors.

Acknowledgements. Work supported by grants from the Arthritis Research Campaign.

References

1. O'Rahilly R, Gardner E (1978) The embryology of movable joints. In: Sokoloff L (Ed) The joints and synovial fluid. Vol 1 Academic press, New York pp 49–103
2. Solursh M (1986) Environmental regulation of limb chondrogenesis. In: Kuettner KE, Schleyerbach R, Hascall VC (Eds) Articular cartilage biochemistry. Raven Press, New York pp 145–161
3. Helminen HJ, Kiviranta I, Saamanen AM et al. (1991). In: Kuettner KE, Schleyerbach R, Peyron JG, Hascall VC (Eds) Articular cartilage and osteoarthritis. Raven Press, New York pp 501–510

4. Lanyon LE (1987) Functional strain in bone tissue as an objective, and controlling stimulus for adaptive bone remodelling. J Biomech 20 : 1083–1093
5. Henriksson J, Hickner RC (1994) Training induced adaptations in skeletal muscle. In: Harries M, Williams C, Stanish WD, Michaeli LJ (Eds) Oxford Textbook of Sports Medicine. Oxford Medical Publications, Oxford pp 27–45
6. Kuettner K, Goldberg VM (Eds) (1995) Osteoarthritic disorders. American Academy of Orthopaedic Surgeons, Rosemont pp 21–25
7. Nuki G (Ed) (1980) The aetiopathogenesis of osteoarthrosis. Pitman Medical, London
8. Nuki G (1998) Osteoarthritis: a problem of joint failure (in press)
9. Brandt KD, Lohmander LS, Doherty M (1998) Pathogenesis of osteoarthritis. Introduction: the concept of osteoarthritis as failure of the diathrodial joint. In: Brandt KD, Lohmander LS, Doherty M (Eds) Osteoarthritis. Oxford University Press, Oxford pp 70–74
10. Mankin HJ, Brandt KD, Shulman LE (1986) Workshop on aetiopathogenesis of osteoarthritis: proceedings and recommendations. J Rheumatol 13 : 1130–1160
11. Altman RD (1995) The classification of osteoarthritis. J Rheumatol 22 (Suppl 43): 42–43
12. Doherty M, Watt I, Dieppe PA (1983) Influence of primary generalised osteoarthritis on development of secondary osteoarthritis. Lancet 2 : 8–11
13. Roos H, Adalberth T, Lohmander LS (1996) Osteoarthrosis after meniscectomy. Ann Rheum Dis 55 : 692
14. Oliveria SA, Felson DT, Reed JI et al. (1995) Incidence of symptomatic hand, hip and knee osteoarthritis among patients in a health maintenance organisation. Arthritis Rheum 38 : 1134–1141
15. Hardingham TE, Venn G, Bayliss MT (1991) Chondrocyte responses in cartilage and in experimental osteoarthritis. Brit J Rheumatol 30 (Suppl 1): 32–37
16. Roughley PJ, White RG, Magny MC et al. (1993) Non-proteoglycan forms of biglycan increase with age in human articular cartilage. Biochem J 295 : 421–427
17. Holmes MW, Bayliss MT, Muir H (1988) Hyaluronic acid in human articular cartilage. Age-related changes in content and size. Biochem J 250 : 433–441
18. Kempson GE (1975) Mechanical properties of articular cartilage and their relationship to matrix degradation and age. Ann Rheum Dis 32 (Suppl 2): 11–113
19. Roth V, Mow VC (1980) The intrinsic tensile behaviour of the matrix of bovine articular cartilage and its variation with age. J Bone Joint Surg 62 A: 1102–1117
20. Kempson GE, Muir H, Pollard C et al. (1973) The tensile properties of the cartilage of human femoral condyles related to the content of collagen and glycosaminoglycans. Biochim Biophys Acta 297 : 456–472
21. Wachtel E, Maroudas A, Schneiderman R (1995) Age related changes in collagen packing of human articular cartilage. Biochim Biophy Acta 1243 : 239–243
22. Kirk JA, Ansell BM, Bywaters EGL (1967) The hypermobility syndrome. Ann Rheum Dis 26 : 419–425
23. Bird HA, Tribe CR, Bacon PA (1978) Joint hypermobility leading to osteoarthrosis and chondrocalcinosis. Ann Rheum Dis 37 : 203–211
24. Bridges AJ, Smith E, Reid J (1992) Joint hypermobility in adults referred to rheumatology clinics. Ann Rheum Dis 51 : 793–796
25. Harper P, Nuki G (1980) Genetic factors in osteoarthrosis. In: Nuki G (Ed). The aetiopathogenesis of osteoarthrosis. Pitman Medical, London pp 184–201
26. Jonsson H, Valtysdottir ST, Kjartansson O et al. (1996) Hypermobility associated with osteoarthritis of the thumb base. A clinical and radiological subset of hand osteoarthritis. Ann Rheum Dis 55 : 540–543
27. Wright V (1990) Post-traumatic osteoarthritis – a medico-legal minefield. Brit J Rheumatol 29 : 424–478
28. Felson DT (1990) The epidemiology of knee osteoarthritis: results from the Framingham Osteoarthritis Study. Seminars Arthritis Rheum 20 : 42–50
29. Harris WH (1969) Traumatic arthritis of the hip after dislocation and acetabular fractures: treatment by mold arthroplasty. J Bone Joint Surg 51 A: 737–755

30. Jacobsen K (1977) Osteoarthrosis following insufficiency of the cruciate ligaments in man. Acta Orthopaedica Scand 48:520–526
31. Tirgari M, Vaughan LC (1975) Arthritis of the canine stifle joint. Vet Rec 96:394–399
32. Pond MJ, Nuki G (1973) Experimentally-induced osteoarthritis in the dog. Ann Rheum Dis 32:387–388
33. Chantraine A (1985) Knee joint in soccer players: osteoarthritis and axis deviation. Med Sci Sports Exercise 17:434–439
34. Roos H, Lindberg H, Gardsell P (1994) The prevalence of gonarthrosis in former soccer players and its relation to meniscectomy. Am J Sports Med 22:219–222
35. Rall KL, McElroy GL, Keats TE (1964) A study of long-term effects of football injury to the knee. Mo Med 61:435–438
36. Harris PA, Hart DJ, Jawad S et al. (1994) Risks of osteoarthritis associated with running: a radiological survey of ex-athletes. Arthritis Rheum 37:S369
37. Vingard E, Alfredsson L, Goldie I et al. (1993) Sports and osteoarthrosis of the hip. An epidemiological study. Am J Sports Med 21:195–200
38. Paranen J, Ala-Ketola L, Peltokallio P et al. (1975) Running and primary osteoarthritis of the hip. Brit Med J 1:424–425
39. Kujala VM, Kettunen J, Paananen H et al. (1995) Knee osteoarthritis in former runners, soccer players, weight lifters and shooters. Arthritis Rheum 38:539–546
40. Spector TD, Harris PA, Hart DJ et al. (1996) Risks of osteoarthritis associated with long-term weight-bearing sports: a radiographic survey of the hips and knees in female ex-athletes and population controls. Arthritis Rheum 39:988–995
41. Buckwalter JA, Lane NE (1997) Athletics and osteoarthritis. Am J Sports Med 25:873–881
42. Cooper C, MacAlindon T, Egger P et al. (1994) Occupational activity and osteoarthritis of the knee. Ann Rheum Dis 53:90–93
43. Anderson JAD, Duthie JJR, Moody BP (1962) Social and economic effects of rheumatic diseases in a mining population. Ann Rheum Dis 21:342–352
44. Partridge REH, Duthie JJR (1968) Rheumatism in dockers and civil servants. Ann Rheum Dis 27:559–568
45. Vingard E, Alfredsson L, Goldie I et al. (1991) Occupation and osteoarthrosis of the hip and knee: a register based cohort study. Int J Epidemiol 20:1025–1031
46. Croft P, Coggon D, Cruddas M et al. (1992) Osteoarthritis of the hip: an occupational disease in farmers. Brit Med J 304:1269–1272
47. Anderson JJ, Felson DT (1988) Factors associated with osteoarthritis of the knee in the first national health and nutrition examination survey (HANES-1). Am J Epidemiol 128:179–189
48. Felson DT, Hannan MT, Maimark A et al. (1991) Occupational physical demands, knee bending and knee osteoarthritis: results from the Framingham study. J Rheumatol 18:1587–1592
49. Lawrence JS (1961) Rheumatism in cotton operatives. Br J Ind Med 18:270–276
50. Hadler NM, Gillings DB, Imbus R et al. (1978) Hand structure and function in an industrial setting. Arthritis Rheum 21:210–220
51. Felson DT, Chaisson CE (1997) Understanding the relationship between body weight and osteoarthritis. Bailliere's Clin Rheumatol 11 (4):671–681
52. MacAlinden T, Zhang Y, Hannan MT et al. (1996) Are risk factors for patellofemoral and tibiofemoral knee osteoarthritis different? J Rheumatol 23:332–337
53. Cicuttini FM, Baker JR, Spector TD (1996) The association of obesity with osteoarthritis of the hand and knee in women: a twin study. J Rheumatol 23:1221–1226
54. Felson DT, Zhang Y, Hannan MT et al. (1997) Risk factors for incident radiographic osteoarthritis in the elderly: the Framingham study. Arthritis Rheum 40:728–733
55. Hannan MT, Anderson JJ, Zhang Y et al. (1993) Bone mineral density and knee osteoarthritis in elderly men and women: the Framingham study. Arthritis Rheum 36:1671–1680
56. Radin EL, Paul IL, Lovy M (1970) A comparison of the dynamic force transmitting properties of subchondral bone and articular cartilage. J Bone Joint Surg 52 A:444–456

57. Finlay JB Repo RU (1978) Cartilage impact *in-vitro*: effect of bone and cement. J Biomechanics 11 : 379 – 388

58. Redler I, Mow VC, Zimny MC et al. (1975) The ultrastructure and biomechanical significance of the tidemark of articular cartilage. Clin Orthopaedics and Related Research 112: 357 – 362

59. Radin EL, Rose RM (1986) Role of subchondral bone in the initiation and progression of cartilage damage. Clin Orthopaedics and Related Research 213 : 34 – 40

60. Brown TD, Radin EL, Martin RB et al. (1984) Finite element studies of some juxta-articular stress changes due to localised subchondral stiffening. J Biomechanics 17 : 11 – 24

61. Hoshino A, Wallace WA (1987) Impact absorbing properties of the human knee. J Bone Joint Surg 69 B: 807 – 811

62. Foss MVL, Byers PD (1972) Bone density, osteoarthrosis of the hip and fracture of the upper end of the femur. Ann Rheum Dis 31 : 259 – 264

63. Dequeker J (1985) The relationship between osteoporosis and osteoarthritis. Clinics in the Rheumatic Diseases 11 : 271 – 296

64. Vertraeten A, Van Erman H, Haghebaert G et al. (1991) Osteoarthrosis retards the development of osteoporosis. Clin Orthopaedics and Related Research 264 : 169 – 177

65. Pogrund H, Rutenberg M, Makin M et al. (1982) Osteoarthritis of the hip joint and osteoporosis: a radiological study in a random population sample in Jerusalem. Clin Orthopaedics and Related Research 164 : 130 – 135

66. Murray RO (1965) The aetiology of primary osteoarthritis of the hip. Brit J Radiol 38 : 810 – 824

67. Stulberg SD, Harris WH (1974) Acetabular dysplasia and development of osteoarthritis of the hip. In: Harris WH (Ed) The hip. Proceedings of the second open scientific meeting of the hip society. Mosby, St Louis pp 82 – 93

68. Cooperman DR, Wallenstein R, Stulbert SD (1983) Acetabular dysplasia in the adult. Clin Orthop 175 : 79 – 85

69. Croft P, Cooper C, Wickham C et al. (1991) Osteoarthritis of the hip and acetabular dysplasia. Ann Rheum Dis 50 : 308 – 310

70. Palotie A, Vaisanen P, Ott J et al. (1989) Predisposition to familial osteoarthritis linked to type II collagen gene. Lancet 1 : 924 – 927

71. Knowlton RG, Katzenstein PL, Moskowitz RW et al. (1990) Genetic linkage of a polymorphism of the type II collagen gene (COL21A) to primary osteoarthritis associated with mild chondrodysplasia. New Eng J Med 322 : 526 – 530

72. Jimenez SA, Williams CJ, Karasick D (1998) Hereditary osteoarthritis. In: Brandt KD, Doherty M, Lohmander LS (Eds) Osteoarthritis. Oxford University Press, Oxford pp 931 – 49

73. Jacenko O, Olsen BR (1995) Transgenic mouse models in studies of skeletal disorders. J Rheumatol 22 (Suppl 43): 39 – 41

74. McIntosh I, Abbott MH, Francomano CA (1995) Concentration of mutations causing Schmid metaphyseal chondrodysplasia in the c-terminal non-collagenous domain of type X collagen. Human mutation 5 : 121 – 125

75. Briggs MD, Hoffman SMG, King LM et al. (1995) Pseudoachondroplasia and multiple epiphyseal dysplasia due to mutations in the cartilage oligomeric matrix protein gene. Nature Genetics 10 : 330 – 336

76. O'Connor BL, Palmoski MJ, Brandt KD (1985) Neurogenic acceleration of degenerative joint lesions. J Bone Joint Surg 67-A: 562 – 571

77. Barrett DS, Cobb AG, Bentley G (1991) Joint proprioception in normal, osteoarthritic and replaced knees. J Bone Joint Surg 73-B: 53 – 56

78. Radin EL, Yang KH, Reiger C et al. (1991) Relationship between lower limb dynamics and knee joint pain. J Orthop Res 9 : 398 – 405

79. Urban JPG, Hall AC (1994) The effects of hydrostatic and osmotic pressures on chondrocyte metabolism. In: Mow VC, Guilak F, Tran-Son Tay R, Hochmuth RM (Eds) Cell mechanics and cellular engineering. Springer Verlag, New York pp 348 – 419

80. Mow VC, Ratcliffe A, Poole AR (1992) Cartilage and diarthrodial joints as paradigms for hierarchical materials and structures. Biomaterials 13 : 67 – 97

81. Stockwell RA (1991) Cartilage failure in osteoarthritis: relevance of normal structure and function. A review. Clinical Anatomy 4:161–191
82. Hodge WA, Fijan RS, Carlson KL et al. (1986) Contact pressures in the human hip joint measured *in vivo*. Proc Natl Acad Sci (USA) 83:2879–2883
83. Armstrong CG, Bahrani AS, Gardner DL (1980) Changes in deformational behaviour of human hip cartilage with age. J Biomech Eng 102:214–220
84. Parkkinen JJ, Ikonen J, Lammi MJ et al. (1993) Effects of cyclic hydrostatic pressure on proteoglycan synthesis in cultured chondrocytes and articular cartilage explants. Arch Biochem Biophy 300:458–465
85. Sah RL, Grodzinsky AJ, Plaas AHK et al. (1992) Effects of static and dynamic compression on matrix metabolism in cartilage explants. In: Kuettner K, Schleyerbach R, Peyron J, Hascall VC (Eds) Articular cartilage and osteoarthritis. Raven Press, New York pp 373–392
86. Hall AC, Urban JPG, Gehl GA (1991) The effects of hydrostatic pressure on matrix synthesis in articular cartilage. J Orthop Res 9:1–10
87. Saamanen A-M, Tammi J, Jurvelin I et al. (1990) Proteoglycan alterations following immobilisation and remobilisation in the articular cartilage of young canine knee (stifle) joint. J Orthop Res 8:863–873
88. Kiviranta I, Jurvelin J, Tammi M et al. (1987) Weightbearing controls glycosaminoglycan concentration and thickness of articular cartilage in knee joints of young Beagle dogs. Arthritis Rheum 30:801–808
89. Veldhuijzen JP, Bourret LA, Rodan GA (1979) *In vitro* studies of the effect of intermittent compressive forces on cartilage cell proliferation. J Cell Physiol 98:299–306
90. Wright MO, Stockwell RA, Nuki G (1992) Response of plasma membrane to applied hydrostatic pressure in chondrocytes and fibroblasts. Connect Tissue Res 28:49–70
91. Wright MO, Jobanputra P, Bavington C, Salter DM, Nuki G (1996) Effects of intermittent pressure-induced strain on the electrophysiology of cultured human chondrocytes: evidence for the presence of stretch-activated ion channels. Clinical Science 90:61–71
92. Wright MO, Jobanputra P, Bavington C, Salter DM, Nuki G (1995) Intracellular signal transduction pathways in human chondrocytes stimulated by intermittent pressurisation. J Bone Joint Surg 29-A: 88
93. Nuki G, Bavington C, Jobanputra P et al. (1994) Stretch-activated ion channels in human chondrocytes and proteoglycan synthesis following cyclical pressurisation of chondrocytes. Osteoarthritis and Cartilage 2:533
94. Wright MO, Nishida K, Bavington C et al. (1997) Hyperpolarisation of cultured human chondrocytes following cyclical pressure-induced strain: evidence of a role for $\alpha5\beta1$ integrin as a chondrocyte mechanoreceptor. J Orthopaed Res 15:742–747
95. Millward-Sadler SJ, Wright MO, Nishida K et al. (1998) Integrin-regulated secretion of interleukin-4: a novel pathway of mechanotransduction in human articular chondrocytes. Submitted for publication
96. Lin H, Bavington C, Goldring MB et al. (1998) P38 MAP Kinase controls the accelerated proteoglycan synthesis that follows cyclical strain in immortalised human chondrocytes. Brit J Rheumatol 37(Suppl 1): 18

4.2
Role of Biomechanical Factors

P. Ghosh

4.2.1
Introduction

Degeneration of articular cartilage, subchondral bone sclerosis and remodelling are well established hallmarks of osteoarthritis (OA) but the etiologic factors responsible are still the subject of debate. Numerous epidemiological studies have shown that certain occupations which involve long-term repetitive joint usage can increase the risk of cartilage failure and OA [1-14]. However, it is often difficult, if not impossible, to separate the mechanical contribution to OA from the influences of age, cultural habits, genetic, hormonal or other unknown factors, all of which can impinge on the onset and rate of disease progression to varying degrees. Where appropriate stratifications and normalisation for confounding variables has been undertaken, occupations such as farming [3, 5, 13], ballet dancing [2] and heavy construction work [1, 8, 11, 12, 14] emerge as risks for OA. Regular participation in certain sports, such as soccer [15-17] skiing, racquet sports and some track and field activities [17-20], have all been shown to be associated with OA in later life. But again it is a problem to clearly distinguish cartilage degeneration related directly to these sporting activities from secondary cartilage changes arising from injury to other joint tissues, such as the menisci or ligaments. Injury to and rupture of the menisci and anterior cruciate ligament (ACL) are relatively common events in joints of competitive soccer players [21]. Studies of the kinetics of release into synovial fluid of cartilage-derived proteoglycans (PGs) in a group of these individuals showed that the concentration was markedly elevated a few hours after injury and although the levels declined with time, they remained above normal for several years thereafter [22]. Radiological evidence of OA did not appear in these patients for 15 years post injury, highlighting the long lead time between an initial joint injury altering cartilage metabolism and the appearance of clinical signs of OA [21]. Since the knee joint meniscus is a weight-bearing tissue which has an important mechanical role in normal joint function [23-25], its mechanical failure due to injury results in the imposition of abnormally high contact stresses on articular cartilage. These stresses may accelerate its degeneration and development of OA [26, 27].

4.2.2
Cartilage and Exercise: Long Distance Running

4.2.2.1
Human Investigations

Long distance running as a risk factor for OA has attracted particular attention in recent years because of the popularity of jogging as a form of exercise.

Retrospective and prospective studies [19, 28–35] have shown that middle distance and marathon runners do not exhibit higher symptomatic or radiologic evidence of OA than non-running cohorts. However, many of these studies had weaknesses in experimental design (eg. inadequate numbers for statistical analysis, incomplete or invalid methods of diagnosis or assessment of OA) and their conclusions have therefore been questioned [19]. Some of these methological deficiencies were redressed in the longitudinal studies undertaken by Lane et al. [29–32] where non-elite veteran runners were evaluated over 2, 5 and 9 years follow-up periods. In a group of these runners with an average age of 65 years, they reported that the incidence of radiological assessed OA was no greater than in non-running age-matched controls. However, females of the group showed higher subchondral sclerosis and in both males and females osteophytes were more common in the runners. Furthermore, it could be argued that individuals of this age who continued running were a self-selected group. Nevertheless, it was concluded by Lane et al. [29, 30] and Lequesne et al. [19] that non-competitive (non-elite) running was not a risk for OA.

Collectively, these epidemiological studies indicate that for individuals with well aligned "healthy" joints, long distance running is not a definite cause of cartilage degeneration and subsequent OA providing the level of running was non-competitive.

4.2.2.2
Animal Models

More direct support for this conclusion has been provided by experiments undertaken with animals. Animal models offer many advantages over epidemiological or radiological investigations conducted with human subjects. Animals of similar weight, sex and genetic stock may be used and randomly assigned to exercised and non-exercised groups. The type and level of exercise to be undertaken by the animal may also be predetermined and the duration of the experiment varied. Moreover, animals may be euthanased at the completion of the experiments and joint examined for qualitative and quantitative changes at specific tissue sites and correlations sought with the experimental protocol used.

Beagles. In a recent study reported by Newton et al. [36] skeletally mature young adult beagles were trained to run at 3.3 km/h on a level treadmill for 75 minutes a day for 5 days a week carrying an external average load of 11.5 kg (130% body weight). A matched non-exercised non-weight carrying control group were housed in dog runs with an area of 4 square meters. Both groups were sacrificed 527 weeks after initiating the exercise protocol and knee joint cartilage, ligaments and menisci examined histologically. Surprisingly, it was found that this level of "lifelong" physical activity failed to provoke degenerative changes in joint tissues in the exercised dogs. Menisci and ligaments appeared normal while articular cartilage exhibited no evidence of fibrillation, loss of PGs or osteophytosis. The material properties of the cartilages of the exercised and non-exercised groups as determined biomechanically were also found to be indistinguishable. In another study in which immature beagles were subjected to a non-strenuous exercise program (4 km/day on a treadmill inclined at 15°) for 15 weeks, it was observed that the thickness and PG content of patella and femoral cartilage increased relative to a non-exercised control group [37, 38]. However, a larger proportion of PGs which accumulated in the cartilages of the exercised animals failed to aggregate with hyaluronan and contained more chondroitin 6-sulphate than the PGs isolated from the non-exercised group [39]. It was postulated that this level of exercise accelerated the maturation of matrix deposited in the cartilage of these animals. In a subsequent study, again with young beagles, the exercise program was increased to 20 km/day for 15 weeks [40]. Under these more vigorous conditions, evidence of cartilage degeneration became apparent as shown by the loss of collagen, increased water content and reduced ratio of chondroitin-6 to chondroitin-4- sulphate in cartilage from the lateral femoral condyles of these animals. Extending the distance exercised by the beagles to 40 km/day confirmed that high endurance running (15–52 weeks) promoted loss of PGs from the cartilage extracellular matrix [41, 42]. Site-specific analysis of glycosaminoglycans in different joint regions revealed that the loss occurred primarily at the summits of the femoral condyles, particularly in the cartilage superficial zones [42, 43]. Further support for the disruption of cartilage matrix assembly by this high level of running activity was provided by the observed decreased birefringence of the collagen fibres [42, 44].

Horses. We have confirmed, using standard bred horses, that sustained strenuous exercise can induce metabolic changes in cartilage PGs in carpal joints [45]. In this study the relative effects of moderate or strenuous exercise on the synthesis and degradation of the large aggregating PGs (aggrecan) and two small dermatan sulphate-containing proteoglycans, DS-PGII (decorin) and DS-PGI (biglycan) were investigated. Cartilage explants were taken at necropsy from three weight-bearing regions of the third carpal bone, which are common sites of OA lesions in sporting horses [46] (Fig. 1). Twelve adult horses (aged three to

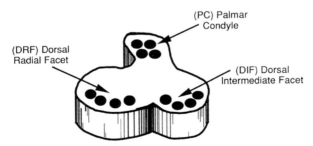

Fig. 1. Schematic representation of the third carpal bone of the horse showing the three regions analysed. Full-depth 2 mm cartilage plugs (shown as *solid circles*) were sampled from the dorsal radial facet (DRF), palmar condyle (PC) and dorsal intermediate facet (DIF) regions and established in culture. Osteochondral plugs from similar sites of contralateral joints were also taken for histological investigations

five years) that were free from clinical and radiographic evidence of disease of the middle carpal joint at entry were used for the study. Animals were subjected to an eight week moderate exercise program consisting of running 2,000 meters at 6 m/s three days a week increasing to 4000 metres for eight weeks. The horses were then randomly assigned to one of two groups. Group A continued the moderate exercise as before while the program for Group B was increased to 4000 metres at 8 m/s, four days/week for 17 weeks. The horses of both groups were then rested for 16 weeks before euthanasia and collection of both carpal joints for study. Osteochondral plugs were sampled from the dorsal radial facet, dorsal intermediate facet and palmar condyle of the third carpal bone (Fig. 1) for histological examination. From the other joint full depth articular explants were removed from the same regions and established in culture. After 72 hours, media containing $^{35}SO_4^{2-}$ was added to the explant cultures for 48 hours to radiolabel newly synthesised PGs. Explants were removed and 3 out of 4 explants extracted with 4 M guanidinium hydrochloride. Media and the remaining unextracted explant were digested with papain and sulphated glyco-saminoglycans and radioactivity determined. The extracts from the cartilage explants were subjected to hydrophobic and anion exchange chromatography to separate aggrecan from the dermatan sulphate containing PGs, decorin and biglycan. The proportions of ^{35}S incorporated into these individual PG species was quantitated by SDS-PAGE followed by phosphor screen autoradiography.

Histological examination of cartilage from the carpal joints of both strenuously and moderately exercised groups showed superficial cartilage depressions accompanied by disruption of calcified cartilage and the tidemark in the radial facet of the third carpal bone but not in the other regions. However, there were no apparent differences between these histological changes in cartilages from group A and B animals. In explant cultures from the strenuously exercised group, more PGs were released into media from cartilage of the DRF region than in the same region of moderately exercised animals, suggesting enhanced catabolism of cartilage in the strenuous exercise group. Extracts of cartilage explants from the DRF region, after purification and quantitation of PGs by phosphor autoradiography, showed that the incorporation of ^{35}S into aggrecan PGs was less in tissues from the strenuously exercised animals than in the same region of the moderately exercised group (Fig. 2). In contrast, decorin synthesis was elevated and biglycan synthesis remained unchanged (Fig. 2).

These data indicated that in joint regions of the horse carpal joint normally subjected to high contact stress (DRF), strenuous running activity altered chondrocyte metabolism of PGs. The synthesis of aggrecan was decreased while the synthesis of the DS-containing PG, decorin, was elevated.

The functional role of decorin in connective tissues is still the subject of investigation, however, it would appear that it plays a central role in collagen macromolecular assembly and organisation [47], cell proliferation [48], and the modulation of the activities of growth factors such as TGF-β [49]. Addition of decorin to collagen gels was observed to lead to the deposition of more uniformly thin fibrils than in the absence of this PG [50]. Moreover, the decorin was shown to be associated with d bands of the collagen fibrils [50, 51a]. In periparturient uterine cervical tissue, loosening of the collagen network has

Fig. 2.
Synthesis of (*A*) aggrecan, (*B*) decorin, (*C*) biglycan proteoglycans in explant cartilage cultures from different regions (Fig. 1) of carpal bones from moderately exercised (*black bars*) and strenuously exercised (*hatched bars*) horses. Results are shown as DPM-^{35}S/µg DNA (as means ± SE). Note the decreased synthesis of aggrecan and increased synthesis of decorin in cartilages of the strenuously exercised group

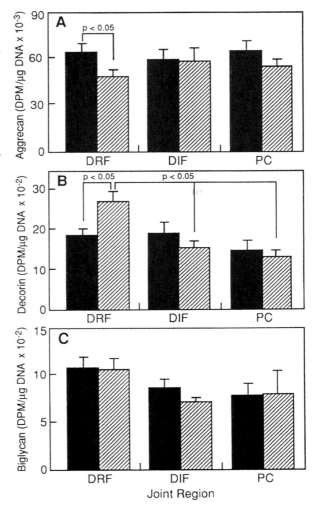

been shown to correlate with increased decorin levels [51]. From these studies, it would appear that an important function of decorin is in orchestrating the repair and remodelling of connective tissues. The enhanced synthesis of decorin by chondrocytes in the cartilage of strenuously exercised horse joints could therefore be interpreted to indicate that this PG (and perhaps other leucine rich PGs) are messengers released by traumatised chondrocytes in response to mechanical overload. This hypothesis is supported by *in vitro* and *in vivo* studies which have demonstrated increased production of decorin by chondrocytes subjected to supraphysiological mechanical stresses. Korver et al. [52] reported a three fold increase in decorin synthesis in cartilage explants subjected to *in vitro* cylic loading for seven days. Similar results were obtained by Visser et al. (1994) using both immature [53] and mature articular cartilage [54]. In a model of early (hypertrophic) OA induced in dogs by transection of the ACL, Douradoi et al. [55] observed increased mRNA levels for biglycan, decorin and fibromodulin in cartilage of the destabilised joints. Meniscectomy in sheep joints has been shown to increase focal stress on cartilage and induced OA. In this model, decorin synthesis was increased in cartilage regions subjected to high contact stresses [56, 57].

4.2.3
Cartilage and Injury: Meniscectomy

As already mentioned, the knee joint menisci have an important role in normal joint function. Menisci are weight bearing structures which increase tibial-femoral congruence, increase lateral stability and improve synovial fluid distribution and nutrient exchange with articular cartilage [23, 24]. Total or partial meniscectomy, which is often necessary if a meniscus is torn and symptomatic, is therefore not a benign procedure since it leads to the imposition of high focal stresses on articular cartilage which generally degenerate [27]. This sequela has been observed clinically [58 – 60] and in animal models where meniscectomy has been used to induce OA [61, 62].

We initially used medial meniscectomy in dogs [63] and sheep [64 – 69] to produce degenerative changes in articular cartilage. However, more recent studies [45, 56, 69, 70] have shown that lateral meniscectomy provides a more rapidly progressive OA model than medial meniscectomy. Using lateral meniscectomy (Fig. 3) as a model of traumatic OA, we have investigated the cartilaginous and subchondral bone changes which evolved in different topographical regions of sheep joints (Fig. 4) as a function of time and different post-operative regimens. Six months following meniscectomy, the aggregate histological scores for cartilage degeneration as defined by a modified Mankin system, were elevated in the lateral femoral condyles (FUL), unprotected (TUL), and previously protected (by the lateral meniscus) (TPL) regions of the tibial plateau [45] (Fig. 5). Typical histological sections illustrating the changes induced in cartilage and the subchondral bone plate in this model are collected in Fig. 6. Cartilage fibrillation, loss of matrix PGs as indicated by reduce staining with Toluidine blue, cell death and cloning were universal features of this model. Beneath areas of cartilage depletion, capillaries in the subchondral bone were noted to invade and penetrate the calcified cartilage accompanied by advancement of the tide mark and thickening of the subchondral cancellous bone (Fig. 6). In a subsequent study, where joint tissues were examined 3 and 9 month post-meniscectomy [71], it was observed that bone remodelling and increased bone mineral density appeared to be secondary to the failure of the articular cartilage. Investigations of PG synthesis in cartilages from meniscectomized ovine joints revealed elevated synthesis of the DS-PGs in those regions subjected to the abnormally high mechanical stresses introduced by the excision of the lateral meniscus [56]. These regions (Fig. 5) included the lateral femoral (FUL) condyles and tibial plateaux (TUL and TPL) although the cartilages of the medial tibial plateau (TUM) also showed increased synthesis of

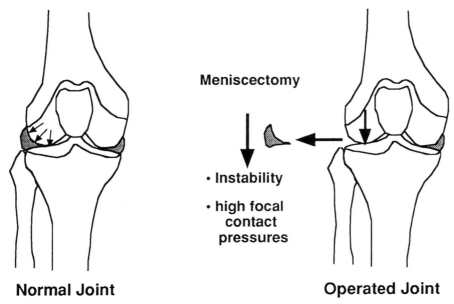

Fig. 3. Schematic representation of the knee joint showing how lateral meniscectomy increases the intensity of focal stresses on articular cartilage and subchondral bone

Fig. 4.
Diagram of the ovine knee
joint identifying topographical regions analyzed for cartilage and subchondral bone
changes associated with
altered mechanical loading
following meniscectomy

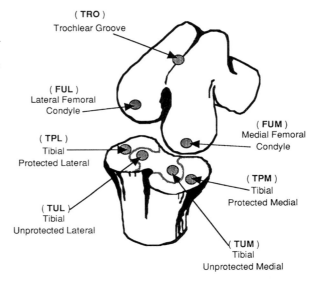

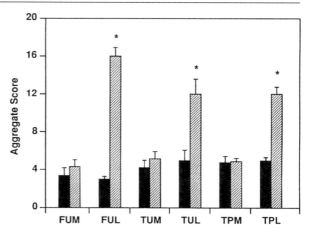

Fig. 5.
Aggregate histological scores using a modified Mankin scoring system [45] for different topographical regions (see Fig. 4) of ovine joints with (*hatched bars*) and without (*black bars*) lateral meniscectomy. Note the high scores for tissues of the lateral compartment (FUL, TUL, TPL) of meniscectomized joints. *, $p < 0.05$ between control and meniscectomized groups

these PG species. By means of Western blotting [56] and in situ hybridization [70] it was confirmed that decorin was the major DS-PG which was up-regulated in the cartilages subjected to high focal stresses. The levels were highest in the middle and deep zones of these cartilages [70]. Such observations were consistent with the report of Poole et al. [72] who showed that decorin levels in human OA cartilage were high in the deep zone.

Concomitant with increased DS-PG synthesis in high weight bearing regions of the meniscectomized ovine joints was increased aggrecan catabolism, as shown by the release of these fragments into media from cultures of the same cartilage explants [56]. Parallel experiments [73] using extracts of cartilage from cartilages of the lateral compartment of meniscectomized joints revealed that levels of matrix metalloproteinases (MMPs) were elevated in high weight-bearing regions (Fig. 7).

Although it is well established that MMPs can degrade most cartilage components, including aggrecan [74], there is presently some debate as to whether the interglobular domain (IGD) G1-G2 region of aggrecan, is initially cleaved by MMPs or another class of proteinase, aggrecanase [75]. This debate rests on the finding that G1-G2 cleavage fragments released from cartilage into synovial fluid [75, 76] or culture media of cartilage explants [77] were not generated by the proteolytic action of MMPs as determined using monoclonal antibodies which identify specific amino acid sequences (see Chapter 5.4 for further details). As indicated in Fig. 8, the monoclonal antibody (MAb) BC-3 recognises the aggrecanase cleavage site on G1-G2 attached to the glycosaminoglycan containing end of aggrecan. This fragment is released from cartilage into synovial fluid (or culture media) and its presence has been used to indict aggrecanase as the catabolic mediator of aggrecan [75–77]. Using explant culture of cartilage from the lateral region of meniscectomized sheep joints, we have found, using MAbs and Western blotting, that the culture media contained material that reacted positively with MAb BC-3 (Fig. 9). These data suggest that the proteolytic cleavage of the G1-G2 domain of aggrecan in cartilages of ovine joints subjected to the high focal stresses introduced by meniscectomy is similar to the re-

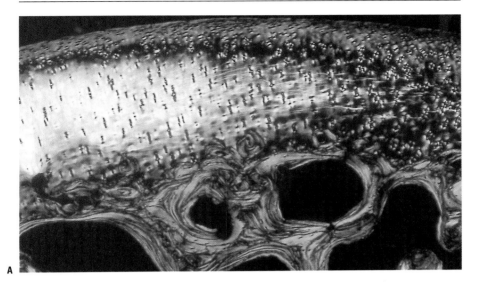

A

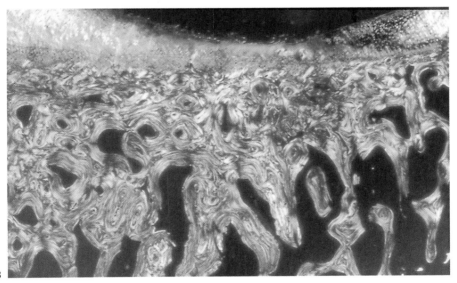

B

Fig. 6A–B. Stained histological coronal sections derived from laterally meniscectomized ovine joints. **A** Normal cartilage and bone of medial femoral condyle stained with Toluidine blue/fast green and photographed with crossed-polarizers showing intact full-depth cartilage (*green*) and well organized trabeculae of the cancellous bone (violet) (M ×16). **B** Lesion region on lateral tibial plateau viewed and stained in as **A** showing erosion of cartilage (green) down to calcified cartilage with loose collagen fibres remaining on the top in the defect (violet). Note that the subchondral bone is markedly thickened with deposition of woven bone (violet) and decreased marrow space (M ×16)

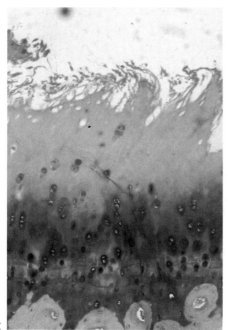

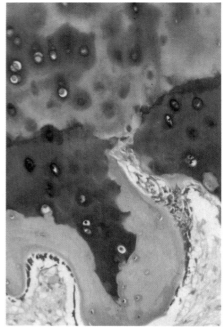

C   D

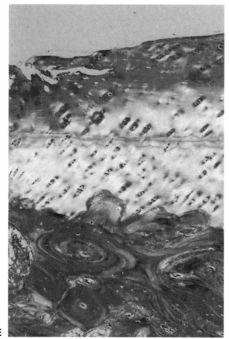

Fig. 6 C – E.
(C) Toluidine blue/fast green stained section
of a central lesion of lateral tibial plateau
showing fibrillation and loss of cartilage
down to the middle zone, depletion of
matrix proteoglycans (decreased blue) and
decline in chondrocyte numbers (M × 50).
(D) Higher magnification (M × 100) of
Toluidine blue/fast green staining section of
lateral tibial plateau lesion area showing
penetration of calcified cartilage by a subchondral blood vessel indicating early
endochondral ossification of cartilage.
(E) Polarized Masson Trichrome stained
section of lateral tibial plateau showing
multiple tidemarks (as 3 wavy red bands) in
the calcified cartilage (yellow) region of the
periphery of the lesion. Note also the
thickened subchondral bone which appears
E   in red under these conditions (M × 50)

Fig. 7 A, B.
Relative levels of active
forms of matrix metallo-
proteinases in different
regions (see Fig. 4) of control (*open bars*) and laterally
meniscectomized (hatched
bars) sheep joints. The MMP
activity in these cartilages
was determined using **A**
gelatin zymography for
MMP-2 and **B** Western blotting for MMP-3. Regions,
FUL, TUL and TPL, where
focal stresses on cartilage
were highest showed
elevated levels of MMPs

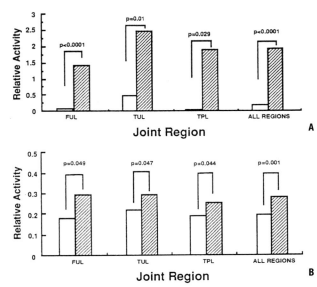

Fig. 8. Cleavage of the interglobular domain (G1-G2) of aggrecan releases fragments from cartilage into synovial fluid or culture media. Matrix metalloproteinases cleave at a different G1-G2 site to aggrecanase. The terminal amino-acid sequences generated by cleavage along G1-G2 by these two classes of proteinases can be recognised by monoclonal antibodies (MAb). These MAb have therefore been used to identify the proteinases responsible for turnover of aggrecan G1-G2 region in cartilage. MMP = matrix metalloproteinase, G1 – globular domain 1, G2 = globular domain 2, G3 = globular domain 3, KS = keratan sulphate region, CS-1 = chondroitin sulphate region-1, CS-2 = chondroitin sulphate region-2

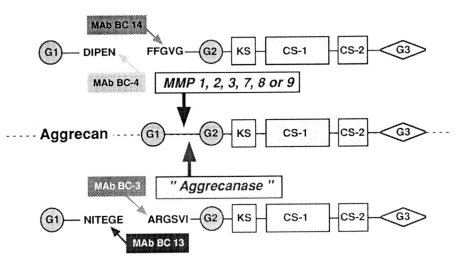

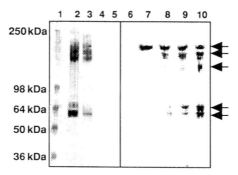

Fig. 9. Full-depth cartilage plugs (see Fig. 4) taken from different regions of the stifle joints of sheep which had been meniscectomized or sham operated, where initiated in explant culture. PG fragments which were released into the culture medium were analysed on Western blots with the monoclonal antibody BC-3 which recognises aggrecan fragments with the N-terminal ARGSVIL (aggrecanase cleavage site). Media samples of explant cultures from degenerate regions of meniscectomized joints showed clear immuno-reactivity with the MAb BC-3 while those from the same regions of control joints did not. The BC-3 positive bands migrated as a triplet with apparent M_r of ~ 120, 140 and 180 kDa and a doublet of ~ 89 kDa. *Lane 1*, globular protein standards, *lanes 2, 3*, extracts from ovine cartilage from meniscectomized joint, *lanes 4, 5*, extracts of same regions as 2, 3 but from control joint. *Lanes 6–10* were a time course digestion of ovine fetal aggrecan with purified ovine AC serine proteinase: *lane 6 = 0 h, lane 7 = 1 h, lane 8 = 2 h, lane 9 = 4 h* and *lane 10 = 24 h* digestion. *Arrows* indicate BC3 positive bands

ported proteolysis of aggrecan in human OA cartilage [75]. The question of whether aggrecanase acts independently of MMPs may be dependent on the pools of PGs available at the sites of proteolysis, *eg.* in the pericellular or interterritorial matrix [76]. More recently an alternative pathway has been postulated by Imai et al. [78], invoking membrane-type I matrix metalloproteinase (MTI-MMP) as a critical activator. Levels of MTI-MMP are up-regulated in OA cartilage and correlate with the activation of pro-MMP-2, a potent mediator of cartilage destruction.

4.2.4
Biomechanical Factors and OA

Although many questions still remain unanswered, the aforementioned studies have provided some insight into how biomechanical factors may contribute to the pathobiology of OA. It is clear that the chondrocyte is capable of sensing its mechanical environment and responding by synthesizing an extracellular matrix which is most suited to dissipate the stresses imposed upon it, thereby protecting it from injury. Thus in young adult animals, moderate exercise was found to promote the synthesis of an aggrecan-rich matrix which could readily accommodate the increased stresses imposed on their joints. This adaptive or hypertrophic phase of the chondrocyte response may continue for some years, provided the level of mechanical stress remains fairly uniform and the chondrocyte population within the cartilage are metabolically capable of sustaining the biosynthetic demands required of them. However, if this balance is disturbed either by increasing the level and duration or the loading or changing the normal mechanics of the joint complex through injury or surgery, or if the ability of the chondrocyte to respond to these additional stresses is diminished through ageing or chemical injury then significant cellular and matrix changes to the cartilage can follow.

The finding in our sheep experiments that aggrecan synthesis was diminished while DS-PG synthesis was increased in regions of joint cartilage subjected to high contact stress is consistent with altered phenotypic expression by chondrocytes in these regions. Similar conclusions have been reached by Aigner and Dudhia [79] who noted that type II collagen expression was decreased and type III and type X collagen increased in chondrocytes in the superficial zone of OA cartilage where mechanical loading was high. The meniscectomy model also showed that concomitant with this altered chondrocyte biosynthetic response was increased catabolism of the extracellular matrix. This was most evident in focal cartilage lesions where MMP (Fig. 7) and aggrecanases (Fig. 9) levels were elevated. Since synovial inflammation was minimal in this animal model [57], we postulate that these proteinases originated from the chondrocytes themselves.

How mechanical stress up-regulates chondrocyte resorption of its extracellular matrix is presently unknown but the process is most probably mediated by prostanoids, cytokines such as Il-1β or TNF-α, or oxygen-derived free radicals including nitric oxide (NO$^\bullet$). However, it should be noted that once synovitis becomes established within the joint, synovial cells and infiltrating leukocytes are major sources of these mediators and these too can promote expression of additional anabolic and catabolic activities by chondrocytes [80–82].

An early study by Chrisman et al. [83] provided evidence that traumatic injury to cartilage can stimulate the production of the prostaglandin precursor, arachidonic acid. In these experiments, a weighted pendulum was made to swing directly on to the surface of femoral cartilage of anaesthetized dogs. It was estimated that the mechanical load imparted to the cartilage in this model was approximately 70 Newtons which was considered to be equivalent to stress received to a knee in an automobile dashboard injury. After 25 impactions it was found that the arachidonic acid content of impacted cartilage increased to 2–4 times that of non-impacted cartilage. The arachidonate was considered to be derived from the membranes of "injured" chondrocyte by the action of phospholipases. Arachidonate is known to be rapidly converted to eicosanoids by the cyclooxygenase pathway [83]. Prostanoids and PG-E$_2$ in particular, have been shown to interact with chondrocyte receptors [84] and alter gene expression [85]. However, whether this interaction stimulates or down-regulates production of proteinases such as MMPs or aggrecanase remains controversial. Early studies [86, 87] suggested that PGE$_2$ increases MMP production and caused degradation of cartilage. But this conclusion is contrary to other studies which show that PGE$_2$ is both anabolic and protects matrix integrity by down-regulating cytokine production by chondrocytes [85]. These conflicting experimental findings may be attributed to the different concentration of PGE$_2$ used in these studies, since the effects of PGE_2 on chondrocytes is known to be biphasic [85].

It is currently accepted that interleukin-1 (IL-1) is a prime up-regulator of MMP gene expression by chondrocytes (see review by [80, 81]). IL-1β and tumour necrosis factor α (TNF-α) also down-regulate production of endogenous inhibitors of MMPs, the TIMPs [81] as well as the synthesis of PGs and collagens [82]. IL-1β has been shown in a variety of mammalian species to promote nitric oxide free-radical generation by stimulating gene expression and levels of inducible nitric oxide synthase (iNOS) in chondrocytes [88].

Nitric oxide free-radicals have profound effects on chondrocyte biosynthesis of matrix components. Both aggrecan and type II collagen synthesis are suppressed and it can induce chondrocytes to undergo apoptosis [88]. Preliminary studies also suggest that MMP production may be up-regulated by this radical.

Chondrocytes can secrete IL-1β in response to treatment with LPS or other cytokines [89]. It is feasible therefore, that mechanical injury to chondrocytes could generate small amounts of IL-1β whose effects on other chondrocytes would be amplified by autocrine and paracrine pathways induced by this cytokine leading to the release of mediators of matrix destruction. Given that all these mediators have been detected in OA cartilage (see reviews by [80, 81, 88]) it is highly likely that they are implicated in mechanically-induced cartilage hypertrophy and resorption.

4.2.5
Summary and Conclusions

From the above considerations, it is clear that chondrocytes, the living elements of cartilage, can readily adapt to the changing mechanical demands placed upon them over a lifetime of weight-bearing activities. However, their ability to react to these mechanical demands may be modified by other factors which influence cellular functions. Examples of such factors could include: genetic defects inherited or accumulated through ageing, endocrine and paracrine factors (hormones, growth factors, cytokines, etc.) all of which can influence cell metabolism and macromolecular synthesis. Furthermore, even in the absence of these non-mechanical contributions the chondrocyte can still fail when subjected to supraphysiological stresses for long periods of time.

For the most part, the non-mechanical influences on chondrocyte metabolism and function are described elsewhere in this publication and therefore are not discussed here. However, the induction of mechanically-induced changes in chondrocyte metabolism was reviewed and potential mechanisms identified. In general terms, these studies showed that chondrocytes respond positively to dynamic loads below the threshold which causes cellular necrosis. Maintenance of this level of mechanical insult, for as yet to be determined periods of time, stimulates chondrocytes to divide and enter a hypertrophic phase in where differentiation and/or clonal selection of chondrocyte populations more capable of tolerating the new mechanical environment accumulate in the tissue.

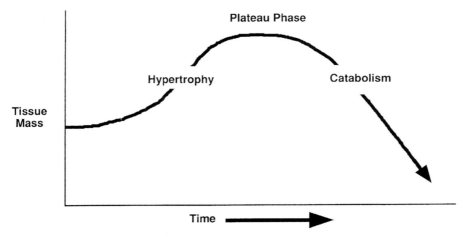

Fig. 10. A simplified diagrammatic representation of the temporal relationship between supraphysiological loading of cartilage and the metabolic response of resident chondrocytes. The end stages, i.e., where the catabolic processes are well established generally corresponds to the symptomatic stage of osteoarthritis

These hypertrophic chondrocytes may be considered to be at the terminal stage of differentiation and as such their expression of important matrix genes is altered. Thus, aggrecan PGs and type II collagen synthesis become repressed while decorin and types I, III and X collagen synthesis by these cells are up-regulated. The decline in aggrecan and type II collagen levels in the extracellular matrix due to the imbalance between synthesis and degradation renders the cartilage biomechanically inadequate and less capable of dissipating the mechanical stresses imposed upon the cell. As a consequence, the chondrocyte becomes "deshielded" and may be further mechanically driven to a catabolic state where excess proteolytic activity and secretion of autocrine/paracrine factors predominate. Matrix destruction ensues and clinical signs of OA may become manifest. This hypothesis is summarised in Fig. 10 and while it is undoubtedly an over simplification of a very complex issue, it is nevertheless consistent with current concepts of cartilage pathobiology.

References

1. Anderson JAD (1984) Arthrosis and its relation to work. Scand J Work Environ Health 10:429–433
2. Andersson S, Hessel T, Noren A, et al. (1989) Degenerative joint disease in ballet dancers. Clin Orthop 238:233–236
3. Axmacher B, Lindberg H (1993) Coxarthrosis in farmers. Clin Orthop 287:82–86
4. Cooper C, McAlindon T, Coggon D, et al. (1994) Occupational activity and osteoarthritis of the knee. Ann Rheum Dis 53:90–93
5. Croft P, Coggon D, Cruddas M, et al. (1992) Osteoarthritis of the hip: An occupational disease in farmers. Br Med J 304:1269–1272

6. Danielsson L, Lindberg H, Nilsson B (1984) Prevalence of coxarthrosis. Clin Orthop 191: 110–115
7. Felson DT (1994) Do occupation-related physical factors contribute to arthritis? Bailliére's Clin Res 8:63–77
8. Felson DT, Hannan MT, Naimark A, et al. (1991) Occupational physical demands, knee bending, and knee osteoarthritis: Results from the Framingham study. J Rheumatol 18: 1587–1592
9. Hadler NM, Gillings DB, Imbus HR, et al. (1978) Hand structure and functions in an industrial setting: Influence of three patterns of stereotype repetitive usage. Arthritis Rheum 21:210–220
10. Lawrence JS (1955) Rheumatism in coal miners. III: Occupational factors. Br J Ind Med 12:249–251
11. Lindberg H, Montgomery F (1987) Heavy labor and the occurrence of gonarthrosis. Clin Orthop 214:235–236
12. Partridge REH, Duthie OR (1968) Rheumatism in dockers and civil servants: A comparison of heavy manual and sedentary workers. Ann Rheum Dis 27:559–568
13. Thelin A (1990) Hip joint arthrosis: An occupational disorder among farmers. Am J Ind Med 18:339–343
14. Vingard E, Alfredsson L, Goldie I, et al. (1991b) Occupation and osteoarthrosis of the hip and knee. Int T Epidemiol 20:1025–1031
15. Klunder KB, Rud B, Hansen J (1980) Osteoarthritis of the hip and knee joint in retired football players. Acta Orthop Scand 51:925–927
16. Lindberg H, Roos H, Gardsell P (1993) Prevalence of coxarthrosis in former soccer players. Acta Orthop Scand 64:165–167
17. Vingard E, Alfredsson L, Goldie I, et al. (1993) Sports and osteoarthrosis of the hip. Am J Sports Med 21:195–200
18. Kujala U, Kaprio J, Srna S (1994) Osteoarthritis of weight bearing joints of lower limbs in former elite male athletes. Br Med J 308:231–234
19. Lequesne MG, Dang N, Lane NE (1997) Sport practice and osteoarthritis of the limbs. Osteoarthritis Cart 5:75–86
20. Marti B, Knobloch M, Tschopp A, et al. (1989) Is excessive running predictive of degenerative hip disease? Controlled study of former elite athletes. Br Med J 299:91–93
21. Roos H (1994) Exercise, knee injury and osteoarthrosis. Doctoral Dissertation, University of Lund, Sweden
22. Lohmander LS, Dahlberg L, Ryd L, Heinegård D (1989) Increased levels of proteoglycan fragments in knee joint fluid after injury. Arthritis Rheum 32:1434–1442
23. Kurosawa H, Fukudayashi T, Makajima H (1980) Load bearing mode of the knee joint: Physical behaviour of the knee joint with or without menisci. Clin Orthop 149:283–290
24. Seedhom BB, Hargreaves DJ (1979) Transmission of the load in the knee joint with special reference to the role of the menisci. Eng Med 8:220–228
25. Shrive NG, O'Connor JJ, Goodfellow JW (1978) Weight bearing in the knee joint. Clin Orthop 131:279–287
26. De Haven KE (1985) Meniscectomy versus repair: Clinical experience. In: Mow VC, Arnosky SR, Jackson DW (eds) Knee meniscus basic and clinical foundations. Raven Press, NY, pp 131–139
27. Helfet AJ (1959) Mechanism of derangements of the medial semi-lunar cartilage and their management. J Bone Joint Surg (Br) 41B:319–355
28. Konradsen L, Hansen EMB, Sondergaard L (1990) Long distance running and osteoarthrosis. Am J Sports Med 18:379–381
29. Lane NE, Buckwalter JA (1993a) Exercise: A cause of osteoarthritis? Rheum Dis Clin North Am 19:617–633
30. Lane NE, Michel B, Bjorkengren A, et al. (1993b) The risk of osteoarthritis with running and ageing: A 5-year longitudinal study. J Rheumatol 20:461–468
31. Lane NE, Bloch DA, Jones HH, et al. (1986) Long-distance running, bone density, and osteoarthritis. J Am Med Assoc 255:1147–1151

32. Lane NE, Bloch DA, Wood PD, et al. (1987) Aging, long-distance running, and the development of musculoskeletal disability. Am J Med 82:772–780
33. Panush RS, Schmidt C, Caldwell JR, et al. (1986) Is running associated with degenerative joint disease. J Am Med Assoc 255:1152–1154
34. Puranen J, Ala-Keltola L, Peltokallio P, et al. (1975) Running and primary osteoarthritis of the hip. Br Med J 285:424–425
35. Sohn RS, Lyle MJ (1987) The effect of running on the pathogenesis of osteoarthritis of the hips and knees. Clin Orthop 198:106–109
36. Newton PM, Mow VC, Gardner TR, et al. (1997) The effect of life-long exercise on canine articular cartilage. J Sports Med 25:292–287
37. Kiviranta I, Jurvelin J, Tammi M, Säämänen AM, Helminen HJ (1987) Weight bearing controls glycosaminoglycan concentration and articular-cartilage thickness in the knee joints of young beagle dogs. Arthritis Rheum 30:801–809
38. Kiviranta I, Tammi M, Jurvelin J, et al. (1988) Moderate running exercise augments glycosaminoglycans and thickness of articular cartilage in the knee joint of young beagle dogs. J Orthop Res 6:188–195
39. Säämänen A-M, Kiviranta I, Jurvelin J, Helminen HJ, Tammi M (1994) Proteoglycan and collagen alterations in canine knee articular cartilage following 20 km daily running exercise for 15 weeks. Connect Tissue Res 30:191–201
40. Kiviranta I, Tammi M, Jurvelin J, et al. (1992) Articular cartilage thickness and glycosaminoglycan distribution in the canine knee joint after strenuous running exercise. Clin Orthop 283:302–308
41. Arokoski J, Kiviranta I, Jurvelin J, et al. (1993) Long-distance running causes site-dependent decrease of the cartilage glycosaminoglycan content in the knee joint of beagle dogs. Arthritis Rheum 36:1451–1459
42. Arokoski J, Jurvelin J, Kiviranta I, et al. (1994) Softening of the lateral condylar articular cartilage in the canine knee joint after long distance (up to 40 km/day) running training lasting one year. Int J Sports Med 15:254–260
43. Helminen HJ, et al. (1992) Subchondral bone and articular cartilage responses to long distance running training (40 km per day) in the beagle knee joint. Eur J Exp Musculoskel Res 1:145–154
44. Arokoski J, Hyttinen MM, Lapvetelainen T, et al. (1996) Decreased birefringence of the superficial zone collagen network in the canine knee (stifle) articular cartilage after long distance running training, detected by quantitative polarized light microscopy. Ann Rheum 55:253–264
45. Little C, Smith S, Ghosh P, Bellenger C (1997) Histomorphological and immunohistochemical evaluation of joint changes in a model of osteoarthritis induced by lateral meniscectomy in sheep. J Rheumatol 24:2199–2209
46. McIlwraith CW (1982) Current concepts in equine degenerative joint disease. J Am Vet Med Assoc 180:239–250
47. Brown DC, Vogel KG (1989) Characteristics of the *in vitro* interaction of a small proteoglycan (PG II) of bovine tendon with type I collagen. Matrix 9:468–478
48. Kresse H, Hausser H, Schönherr E (1993) Small proteoglycans. Experientia 49:403–416
50. Yamaguchi Y, Mann DM, Ruoslahti E (1990) Negative regulation of transforming growth factor-β by the proteoglycan decorin. Nature 346:281–284
51. Rechberger T, Woessner (Jr) JF (1993) Collagenase, its inhibitors, and decorin in the lower uterine segment in pregnant women. Am J Obstet Gynecol 168:1598–1603
51a. Vogel KG, Trotter JA (1987) The effect of proteoglycans on the morphology of collagen fibrils formed in vitro. Collagen Rel Res 7:105–114
52. Korver THV, van de Stadt RJ, Kiljan E, van Kampen GP, van der Korst JK (1992) Effects of loading on the synthesis of proteoglycans in different layers of anatomically intact articular cartilage in vitro. J Rheumatol 19:905–912
53. Visser NA, Vankampen GP, Dekoning MH, Vanderkorst JK (1994a) Mechanical loading affects the synthesis of decorin and biglycan in intact immature articular cartilage in vitro. Int J Tiss Reac 16:195–203

54. Visser NA, Vankampen GP, Dekoning MH, Vanderkorst JK (1994b) The effects of loading on the synthesis of biglycan and decorin in intact mature articular cartilage in vitro. Connect Tissue Res 30:241–250

55. Dourado GS, Adams ME, Matyas JR, Huang D (1996) Expression of biglycan, decorin and fibromodulin in the hypertrophic phase of experimental osteoarthritis. Osteoarthritis Cart 4:187–196

56. Little CB, Ghosh P, Bellenger CR (1996) Topographic variation in biglycan and decorin synthesis by articular cartilage in the early stages of osteoarthritis: An experimental study in sheep. J Orthop Res 14:433–444

57. Little CB, Ghosh P, Rose R (1997) The effect of strenuous versus moderate exercise on the metabolism of proteoglycans in articular cartilage from different weight-bearing regions of the equine third carpal bone. Osteoarthritis Cart 5:161–172

58. Appel H (1970) Late results after meniscectomy in the knee joint. A clinical and roentgenological follow-up. Acta Orthop Scand 133(Suppl):89–99

59. Johnson RJ, Kettelkamp DB, Clark W, Leaverton P (1974) Factors affecting late results after meniscectomy. J Bone Joint Surg (Am) 56:719–729

60. Tapper EM, Hoover NW (1969) Late results after meniscectomy. J Bone Joint Surg (Am) 51 A:517–526

61. Colombo C, Butler M, O'Byrne E, Hickman L, Swartzendruber D, Selwyn M, Steinetz B (1983) Development of knee joint pathology following lateral meniscectomy and section of the fibular collateral and sesamoid ligaments. Arthritis Rheum 26:875–886

62. Cox JS, Cordell LD (1977) The degenerative effects of medial meniscus tears in dogs' knees. Clin Orthop 125:236–242

63. Ghosh P, Sutherland JM, Taylor TKF, Petti GD, Bellenger CR (1983) The effects of postoperative joint immobilisation on articular cartilage degeneration following meniscectomy. J Surg Res 35:461–472

64. Armstrong S, Read R, Ghosh P (1994) The effects of intraarticular hyaluronan on cartilage and subchondral bone changes in an ovine model of early osteoarthritis. J Rheumatol 21:680–688

65. Ghosh P, Sutherland, Bellenger C, et al. (1990) The influence of weight-bearing exercise on articular cartilage of meniscectomised joints. Clin Orthop 252:101–113

66. Ghosh P, Read R, Armstrong S, Wilson D, Marshall R, McNair P (1993a) The effects of intra-articular administration of hyaluronan in a model of early osteoarthritis in sheep. I. Gait analysis, radiological and morphological studies. Sem Arthritis Rheum 22(Suppl 1): 18–30

67. Ghosh P, Read R, Numata Y, Smith S, Armstrong S, Wilson D (1993b) The effects of intra-articular administration of hyaluronan in a model of early osteoarthritis in sheep. II. Biochemical Studies. Sem Arthritis Rheum 22(Suppl 1):31–42

68. Ghosh P, Wells C, Numata Y, Read R, Armstrong S (1993c) The effects of orally administered tiaprofenic acid on the biosynthesis of proteoglycans in ex vivo cartilage cultures from joints of animals with early osteoarthritis. Curr Therap Res 54:703–713

69. Ghosh P, Numata Y, Smith S, Read R, Armstrong S, Johnson K (1993d) The metabolic response of articular cartilage to abnormal mechanical loading induced by medial or lateral meniscectomy. Joint Destruction in Arthritis and Osteoarthritis AAS 39: 89–93

70. Ghosh P, Xu Q, Little C, Robinson B (1997) Up-regulation of decorin mRNA in cartilage of an ovine model of osteoarthritis. Trans Orthop Res Soc 22:171

71. Ghosh P, Xu A, Hwa S-Y, Burkhardt D, Little C (1998a) Evaluation of the protective effects of diacerhein on cartilage and subchondral bone in an ovine model of osteoarthritis. La Revue du Praticien (in press)

72. Poole AR, Rosenberg LC, Reiner A, Ionescu M, Bogoch E, Roughley PJ (1996) Contents and distribution of the proteoglycans decorin and biglycan in normal and osteoarthritic human articular cartilage. J Orthop Res 14:681–689

73. Ghosh P, Xu A, Little C (1998b) Modulation of matrix metalloproteinase activities in osteoarthritic cartilage by calcium xylopyranose polysulphate (submitted for publication)

74. Birkedal-Hansen H, Moore WGI, Bodden MK, Windsor LJ, Birkedal-Hansen B, DeCarlo A, Engler JA (1993) Matrix metalloproteinases: A review. Crit Rev Oral Biol 4:197–250

75. Sandy JD, Flannery CR, Neame PJ, Lohmander LS (1992) The structure of aggrecan fragments in human synovial fluids. Evidence for the involvement in osteoarthritis of a novel proteinase which cleaves the Glu373- Ala374 bond in the interglobular domain. J Clin Invest 89:1512–1516

76. Lark MW, Gordy JT, Weidner JR, Ayala J, Kimura JH, Williams HR, Mumford RA, Flannery CR, Carlson SS, Kwata M (1995) Cell-mediated catabolism of aggrecan. Evidence that cleavage at the "Aggrecanase" site (Glu373-Ala374) is a primary event in proteolysis of the interglobular domain. J Biol Chem 270:2550–2556

77. Buttle DJ, Fowles A, Ilic MZ, Handley CJ (1997) Aggrecanase activity is implicated in tumor necrosis factor alpha mediated cartilage aggrecan breakdown but is not detected by an *in vitro* assay. J Cl Path M 50:153–159

78. Imai K, Ohta S, Matsumoto T, Fujimoto N, Sato H, Seiki M, Okada Y (1997) Expression of membrane type 1 matrix metalloproteinase and activation of progelatinase A in human osteoarthritic cartilage. Am J Path 151:245–256

79. Aigner T, Dudhia J (1997) Phenotypic modulation of chondrocytes as a potential therapeutic target in osteoarthritis: A hypothesis. Ann Rheum Dis 56:287–291

80. Brinckerhoff CE (1992) Regulation of metalloproteinase gene expression: Implications for osteoarthritis. CRC Crit Rev Euk Gene Exp 2:145–164

81. Pelletier J-P, Roughley PJ, Dibattis JA, McCollum R, Martel-Pelletier J (1991) Are cytokines involved in osteoarthritic pathophysiology. Semin Arth Rheum 20:12–25

82. Saklatvala J (1992) Regulation of chondrocytes by cytokines. In: Adolphe M (ed) Biological regulation of the chondrocytes. CRC Press, Boca Raton, Fl, USA, pp 191–204

83. Chrisman OD, Ladenbauer-Bellis IM, Panjabi M, et al. (1981) The relationship of mechanical trauma and the early biochemical reactions of osteoarthritic cartilage. Clin Orthop 161:275–284

84. de Brum-Fernandes AJ, Morisset S, Bkaily G, Patry C (1996) Characterization of the PGE2 receptor subtype in bovine chondrocytes in culture. Br J Pharmacol 118:1597–1604

85. Di Battista JA, Doré S, Martel-Pelletier J, Pelletier J-P (1996) Prostaglandin E2 stimulates incorporation of proline into collagenase digestible proteins in human articular chondrocytes: Identification of an effector autocrine loop involving insulin-like growth factor I. Mol Cell Endocrinol 123:27–35

86. Fulkerson JP, Ladenbauer-Bellis I-M, Chrisman OD (1979) In vitro hexosamine depletion of intact articular cartilage by E-prostaglandins. Prevention by chloroquine. Arthritis Rheum 22:1117–1121

87. Teitz CC, Chrisman OD (1975) The effects of salicylate and chloroquine on prostaglandin-induced articular damage in rabbit knees. Clin Orthop 108:264–274

88. Evans CH, Watkins SC, Stefanovic-Racic M (1996) Nitric oxide and cartilage metabolism. Methods Enzymol 269:75–88

89. Tiku K, Thakker-Varia S, Ramachandrula A, Tiku ML (1992) Articular chondrocytes secrete IL-1, express membrane IL-1, and have IL-1 inhibitory activity. Cell Immunol 140:1–20

4.3
Genetic and Metabolic Aspects

C. J. WILLIAMS and S. A. JIMENEZ

4.3.1
Overview

Although osteoarthritis (OA) is frequently a manifestation of mechanical or inflammatory/immunologic events, there is compelling evidence that several distinct forms are inherited as Mendelian traits. In general, the heritable osteoarthropathies can be sub-divided into conditions such as primary generalized osteoarthritis (PGOA) and some metabolic joint diseases including the crystal-associated arthropathies, and precocious osteoarthritis that is a consequence of an underlying osteochondrodysplasia. It is this latter group which has been the easier to study and in which most of the successful identification of gene mutations responsible for the disease phenotype has been accomplished to date. This review of heritable arthropathies is designed to illustrate the significant progress that has been made in our understanding of the genetics of these diseases and to demonstrate the appropriateness of a molecular genetic approach toward understanding the etiopathogenesis of the metabolic joint diseases such as calcium pyrophosphate dihydrate crystal deposition disease (CPPDD).

4.3.2
Hereditary OA: Historical Perspective and Phenotypic Spectrum

In 1803, Heberden described "little hard knots, about the size of a small pea" in the dorsal aspect of the distal interphalangeal joints of the hands. This obvious trait made it possible for him to distinguish OA from other forms of arthritis, including gout [1]. Haygarth expanded the clinical description of Heberden's nodes to include their association with the simultaneous involvement of other joints [2] and Bouchard further described bony enlargements of the proximal interphalangeal joints of the hands (Bouchard 1982). These characteristic "Heberden's and Bouchard's nodes" provided a means by which Osler was able to separate "arthritis deformans" from "hypertrophic arthritis" (Osler 1909). In 1953, Stecher and Hersh documented the familial occurrence of Heberden's nodes and concluded that the lesions were inherited in an autosomal dominant manner with a strong female sex bias [3]. Other studies rapidly followed in which familial cases of Heberden's and Bouchard's nodes associated with degenerative disease of other joints, were identified [4–10]; based on the clinical presentation and HLA typing several of these studies suggested a polygenic inheritance, rather than a single gene defect [11, 12].

The phenotypic spectrum of hereditary OA is quite varied encompassing mild disorders, which do not become clinically apparent until late adult life, to very severe forms that manifest early in childhood. Traditionally, all these forms have been classified as secondary OA. However, it is now known that several of

Table 1. Differences between hereditary OA and secondary OA

	Hereditary OA	Secondary OA
Etiology	Mutations in genes expressed in articular cartilage	Various hereditary or acquired diseases
Pathogenesis	Alterations in structural or functional components of articular cartilage	Secondary effects to diseases not exclusively affecting articular cartilage
Therapy	Possible gene therapy to correct gene defect	Treatment of primary disease

these phenotypes are caused by mutations in the genes that code for extracellular matrix macromolecules of articular cartilage. As a result, the structural integrity of the cartilage matrix may be compromised, or the regulation of chondrocyte proliferation or gene expression may be deranged. Thus, these hereditary disorders represent a truly distinct sub-group of OA that is different from secondary OA. Hereditary OA disorders include PGOA, the familial crystal-associated arthropathies, several osteochondrodysplasias (OCD), and the multiple epiphyseal dysplasias (MED). Mutations in cartilage extracellular matrix gene products have already been identified in several MEDs, and OCDs. In the discussion of the dysplastic syndromes below, we will concentrate on those disorders in which precocious onset of OA is a common clinical feature of the syndrome, and in which mutations in candidate genes have already been identified. For the crystal-associated arthropathies, progress has been made in defining loci that are linked to these phenotypes, and in some cases, gene mutations have been identified. However, for the calcium crystal arthropathies, no gene mutations have yet been described. Additional likely "candidate genes" for hereditary OA phenotypes may include proteoglycans and other non-collagenous cartilage proteins, growth factors and their receptors, and other regulatory proteins or enzymes that are involved in cartilage-specific functions.

As described above, the distinction between hereditary OA and secondary OA is not an artificial one since it is based on clear-cut differences in their etiology and pathogenesis, as well as in their course of evolution and prognosis (see Table 1). Furthermore, there are clear differences in the therapeutic approaches for these two forms of OA. Whereas in secondary OA treatment must be directed toward the primary disease, in hereditary OA the ideal treatment would be the correction of the causative gene mutation. Progress toward this end is underway in several laboratories and the prospects for gene therapy appear plausible in the near future.

4.3.3
Chondrodysplasias/Osteochondrodysplasias and Inherited Osteoarthritis

The chondrodysplasias/osteochondrodysplasias (CD/OCD) are a group of clinically heterogeneous hereditary disorders characterized by abnormalities in

Table 2. Heritable dysplasias associated with premature onset of OA

Disorder	Locus	Inheritance	Mutated Gene	Type of Mutation
Precocious OA with late-onset SED (OAP)[a]	12q13.1-q13.2	AD	COL2A1	Base substitution, splice site, deletion
Stickler syndrome (STL1)	12q13.1-q13.2	AD	COL2A1	Base substitution; splice site
Stickler syndrome (STL2)	6p21.3	AD	COL11A2	Splice site; deletion
Stickler syndrome	1p21	AD	COL11A1	Base substitution
Wagner syndrome	12q13.1-q13.2	AD	COL2A1	Base substitution
OSMED	6p21.3	AR	COL11A2	Base substitution
Marshall syndrome	1p21	AD	COL11A1	Splice site
Kniest dysplasia	12q13.1-q13.2	AD	COL2A1	Splice site; deletion
MED (EDM 1)	19p13.1	AD	COMP	Base substitution; (deletion in PASCH)
MED (EDM 2)	1p32.2-p33	AD	COL9A2	Splice site
MCD Schmid (MCDS)	6q21-q22.3	AD	COL10A1	Base substitution; deletion
MCD Jansen (MCDJ)	3p21.2-p21.3	AD	PTHR1	Base substitution

AD, autosomal dominant; AR, autosomal recessive.
[a] Locus symbol.

the growth and development of articular and growth plate cartilages. Among the CD/OCD, several distinct entities are more likely to result in premature OA. The term "chondrodysplastic rheumatism" has been coined to refer to these forms of OA [13]. Those CD/OCD that are frequently accompanied by the premature onset and often severe clinical course of osteoarthritis include the spondyloepiphyseal dysplasias, Stickler syndrome and its variants, Kniest dysplasia, the multiple epiphyseal dysplasias, the metaphyseal chondrodysplasias, and some oto-spondylomegaepiphyseal dysplasias (see below). The CD/OCD present with radiological changes that make them distinct from the non-dysplastic forms of inherited osteoarthritis. Also, expression of the phenotype occurs relatively early in life; most are inherited as dominant traits and are fully penetrant. These characteristics facilitate the distinction of the phenotypes and identification of affected families. A summary of the genetic characteristics of various chondro- and osteochondrodysplasias that give rise to precocious (and often severe) OA is depicted in Table 2.

4.3.3.1
Spondyloepiphyseal Dysplasia (SED)

The SED comprise a heterogeneous group of autosomal dominant disorders characterized by abnormal development of the axial skeleton and severe alterations of the epiphyses of the long bones often resulting in dwarfism. Congenital

SED is an autosomal dominant disorder and is usually clinically severe, with marked shortening of the trunk and, to a lesser extent, of the extremeties [14–18]. However, in the late-onset form, the phenotype is often far less severe and may not be clinically apparent until affected individuals present with severe OA in adolescence. Deformity of the lumbar spine may be manifested with disc space narrowing, platyspondyly and mild kyphoscoliosis. There may be mild epiphyseal abnormalities in peripheral joints and early degenerative changes are present in multiple joints. The most constant features of peripheral joint involvement include flattening of the articular surfaces of the ankles and the knees, and shallowness of the femoral intercondylar notches. Deformities of the femoral head and neck are commonly observed and hip OA may develop in adolescence, worsening in early adulthood.

Since type II collagen is the major constituent of hyaline cartilage, the gene which codes for it, COL2A1, was originally suspected in the development of chondrodysplasias such as SED. Initial descriptions of genetic linkage between the phenotype of precocious OA/late-onset SED and the type II procollagen gene (COL2A1) were made in 1989 and 1990 [19, 20]. The first report of a COL2A1 mutation in a precocious OA/mild SED kindred was a heterozygous Arg519 → Cys base substitution [21]. Four additional families with an identical mutation have now been identified [22]. A second dominant Arg → Cys base substitution, at position 75 of the type II collagen triple helix, has been identifed in another kindred with precocious OA and mild SED [23], although the SED phenotype in the affected members of the family carrying this mutation is not identical to that seen in the Arg519 mutation kindreds. However, like the Arg519 mutation, the Arg75 mutation has been shown to exist in an additional, presumably unrelated, family [24]. Other kindreds with mild chondrodysplasias and precocious osteoarthritis have also been found to display mutations in COL2A1; these mutations include a dominant Gly976 → Ser mutation [23] and a Gly493 → Ser heterozygous base substitution [25]. Interestingly, several other point mutations near to these positions have been reported in the more severe phenotypes of SED congenita and achondrogenesis II/hypochondrogenesis (see [26] for review), and the term "type II collagenopathies" has been used to describe hereditary cartilage diseases in which the primary defects are mutations in COL2A1 [27]. Clearly, the position and nature of the substituted amino acid ultimately affects the severity of the phenotype in these dominant disorders.

4.3.3.2
Stickler Syndrome and Its Variants

The classic form of Stickler syndrome was originally described in 1965 and was termed hereditary arthro-ophthalmopathy [28]. It is characterized by prominent ocular involvement and severe degenerative joint disease which often develops in the third or fourth decade. It is an autosomal dominant condition with a prevalence of approximately 1 in 10,000 births. Associated clinical symptoms include myopia, progressive sensorineural hearing loss, cleft palate and mandibular hypoplasia (Pierre-Robin anomaly), and epiphyseal dysplasia.

Radiographic studies of affected joints from patients with Stickler syndrome in the neonatal period show enlarged epiphyses, particularly of the proximal femur and distal tibia. With growth, epiphyseal dysplasia develops with irregular ossification of the epiphyses and subsequent progressive degenerative changes. In the spine, there is often mild irregular platyspondyly with endplate irregularity and anterior wedging.

COL2A1 was also a likely candidate gene in early studies of the molecular defect in Stickler syndrome because of its expression both in articular cartilage and the vitreous of the eye. Linkage analyses of several Stickler syndrome kindreds showed that the disease is linked to COL2A1 in some, but not all, affected families [29–31]. The mutations in COL2A1 that have been identified in Stickler kindreds have resulted in the generation of a stop codon in the coding region of COL2A1 due to base substitution, or from frame shifts caused by insertions, deletions, or splice site mutation (for review see [26]). Of historical interest is the fact that the COL2A1 mutation in the original kindred described by Stickler in 1965 was shown to result from a base substitution in the 3′ splice acceptor site of intron 17 and the utilization of a cryptic splice site in exon 18, giving rise to a deletion of 16 basepairs of exon 18. The resultant frame shift eventually generates a stop codon [32]. The form of Stickler syndrome that is caused by mutations in COL2A1 is now referred to as type 1 (MIM 108 300; locus symbol: STL1)

The clinical spectrum of Stickler syndrome is varied, and different subset phenotypes have now been distinguished. Among these is Wagner syndrome (MIM 143 200), which is characterized by predominant ocular involvement and virtually no osteoarticular alterations. Nonetheless, in a patient with Wagner syndrome, a COL2A1 dominant mutation (Gly67 → Asp) was detected [33]. Why this particular substitution in COL2A1 would compromise the function of vitreous tissue but not hyaline cartilage is unclear. Another variant of Stickler syndrome was also recently described in a Dutch kindred that displayed all the features of classical Stickler syndrome except ocular involvement. In this case, linkage to the COL2A1 locus was excluded and other cartilage-expressed extracellular matrix proteins were examined, including the genes for type XI collagen. This collagen is closely associated with type II collagen in the thin fibrils of hyaline cartilage. Brunner et al. demonstrated that the phenotype in the Dutch family was linked to the COL11A2 locus [34]. The dominant mutation was shown to be a splice site abnormality that resulted in a 54 basepair in-frame deletion, and the subsequent deletion of an exon [35]. This finding made COL11A2 the second locus in Stickler syndrome and this phenotype is now referred to as Stickler syndrome type II (MIM 184 840; locus symbol: STL2). The role of COL11A2 in the etiopathogenesis of non-ocular Stickler syndrome has been confirmed by the finding of a second, unrelated family with clinical manifestations similar to the Dutch family, in which the observed phenotype is caused by a heterozygous 27 basepair deletion in the COL11A2 gene (Sirko-Osadsa et al. 1998). Finally, a third locus for Stickler syndrome has now been identified in a family with a variant of Stickler syndrome exhibiting vitreoretinal changes that were phenotypically distinct from those seen in classic Stickler syndrome. In affected members of this family, a heterozygous base substitution in the COL11A1 gene (Gly97 → Val) was detected [36]. It has been postulated that mutations in COL11A2 lead to the Stickler syndrome variant that displays no ocular involvement, whereas mutations in COL11A1 lead to a Stickler syndrome variant with ocular changes that are distinct from classic Stickler syndrome. Clearly, more cases will need to be examined to determine if this phenotype/genotype trend is confirmed.

Marshall syndrome has long been the subject of controversy concerning its nosologic relationship to classic Stickler syndrome. It has now been classified as a distinct phenotype, in large part due to a greater degree of facial skeletal deformity. Marshall syndrome, however, displays substantial clinical overlap with classic Stickler syndrome especially with regard to joint manifestations. A family with Marshall syndrome has recently been described in which early onset (4th decade) symptomatic osteoarthritis affecting the knees and lumbosacral spine was present. Radiographic findings included narrowed joint spaces, with osteophytic degeneration in the hips and knees. Interestingly, in this family the clinical phenotype was associated with a splicing defect in the COL11A1 gene, causing the deletion of 18 amino acids from the triple helical domain of the $\alpha 1$(XI) collagen chain [37]. These results suggest that Marshall syndrome and Stickler syndrome associated with COL11A1 mutations are allelic; however, the differences in the severity of their respective phenotypes would suggest that COL11A1 mutations in Marshall syndrome are more disruptive to protein structure that those in Stickler syndrome.

4.3.3.3
Other Osteochondrodysplasias (OCD)

Another OCD that exhibits precocious and severe OA, and in which a mutation in an extracellular matrix protein has been demonstrated, is a recessive disorder that closely resembles otospondylomegaepiphyseal dysplasia (OSMED; MIM 215150). This phenotype was described in another Dutch family in which severe degenerative joint changes, resembling osteoarthritis, presented in early adulthood and occurred predominantly in the hips, knees, elbows and shoulders. There was also increased lumbar lordosis and prominent interphalangeal joints. The affected members had distinctive facial features and sensorineural hearing loss; however, no ocular abnormalities were observed. In this family, linkage to COL11A2, the gene coding for the alpha 2 chain of type II collagen, was demonstrated. The mutation was shown to be a G to A transition that converted a glycine codon to an arginine codon in both alleles of the gene. The mutation occurred in a gly-X-Y triplet of the helical region of type XI collagen [35] and is a rare example of a recessive mutation in the OA/dysplasia syndromes.

Kniest dysplasia (MIM 156550) is a disorder characterized by an autosomal dominant pattern of inheritance displaying shortening of the trunk and limbs, flattening of the face and nosebridge, protuberance of the eye globes and severe joint abnormalities [38, 39]. The joints are usually very large at birth and continue to enlarge during childhood and early adolescence. Myopia, hearing loss, cleft palate, and clubfoot are common, and the majority of affected individuals develop severe, premature degenerative joint disease which is prominent in the knees and hips. On radiographs, the vertebral bodies are flat, irregular and markedly elongated; the findings in the spine include irregular platyspondyly and anterior wedging. The long bones are dumb-bell shaped with marked delay in epiphyseal ossification and the metaphyses display irregularity with cloud-like defects on both sides of the epiphyseal plate. The joints in the hands display flattened and squared epiphyses with joint space narrowing. The articular cartilage is soft and has decreased resiliency, and, histologically, shows large cystic lesions giving a typical appearance that has been compared to that of Swiss cheese. Since large inclusions in the rough endoplasmic reticulum have been found to contain the carboxyl propeptide of type II collagen, it was originally suggested that the disorder results from abnormalities in the processing of type II procollagen [40]. We now know that most of the cases of Kniest dysplasia that have been studied to date demonstrate mutations in the gene that codes for type II procollagen. These mutations include splicing defects resulting in deletions and exon skipping, and partial gene deletions [41–44].

4.3.4
Multiple Epiphyseal Dysplasias (MED)

The MED are a heterogeneous group of disorders characterized by alterations in epiphyseal growth that subsequently cause irregularity and fragmentation of the epiphyses of multiple long bones. Characteristically, spinal alterations are minimal (limited to the occurrence of irregular end-plates with varying degrees of flattening of vertebral bodies) or absent. The epiphyseal abnormalities often result in precocious, crippling OA of both weight-bearing and non-weight bearing joints. MED is inherited in an autosomal dominant manner with a high degree of penetrance. These diseases include various phenotypes such as those described by Fairbanks [45] and Ribbing [46]. The MEDs are characterized by abnormalities in the development of the epiphyseal growth plates of long bones. These abnormalities are usually multiple and symmetric, particularly involving the knees, hips, hands, wrists and shoulders. Most of the affected individuals develop symptoms in early childhood with pain and stiffness in multiple joints, and abnormal gait. These symptoms become progressively more severe and joint alterations evolve relentlessly into severe degenerative arthritis. Although there is no marked dwarfism, affected individuals are usually shorter than their unaffected siblings. There are no ocular or retinal abnormalities. Characteristic radiographic features include irregularity of multiple epiphyses predominantly at the knees, hips, and shoulders. Centers of ossification are fragmented and irregular and appear later than usual. The capital femoral epiphyses are nearly always involved and the femoral heads become subsequently more flattened.

As abnormalities in the epiphyseal growth plate are the hallmark of MED, it was suspected that a defect in one of the genes encoding growth plate cartilage macromolecules may be responsible for the disease. We now know that there are at least three loci that are linked to the MED phenotype. Linkage analyses of some families with MED, and of the clinically related pseudoachondroplasia

(PSACH) syndrome, excluded the genes for collagen types II and VI, chondroitin sulfate proteoglycan core protein, and cartilage link protein [47, 48]. However, close linkage of these two diseases to the pericentromeric region of chromosome 19 was observed in some families [49, 50]. Subsequent studies identified mutations in the gene encoding the cartilage oligomeric protein (COMP) in three patients affected with MED/pseudoachondroplasia (locus symbol: EDM 1; [51]). Because the three mutations occurred in a region of the gene encoding the calcium binding domain in COMP, it is likely that the calcium binding function of the protein is essential for the normal development of growth plate cartilage. In a Dutch family, linkage to a region of chromosome 1 containing one of the genes for type IX collagen (locus symbol EDM 2) was demonstrated [52]. In this family, a heterozygous splice site mutation in COL9A2 was demonstrated [53]; the mutation resulted in exon skipping and an in-frame loss of 12 amino acids. Although type IX collagen was known to be located on the surface of type II collagen fibrils, the finding of a mutation associated with a disease phenotype for this particular collagen was the first evidence of its role in maintaining the integrity of hyaline cartilage. Further genetic heterogeneity of MED was demonstrated when a family with the Fairbanks type MED did not show linkage of their disease phenotype to either the EDM 1 or EDM 2 loci [54]; no other locus linked to the observed phenotype has yet been identified in this family.

4.3.5
Metaphyseal Chondrodysplasias (MCD)

The metaphyseal chondrodysplasias [55–57] are another family of heritable cartilage disorders that may present with precocious OA. These disorders are heterogeneous (over 150 types have been described) and are characterized by intrinsic alterations of metaphyseal bone. Clinical features include short stature with short limbs, bowed legs, and a waddling gait. There may also be manifestations reflecting abnormalities in other organ systems such as the immune and digestive systems. The growth plate cartilage is highly disorganized, displaying clusters of proliferating and hypertrophic chondrocytes surrounded by thickened septa and disorganized matrix, with unmineralized cartilage extending into the subchondral bone.

Three of the most well-characterized syndromes within this group are the Jansen, Schmid and McKusick types. The skeletal abnormalities are similar in all three groups but they differ in their degree of severity (Jansen > McKusick > Schmidt). The Schmid type (locus symbol: MCDS) is the most common and displays an autosomal dominant mode of inheritance. The radiographic features include coxa vara, shortening and bowing of the tubular bones, and cupping and fraying of the metaphyses with more pronounced proximal than distal femoral involvement. The most prominent alterations occur in the growth plates of long bones which are irregular, disorganized, and markedly widened, especially at the knees.

To date, at least 17 mutations in the gene for type X collagen have been characterized in the Schmid type metaphyseal chondrodysplasia. Type X collagen is expressed almost exclusively in hypertrophic chondrocytes of the growth plate and probably plays a role in endochondral ossification [58]. Thus, the gene encoding this collagen type (COL10A1) has been an obvious candidate. All of the mutations identified have been in the region of the gene that codes for the carboxyl terminus of the protein and include missense, nonsense, and deletion mutations (for review, see [26]). The carboxyl terminus of the protein is important for chain association and the mutations presumably decrease the amount of type X collagen that is synthesized and secreted by hypertrophic chondrocytes.

In Jansen metaphyseal chondrodysplasia (locus symbol: MCDJ), hypercalcemia was noted in childhood cases [59]. A number of biochemical indices of bone turnover were assessed and, despite hypercalcemia, elevated urinary phosphate and suppressed values of parathyroid hormone and PTH-related peptide were found. In 1994, Karaplis et al. disrupted the gene encoding PTH-related peptide in murine embryonic stem cells by homologous recombination. Mice homozygous for the null allele died postnatally and exhibited widespread abnormalities in subchondral bone development. Cartilage growth was disturbed and chondrocyte proliferation was decreased [60]. These findings suggested that PTH-related pathways were probably the cause of Jansen type metaphyseal chondrodysplasia. In 1995, Schipani et al. demonstrated the first heterozygous mutation in the PTH receptor gene in a patient with this disorder [61]. The mutation was a *de novo* His223 to Arg substitution which led to ligand-independent cAMP accumulation, thus indicating that the His223 residue has a critical role in signal transduction [62]. Two other Jansen patients were found to harbor the same mutation and a third patient displayed a novel Thr410 to Pro mutation. Interestingly, in two patients with radiologic evidence of the Jansen type metaphyseal chondrodysplasia, but with less severe hypercalcemia, no receptor mutations were detected [63], suggesting the potential for locus heterogeneity.

4.3.6
Primary Generalized OA (PGOA)

The most common form of inherited, non-dysplastic OA is PGOA which was first described as a discrete clinical entity in 1952 [4]. PGOA is characterized by the development of Heberden's and Bouchard's nodes and premature degeneration of the articular cartilage of multiple joints [7, 10]. Typically, the clinical and radiologic features have a precocious onset and accelerated progression. The loss of articular cartilage in PGOA is concentric or uniform, particularly in the knees and hips [5, 64, 65]. This pattern of cartilage loss is not constant and the radiographic appearance of affected joints is indistinguishable from that of non-hereditary OA, except for its premature occurrence, increased severity, and rapid progression. In the hand, the pattern of distribution favors the distal and proximal interphalangeal joints, with prominent bone reaction resulting in formation of Heberden's and Bouchard's nodes, and with frequent involvement of the first carpometacarpal joint. Degenerative changes of the hip typically develop early in adult life. The femoral heads tend to become flattened as the disease progresses. Sclerosis, pseudocysts, and femoral head deformity are seen with advanced disease and usually occur more rapidly than in sporadic OA.

Although there is controversy regarding the etiopathogenesis of PGOA, multiple studies have shown that a genetic predisposition plays an important role in its development and progression [5–8, 66]. One study found that Heberden's and Bouchard's nodes were present in 36% of the relatives of males and in 49% of relatives of females with PGOA in comparison to expected frequencies in the general population of 17% and 26%, respectively [7]. The frequency of nodal generalized OA increased to 45% if only first degree female relatives of individuals with nodal OA were studied. The familial pattern of PGOA is also supported by studies that examined the inheritance of various genetic markers in affected individuals with PGOA and in their non-affected relatives. For example, a genetic predisposition to the disease was suggested by the demonstration of an increased frequency of the HLA A1 B8 haplotype [12, 67], and of the MZ isoform of αl antitrypsin [67]. More recently, the relative contribution of genetic and environmental factors to OA affecting the hands and knees was investigated employing a classic twin study [68]. In this study, 130 identical and 120 non-identical female twins were examined radiographically for the presence of OA changes in hands and knees. The results demonstrated a clear genetic influence on the development of PGOA with a calculated score for heritability influence ranging from 40 to 70%, independent of known environmental or demographic confounders. The concordance of radiographic changes of OA at all sites examined was consistently two-fold higher in identical twins compared to the non-identical pair, providing convincing evidence for the hereditary nature of the disease. Finally, in a recent study of nodal arthritis, evidence for earlier disease onset, increased severity of disease in offspring, and negative correlation between the age of disease onset and parental age at conception, suggested that genetic anticipation may occur in nodal OA of the hands [69]. Since the mechanism for genetic anticipation is expansion of trinucleotide repeats (likely due to somatic and/or germline mitotic instability), the authors suggested that a search of trinucleotide repeat regions may be warranted.

4.3.7
Etiology of Metabolic Joint Diseases: Crystal-Associated Arthropathies

Among the crystal-associated arthropathies, the deposition of uric acid crystals and calcium-containing crystals in joint spaces has been shown to occur as familial conditions. However, the contribution of heredity to these relatively common arthropathies remains unclear. For example, gout is probably the most common cause of joint inflammation; however, gout is actually a heterogeneous group of disorders that results when the end products of purine metabolism supersaturate extracellular fluids. The monosodium urate crystals that precipitate from these fluids can deposit in a variety of connective tissues. Hyperuricemia can be caused by increased biosynthesis or urate production resulting from a variety of inherited disorders such as hypoxanthine guanine phosphoribosyl transferase (HPRT) deficiency (locus

Table 3. Heritable Crystal-associated Arthropathies

Disorder	Locus	Inheritance	Mutated Gene	Type of Mutation
Gout (HPRT-related)[a]	Xq27	X-linked	HPRT1	Base substitution, deletion
Gout (PRPS-related)	Xq22-q24	X-linked	PRPS1	Base substitution
primary CPPDD (CCAL1)	5p15.1-p15.2	AD	?	?
precocious OA/CPPDD (CCAL2)	8q	AD	?	?

AD, autosomal dominant.
[a] Locus symbol.

symbol: HPRT1) or phosphoribosyl pyrophosphate synthetase (locus symbol: PRPS1) superactivity. Both these disorders are inherited as X-linked traits. However, inherited disorders caused by deficiencies of these two enzymes are rare, and most cases of hyperuricemia result from non-hereditary clinical disorders that lead to purine over-production or decreased renal clearance of urate. Likewise, those arthropathies that are associated with the deposition of calcium pyrophosphate dihydrate and/or basic calcium phosphate crystals may occur as late-stage events in the course of degenerative joint disease, or as arthropathies secondary to other metabolic disorders. Nevertheless, in an effort to be consistent with our focus on genetic aspects of OA, the discussion below will concentrate on the etiology of heritable metabolic joint disorders that are characterized by the deposition of crystalline species, including monosodium urate, calcium pyrophosphate dihydrate and hydroxyapatite, in the joint space. A summary of genetic characteristics of some heritable crystal-associated arthropathies is shown in Table 3.

4.3.7.1
Gout

In its most severe form, an absolute deficiency of HPRT results in Lesch-Nyhan syndrome, with features that include mental retardation, spastic cerebral palsy, and self-destructive behavior, in addition to hyperuricemia [70]. However, multiple reports of partial HPRT deficiency have documented a phenotype that is referred to as HPRT-related gout. One of the earliest reports of this phenotype described 5 male patients in two families. In one family, two brothers displayed nephrolithiasis at the ages of 6 and 7 years, followed by gouty arthritis at the age of 13 years. In the second family, acute gouty arthritis began between the ages of 20 and 31 years in the three affected brothers [71]. With the advent of molecular techniques, it has become clear that most cases of HPRT-related gout result from base substitution mutations in the HPRT1 gene (see [72] and [73] for a review of HPRT1 mutations that cause human disease). In one case, however, the phenotype resulted from a 13 basepair deletion in the 5' untranslated region of the HPRT1 gene [74]. This deletion included the first nucleotide of the initiation codon, leading to inappropriate downstream, in-frame initiation. Because of a lack of information about the three dimensional structure of the HPRT protein, it is difficult to determine structure-function correlations that result from various mutations, but clearly some mutations have far more devastating functional consequences than others.

PRPS1 superactivity, described in 1972 as a familial disorder associated with gout [75], may be due to defects in the allosteric regulation of phosphoribosyl pyrophosphate synthetase (PRPS), or due to an inherited catalytic superactivity. With respect to the former mechanism, at least 8 allelic variants of the disorder have been reported. Each variant resulted from a base substitution that changed the amino acid encoded by PRPS1 messenger RNA [72, 76–78]. In some cases, the functional consequence of the mutation extended beyond gouty arthritis symptoms to include neurodevelopmental anomalies [76]. In the latter mechanism, where regulation of enzyme activity by nucleotide inhibitors is normal, as are affinities for substrates and activators, there are no detectable alterations in the coding sequence for PRPS1. It appears, therefore, that the catalytic superactivity of PRPS may reflect increased intracellular concentrations of the normal PRPS1 isoform, suggesting that a pre- or post-translational mechanism may be responsible for regulating expression of PRPS in affected (and mutation-free) patients [78].

4.7.3.2
Calcium Pyrophosphate Dihydrate Deposition Disease (CPPDD)

In 1958, Zitnan and Sitaj presented case studies of 27 patients with what they referred to as articular chondrocalcinosis [79, 80]. Most of the patients were members of five families, suggesting that the disease had a strong hereditary component. McCarty and Hollander later reported on two cases of non-urate associated crystal deposition in the joints of patients thought to have gout [81]. Radiographic examination of the joints in these and other patients revealed distinctive and abnormal calcifications in and around hyaline articulate cartilage and fibrocartilage of numerous joints. The arthropathy of CPPDD (calcium pyrophosphate dihydrate crystal deposition disease) radiographically resembles non-hereditary, sporadic OA but its distribution is distinctive; it occurs in sites less commonly involved in the usual form of OA such as the metacarpophalangeal, radioscaphoid, and patellofemoral articulations [82]. Subchondral cysts are more common, frequently being numerous and large.

Following the initial description of CPPDD in the five Czech families, multiple ethnic series were reported from throughout the world [84–96]. Most familial cases appeared to be inherited in an autosomal dominant manner with precocious onset and severe clinical expression. The radiographic features included crystal deposition in the knee, symphysis pubis, and triangular fibrocartilage of the wrist [82, 97].

Although most familial cases of chondrocalcinosis display crystal deposition prior to the onset of degenerative joint disease, the disorder may present idiopathically as a secondary consequence to a variety of diseases including advanced osteoarthritis and several metabolic disorders such as hypophosphatasia, hypomagnesemia, hemochromatosis and hyperparathyroidism. The mechanisms responsible for the deposition of the CPPD crystals are not known, although some studies have reported that structural changes in articular cartilage extracellular matrix might promote crystal formation [98, 99]. In support of this suggestion are results of a study of articular cartilage from a Swedish patient with familial CPPDD showing decreased collagen content in the middle zone of the cartilage matrix with some fragmentation of the collagen fibers [98, 99]. Since these changes were in crystal-free areas of the matrix, it was postulated that a matrix abnormality may predispose the tissue to CPPD deposition and to its degeneration. In addition, other abnormalities in the organic matrix have been reported in sporadic cases of CPPDD [100, 101]. In light of these reports, genes encoding cartilage extracellular matrix proteins have been considered as candidate genes for chondrocalcinosis. In a large family from the Chiloe Islands with a clinical phenotype of severe, precocious osteoarthritis with ankylosis, late-onset spondyloepiphyseal dysplasia, and chondrocalcinosis in multiple joints and fibrocartilages, a heterozygous mutation in the COL2A1 gene that resulted in an Arg75 to Cys substitution in the gene product was identified [102, 103]. However, it appears that in this family, the chondrocalcinosis phenotype was a secondary consequence of the advanced and severe osteoarthritis.

It has also been suggested that the inorganic composition of the matrix may affect CPPD formation. For example, hypomagnesemia has been associated with chondrocalcinosis by decreasing pyrophosphatase action, thereby decreasing crystal dissolution [104]. Likewise, elevated levels of inorganic phosphate have been observed in the synovial fluids of patients with CPPDD [105]. This and other observations have led to the suggestion that abnormal local metabolism of inorganic pyrophosphate (PPi) in cartilage may occur in CPPDD patients [105, 106]. A chondrocyte nucleoside triphosphate pyrophosphohydrolase (NTPPPH) that may play a role in the extracellular generation of inorganic pyrophosphate at the site of crystal deposition has been characterized [107–110]. The activity of this enzyme was elevated in sporadic cases of CPPDD; however, elevated levels of NTPPPH activity were not observed in the familial form of the disease [111]. Nonetheless, increased levels of inorganic pyrophosphate have been observed in cultured fibroblasts and lymphoblasts of patients affected with familial CPPDD [112, 113], thus perpetuating the suspicion that abnormalities in pyrophosphate metabolism may give rise to abnormal crystal deposition in these families.

In recent years, genetic linkage analysis has been undertaken to map the disease gene(s) for familial CPPDD. A study of a large family from Maine, in which the CPPDD phenotype appeared to occur as a secondary consequence to severe, non-dysplastic osteoarthritis, excluded linkage to the COL2A1 locus; in this family, genetic linkage was demonstrated between the disease phenotype and a locus on the long arm of chromosome 8 (MIM 600668; Locus symbol:

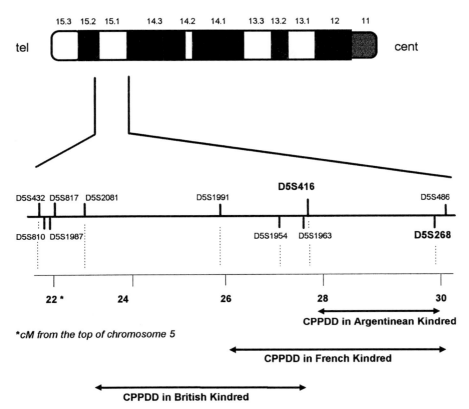

Fig. 1. Ideogram of the short arm of chromosome 5 showing CPPDD interval for the Argentinean, French and British kindreds. Sex-averaged distances between markers are shown in centiMorgans (cM)

CCAL2; [114]). A study conducted on a British family with a phenotype of primary chondrocalcinosis and childhood seizures demonstrated genetic linkage to a chromosomal interval in the region of 5p15 (MIM 118 600; Locus symbol: CCAL1; [115]). Williams et al. have reported that the CCAL1 locus in a large Argentinean kindred resides just proximal to that reported by Hughes et al., in the 5p15.1 locus ([116]; see Fig. 1); this observation has been confirmed in a genetic linkage study of a large French kindred previously described [86]. The results of all these studies indicate that familial CPPDD is a clinically and genetically heterogeneous disease and that mutations in at least three different genes may eventually lead to the expression of the disease.

4.3.7.3
Hydroxyapatite Deposition Disease

The basic calcium phosphate (BCP) crystal deposition diseases have been difficult to study because of lack of diagnostic tests and the considerable heterogeneity of crystal species that characterize these disorders (see [117] for review). The crystals can be found in joint fluid and in cartilage and synovial tissue and their presence can give rise to acute painful and inflammatory attacks that resemble gout. Several clinical studies have reported that basic calcium phosphate crystals can be found in the joint fluid of 30 % to 60 % of patients with OA of the knee [118 – 120] and the presence of the crystals correlated with the degree of joint deterioration [120]. Although BCP crystal deposition has been associated with many articular and periarticular conditions, the Milwaukee shoulder syndrome [121] is a peculiar arthropathy that frequently manifests BCP crystal deposition. The most common radiographic features of this arthropathy include glenohumeral joint degeneration and soft tissue calcification. Aggregates of BCP crystals are found in synovial fluids. There has been one report in the literature of an Italian-Argentinean kindred with familial Milwaukee shoulder syndrome. In this case, X-ray diffraction analyses of aspirated synovial fluids from two affected family members confirmed the presence of calcium pyrophoshate dihydrate and hydroxyapatite crystals [122]. Genetic linkage analyses in this family have excluded several cartilage extracellular matrix components, as well as some loci that are important in cartilage development, as the disease gene (Serrano de la Peña L., pers. commun.). A genome-wide screen will need to be undertaken in order to identify the genetic locus that is linked to the phenotype in this family.

Hydroxyapatite deposition disease (HADD) is, as its name implies, due to the deposition of hydroxyapatite crystals in articular cartilage and joint fluids [123 – 131]. In the familial form of the disease (MIM 118 610), the mode of inheritance is that of an autosomal dominant pattern with full penetrance. This disorder results in periarticular disease in the form of tendinitis or bursitis and, less frequently, true articular disease [126, 132, 133]. Calcium hydroxyapatite deposits in bursae and tendon sheaths are radiographically visible either as poorly defined linear densities or as dense, homogeneous, well-delineated masses. The most common locations of HADD are the shoulder, hip and wrists. In the shoulder, calcifications are visible in the rotator cuff and adjacent bursae. Calcification of the supraspinatus tendon is common and occurs in close proximity to the greater trochanter and surrounding bursa. Triceps tendon calcification at its insertion on the olecranon is occasionally observed. In the wrist, both flexor and extensor tendon calcifications can be seen. Calcific tendinitis may also occur in the neck, within the longus colli muscle tendon; it is visualized below the anterior arch of C1 and is accompanied by retropharyngeal soft tissue swelling.

Generally, the clinical manifestations of HADD are essentially identical to those of CPPDD except for the nature of the crystalline material that is deposited in the tissues. The effects of hydroxyapatite crystal deposition on the structural integrity of articular cartilage have not been defined to date. One study examined the formation of hydroxyapatite crystals in normal and OA articular cartilage [134] and another study described the ultrastructural alterations in articular cartilage matrix in HADD [135]. The results indicated the occurrence of severe structural alterations in the extracellular matrix in areas of crystal deposits but there was no indication of ultrastructural abnormalities in collagen fibers or matrix in crystal free regions.

Genetic linkage analyses in families with HADD have been more limited. A recent linkage study of a large Argentinean family with HADD associated with SED excluded several candidate genes including types II and X collagens [136]. However, no linkage to a chromosomal location has been described to date in this or in other HADD families [131].

4.3.8
Summary

The studies reviewed in this chapter provide conclusive demonstration that certain forms of OA are inherited and are caused by mutations in a variety of genes. Most of the chondrodysplasia/osteochondrodysplasia syndromes display mutations in genes which encode structural proteins that are found in cartilage, including collagen types II, IX, X, and XI and COMP. However, as demonstrated in studies of Jansen-type MCD, mutations in genes that encode molecules for growth factors and their receptors, as well as other yet-to-be-described mutated genes, may also be implicated in the compromise of cartilage that leads to degenerative joint disease. Further study of other forms of familial OA, employing the techniques of molecular genetics now available or being developed, will allow the definition of the exact molecular cause of those disorders. An excellent example of this approach is currently underway in the study of familial chondrocalcinosis; here the tools of "reverse genetics" are being used to define chromosomal loci that are linked to the disease phenotype. Where loci have been identified (see Table 3), the tools of positional cloning will be utilized to identify the disease gene. Eventually, these studies may lead to a classification of OA and related disorders that is based on their exact causative gene defects, rather than on their vastly variable clinical and radiographic phenotypes. Also, these studies may lead to the development of simple DNA tests that will permit definitive diagnosis of molecular defects in individual patients in whom it may be possible to initiate preventive therapy. The ultimate expectation is that studies of heritable forms of OA will help define the range of components that constitutes the complex milieu of cartilage and synovial tissues, and that this insight will reveal new therapeutic opportunities for the treatment of primary OA.

References

1. Heberden W (1803) Commentaries on the history and cure of diseases. (2nd ed). T Payne, London
2. Haygarth J (1805) A clinical history of diseases. Cadell and Davies, London, pp 147–168
3. Stecher RM, Hersh H (1994) Heberden's nodes: the mechanisms of inheritance in hypertrophic arthritis of the fingers. J Clin Invest 23:699–704

4. Kellgren, JH, Moore R (1952) Generalized osteoarthritis and Heberden's nodes. Br Med 1:181–187
5. Stecher RM, Hersh AH, Hauser H (1953) Heberden's nodes: The family history and radiographic appearance of a large family. Am J Hum Genet 5:46–69
6. Allison AC, Blumberg BS (1958) Familial osteoarthropathy of the fingers. J Bone Joint Surg 40 B:538–540
7. Kellgren JH, Lawrence JS, Bier F (1963) Genetic factors in generalized osteoarthritis. Ann Rheum Dis 22:237–255
8. Nuki G (1983) Osteoarthritis: Some genetic approaches. J Rheumatol Suppl 9:29–31
9. Crain DC (1961) Interphalangeal osteoarthritis characterized by painful inflammatory episodes resulting in deformity of the proximal and distal articulations. J Am Med Assoc 175:1049–1051
10. Buchanan WW, Park WM (1983) Primary generalized osteoarthritis: definition and uniformity. J Rheum suppl 9:4–6
11. Lawrence JS (1977) Rheumatism in populations. Heinemann Medical Books, London
12. Lawrence JS, Gelsthorpe K, Morell G (1983) Heberden's nodes and HLA markers in generalized osteoarthritis. J Rheumatol suppl 9:32–33
13. Kahan MF, Jurman SH, Bourgeois P (1977) Le rhumatisme chondroplastique. A propos de 50 cas. Ann Med Interne (Paris) 128:857–860
14. Spranger J (1976) The epiphyseal dysplasias. Clin Orthoped and Rel Res 114:46–59
15. Rimoin DL, Lachman RS (1990) The chondrodysplasias. In: Emery AEH, Rimoin DL (eds) Principles and practice of medical genetics. Churchill Livingstone, New York, pp 507–895
16. Horton WA, Hecht JT (1993) The chondrodysplasias. In: Royce PM, Steinman B (eds) Connective tissue and its heritable disorders. Wiley-Liss, New York, pp 641–675
17. Pyeritz RE (1993) Heritable and developmental disorders of connective tissue and bone. In: McCarty DJ, Koopman WJ (eds) Arthritis and allied conditions (12th ed). Lea and Febiger, Philadelphia, pp 1483–1509
18. Byers PH (1994) Molecular genetics of chondrodysplasias, including clues to development, structure and function. Curr Opin in Rheumatol 6:345–350
19. Palotie A, Vaisanen P, Ott J, Ryhanen L, Elima K, Vikkula M, Cheah K, Vuorio E, Peltonen L (1989) Predisposition to familial osteoarthritis linked to type II collagen gene. Lancet i: 924–927
20. Knowlton RG, Katzenstein PL, Moskowitz RW, Weaver EJ, Malemud CJ, Pathria IMN, Jimenez SA, Prockop DJ (1990) Genetic linkage of a polymorphism in the type II collagen gene (COL2A1) to primary osteoarthritis associated with a mild chondrodysplasia. New Eng J Med 322:526–530
21. Ala-Kokko L, Baldwin CT, Moskowitz RW, Prockop DJ (1990) Single base mutation in the type II procollagen gene (COL2A1) as a cause of primary osteoarthritis associated with a mild chondrodysplasia. Proc Natl Acad Sci USA 87:6565–6568
22. Bleasel JF, Holderbaum D, Brancolini V, Moskowitz RW, Considine EL, Prockop DJ, Devoto M, Williams CJ (1998) Five families with Arginine 519 to cysteine mutation in COL2A1: evidence for three distinct founders. Hum Mut 12:172–176
23. Williams CJ, Rock M, Considine E, McCarron S, Gow P, Ladda R, McLain D, Michels VM, Murphy W, Prockop DJ, Ganguly A (1995) Three new point mutations in type II procollagen (COL2A1) and identification of a fourth family with the COL2A1 Arg519 → Cys base substitution using conformation sensitive gel electrophoresis. Hum Molec Genet 4:309–312
24. Bleasel JF, Bisagni-Faure A, Holderbaum D, Vacher-Lavenu M-C, Haqqi TM, Moskowitz RW, Menkes CJ (1995) Type II procollagen gene (COL2A1) mutation in exon 11 associated with spondyloepiphyseal dysplasia, tall stature, precocious osteoarthritis. J Rheumatol 22:255–261
25. Katzenstein PL, Campbell DF, Machado MA, Horton WA, Lee B, Ramirez F (1992) A type II collagen defect in a new family with SED tarda and early-onset osteoarthritis. Arthritis Rheum 35:S31

26. Kuivaniemi H, Tromp G, Prockop DJ (1997) Mutations in fibrillar collagens (types I, II, III, and XI), fibril-associated collagen (type IX), and network forming collagen (type X) cause a spectrum of diseases in bone, cartilage, and blood vessels. Hum Mut 9:300–315

27. Spranger J, Winterpacht A, Zabel B (1994) The type II collagenopathies: a spectrum of chondrodysplasias. Eur J Pediatr 153:56–65

28. Stickler GB, Belau PG, Farrell FJ, Jones JD, Pugh DG, Steinberg AG, Ward LE (1965) Hereditary progressive Arthro-Ophthalmopathy. Mayo Clin Proc 40:433–455

29. Francomano CA, Liberfarb RM, Hirose T, Maumenee IH, Streeten EA, Meyers DA, Pyeritz RE (1987) The Stickler syndrome: evidence for close linkage to the structural gene for 2 type II collagen. Genomics 1:293–296

30. Knowlton RG, Weaver EJ, Struyk AF (1989) Genetic linkage analysis of hereditary Arthro-ophtalmopathy (Stickler Syndrome) and the type II procollagen gene. Am J Hum Genet 45:681–688

31. Bonaventure J, Philippe C, Plessis G, Vigneron J, Lasselin C, Maroteaux P, Gilgenkrantz S (1992) Linkage study in a large pedigree with Stickler syndrome: exclusion of COL2A1 as the mutant gene. Hum Genet 90:164–168

32. Williams CJ, Ganguly A, McCarron S, Considine E, Michels VV, Prockop DJ (1996) An A-2 → G transition at the 3' acceptor splice site of IVS17 characterizes the COL2A1 gene mutation in the original Stickler kindred. Am J Med Genet 63:461–467

33. Korkko J, Ritvaniemi P, Haataja L, Kaariainan H, Kivirikko K, Prockop DJ, Ala-Kokko L (1993) Mutation in type II procollagen (COL2A1) that substitutes aspartate for glycine 67 and that causes cataracts and retinal detachment. Evidence for molecular heterogeneity in the Wagner syndrome and the Stickler syndrome (arthro-ophthalmopathy). Am J Hum Genet 53:55–61

34. Brunner HG, von Beersum SE, Warman ML, Olsen BR, Ropers HH, Mariman EC (1994) A Stickler syndrome gene is linked to chromosome 6 near the COL11A2 gene. Hum Mol Genet 3:1561–1564

35. Vikkula M, Mariman ECM, Lui VCH, Zhidkova NI, Tiller GE, Goldring MB, van Beersum SE, de Waal Malefijt MC, van den Hoogen FH, Ropers HH, et al. (1995) Autosomal dominant and recessive osteochondrodysplasias associated with the COL11A2 locus. Cell 80:431–437

36. Richards AJ, Yates JR, Williams R, Payne SJ, Pope FM, Scott JD, Snead MP (1996) A family with Stickler syndrome type 2 has a mutation in the COL11A1 gene resulting in the substitution of glycine 97 by valine in alpha 1 (XI) collagen. Hum Molec Genet 5:1339–1343

37. Griffith AJ, Sprunger LK, Sirko-Osadsa A, Tiller GE, Meisler MH, Warman ML (1998) Marshall syndrome associated with a splicing defect at the COL11A1 locus. Am J Hum Genet 62:816–823

38. Kniest W, Lieber B (1977) Kniest syndrom. Monatsschrift kinderheilkunde 125:970–973

39. Maroteaux P, Spranger J (1973) La maladie de Kniest. Arch Francaises de Pediatrie 30:735–750

40. Poole AR, Pidoux I, Reine A, Rosenberg L, Hollister D, Murray L, Rimoin D (1988) Kniest dysplasia is characterized by an apparent abnormal processing of the C-propeptide of type II cartilage collagen resulting in imperfect fibril assembly. J Clin Invest 81:579–589

41. Bogaert R, Wilkin DJ, Wilcox WR, Lachman R, Rimoin D, Cohn DH, Eyre DR (1994) Expression in cartilage of a seven amino acid deletion in type II collagen from two unrelated individuals with Kniest dysplasia. Am J Hum Genet 55:1128–1136

42. Winterpacht A, Hilbert M, Schwarze U, Mundlos S, Spranger J, Zabel BU (1993) Kniest and Stickler dysplasia phenotypes caused by collagen type II gene (COL2A1) defects. Nat Genet 3:323–326

43. Mortier GR, Wilkin DJ, Fenandes R, Eyre D, Rimoin DL, Cohn DH (1995) Five new COL2A1 mutations in the type II collagen diseases. Am J Hum Genet 57 S:A221

44. Wilkin DJ, Weis MA, Gruber HE, Rimoin DL, Eyre DR, Cohn DH (1993) An exon skipping mutation in the type II collagen gene (COL2A1) preduces Kniest dysplasia. Am J Hum Genet 53:A210

45. Fairbanks T (1947) Dysplasia epiphysialis multiplex. Brit J Surg 34:224–232

46. Ribbing S (1937) Studien über hereditäre multiple Epiphysenusstörungen. Acta Radiol. Supplementum 34
47. Weaver EJ, Summerville GP, Yeh G, Hervada-Page M, Oehlman R, Rothman R, Jimenez SA, Knowlton RG (1993) Exclusion of type II and type VI procollagen gene mutations in a five-generation family with multiple epiphyseal dysplasia. Am J Med Genet 45:345–352
48. Hecht JT, Blanton SH, Wang Y, Daigier SP, Horton WA, Rhodes C, Yamada Y, Francomano CA (1992) Exclusion of human proteoglycan link protein (CRTLl) and type II collagen (COL2A1) genes in pseudoachondroplasia. Am J Med Genet 44:420–424
49. Hecht JT, Francomano CA, Briggs MD, Deere M, Conner B, Horton WA, Warman M, Cohn DH, Blanton SH (1993) Linkage of typical pseudoachondroplasia to chromosome 19. Genomics 18:661–666
50. Oehlmann R, Summerville GP, Yeh G, Weaver EJ, Jimenez SA, Knowlton RG (1994) Genetic linkage mapping of multiple epiphyseal dysplasia to the pericentromeric region of chromosome 19. Am J Hum Gen 54:3–10
51. Briggs MD, Hoffinan SMG, King LM, Olsen AM, Mohrenweiser H, Leroy JG, et al. (1995) Pseudo achondroplasia and multiple epiphyseal dysplasia due to mutations in the cartilage oligomeric matrix protein gene. Nature Genet 10:330–336
52. Briggs MD, Choi H, Warman ML, Laughlin JA, Wordsworth P, Sykes BC, Irven CM, Smith M, Wynne-Davies R, Lipson MH, et al. (1994) Genetic mapping of a locus for multiple epiphyseal dysplasia (EDM 2) to a region of chromosome 1 containing a type IX collagen gene. Am J Hum Genet 55:678–684
53. Muragaki Y, Mariman ECM, van Beersum SEC, Perala M, van Mourik JBA, Warman ML, Olsen BR, Hamel BCJ (1996) A mutation in the gene encoding the 2 chain of the fibril-associated collagen IX, COL9A2, causes multiple epiphyseal dysplasia. Nature Genet 12:103–105
54. Deere M, Halloran-Blanton S, Scott CI, Langer LO, Pauli RM, Hecht JT (1995) Genetic Heterogenity in Multiple Epiphyseal Dysplasia. Am J Hum Genet 56:698–704
55. Sutcliffe J, Stanley P (1973) Metaphyseal chondrodysplasias. Prog Ped Radiol 4:250–269
56. Kozlowski K (1976) Metaphyseal and spondylometaphyseal chondrodysplasias. Clin Orthoped 114:83–93
57. Lachman RS, Rimoin DL, Spranger J (1988) Metaphyseal chondrodysplasia, Schmid type. Clinical and radiographic delineation with a review of the literature. Ped Radiol 18:93–102
58. Jacenko O, LuValle P, Olsen BR (1993) Spondylometaphyseal dysplasia in mice carrying a dominant negative mutation in a matrix protein specific for cartilage-to-bone transition. Nature 365:56–61
59. Lenz W (1969) Discussion. Birth Defects Orig Art Ser 4:71–72
60. Karaplis AC, Luz A, Glowacki J, Bronson RT, Tybulewicz VLJ, Kronenberg HM, Mulligan RC (1994) Lethal skeletal dysplasia from targeted disruption of the parathyroid hormone-related peptide gene. Genes Dev 8:277–289
61. Schipani E, Kruse K, Juppner H (1995) A constitutively active mutant PTH-PTHrP receptor in Jansen-type metaphyseal chondrodysplasia. Science 268:98–100
62. Schipani E, Jensen GS, Pincus J, Nissenson RA, Gardella TJ, Juppner H (1997) Constitutive activation of the cyclic adenosine 3′,5′-monophosphate signaling pathway by parathyroid hormone (PTH)/PTH-related peptide receptors mutated at the two loci for Jansen metaphyseal chondrodysplasia. Mol Endocrinol 11:851–858
63. Schipani E, Langman CB, Parfitt AM, Jensen GS, Kikuchi S, Kooh SW Cole WG, Juppner H (1996) Constitutively activated receptors for parathyroid hormone and parathyroid hormone-related peptide in Jansen metaphyseal chondrodysplasia. N Engl J Med 335:708–714
64. Kellgren JH, Lawrence JS (1957) Radiologic assessment of osteoarthritis. Ann Rheum Dis 16:494–502
65. Marks JS, Stewart IM, Hardinge K (1979) Primary osteoarthritis of the hip and Heberden's nodes. Ann Rheum Dis 38:107–111
66. Harper P, Nuki G (1980) Genetic factors in osteoarthritis. In: Nuki G (ed) The Aetiopathogenesis of Osteoarthritis, Pitman, Tunbridge Wells, England, pp 184–201

67. Pattrick M, Manhire A, Ward AM, Doherty M (1989) HLA-AB antigens and α1-antitrypsin phenotypes in nodal generalized osteoarthritis and erosive arthritis. Ann Rheum Dis 48:470–475
68. Spector TD, Cicuttini F, Baker J, Loughlin JA Hart DJ (1996) Genetic influences on osteoarthritis in females: A twin study. Brit Med J 312:940–943
69. Wright GD, Regan M, Deighton CM, Doherty M (1997) Genetic anticipation in nodal osteoarthritis. Arthritis Rheum 40:S320
70. Lesch M, Nyhan WL (1964) A familial disorder of uric acid metabolism and central nervous system function. Am J Med 36:561–570
71. Kelley WN, Rosenbloom FM, Henderson JF, Seegmiller JE (1967) A specific enzyme defect in gout associated with over-production of uric acid. Proc Natl Acad Sci (USA) 57:1735–1739
72. Roessler BJ, Palella TD, Heidler S, Becker MA (1991) Identification of distinct PRPS1 mutations in two patients with X-linked phosphoribosylpyrophosphate synthetase superactivity. Clin Res 39:267 A
73. Renwick PJ, Birley AJ, McKeown CME, Hulten M (1995) Southern analysis reveals a large deletion at the hypoxanthine phosphoribosyl transferase locus in a patient with Lesch-Nyhan syndrome. Clin Genet 48:80–84
74. Gibbs RA, Nguyen P-N, McBride LJ, Koepf SM, Caskey CT (1989) Identification of mutations leading to Lesch Nyhan syndrome by automated direct DNA sequencing of in vitro amplified cDNA. Proc Natl Acad Sci (USA) 86:1919–1923
75. Sperling O, Eliam G, Persky-Brosh S, DeVries A (1972) Accelerated erythrocytes 5-phosphoribosyl-1-pyrophosphate synthesis: a familial abnormality associated with excessive uric acid production and gout. Biochem Med 6:310–316
76. Roessler BJ, Nosal JM, Smith PR, Heidler SA, Palella TD, Switzer RL, Becker MA (1993) Human X-linked phosphoribosylpyrophosphate synthetase superactivity is associated with distinct point mutations in the PRPS1 gene. J Biol Chem 268:26476–26481
77. Becker MA, Smith PR, Taylor W, Mustafi R, Switzer RL (1995) The genetic and functional basis of purine nucleotide feedback-resistant phosphoribosylpyrophosphate synthetase superactivity. J Clin Invest 96:2133–2141
78. Becker MA, Taylor W, Smith PR, Ahmed M (1996) Overexpression of the normal phosphoribosylpyrophosphate synthetase 1 isoform underlies catalytic superactivity of human phosphoribosylpyrophosphate synthetase. J Biol Chem 271:19894–19899
79. Zitnan D, Sitaj S. (1958) Mnohopocentna familiarna kalcifikacin articularnych chrupiek. Bratisl Lek Listy 38:217–228
80. Zitnan D, Sitaj S (1963) Chondrocalcinosis articularis. Section I. Clinical and radiologic study. Ann Rheum Dis 22:142–169
81. McCarty D, Hollander JL (1961) Identification of urate crystals in gouty synovial fluid. Ann Intern Med 54:45–456
82. Riestra JL, Sanchez A, Rodriguez-Valverde V, Alonso JL, de la Hera M, Merino J (1988) Radiographic features of hereditary articular chondrocalcinosis. A comparative study with the sporadic type. Clin Exp Rheumatol 6:369–372
83. Moskowitz RW, Katz D (1964) Chondrocalcinosis (pseudogout syndrome). A family study. JAMA 188:867–871
84. Louyot P, Peterschmitt J, Barthelme P (1964) Chondrocalcinose articulaire diffuse familiale. Rev Rhum 31:659–663
85. Reginato AJ, Hollander JL, Martinez V, Valenzuela F, Schiapachasse V, Covarrubias E et al. (1975) Familial chondrocalcinosis in the Chiloe Islands, Chile. Ann Rheum Dis 34:260–268
86. Gaucher A, Faure G, Netter P, Pourel J, Raffoux C, Streiff F, Tongio MM, Mayer S (1977) Hereditary diffuse articular chondrocalcinosis. Dominant manifestation without close linkage with the HLA system in a large pedigree. Scand J Rheum 16:217–221
87. Gaudreau A, Camerlain M, Piborot ML, Beauregard G, Lebiun A, Petitclerc C (1981) Familial articular chondrocalcinosis in Quebec. Arthritis Rheum 24:611–615
88. Bjelle AO (1982) Pyrophosphate arthropathy in two Swedish families. Arthritis Rheum 25:66–74

89. Sakaguchi M, Ishikawa K, Mizuta H, Kitagawa T (1982) Familial pseudogout with destructive arthropathy. Ryumachi 22:4–13
90. Richardson BC, Chafetz NI, Ferrell LD, Zulman JI, Genant HK (1983) Hereditary chondrocalcinosis in a Mexican-American family. Arthritis Rheum 26:1387–1396
91. Fernandez-Dapica MP, Gomez-Reino J (1986) Familial chondrocalcinosis in the Spanish population. J Rheumatol 13:631–633
92. Rodriguez-Valverde V, Zuffiga M, Casanueva B, Sanchez S, Merino J (1988) Hereditary articular chondrocalcinosis. Clinical and genetic features in 13 pedigrees. Am J Med 84:101–106
93. Balsa A, Martin-Mola E, Gonzalez T, Cruz A, Ojeda S, Gijon-Banos J (1990) Familial articular chondrocalcinosis in Spain. Ann Rheum Dis 49:531–535
94. Eshel G, Gulik A, Halperin N, Avrahami E, Schumacher Jr, HR, McCarty DJ, Caspi D (1990) Hereditary chondrocalcinosis in an Ashkenazi Jewish family. Ann Rheum Dis 49:528–530
95. Doherty M, Hamilton E, Henderson J, Misra H, Dixey J (1991) Familial chondrocalcinosis due to calcium pyrophosphate dihydrate crystal deposition in English families. Br J Rheum 30:10–15
96. Hamza M, Meddeb N, Bardin T (1992) Hereditary chondrocalcinosis in a Tunisian family. Clin Exp Rheumatol 10:43–49
97. Ryan LM, McCarty DJ (1993) Calcium pyrophosphate crystal deposition disease; Pseudogout; Articular Chondrocalcinosis, In: Arthritis and Allied Conditions, Lea & Febiger, Philadelphia, PA, pp 1835–1855
98. Bjelle AO (1972) Morphological study of articular cartilage in pyrophosphate arthropathy (chondrocalcinosis articularis or calcium pyrophosphate dihydrate crystal deposition disease). Ann Rheum Dis 31:449–456
99. Bjelle AO (1981) Cartilage matrix in hereditary pyrophosphate arthropathy. J Rheumatol 8:959–964
100. Ishikawa K, Masuda I, Ohira T, Kumamoto-Shi, Yokoyama M, Kitakyushu-Shi (1989) A histological study of calcium pyrophosphate dihydrate crystal-deposition disease. J Bone Joint Surg 71:875–886
101. Masuda I, Ishikawa I, Usuku G (1991) A histologic and immunohistochemical study of calcium pyrophosphate dihydrate crystal deposition disease. Clin Orthop 263:272–287
102. Williams CJ, Considine EL, Knowlton RG, Reginato A, Neumann G, Harrison D, Buxton P, Jimenez SA, Prockop DJ (1993) Spondyloepiphyseal dysplasia and precocious osteoarthritis in a family with an Arg75 → Cys mutation in the procollagen type II gene (COL2A1). Hum Genet 92:499–505
103. Reginato AJ, Passano GM, Neumann G, Falasca GF, Diaz-Valdez M, Jimenez SA, Williams CJ (1994) Familial spondyloepiphyseal dysplasia tarda, and precocious osteoarthritis associated with an Arginine 75 → Cysteine mutation in the procollagen type II gene in a kindred of Chiloe Islanders. I. Clinical, Radiographic, and Pathologic findings. Arthritis Rheum 37:1078–1086
104. Bennett RM, Lehr JR, McCarty DJ (1975) Factors affecting the solubility of calcium pyrophosphate dihydrate crystals. J Clin Invest 56:1571–1579
105. Silcox DC, McCarty D (1974) Elevated inorganic pyrophosphate concentrations in synovial fluid in osteoarthritis and pseudogout. J Lab Clin Med 83:518–531
106. Altman RD, Muniz OE, Pita JC, Howell DS (1973) Articular chondrocalcinosis: Microanalysis of pyrophosphate (PPi) in synovial fluid and plasma. Arthritis Rheum 16:171–178
107. Howell DS, Martel-Pelletier J, Pelletier J-P, Morales S, Muniz O (1984) NTP pyrophosphohydrolase in human chondocalcinotic and osteoarthritic cartilage. II. Further studies on histologic and subcellular distribution. Arthritis Rheum 27:193–196
108. Ryan LM, Wortmann RL, Karas B, McCarty DJ (1984) Cartilage nucleoside triphosphate (NTP) pyrophosphohydrolase. I. Identification as an ecto-enzyme. Arthritis Rheum 27:404–408

109. Ryan LM, Wortmann RL, Karas B, McCarty DJ (1985) Cartilage nucleoside triphosphate (NTP) pyrophosphohydrolase. II. Role in extracellular pyrophosphate generation and nucleotide metabolism. Arthritis Rheum 28:413–419

110. Muniz O, Pelletier J-P, Martel-Pelletier J, Morales S, Howell DS (1984) NTP pyrophosphohydrolase in human chondrocalcinotic and osteoarthritic cartilage. I. Some biochemical characteristics. Arthritis Rheum 27:186–192

111. Ryan LM, Wortmann RL, Karas B, Lynch MP, McCarty DJ (1986) Pyrophosphohydrolase activity and inorganic pyrophosphate content of cultured human skin fibroblasts. Elevated levels in some patients with calcium pyrophosphate dihydrate deposition disease. J Clin Invest 77:1689–1696

112. Lust G, Faure G, Netter P, Gaucher A, Seegmiller JE (1981) Increased pyrophosphate in fibroblasts and lymphoblasts from patients with hereditary diffuse articular chondrocalcinosis. Science 214:809–810

113. Lust G, Faure G, Netter P, Gaucher A, Seegmiller JE (1981 a) Evidence of a generalized metabolic defect in patients with hereditary chondrocalcinosis: Increased inorganic phosphate in cultured fibroblasts and lymphoblasts. Arthritis Rheum 24:1517–1522

114. Baldwin CT, Farrar LA, Dharmavaram R, Jimenez SA, Anderson L (1995) Linkage of early-onset osteoarthritis and chondrocalcinosis to human chromosome 8q. Am J Hum Genet 56:692–697

115. Hughes AE, McGibbon D, Woodward E, Dixey J, Doherty M (1995) Localisation of a gene for chondrocalcinosis to chromosome 5p. Hum Mol Genet 4:1225–1228

116. Williams CJ, Hardwick LJ, Butcher S, Considine E, Nicod A, Walsh S, Prockop DJ, Caeiro F, Marchegiani R, Reginato A, Brancolini V, Devoto M, Carr A, Lathrop M, Wordsworth BF (1996 a) Linkage of chondrocalcinosis to chromosome 5p15.1–p15.2 an a large Argentinean kindred. Am J Hum Genet S59:A242

117. Halverson PB, McCarty DJ (1993) Basic calcium phosphate crystal deposition diseases. In: McCarty DJ, Koopman WJ (eds), Arthritis and Allied Conditions, 12th edition, Lea and Febiger, Philadelphia, pp 1857–1872

118. Dieppe PA, Crocker PR, Corke CF, Doyle DV, Huskisson EC, Willoughby DA (1979) Synovial fluid crystals. Q J Med 192:533–553

119. Gibilisco PA, Schumacher HR, Hollander JL, Soper KA (1985) Synovial fluid crystals in osteoarthritis. Arthritis Rheum 28:511–515

120. Halverson PB, McCarty DJ (1986) Patterns of radiographic abnormalities associated with basic calcium phosphate and calcium pyrophosphate dihydrate crystal deposition in the knee. Ann Rheum Dis 45:603–605

121. Halverson PB, Carrera GF, McCarty DJ (1990) Milwaukee shoulder syndrome: Fifteen additional cases and a description of contributing factors. Arch Intern Med 150:677–682

122. Pons-Estel B, Sacnum M, Gentiletti S, Battagliotti C, Williams C (1994) Familial chronic shoulder destructive arthropathy (ChSDA), calcium pyrophosphate and apatite deposition. Arthritis and Rheum 37 S:414

123. Sharp J (1954) Heredo-familial vascular and articular calcifications. Ann Rheum Dis 13:15–16

124. Zaphiropoulos G, Graham R (1973) Recurrent calcific periarthritis involving multiple sites. Proc R. Soc Med 66:351–352

125. Cannon RB, Schmid FR (1973) Calcific periarthritis involving multiple sites in identical twins. Arthritis Rheum 16:393–395

126. Dieppe PA, Huskisson EC, Crocker P, Willoughby DA (1976) Apatite deposition disease: a new arthropathy. Lancet I:266–269

127. Marcos JC, De Benyacar MA, Garcia-Morteo O, Arturi AS, Maldonado-Cocco JR, Morales VH, et al. (1981) Idiopathic familial chondrocalcinosis due to apatite crystal deposition. Am J Med 71:557–564

128. Hajiroussou VJ, Webley M. (1986) Familial calcific periarthritis. Ann Rheum Dis 42:469–470

129. Caspi D, Rosembach TO, Yaron M, McCarty DJ, Graff E (1988) Periarthritis associated with basic calcium phosphate crystal deposition and low level of alkaline phosphatase. Report of three cases from one family. J Rheumatol 15:823–827
130. Fernandez-Dapica MP, Gomez-Reino J, Reginato AJ (1993) Familial periarticular calcification in a Spanish kindred. Rev. Espanola Rheum 20:403
131. Ferri S, Zanardim M, Barozzi L, Williams C, Reginato AJ (1994) Familial apatite deposition disease (FADD) in a Northern-Italian Kindred. Arthritis Rheum 37:S413
132. Schumacher HR, Smolyo AP, Tse RL, Maurer K (1977) Arthritis associated with apatite crystals. Ann Intern Med 87:411–416
133. Halverson PB (1992) Arthropathies associated with basic calcium phosphate crystals. Scanning Microscopy 6:791–797
134. Ali SY, Griffiths S (1983) Formation of calcium phosphate crystals in normal and osteoarthritic cartilage. Ann Rheum Dis suppl 42:45–58
135. Ohira T, Ishikawa K (1987) Hydroxyapatite deposition in osteoarthritic articular cartilage of the proximal femoral head. Arthritis Rheum 30:651–660
136. Marcos JC, Arturi AS, Babini C, Jimenez SA, Knowlton R, Reginato AJ (1995) Familial hydroxyapatite chondrocalcinosis with spondyloepiphyseal dysplasia: Clinical course and absence of genetic linkage to the type II procollagen gene. J Clin Rheumatol 1:171–178

4.4
Biochemical Factors in Joint Articular Tissue Degradation in Osteoarthritis

J. MARTEL-PELLETIER, J. DI BATTISTA and D. LAJEUNESSE

4.4.1
Introduction

Osteoarthritis (OA) is an idiopathic disease characterized by a degeneration of articular cartilage. A breakdown of the cartilage matrix leads to development of fibrillation, fissures, the appearance of gross ulcerations, and disappearance of the full thickness surface of the joint. This is accompanied by hypertrophic bone changes with osteophyte formation and subchondral plate thickening. Moreover, at the clinical stage of the disease, changes caused by OA involve not only the cartilage, but also the synovial membrane, where an inflammatory reaction is often observed.

Although the etiology of OA is not yet known and likely multifactorial, the progression of this disease is generally divided into three stages [1]. Stage I involves the proteolytic breakdown of the cartilage matrix. Stage II occurs when there is fibrillation and erosion of the cartilage surface, accompanied by a release of breakdown products into the synovial fluid. During Stage III, synovial inflammation begins, when synovial cells ingest the breakdown products through phagocytosis, and produce proteases and pro-inflammatory cytokines.

In this review, we will focus our attention on current knowledge of the major factors participating in the degeneration of OA articular joint tissues. Firstly, emphasis will be placed on the possibility of an interaction between subchondral bone and cartilage as an integral part of the disease, leading and/or contributing to cartilage destruction in OA; do changes in one cause alterations of the other? We will then address the biochemical agents involved in the destruction of cartilage and the synovial membrane, followed by a brief survey of the intracellular signaling cascades of the most important pro-inflammatory cytokines, interleukin-1 beta (IL-1β) and tumour necrosis factor-alpha (TNF-α).

4.4.2
Subchondral Bone

In addition to degeneration of the articular cartilage, OA involves changes in the surrounding bone, and the recently expanded body of knowledge concerning the subchondral bone provides the basis upon which we may assert that this tissue is intimately involved in the pathology of OA. Indeed, it is suggested that the thickening of the subchondral bone plate may induce and/or participate in the progression of OA [2, 3]. The following hypothesis may explain the relationship between OA and subchondral bone alterations (Fig. 1). As OA progresses, the articular cartilage, which is subjected to mechanical as well as chemical stresses, slowly erodes due to an imbalance in repair and loss of cartilage. In particular, the mechanical stress on weight–bearing joints may contribute to increased microfractures in the subchondral bone plate and overlying cartilage. As articular cartilage slowly erodes, sclerosis of the subchondral bone also progresses, and subchondral bone stiffness increases in this tissue, possibly contributing to further mechanical disturbances of the cartilage.

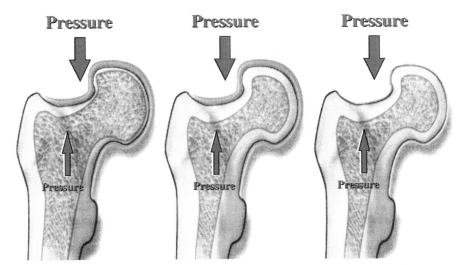

Fig. 1. Schematic view of progressive alterations of cartilage and subchondral bone of articular joints in OA. The mechanical stress on articular joints may contribute to increased microfractures in subchondral bone and cartilage. As cartilage slowly erodes, sclerosis of the subchondral bone also progresses, and subchondral bone stiffness increases. This probably contributes to further mechanical disturbances of the cartilage. Whether bone sclerosis initiates or is involved in the progression of cartilage loss remains under debate

Whether bone sclerosis initiates or is involved in the progression of cartilage loss, however, remains a matter of debate.

Roentgenographic changes in the subchondral cancellous bone, such as sclerosis and cyst formation, are observed in patients with OA, yet have generally been considered secondary. One of the mechanisms of initiation of OA, however, may be a steep stiffness gradient in the underlying subchondral bone [2, 3] as the integrity of the overlying articular cartilage depends on the mechanical properties of its bony bed. Evidence from a primate animal model (Macaca fascicularis) of OA indicates that alterations of the bony bed may precede the changes in cartilage [4, 5]. Evidence for and against this hypothesis has recently emerged from both animal model studies [6–8] and clinical trials [9–12], hence fueling further debate. Trabecular thickening in subchondral bone is not always accompanied by increased bone mineralization, but rather by osteoid volume increases [12]. This is an indication of abnormal mineralization [13], suggesting that a disregulation of bone remodeling may be an integral part of OA. This would support the concept of a bone cell defect in this disease, which in fact may be a more generalized bone metabolic disease, as suggested by Dequeker's group [14, 15].

4.4.2.1
Bone Cell Physiology

The bone is not a static organ as it undergoes continuous renewal. This dynamic process, termed bone remodeling, is a complex sequence of bone resorption/mineralization, and the mechanisms involved in these events remain undefined. While osteoclasts resorb bone [16], osteoblasts secrete proteins forming the basic organic matrix for bone mineralization. Bone formation and resorption do not occur randomly throughout the skeleton, but follow a programmed sequence at discrete loci called bone remodeling units [17]. At the beginning of a cycle, osteoclasts appear on a previously inactive surface. Within two weeks, osteoclasts construct a tunnel in cortical bone, or a lacuna at the surface of trabecular bone. The activation frequency of new bone-remodeling units determines the rate of bone turnover. Resorption and formation phases are tightly coupled in normal young adults, and bone mass is maintained. The hormonal control of resorption, at least for parathyroid hormone (PTH) and prostaglandin E_2 (PGE$_2$), directly indicates a signal transduction within osteoblasts, as the exposure of isolated osteoblasts to PTH or PGE$_2$ releases a factor(s) that stimulates osteoclastic bone resorption. However, there are currently more than 12 known local or systemic regulators of bone growth, including PTH, 1,25 $(OH)_2D_3$, calcitonin, growth hormone, glucocorticoids, thyroid hormone, insulin and insulin-like growth factor–1 and 2 (IGFs), estrogens, PGE$_2$ and androgens, that effect bone remodeling [18, 19].

Bone cells release a number of proteins/cytokines involved in cell signaling and endocrine regulation. Proteins produced by osteoblasts include bone matrix proteins such as collagen, osteopontin, osteocalcin and bone sialoprotein [20–23]. These cells also release proteases, in both active and latent forms, that are involved in the process of bone remodeling. These include metalloproteases (MMP) [24–26] and members of the PA/plasmin system [27–29]. The cytokines released by osteoblasts can act both locally via autocrine mechanisms, or in a paracrine fashion on local cells (other osteoblasts, lining cells or osteoclasts) [30, 31]. These signaling pathways are "static", which is to say they act to promote chemical signals within the bone milieu.

Whether these signals are regulated by mechanical stresses, or if other chemical signals result from these stresses remains under debate. Repeated mechanical stresses are however known to act on local bone cell proliferation and/or protein synthesis. *In vivo* mechanical loading modifies bone strength, and is capable of activating osteoblasts [32]. Indeed, it can increase cyclic nucleotide levels [33, 34], prostaglandin production [33, 35], and morphological changes associated with the remodeling of bone tissue [32]. *In vitro*, mechanical stresses (mechanical stretch of culture dishes and/or applied pressure in bone organ culture) can increase the proliferation of osteoblasts in culture [36]. This can also promote the expression of a number of mRNA for bone proteins involved in osteoid formation and mineralization [36, 37] local growth factor release such as IGF-1 and IGF-2 [38] and integrin and non-integrin adhesion molecules [39]. The effect of mechanical loading is also related to sex, as cumulative effects of loading and estrogens are observed in males, and enhanced effects are observed in females in the presence of estrogens alone [40, 41]. This may indicate an indirect relationship to OA as this pathology is related to gender and obesity. Signal transduction of mechanical loading/stresses may be carried out via mechanosensitive ion channels, and ion channels have been linked to early events in bone cell metabolism [42–44]. There are absolutely no data in OA studies, however, on this particular point.

4.4.2.2
Possible Causes of Subchondral Bone Sclerosis in OA

Opposing concepts can explain a stiffening of the subchondral bone. In subchondral bone, the healing of trabecular microfractures, which are present due to repetitive impulsive loading of the joint and remodeling of the bony internal architecture to better resist these stresses, can generate a stiffer bone that is no longer an effective shock absorber [2, 3]. Conversely, subchondral bone stiffness may be part of a more generalized bone alteration leading to increased bone mineral density/volume. OA is generally not seen in osteoporosis patients [45, 46], while osteopetrosis, a condition associated with bone sclerosis [47], can present with OA in those patients who reach adulthood despite their osteopetrotic condition [48]. Lajeunesse et al. [49] recently showed that, in addition to an osteoclast defect, human malignant osteopetrosis may be due to an osteoblast defect as measured in primary osteoblast cell cultures showing reduced production of osteocalcin (a bone-specific protein) and of macrophage colony-stimulating factor (a stimulator of bone resorption). Hence, the relatively soft osteoporotic bone would act as an excellent shock absorber, easily sustaining the compression fracture of its relatively weak structure. Moreover, primary OA and primary osteoporosis rarely coexist [46, 50, 51]. Finally, OA patients have a better preserved bone mass [52–54] independently of body weight [55–57] suggesting that a bone disease may initiate OA. In animal models with mild to moderate OA, increased bone density and osteoid volume are often more severe than cartilage changes [4, 5, 7, 8]. In a primate animal model, the severity of cartilage fibrillation and loss generally exceeds bone changes only in advanced OA [4].

Three hypotheses may explain bone sclerosis. This condition may be due to a "field" or systemic effect. Hence, OA may be the result of a primary cartilage disease/dysfunction (or from another non-bone origin) or systemic hormonal alterations that promote changes locally in subchondral bone. Minor systemic endocrine changes between OA and primary osteoporosis have however been noted, and serum concentrations of calciotropic hormones are within normal limits in OA patients [58, 59]. Moreover, short-term $1,25(OH)_2D_3$ therapy in postmenopausal women with osteoporosis or OA revealed no difference in calcium metabolism [60]. Alternately, it could result from a cellular defect of osteoblasts that perturb local bone remodeling/mineralization. Indeed, although within normal limits, intact PTH levels are somewhat higher in OA than in osteoporosis patients [59]. We have recently reported a resistance to PTH-stimulation in OA osteoblast-like cells *in vitro* [61]. Lastly, combined with cellular alterations, mechanical stresses may lead to bone sclerosis. Subchondral bone sclerosis in OA indicates both an increase in bone volume fraction and alterations in other microstructural characteristics. OA subchondral bone contains fewer, widely spaced, thicker than normal trabeculae [62]. Moreover, Kamibayashi et al. [62] have defined highly localized regional differences by depth from the articular surface, and from anterior to posterior across the medial condyle, variations that may significantly affect the biomechanical competence of bone, and disrupt bone remodeling, especially in weight bearing joints.

4.4.2.3
Evidence for a Role of Abnormal Osteoblasts in OA

Indirect evidence of perturbed osteoblast function in OA has been reported. Gevers and Dequeker [63] have shown elevated serum osteocalcin levels in women with hand OA, and elevated osteocalcin in cortical bone explants, implying that a bone disease may be part of OA. OA has been associated with a thickening of subchondral bone, and also with an abnormally low mineralization pattern of the femoral head, identified in OA patients at autopsy [12]. In an animal model, a striking increase in the bone fraction, measured by computer tomography, was observed at the subchondral level in guinea pigs with surgically-induced OA [64]. An imbalance in collagen and non-collagen protein production (such as osteocalcin) can lead to an increase in bone volume without a concomitant increase in bone mineralization pattern. In this respect, it is also important to note that Shimizu et al. [109] have shown, using a large number of patients, that the progression of joint cartilage degeneration is associated with intensified remodeling of the subchondral bone and increased bone stiffness. This is strongly indicative of a cellular bone defect in OA. Hannan et al. [65] have suggested that the relationship between osteophytes and femoral bone mineral density is a sign that a primary attribute of bone formation may underlie the pathophysiology of OA. Indeed, the proliferation of defective bone cells may result in an increased stiffness, not an increase in bone mineral density, an hypothesis also proposed by Li and Aspden [66].

The hypothesis that abnormal OA osteoblasts directly influence cartilage metabolism has recently been put forward by Westacott et al. [67]. These authors have shown that conditioned media from primary osteoblasts of OA patients versus subjects without arthritis significantly altered glycosaminoglycan release from normal cartilage *in vitro*, while cytokine release from these cells remained intact [67]. Hilal et al. [61] have recently reported that *in vitro* primary cultures of osteoblasts prepared from human OA subchondral bone plates show an altered metabolism, and that the uPA/plasmin system activity and IGF-1 levels are elevated in these cells. This increase in protease activity by OA subchondral bone cells may consequently explain the observations of Westacott et al. [67].

Whether these changes in subchondral bone cells are responsible for OA or contribute to its progression is not definitively known. Indeed, using a cruciate-deficient dog model of OA, Dedrick et al. [7] have reported that a thickening of the subchondral bone is not required for the development of cartilage changes in this model. In contrast, they suggested that these bony changes contribute to the progression of cartilage degeneration, an hypothesis that could be reconciled with the results of Westacott et al. [67]. The results of Dedrick et al. [7], however, are not supported by those of Saïed et al. [68] who, using 50 MHz echography for assessing initial and progressive morphological and structural changes of articular cartilage and bone in experimental OA induced by intra-articular injection of mono-iodo-acetic acid in the knee joint of rats, have shown that the initial changes in cartilage occur simultaneously with bone changes as early as three days following the injection.

Osteoblasts secrete a number of growth factors and cytokines that are involved in local remodeling of bone tissues, and these could also contribute to remodeling of the overlying cartilage in weight-bearing joints after seeping through microcracks in the calcified layer of articular cartilage [69]. Moreover, bone cell products are detected in synovial fluid, hence are secreted into the joint space [70]. Since Westacott et al. have shown that OA osteoblasts may secrete a product(s) that promote cartilage degradation *in vitro* [67], this suggests that abnormal osteoblasts may trigger the local remodeling of articular cartilage. Transforming growth factor-beta (TGF-β) and bone morphometric proteins (BMPs, other members of the TGF family) produced by osteoblasts and chondrocytes can all modify bone and cartilage remodeling in the joint space [71–73]. Our recent observation that TGF-β levels are elevated in OA subchondral bone explants as compared to normal samples [74] may provide a clue to the role for this growth factor in OA. Insulin-like growth factors (IGFs), also produced by osteoblasts [75, 76], are elevated in OA osteoblast-like cell cultures [61] and affect cartilage metabolism [77]. TGF-β, IGFs, BMPs and cytokines produced by osteoblasts in the subchondral bone plate may all influence the production of collagenases and other proteolytic pathways in cartilage, that in turn may ultimately promote matrix remodeling/degradation. Macrophage colony-stimulating factor (M-CSF) is produced locally by osteoblasts, and abnormally low production of M-CSF by primary human osteoblasts has been detected in human osteopetrosis [49]. Whether OA osteoblasts produce less M-CSF than normal cells, thereby contributing to subchondral bone thickening, is currently unknown. Recent data also suggests that the vitamin D receptor (VDR) genotype is involved in the pathogenesis of OA via a possible role in osteophyte formation [78]. Given that the VDR is expressed by osteoblasts and that it regulates the expression of a number of proteins/factors synthesized by these cells, this may also partly explain the role of OA osteoblasts in this disease and on the release of a product(s) involved in cartilage damage/loss.

4.4.2.4
Working Hypothesis to Subchondral Bone and Cartilage Remodeling in OA

Taking all these observations into consideration, our laboratories [61,74] have proposed the following hypothesis (Fig. 2). At the onset of or during the OA process, enhanced bone remodeling at the subchondral bone plate, coupled with repetitive impulse loading leading to local microfractures and/or an imbalance of the IGF/IGFBP system due to an abnormal response of subchondral osteoblasts, promotes subchondral bone sclerosis. This in turn may also create local microfractures of the overlying cartilage and promote cartilage matrix damage.

This damage would normally be repaired by local synthesis or release of IGF-1 and IGFBP that stimulate matrix formation in the cartilage. However, at the same time, the IGF system would also promote subchondral bone cell growth and subchondral bone matrix deposition. This general hypothesis implies that the anabolic activity of the IGF system, which could be locally regulated by the PA/plasmin system, is enhanced in subchondral bone, while the local activation of the PA/plasmin system in cartilage promotes local cartilage

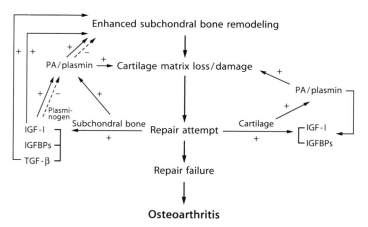

Fig. 2. Hypothetical schematics of the local biochemical processes in both subchondral bone and cartilage leading to cartilage loss/damage and to OA

alteration [79]. However, IGF-1 in OA osteoblast prevents the positive feedback loop of plasmin on PA, hence could refrain remodeling in this tissue ultimately leading to bone sclerosis [77]. Thus, in bone and cartilage, the local induction of IGF-1 and the protease regulatory system would promote both cartilage damage and subchondral bone plate thickening, this last pathway leading to further cartilage damage. The imbalance in the repair capacity and damage of the cartilage due to subchondral plate thickening would then lead to progressively altered cartilage matrix, and eventually to OA. Hence, this would also explain the slow progression of the disease.

4.4.3
Cartilage and Synovial Membrane

4.4.3.1
Enzymes/Enzyme Inhibitors (Fig. 3)

A great deal of attention is focused on identifying the protease responsible for the initial occurrence of matrix digestion. Current knowledge indicates an important involvement of matrix metalloproteases (MMP) (1,80). Of this family, members from three groups in human articular tissue have been identified that are elevated in OA, these being the collagenases, the stromelysins and the gelatinases. In general, collagenase is responsible for the degradation of native collagen; stromelysin for proteoglycans; and gelatinase for the denatured collagen. For proteoglycans, however it is suggested that aggrecanase – another enzyme having MMP properties, but not yet clearly defined – may be responsible for the proteolysis of cartilage proteoglycan aggregates found in the synovial fluid of OA patients [81].

Three collagenases have been identified in human cartilage, and their levels definitely elevated in human OA: collagenase-1 (MMP-1), collagenase-2 (MMP-8) and collagenase-3 (MMP-13). The coexistence of different collagenases in articular tissue is indicative of a specific role for each [82]. Indeed, recent data showing different topographical distributions as well as correlations of these collagenases within pathological cartilage suggest a selective involvement of each collagenase at preferential sites during the disease process. In OA, collagenase-1 and -2 are located predominantly in the superficial and upper intermediate layers, whereas collagenase-3 is found mostly in the lower intermediate and deep layers [82–86]. Moreover, it has been shown in an immunohistochemical study using an OA animal model that the positive staining chondrocyte score for collagenase-3 plateaued, and even declined with the progression of the disease, whereas for collagenase-1, chondrocyte score increased steadily [84]. Interestingly, recent data on these collagenases, combined with those from studies on other target cells, suggest that in OA cartilage, collagenase-1 is involved mostly during the inflammatory process, whereas collagenase-3 is implicated in the remodeling phase of this tissue.

For the second group of MMPs, the stromelysins, three such enzymes have been identified in human, stromelysin-1 (MMP-3), -2 (MMP-10) and -3 (MMP-11). To date, only stromelysin-1 appears to be involved in OA [87–89].

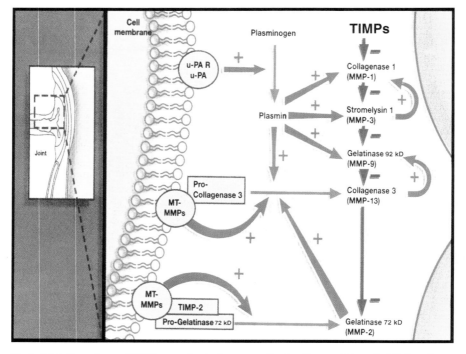

Fig. 3. Metalloproteases/TIMP cascades in human articular tissue. uPA and uPA R refer to urokinase and urokinase receptors respectively, TIMPs are the tissue inhibitors of metalloproteases, MT-MMPs are the membrane type metalloproteases. (+) indicates activation and (–) inhibition. [Reproduced and modified with the permission of Amersham Life Sciences, USA]

Stromelysin-2 could not be detected in OA synovium [88, 89], but was found expressed at very low levels in synovial fibroblasts from rheumatoid arthritis patients [88]. However, the latter enzyme was not affected by IL-1β treatment [88]. Stromelysin-3 was also detected in rheumatoid synovium, and confined to fibroblasts, especially near fibrotic areas [90]. In human articular tissue, two gelatinases have been found, the gelatinase 92 kD (MMP-9) and 72 kD (MMP-2). In human OA, only the gelatinase 92 kD is enhanced [91].

Another group of MMPs, localized at the cell membrane surface, has recently been discovered, and named membrane type MMP (MT-MMP). Four members have been identified, and named MT1-MMP through MT4-MMP.

MT1-MMP was found to be expressed in human articular cartilage [92]. Although MT1-MMP possesses properties of collagenase [93], and both MT1-MMP and MT2-MMP are able to activate the gelatinase 72 kD and collagenase-3 [92, 94, 95], the relevance of these enzymes to OA has yet to be determined.

MMP biologic activity is controlled by physiologically–specific tissue inhibitors (TIMP). There are currently three TIMP known to exist in human joint tissue: TIMP-1, TIMP-2 and TIMP-3 [96–98]. TIMP-4 has been identified and cloned [99], but its involvement in articular joint tissue is not yet known. These molecules specifically bind the active site of the MMP, but some also bind the pro-form of the gelatinase 72 kD (TIMP-2,-3,-4) and pro-gelatinase 92 kD (TIMP-1 and -3) [100, 101]. Studies have shown that, in OA tissue, there is an imbalance in the amount of TIMP and MMP resulting in a relative deficit of the inhibitors [98, 102], which may partially account for the increased level of active MMP in pathologic articular tissues. TIMP-1 and -2 are present in cartilage, and synthesized by chondrocytes [96, 98, 103, 104]. In OA synovium and synovial fluid, only TIMP-1 has been detected [89, 105, 106]. TIMP-3 is found exclusively in the extracellular matrix and not in conditioned media [107]. TIMP-4 has approximately 50% sequence identity with TIMP-2 and TIMP-3, and 38% with TIMP-1 [108]. Moreover, in other target cells, TIMP-4 appears responsible for modulating the cell surface activation of the pro-gelatinase 72 kD, suggesting its importance as a tissue-specific regulator of extracellular matrix remodeling [100].

Another mechanism controlling MMP biological activity is the physiological activators of this family. Enzymes from the serine- and cysteine-dependent protease families, such as the PA/plasmin system and cathepsin B respectively, have been proposed as activators [109, 110], and enhanced levels of urokinase (uPA) and plasmin have been identified in human OA cartilage [79]. Although other cathepsins have been found in the synovial membrane, cathepsin B appears most relevant to MMP activation in cartilage [111, 112]. Several physiologic inhibitors of these two latter protease families have also been detected in human articular tissue, and indeed the plasminogen activator inhibitor-1 (PAI-1) as well as the cysteine protease inhibitory activity, were found at decreased levels in OA articular joint tissue [79, 111]. As for the MMP/TIMP, an imbalance in the levels of these MMP activators and their specific inhibitors appears an important contributing factor in OA articular tissue degradation, and could therefore explain the increased level of biologically active MMP in these pathologic tissues. Other enzymes have also been found to act as MMP activators (Fig. 3); for example, stromelysin-1 activates collagenase-1, collagenase-3 and gelatinase 92 kD; collagenase-3 activates gelatinase 92 kD, MT-MMP activates collagenase-3, and gelatinase 72 kD potentiates the latter activation; MT-MMP also activates gelatinase 72 kD [113–119].

4.4.3.2
Pro-Inflammatory Cytokines and Nitric Oxide (NO)

Despite the profound alterations of proteases in OA which could explain the exhaustive degradation of articular joint tissue, this does not account for the enhanced synthesis and expression of MMP in these pathological tissues. Current evidence suggests that pro-inflammatory cytokines are responsible for this process. They appear to be first produced by the synovial membrane, and diffuse into the cartilage through the synovial fluid. They activate the chondrocytes, which in turn could produce pro-inflammatory cytokines. In OA synovial membrane, it is the synovial lining cells that play a major role as inflammatory effectors. Indeed, these cells can secrete proteases and inflammatory mediators of which IL-1β, TNF-α, IL-6, leukemic inhibitor factor (LIF) and IL-17 appear most relevant to OA.

The OA data in literature strongly support the concept that IL-1β, and perhaps TNF-α, are the major catabolic systems involved in the destruction of joint tissue, and may constitute the *in situ* source of articular tissue degradation [1]. It is still unclear whether IL-1β and TNF-α act independently or in concert to induce the pathogenesis of OA, or if a functional hierarchy exists between these pro-inflammatory cytokines. In animal models, it has been shown that blocking IL-1 or its activity is very effective in preventing cartilage destruction [120, 121], whereas blocking TNF-α results in decreased inflammation [121, 122]. Both these cytokines have been found in enhanced amounts in OA synovial membrane, synovial fluid and cartilage [1, 123 – 127]. In chondrocytes, they have the potential not only to increase the synthesis of proteases – particularly the MMPs and PA, as well as minor collagen types such as I and III – but also to decrease the synthesis of collagen types II and IX, and proteoglycans. These cytokines also stimulate reactive oxygen species and inflammatory mediators like PGE_2. These macromolecular changes in OA cartilage have an important functional impact, as they could result in inadequate tissue repair leading to further cartilage erosion.

The process involved in the inhibition/activation of MMP in OA may also be modulated by these pro-inflammatory cytokines. For instance, the imbalance in the TIMP-1 and MMP levels in OA cartilage may be mediated by IL-1β, as *in vitro* experiments have shown that increasing the concentration of IL-1β produces a decrease in TIMP-1 synthesis, paralleled with an increased MMP synthesis in articular chondrocytes [96]. The PA synthesis is also modulated by IL-1β. *In vitro* stimulation of cartilage chondrocytes using IL-1 revealed a dose-dependent increase in PA, concomitantly with a sharp decrease in PAI-1 synthesis [128]. The potent effect of IL-1 at decreasing PAI-1 synthesis, in combination with an increased PA synthesis, is a powerful mechanism for generating plasmin and activating MMP. In addition to the plasmin role as an enzyme activator, it could also be involved in the degradation of cartilage matrix by direct proteolysis.

IL-1β is primarily synthesized as a 31 kD precursor (pro–IL-1β) devoid of a conventional signal sequence, and released in active form (17.5 kD) [129, 130]. In articular joint tissue including synovial membrane, synovial fluid and cartilage, IL-1β has been found in the active form, and *ex vivo* experiments have demonstrated the ability of the OA synovial membrane to secrete this cytokine [131]. Several serine proteases can process the pro-IL-1β to bioactive forms [132] but in mammals only one protease, belonging to the cysteine-dependent protease family and named IL-1β converting enzyme (ICE or Caspase-1), can specifically generate the mature 17.5 kD cytokine [132, 133]. ICE is a pro-enzyme polypeptide of 45 kD (p45) [132, 133] located in the cellular membrane, and belonging to the family of cysteine aspartate-specific proteases known as caspases. Active ICE is produced following proteolytic cleavage of the pro-enzyme p45, generating two subunits known as p10 and p20, both of which are essential for enzymatic activity [134].

TNF-α occurs in a precursor membrane-bound form (26 kD), and is released from cells by proteolytic cleavage, resulting in a soluble form of 17 kD factor that oligomerizes to form trimers [135, 136]. This appears to occur via a TNF-α converting enzyme (TACE) belonging to a subfamily of the adamalysin (ADAM) [137]. Parenthetically, this enzyme is also required for shedding the TNF receptors (see below). Moreover, Amin et al. [138] have recently reported an upregulation of TACE mRNA in human OA cartilage.

The biological activation of chondrocytes and synovial cells by IL-1 and TNF-α is mediated through association with specific cell-surface receptors, the IL-1R and TNF-R. For each cytokine, two types of receptors have been identified, type I and type II IL-R [139], and TNF-R55 and TNF-R75 [140]. The type I IL-1R and the TNF-R55 appear responsible for signal transduction in articular tissue cells [141–145]. Type I IL-1R has a slightly higher affinity for IL-1β than IL-1α. The type II IL-1R has a greater affinity for IL-1α than IL-1β and it is unclear whether this receptor can mediate IL-1 cell signaling or if it serves to competitively inhibit IL-1 binding to the type I IL-1R. For TNF-R, the affinity constant for TNF-α ranges approximately from $2 - 5 \times 10^{-5}$ M and $0.1 - 7 \times 10^{-10}$ M [146–148] for TNF-R55 and TNF-R75 respectively. The number of type I IL-1R and TNF-R55 is increased in OA chondrocytes and synovial fibroblasts [142–145]. This in turn appears responsible for the higher sensitivity of these cells to stimulation by these cytokines [142]. This process both increases the potential proteolytic enzyme secretion and enhances joint destruction.

IL-6 has also been proposed as a contributor to the OA pathological process by: i) increasing the amount of inflammatory cells in synovial tissue [149]; ii) stimulating the proliferation of chondrocytes; and iii) by inducing an amplification of the IL-1 effects on the increased MMP synthesis and inhibition of proteoglycan production [150]. However, as IL-6 can induce the production of TIMP [151], and not MMP themselves, it is believed that this cytokine is involved in the feedback mechanism that limits enzyme damage.

The LIF is another cytokine of the IL-6 family that is upregulated in OA synovial membrane and fluid, and produced by chondrocytes in response to the pro-inflammatory cytokines IL-1β and TNF-α [152–154]. This cytokine stimulates cartilage proteoglycan resorption, as well as MMP synthesis and NO (see below) cellular production [155]. In OA, however, its role has not yet been clearly defined.

IL-17 is a newly discovered cytokine of 20–30 kD present as a homodimer, and with variable glycosylated polypeptides [156]. The nature of the tissue distribution of the IL-17R appears ubiquitous, and it is not yet known whether all cells expressing IL-17R respond to its ligand. IL-17 upregulates a number of gene products involved in cell activation, including the pro-inflammatory cytokines IL-1β, TNF-α and IL-6, as well as MMP in target cells such as human macrophages [157]. IL-17 also increases the production of NO on chondrocytes [158]. As for the LIF, its role in OA remains undetermined.

In addition, the inorganic free radical NO has been suggested as a factor that promotes cartilage catabolism in OA. Compared to normal, OA cartilage produces a larger amount of NO, both under spontaneous and pro-inflammatory cytokine-stimulated conditions [159]. A high level of nitrite/nitrate has been found in the synovial fluid and serum of arthritis patients [160, 161]. This is the result of an enhanced expression and protein synthesis of the inducible NO synthase (iNOS), the enzyme responsible for NO production [161, 162]. A chondrocyte-specific iNOS cDNA has been cloned and sequenced, and encodes a protein of 131 kD [163]. The deduced amino acid sequence shows about 50% identity and 70% similarity with endothelial and neuronal forms of iNOS.

NO inhibits the synthesis of cartilage matrix macromolecules and enhances MMP activity. Moreover, the elevation of NO production reduces the synthesis of IL-1R antagonist (IL-1Ra, see below) by chondrocytes [159]. As such, an increased level of IL-1, in conjunction with a decreased IL-1Ra level, may cause an over stimulation of OA chondrocytes by this factor, leading to an enhancement of cartilage matrix degradation. Interestingly, *in vivo* therapeutic effects of a selective inhibitor of the iNOS on the progression of lesions in experimental arthritis and OA models have recently been reported [164–166].

4.4.3.3
Inhibitors of Pro-inflammatory Cytokine Production/Activity

Natural inhibitors capable of directly counteracting the binding of the cytokine to cells or reducing the pro-inflammatory level have been identified, and can be divided into three categories based on their mode of action.

The first inhibitor category is a receptor-binding antagonist which interferes with the binding of the ligand to its receptor by competing for the same binding site. Until now, such an inhibitor has been found only for the IL-1 system, and named IL-1Ra [141, 167]. This inhibitor does not bind to IL-1, and therefore is not a binding protein, but rather a competitive inhibitor of IL-1/IL-1R. Moreover, IL-1Ra does not stimulate target cells. IL-1Ra can block many of the effects observed during the pathological process of OA, including prostaglandin synthesis in synovial cells, collagenase production by chondrocytes and cartilage matrix degradation. IL-1Ra is found in different forms, one extracellular and termed the soluble IL-1Ra (IL-1sRa), and two intracellular, the icIL-1RaI and icIL-1RaII [141]. Both the soluble and the icIL-1Ra can bind to the IL-1R, but with about 5-fold less affinity for the latter. Although intensive research is underway, the action of the icIL-1Ra remains elusive. *In vitro* experiments have revealed that an excess of 10–100 times the amount of IL-1Ra is necessary to inhibit the IL-1β activity, whereas 100–2000 times more IL-1Ra is needed *in vivo* [131, 168–170]. This may likely explain the relative deficit of IL-1Ra to IL-1β found in OA synovium, which in turn may cause the increased level of IL-1 activity in this pathological tissue.

The second category is the binding inhibition of the pro-inflammatory cytokine to its receptor by binding to free cytokines. Such molecules exist in humans, two of which are IL-1sR and TNF-sR [171, 172]. These soluble receptors are truncated forms of each receptor – types I and II IL-1sR, and TNF-sR55 and TNF-sR75. The shedded receptor may function as a receptor antagonist because the ligand binding region is preserved, thus being capable of competing with the membrane-associated receptors of the target cells. As well, the shedding of surface receptors may enable target cells to decrease their responsiveness to the ligand.

Recent work suggests that the type II IL-1R serves as the main precursor for shedded soluble receptors. The binding affinity of IL-1sR to both IL-1 and IL-1Ra differs. The type II IL-1sR binds IL–ß more readily than IL-1Ra; in contrast, the type I IL-1sR binds IL-1Ra with high affinity [141, 167, 173]. Hence, the simultaneous addition of both IL-1Ra and type II IL-1sR appears extremely beneficial, while the individual inhibitory effects of both IL-1Ra and type I IL-1sR are abrogated when present concurrently.

For TNF-α, an equivalent to the IL-1Ra has not yet been found; however, both membrane receptors could also be shed from chondrocytes and synovial fibroblasts. *In vivo* both the TNF-sR55 and TNF-sR75 are present in pathological articular tissue [123, 174, 175]. In OA synovial fibroblasts, a statistically significant upregulation in the release of TNF-R75 has been found [144]. The exact role of these TNF-sR in the control of TNF-α action remains under debate, and may depend on the irrelative abundance. It has been suggested that the TNF-sR acts as a receptor antagonist, mediates TNF-α activity, and/or stabilizes TNF-α [176]. Indeed, it has been suggested that at low concentrations these soluble receptors may stabilize the trimeric structure of TNF-α thereby increasing the half life of bioactive TNF-α [177], whereas at high concentrations, TNF-sR may reduce the bioactivity of TNF-α by competing for TNF-α binding with cell-associated receptors [178, 179]. Moreover, it has also been proposed that the TNF-R75 and/or the TNF-sR75 may function as a carrier of TNF-α, and is involved in facilitating the binding of TNF-α to its receptor [180].

Another natural inhibitor able to reduce pro-inflammatory cytokine production and/or activity is the presence in articular tissue of cytokines having anti-inflammatory properties. Four such cytokines, namely TGF-β, IL-4, IL-10 and IL-13, have been identified as able to modulate various inflammatory processes. These processes include a decreased production of pro-inflammatory cytokines such as IL-1ß and TNF-α, as well as some proteases, and an upregulation of the IL-1Ra and TIMP production [181–185]. Of note, it appears that the anti-inflammatory potential of these factors depends greatly on the target cell, even within the articular tissues [186–188]. Moreover, the individual effect on the cellular signaling pathways also varies greatly between them [189].

4.4.4
Signaling Pathways Activated by IL-1β and TNF-α

As mentioned above, IL-1β and TNF-α are the prototypes of pro-inflammatory cytokines involved in OA, and by acting alone or in tandem, both can promote articular joint tissue destruction. We will discuss some signaling pathways activated by the latter two cytokines in chondrocytes and synovial fibroblasts, and how they affect the genetic program of the latter cell types (Fig. 4).

Post-translational modification of proteins by phosphorylation plays an important role in the regulation of many cellular processes including gene expression [190, 191]. Considerable evidence accrued over the years has implicated phosphorylation reactions as the molecular basis for a large number of intracellular signaling cascades. Biological processes that depend on reversible phosphorylation require not only protein kinases but also protein phosphatases, and the cellular concentration of serine/threonine directed kinases (but not tyrosine specific kinases) is approximately equal to that of serine/threonine direct-

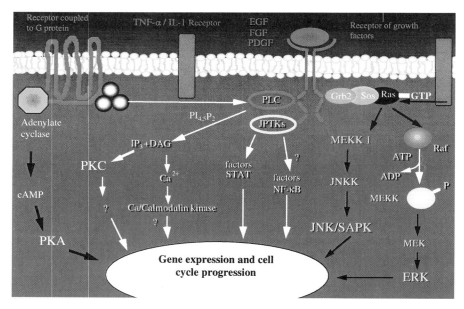

Fig. 4. Signaling pathways identified in human articular chondrocytes activated by various extracellular stimuli. NF-κB, nuclear factor κB; JPTKs, Janus tyrosine kinases SAPK/JNK, c-Jun N-terminal kinase; ERK, extracellular signal-regulated kinase; MAP, mitogen-activated protein; MEK, MAP kinase; MEKK, MEK kinase; PKA, cyclic AMP dependent protein kinase; PKC, calcium/phospholipid dependent protein kinase; PLC, phospholipase C; DAG, diacylglycerol; IP, inositol phosphate

ed phosphatases in cells [191]. Targeted substrate proteins are specifically phosphorylated at cognate sites by protein kinases, and dephosphorylated by substrate-specific phosphatases.

4.4.4.1
IL-1β Activated Signaling Pathways

The precise mechanism by which IL-1β induces target gene expression (e.g. collagenase-1, collagenase-3, cyclooxygenase 2 [COX-2], phospholipase A2 [cPLA2], iNOS, etc.) in chondrocytes and synovial fibroblasts is only partially understood. The cytoplasmic domains of these receptor types have no intrinsic enzymatic (e.g. kinase) activity in contrast to a number of growth factors or other cytokines.

For IL-1β, several post-receptor cytoplasmic signal transduction pathways have been implicated such as those involving protein kinase C (PKC), cAMP-dependent protein kinase A (PKA), MAP kinases ERK1/2, p38, JNK/SAPK and other protein kinases including tyrosine kinases and sphingomyelinase (Smase) [192–197]. IL-1β can also stimulate guanylate cyclase suggesting that cGMP could serve as a second messenger. Liberated as a result of IL-1β induction of iNOS, NO has also been implicated as a second messenger of IL-1 chondrocyte signaling [163, 198].

IL-1 activation of target cell collagenase-1 expression has been convincingly shown to be closely associated with increases in the activity of nuclear AP-1 and JNK/SAPK, and possibly Fos kinase [21, 199–201]. The latter two proline-directed MAP kinases specifically phosphorylate c-Jun and c-Fos, a process necessary for tight DNA binding [202]. The AP-1 protein complex, possibly a heterodimer of c-Fos and c-Jun, binds to a TPA regulatory element (TRE, inducible enhancer sequences) in the promoter region of collagenase-1 gene. This same TRE is known to be responsive to tumour promoting agents such as phorbol esters [203]. Phorbol myristate acetate, a potent phorbol ester, binds specifically to and potently activates PKC, thus giving rise to the association of PKC activation (and IL-1 activation of PKC) and collagenase-1 expression [204].

Interestingly, the increases in AP-1, JNK/SAPK activity, and collagenase-1 expression were found to be contingent on the IL-1 induced generation of reactive oxygen species (ROS) since potent anti-oxidants like N-acetylcysteine (NAC) abrogated the response of chondrocytes to IL-1 [205]. Furthermore, inhibiting endogenous ROS production with diphenyleneiodonium (DPI) also significantly attenuated IL-1 induced AP-1 and collagenase-1 gene expression [205]. Other ROS species stimulated by IL-1, such as NO, have been shown to play a partial role in collagenase-1 gene expression.

As mentioned above, a major IL-1 target gene in human chondrocytes is the iNOS, and indeed, large amounts of NO are released by IL-1 activated chondrocytes. The role of changes in cellular calcium flux as a mediator of IL-1 modulation of target gene expression has been a source of controversy. Increased intracellular Ca^{++} selectively suppresses IL-1-induced NO production by reducing iNOS mRNA stability in human chondrocytes [206]. These data would suggest that IL-1 either suppresses, or has no effect on, calcium metabolism. However, under identical culture conditions, calcium alone mediated increases in COX-2 expression, and combined with IL-1 produced enhanced levels of COX-2 mRNA [206]. In chondrocytes, more recent data indicate that IL-1-induced Ca^{++} signaling is dependent on focal adhesion formation, and that focal adhesions recruit IL-1 receptors by redistribution in the cell membrane [207].

Indeed, IL-1 induction of COX-2 has been shown to be mediated by PKC and NF-κB in mesangial cells [208] although this pathway has never been implicated in chondrocytes and synovial fibroblasts. In human chondrocytes, IL-1β may upregulate COX-2 by inhibiting serine/threonine protein phosphatases like PP-1 and PP-2 A. Specific inhibitors of PP-1 and PP-2 A mimic the effects of IL-1 in terms of COX-2 expression [209]. The inhibition of PP-1/PP-2 A results in a shutdown of the MEKK1/ MEK1/ERK cascade probably due to an increase in PKA activity which is known to inhibit Raf-1, a MEKK1 kinase. In contrast, in addition to an increased level of PKA, there is a concomitant activation of the other proline-directed MAP kinase pathway, namely MEKK1/JNKK/SAPK/JNK. There is circumstantial evidence to implicate a Fos kinase as well, given the prominence of c-Fos in the AP-1 complexes. The accumulated AP-1 factors probably consists partially of c-Fos/c-Jun, c-Jun/JunB and c-Fos/JunB dimers as judged by supershift assays. The AP-1 and CREB/ATF family of transcription factors may be substrates for PP-1/PP-2A in human chondrocytes [209].

Additional studies are underway to identify the regulatory elements in the promoter region of the COX-2 gene that mediate increases in the rate of COX-2 gene transcription following phosphatase inhibition and IL-1 treatment.

4.4.4.2
TNF-α Activated Signaling Pathways

TNF-α induces multiple biological activities and several distinct mechanisms of signal transduction may explain this diversity of action. As mentioned, after being secreted, TNF-α oligomerizes to form trimers [136]. Native TNF-α assumes a triangular pyramidal shape such that each side of the pyramid is formed by a different monomeric subunit. The receptor binding sites are located at the pyramid base permitting the simultaneous binding to more than one receptor.

The multiple biological activities could then first reflect that both the membrane receptors TNF-R55 and TNF-R75 are linked to distinct intracellular second-messengers. Second, these membrane receptors may function as transporters of TNF-α which by itself or complexed to its receptor may exhibit intracellular function. Third, response heterogeneity may be caused by a diversification of post-receptor signal transduction pathways [210]. Following receptor trimerization, a number of intracellular pathways can be triggered by TNF-α. One strategy for transmitting signals from the cell surface to the nucleus is regulated nuclear translocation of transcription factors that are stored as an inactive cytoplasmic complex, first demonstrated for NF-κB [211].

NF-κB consists of at least five members (NF-κB1 p50, NF-κB2 p52, Rel A p65, Rel B, c-Rel) forming complexes. In non-stimulated chondrocytes and synovial fibroblasts, the various NF-κB complexes (e.g. NF-κB1 p50 and Rel A p65) are held in the cytoplasm by interaction with the IκBα/β inhibitors. The latter may function by masking the nuclear translocation sequence within the Rel-homology domain of NF-κB proteins [212]. Following cell stimulation with TNF-α, the NF-κB-IκBα/β complex dissociates and NF-κB dimers are rapidly (within minutes) translocated to the nucleus. The key step in NF-κB activation is the TNF-α-inducible proteolysis of IκBα/β [213], an event that precedes its degradation [214]. Two kinases have recently been identified that specifically phosphorylate IκBα/β, namely IκBα and IκBβ kinases, which are encoded by distinct genes [215]. Once IκBα/β are phosphorylated, they are targeted for degradation by the ubiquitin/proteasome system [214,216]. It is quite likely that COX-2 and IL-1β are but two of several genes modulated, at least in part, by TNF-α-induced NF-κB nuclear translocation.

The regulation of collagenase-1 and cPLA2 by TNF-α in chondrocytes and synovial fibroblasts and other cell types probably involves another signaling pathway distinct from NF-κB. The promoter region of both of these genes harbors critical AP-1 sites, and TNF-α induces AP-1 synthesis [217]. TNF-α activates a phosphatidylcholine (PC)-specific phospholipase (PLC) producing Ca^{++} independent diacylglycerol (DAG) formation and inositol phosphates from phosphatidylcholine [218]. The DAG acts as a second messenger of TNF-α action and activates, among other enzymes involved in signal transduction, acidic shingomyelinase (SMase) and PKC. The activation of the acid SMase by DAG causes a breakdown of sphingomyelin to produce ceramide, which acts as a second messenger mediating a number of cellular responses in many cell types, but has not been confirmed in chondrocytes and synoviocytes [219].

It has been shown that TNF-α can induce PKC-α (principal isoform in chondrocytes and synovial fibroblasts) activation/translocation to membrane fractions in these articular tissue cells resulting in long-term downregulation of cytosolic PKC activity [220]. There is a concomitant increase in nuclear AP-1 activity that follows increases in JNK/SAPK activity. The PKC signaling pathways mainly affect AP-1 activity at two levels: transcriptional and post-transcriptional. First, transcription of the *fos* genes, very low in most non-stimulated cells, is induced in response to TNF-α. The most rapid induction is exhibited by c-*fos*, the expression of which is also highly transient while induction of other fos genes, such as *fra*-1, is somewhat slower and longer lasting [221]. Most of the signals stimulate c-*fos* transcription through the serum response element (SRE) [222]. Induction of fos transcription results in increased synthesis of Fos proteins which combine with pre-existing Jun proteins to form more stable heterodimers and thereby increase the level of AP-1 binding activity. Most of the signals that stimulate AP-1 activity induce c-*jun* transcription, which usually is longer lasting than c-*fos* induction [221]. The persistent induction of c-*jun* is presumably due to the ability of c-Jun to autoregulate its expression by binding to a TRE in the c-*jun* promoter [223]. Expression of *jun*B is also stimulated by TNF-α, while the expression of *jun*D is constitutive [224]. The differential responsiveness and induction kinetics of the various *jun* and *fos* genes result in the formation of different AP-1 complexes at various times after cell stimulation.

TNF-α stimulates the activation of cPLA2 [225–228] resulting in the production of arachidonic acid (AA). Metabolites of AA such as prostaglandins may function as effector molecules in TNF-α cytotoxicity [229], and may be important mediators of inflammation. cPLA2 is phosphorylated on serine residues by PKC and the p42 MAP kinase, and the MAP kinase mediated phosphorylation is essential for receptor-induced cPLA2 activation [230, 231]. The pathway from the TNF-R to cPLA2 is not clear, and the SMase/ceramide cycle may possibly offer a link. Indeed, the TNF/SMase initiated protein phosphorylation cascade stimulates a MAP kinase pathway; as the p42 MAP kinases activate cPLA2, it is conceivable that the ceramide-activated protein kinase is an intermediate in the MAP kinase action pathways [232]. What is clear is that TNF-α activates the p42 and p44 MAP kinases and increases their tyrosine phosphorylation in human articular chondrocytes in culture [233]. Arachidonic acid is metabolized by lipoxygenase (LO) and COX generating eicosanoids and prostaglandins respectively. Lipoxygenase metabolites have been implicated in TNF-α responses such as TNF-α cytotoxicity, induction of the transcription factor c-fos, and the mitochondrial superoxide radical scavenging enzyme manganous superoxide dismutase (MnSOD) [234, 235]. The eicosanoids can be converted into lipoxins and other metabolites, and these lipid peroxidation products are a source of reactive-free radicals [236]. Oxygen radical generation by TNF-α [237, 238] may provide the essential cofactors for the induction c-fos, MnSOD, and TNF-cytotoxicity [239].

A 38 kD protein has been identified as the major tyrosine-phosphorylated protein following lipopolysaccharide (LPS) treatment [240]. Sequence of the cDNA indicated that the 38 kD polypeptide is a new member of the MAPK group [240]. In addition to LPS and IL-1, p38 is activated in response to osmotic shock and by and large responds to the same agonists that activate the JNKs [241]. TNF-α is a powerful stimulator of p38 in human chondrocytes in culture, and is believed to mediate many TNF-α induced processes associated with cartilage catabolism [197].

Recently Rothe et al. [242] identified a novel family of molecules that associate with the cytoplasmic domain of TNF-R75 and may serve as signal transducers. TNF receptor-associated factor 1 (TRAF1) and TRAF2 contain a novel region homology and form homo or heterodimers. The TRAF2 facilitates direct contact with the receptor, whereas the interaction between the TRAF1 and the cytoplasmic domain of TNF-R75 occurs indirectly via formation of TRAF1-TRAF2 heterodimers. The mode of activation of TRAFs, their downstream effectors, and related molecules involved in signaling from other members in the TNF receptor family remain to be elucidated.

4.4.5
Conclusion

Although cartilage degeneration characterizes human OA, there is increasing evidence suggesting that OA changes also involve the participation of the synovial membrane and the subchondral bone.

It is currently suggested that subchondral bone sclerosis may be more intimately related to the progression and/or onset of OA rather than merely a consequence of this disease. Both clinical and laboratory evidence indicates altered subchondral bone metabolism in OA, a situation that may result from abnormal osteoblast behaviour. Coupled with mechanical/chemical stresses, abnormal OA osteoblasts would then accelerate subchondral bone formation, which would enhance the mechanical pressure on the overlying cartilage in supporting joints, promoting further deterioration and cartilage erosion. The role for a local factor(s) produced by osteoblasts (including PA/plasmin and IGF systems) promoting cartilage breakdown and/or increasing subchondral bone turnover is gaining support.

At the clinical stage of the disease, the morphological changes observed in OA include a variable degree of synovial inflammation. The changes in cartilage are believed to relate to a complex network of biochemical factors, resulting in the breakdown of the articular joint tissue. In OA, pro-inflammatory cytokines as well as MMP play a pivotal role in mediating pathophysiological mechanisms.

Cytokines are developmental and homeostatic bioregulators of joint tissues, and are etiopathologically associated with progressive joint destruction. A fundamental axiom of cytokine biology is that they exhibit integrated functionality on several levels including biosynthesis and biological activity. A disturbance in the synthesis of pro-inflammatory cytokines may accelerate the progression of OA. A relative deficit in the production of IL-1Ra coupled with an upregulation of the receptor level, as well as imbalances in the soluble IL-1R or TNF-R and/or anti- and pro-inflammatory cytokines, are additional factors that favor the enhancement of the catabolic effect in OA. Cell signaling by IL-1β and TNF-α occurs through specific membrane receptors. Several post-receptor signal transduction pathways have been implicated for each of the latter cytokines. A better understanding of the specific (unique) IL-1β and TNF-α intracellular signaling cascade or transcription factors in OA articular joint tissue cells will provide additional molecular targets for pharmacological intervention. Indeed, the p38 MAP kinase was discovered to be an intracellular target for molecules that act as cytokine suppressive anti-inflammatory drugs. The current therapeutic strategies of antagonizing IL-1β and TNF-α with either receptor blockade (with IL-1Ra) or molecular quenching (with IL-1R or TNF-R soluble receptors) have also proven to be of value in other arthritic diseases or in animal models of OA.

The current understanding of the factors involved in this disease has evolved greatly during recent years. A better comprehension of the modulating factors as well as the major regulators has and will continue to generate new insights into a more accurate identification of effective targets having therapeutic potential in the treatment of OA. The future holds great promise for the development of new and successful approaches to the treatment of this disease.

References

1. Pelletier JP, Martel-Pelletier J, Howell DS (1997) Etiopathogenesis of osteoarthritis. In: Koopman WJ (ed) Arthritis and Allied Conditions. A Textbook of Rheumatology. 13th ed. Baltimore: Williams & Wilkins p 1969–1984
2. Radin EL, Paul IL, Tolkoff MJ (1970) Subchondral changes in patients with early degenerative joint disease. Arthritis Rheum 13: 400–405
3. Radin EL, Rose RM (1986) Role of subchondral bone in the initiation and progression of cartilage damage. Clin Orthop 213: 34–40
4. Carlson CS, Loeser RF, Jayo MJ, Weaver DS, Adams MR, Jerome CP (1994) Osteoarthritis in cynomolgus macaques: a primate model of naturally occurring disease. J Orthop Res 12: 331–339
5. Carlson CS, Loeser RF, Purser CB, Gardin JF, Jerome CP (1996) Osteoarthritis in cynomolgus macaques. III: Effects of age, gender, and subchondral bone thickness on the severity of disease. J Bone Miner Res 11: 1209–1217
6. Armstrong S, Read R, Ghosh P (1994) The effects of intraarticular hyaluronan on cartilage and subchondral bone changes in an ovine model of early osteoarthritis. J Rheumatol 21: 680–688
7. Dedrick DK, Goldstein SA, Brandt KD, O'Connor BL, Goulet RW, Albrecht M (1993) A longitudinal study of subchondral plate and trabecular bone in cruciate-deficient dogs with osteoarthritis followed up for 54 months. Arthritis Rheum 36: 1460–1467
8. Brandt KD, Myers SL, Burr D, Albrecht M (1991) Osteoarthritic changes in canine articular cartilage, subchondral bone, and synovium fifty-four months after transection of the anterior cruciate ligament. Arthritis Rheum 34: 1560–1570
9. Hulth A (1993) Does osteoarthrosis depend on growth of the mineralized layer of cartilage? Clin Orthop 287: 19–24
10. Shimizu M, Tsuji H, Matsui H, Katoh Y, Sano A (1993) Morphometric analysis of subchondral bone of the tibial condyle in osteoarthrosis. Clin Orthop 293: 229–239
11. Chai BF (1991) Scanning electron microscopic study of subchondral bone tissues in osteoarthritic femoral head. Chung Hua Wai Ko Tsa Chih 29: 573–6–590–1

12. Grynpas MD, Alpert B, Katz I, Lieberman I, Pritzker KPH (1991) Subchondral bone in osteoarthritis. Calcif Tissue Int 49:20–26
13. Puzas JE (1993) Primer on the Metabolic Bone Diseases and Disorders of Mineral Metabolism. 2nd ed. New York: Raven Press
14. Gevers G, Dequeker J, Martens M, Van Audekercke R, Nyssen-Behets C, Dhem A (1989) Biomechanical characteristics of iliac crest bone in elderly women, according to osteoarthritis grade at the hand joints. J Rheumatol 16:660–663
15. Gevers G, Dequeker J, Geusens P, Nyssen-Behets C, Dhem A (1989) Physical and histomorphological characteristics of iliac crest bone differ according to the grade of osteoarthritis at the hand. Bone 10:173–177
16. Raisz LG (1988) Local and systemic factors in the pathogenesis of osteoporosis. N Engl J Med 318:818–828
17. Parfitt AM (1979) Quantum concept of bone remodeling and turnover: implications for the pathogenesis of osteoporosis. Calcif Tissue Int 28:1–5
18. Centrella M, Canalis E (1985) Local regulators of skeletal growth: a perspective. Endocr Rev 6:544–551
19. Simpson E (1984) Growth factors which affect bone. Trends Biochem Sci 527–530
20. Price PA (1985) Vitamin K-dependent formation of bone Gla protein (osteocalcin) and its function. Vitam Horm 42:65–108
21. Lo YYC, Wong JMS, Cruz TF (1996) Reactive oxygen species mediate cytokine activation of c-Jun NH2- terminal kinases. J Biol Chem 271:15703–15707
22. Whitson SW, Harrison W, Dunlap MK, Bowers DE Jr, Fisher LW, Robey PG et al. (1984) Fetal bovine bone cells synthesize bone-specific matrix proteins. J Cell Biol 99:607–614
23. Kream BE, Rowe D, Smith MD, Maher V, Majeska R (1986) Hormonal regulation of collagen synthesis in a clonal rat osteosarcoma cell line. Endocrinology 119:1922–1928
24. Heath JK, Atkinson SJ, Meikle MC, Reynolds JJ (1984) Mouse osteoblasts synthesize collagenase in response to bone resorbing agents. Biochim Biophys Acta 802:151–154
25. Otsuka K, Sodek J, Limeback H (1984) Synthesis of collagenase and collagenase inhibitors by osteoblast-like cells in culture. Eur J Biochem 145:123–129
26 Meikle MC, Bord S, Hembry RM, Reynolds JJ (1994) Rabbit calvarial osteoblasts in culture constitutively synthesize progelatinase-A, and TIMP-1 and TIMP-2. Biochim Biophys Acta 1224:99–102
27. Hoekman K, Lowik CW, van der Ruit M, Bijvoet OL, Verheijen JH, Papapoulos SE (1991) Regulation of the production of plasminogen activators by bone resorption enhancing and inhibiting factors in three types of osteoblast-like cells. Bone & Mineral 14:189–204
28. Fawthrop FW, Oyajobi BO, Bunning RA, Russell RG (1992) The effect of transforming growth factor beta on the plasminogen activator activity of normal human osteoblast-like cells and a human osteosarcoma cell line MG-63. J Bone Miner Res 7:1363–1371
29. Allan EH, Zeheb R, Gelehrter TD, Heaton JH, Fukumoto S, Yee JA et al. (1991) Transforming growth factor beta inhibits plasminogen activator (PA) activity and stimulates production of urokinase-type PA, PA inhibitor-1 mRNA, and protein in rat osteoblast-like cells. J Cell Physiol 149:34–43
30. Horowitz MC, Jilka RL (1992) Colony stimulating factors. In: Gowen M (ed) Cytokines and bone metabolism. Boca Raton: CRC Press pp 185–228
31. Löwik CWGM (1992) Differentiation inducing factors: leukemia inhibitor factor and interleukin-6. In: Gowen M (ed) Cytokines and bone metabolism. Boca Raton: CRC Press; pp 299–324
32. Pead MJ, Skerry TM, Lanyon LE (1988) Direct transformation from quiescence to bone formation in the adult periosteum following a single brief period of bone loading. J Bone Miner Res 3:647–656
33. Somjen D, Binderman I, Berger E, Harell A (1980) Bone remodelling induced by physical stress is prostaglandin E2 mediated. Biochim Biophys Acta 627:91–100
34. Shimshoni Z, Binderman I, Fine N, Somjen D (1984) Mechanical and hormonal stimulation of cell cultures derived from young rat mandible condyle. Arch Oral Biol 29:827–831

35. Yeh CK, Rodan GA (1984) Tensile forces enhance prostaglandin E synthesis in osteoblastic cells grown on collagen ribbons. Calcif Tissue Int 36 Suppl 1 : S67 – S71
36. Cheng MZ, Zaman G, Rawlinson SC, Pitsillides AA, Suswillo RF, Lanyon LE (1997) Enhancement by sex hormones of the osteoregulatory effects of mechanical loading and prostaglandins in explants of rat ulnae. J Bone Miner Res 12:1424 – 1430
37. Harter LV, Hruska KA, Duncan RL (1995) Human osteoblast-like cells respond to mechanical strain with increased bone matrix protein production independent of hormonal regulation. Endocrinology 136:528 – 535
38. Zaman G, Suswillo RF, Cheng MZ, Tavares IA, Lanyon LE (1997) Early responses to dynamic strain change and prostaglandins in bone-derived cells in culture. J Bone Miner Res 12:769 – 777
39. Keles AO, Schaffer JL, Gerstenfeld LC, Graves D, Stashenko P (1994) Modulation of integrin and nonintegrin adhesion molecules in normal human osteoblasts by a spatially uniform biaxial strain *in vitro*. J Bone Miner Res 9 (Suppl 1): S305 (Abstract)
40. Cheng MZ, Zaman G, Rawlinson SC, Suswillo RF, Lanyon LE (1996) Mechanical loading and sex hormone interactions in organ cultures of rat ulna. J Bone Miner Res 11 : 502 – 511
41. Cheng MZ, Zaman G, Rawlinson SC, Pitsillides AA, Suswillo RF, Lanyon LE (1997) Enhancement by sex hormones of the osteoregulatory effects of mechanical loading and prostaglandins in explants of rat ulnae. J Bone Miner Res 12:1424 – 1430
42. Yamaguchi DT, Hahn TJ, Iida-Klein A, Kleeman CR, Muallem S (1987) Parathyroid hormone-activated calcium channels in an osteoblast-like clonal osteosarcoma cell line. cAMP-dependent and cAMP-independent calcium channels. J Biol Chem 262 : 7711 – 7718
43. Moreau R, Hurst AM, Lapointe JY, Lajeunesse D (1996) Activation of maxi-K channels by parathyroid hormone and prostaglandin E2 in human osteoblast bone cells. J Membr Biol 150 : 175 – 184
44. Moreau R, Aubin R, Lapointe JY, Lajeunesse D (1997) Pharmacological and biochemical evidence for the regulation of osteocalcin secretion by potassium channels in human osteoblast-like MG- 63 cells. J Bone Miner Res 12 : 1984 – 1992
45. Urist MR (1960) Observations bearing on the problem of osteoporosis. In: Bodahl K (ed) Bone as a tissue. New York: McGraw Hill pp 18 – 23
46. Dequeker J, Goris P, Uytterhoeven R (1983) Osteoporosis and osteoarthritis (osteoarthrosis). JAMA 249 : 1448 – 1451
47. Marks SC Jr, McGuire JL (1989) Primary bone cell disfunction. In: Tam CS, Heersche JNM, Murray TM (eds) Metabolic Bone Disease: Cellular and Tissue Mechanisms. Boca Raton: CRC Press pp 49 – 61
48. Milgram JW, Jasty M (1982) Osteopetrosis – A morphological study of twenty-one cases. J Bone Joint Surg Am 64 A: 912 – 929
49. Lajeunesse D, Busque L, Ménard P, Brunette MG, Bonny Y (1996) Demonstration of an osteoblast defect in two cases of human malignant osteopetrosis: Correction of the phenotype after bone marrow transplant. J Clin Invest 98 : 1835 – 1842
50. Raymaekers G, Aerssens J, Van den Eynde R, Peeters J, Geusens P, Devos P et al. (1992) Alterations of the mineralization profile and osteocalcin concentrations in osteoarthritic cortical iliac crest bone. Calcif Tissue Int 51 : 269 – 275
51. Verstraeten A, van Ermen H, Haghebaert G, Mijs J, Geusens P, Dequeker J (1991) Osteoarthrosis retards the development of osteoporosis. Clin Orthop 264 : 169 – 177
52. Foss MVL, Byers PD (1972) Bone density, osteoarthrosis of the hip and fracture of the upper end of the femur. Ann Rheum Dis 31 : 259 – 264
53. Roh YS, Dequeker J, Muiler JC (1974) Bone mass is osteoarthrosis, measured *in vivo* by photon absorption. J Bone Joint Surg Am 54 A: 587 – 591
54. Carlsson A, Nillson BE, Westlin NE (1979) Bone mass in primary coxarthrosis. Acta Orthop Scand 50 : 187 – 189
55. Vandermeersch S, Geusens P, Nijs J, Dequeker J (1990) Total body mineral measurements in osteoarthritis, osteoporosis and normal controls. In: Ring EF, editor. Current Research in Osteoporosis and Bone Mineral Measurement. London: British Institute of Radiology pp 49

56. Mokassa Bakumobatane L, Dequeker J, Raymaekers G, Aerssens J (1993) Effects of osteo-arthritis (OA) and body weight on subchondral cancellous bone quality of proximal tibia. Osteoarthritis Cartilage 1 : 55 – 56

57. Hordon LD, Stewart SP, Troughton PR, Wright V, Horsman A, Smith MA (1993) Primary generalized osteoarthritis and bone mass. Br J Rheumatol 32 : 1059 – 1061

58. Geusens P, Dequeker J, Verstraeten A (1983) Age-related blood changes in hip osteo-arthritis patients: a possible indicator of bone quality [letter]. Ann Rheum Dis 42 : 112 – 113

59. Geusens P, Dequeker J, Bouillon R (1990) Salmon calcitonin stimulates PTH (1 – 84) and 1,25-dihydroxyvitamin D_3 in osteoporosis and osteoarthritis. In: Christiansen C, Over-gaard K (eds) Osteoporosis. Copenhagen: Osteopress, ApS pp 368 – 369

60. Geusens P, Vanderschueren D, Verstraeten A, Dequeker J, Devos P, Bouillon R (1991) Short-term course of $1,25(OH)_2D_3$ stimulates osteoblasts but not osteoclasts in osteo-porosis and osteoarthritis. Calcif Tissue Int 49 : 168 – 173

61. Hilal G, Martel-Pelletier J, Pelletier JP, Ranger P, Lajeunesse D (1998) Osteoblast-like cells from human subchondral osteoarthritic bone demonstrate an altered phenotype *in vitro*: Possible role in subchondral bone sclerosis. Arthritis Rheum 41: 891 – 897

62. Kamibayashi L, Wyss UP, Cooke TD, Zee B (1995) Trabecular microstructure in the medial condyle of the proximal tibia of patients with knee osteoarthritis. Bone 17 : 27 – 35

63. Gevers G, Dequeker J (1987) Collagen and non-collagenous protein content (osteocalcin, sialoprotein, proteoglycan) in the iliac crest bone and serum osteocalcin in women with and without hand osteoarthritis. Coll Relat Res 7 : 435 – 442

64. Dedrick DK, Goulet R, Huston L, Goldstein SA, Bole GG (1991) Early bone changes in experimental osteoarthritis using microscopic computed tomography. J Rheum Suppl 27 : 44 – 45

65. Hannan MT, Anderson JJ, Zhang Y, Levy D, Felson DT (1993) Bone mineral density and knee osteoarthritis in elderly men and women. Arthritis Rheum 36 : 1671 – 1680

66. Li B, Aspden RM (1997) Composition and mechanical properties of cancellous bone from the femoral head of patients with osteoporosis or osteoarthritis. J Bone Miner Res 12 : 614 – 651

67. Westacott CI, Webb GR, Warnock MG, Sims JV, Elson CJ (1997) Alteration of cartilage metabolism by cells from osteoarthritic bone. Arthritis Rheum 40 : 1282 – 1291

68. Saïed A, Cherin E, Gaucher H, Laugier P, Gillet P, Floquet J et al. (1997) Assessment of articular cartilage and subchondral bone: subtle and progressive changes in experi-mental osteoarthritis using 50 MHz echography in vitro. J Bone Miner Res 12 : 1378 – 1386

69. Sokoloff L (1993) Microcracks in the calcified layer of articular cartilage. Arch Pathol Lab Med 117 : 191 – 195

70. Sharif M, George E, Dieppe PA (1995) Correlation between synovial fluid markers of cartilage and bone turnover and scintigraphic scan abnormalities in osteoarthritis of the knee. Arthritis Rheum 38 : 78 – 81

71. Ripamonti U, Duneas N, Van Den Heever B, Bosch C, Crooks J (1997) Recombinant transforming growth factor-beta1 induces endochondral bone in the baboon and synergizes with recombinant osteogenic protein-1 (bone morphogenetic protein-7) to initiate rapid bone formation. J Bone Miner Res 12 : 1584 – 1595

72. Lietman SA, Yanagishita M, Sampath TK, Reddi AH (1997) Stimulation of proteoglycan synthesis in explants of porcine articular cartilage by recombinant osteogenic protein-1 (bone morphogenetic protein-7). J Bone Joint Surg Am 79 : 1132 – 1137

73. Erickson DM, Harris SE, Dean DD, Harris MA, Wozney JM, Boyan BD et al. (1997) Recombinant bone morphogenetic protein (BMP)-2 regulates costochondral growth plate chondrocytes and induces expression of BMP-2 and BMP-4 in a cell maturation-dependent manner. J Orthop Res 15 : 371 – 380

74. Martel-Pelletier J, Hilal G, Pelletier JP, Ranger P, Lajeunesse D (1997) Evidence for increased metabolic activity in human osteoarthritic subchondral bone explants. Arthritis Rheum 40: S182 (Abstract)

75. Rosen CJ, Dimai HP, Vereault D, Donahue LR, Beamer WG, Farley J et al. (1997) Circulating and skeletal insulin-like growth factor-I (IGF-I) concentrations in two inbred strains of mice with different bone mineral densities. Bone 21: 217–223
76. Canalis E (1997) Insulin-like growth factors and osteoporosis. Bone 21: 215–216
77. Hilal G, Martel-Pelletier J, Pelletier JP, Duval N, Lajeunesse D (1998) Abnormal regulation of urokinase plasminogen activator by insulin-like growth factor-1 in human osteoarthritic subchondral osteoblasts. Arthritis Rheum 41:S199 (abstract)
78. Uitterlinden AG, Burger H, Huang Q, Odding E, Duijn CM, Hofman A et al. (1997) Vitamin D receptor genotype is associated with radiographic osteoarthritis at the knee. J Clin Invest 1100: 259–263
79. Martel-Pelletier J, Faure MP, McCollum R, Mineau F, Cloutier JM, Pelletier JP (1991) Plasmin, plasminogen activators and inhibitor in human osteoarthritic cartilage. J Rheumatol 18: 1863–1871
80. Dean DD (1991) Proteinase-mediated cartilage degradation in osteoarthritis [Review]. Semin Arthritis Rheum 20: 2–11
81. Sandy JD, Flannery CR, Neame PJ, Lohmander LS (1992) The structure of aggrecan fragments in human synovial fluid. Evidence for the involvement in osteoarthritis of a novel proteinase which cleaves the Glu 373-Ala 374 bond of the interglobular domain. J Clin Invest 89: 1512–1516
82. Martel-Pelletier J, Pelletier JP (1996) Wanted – the collagenase responsible for the destruction of the collagen network in human cartilage. Br J Rheumatol 35: 818–820
83. Moldovan F, Pelletier JP, Hambor J, Cloutier JM, Martel-Pelletier J (1997) Collagenase-3 (matrix metalloprotease 13) is preferentially localized in the deep layer of human arthritic cartilage in situ: *in vitro* mimicking effect by transforming growth factor beta. Arthritis Rheum 40: 1653–1661
84. Fernandes JC, Martel-Pelletier J, Lascau-Coman V, Moldovan F, Jovanovic D, Raynauld JP et al. (1998). Collagenase-1 and collagenase-3 synthesis in early experimental osteoarthritic canine cartilage. An immunohistochemical study. J Rheumatol 25:1585–1594
85. Nguyen Q, Mort JS, Roughley PJ (1992) Preferential mRNA expression of prostromelysin relative to procollagenase and in situ localization in human articular cartilage. J Clin Invest 89: 1189–1197
86. Cole AA, Chubinskaya S, Schumacher B, Huch K, Szabo G, Yao J et al. (1996) Chondrocyte matrix metalloproteinase-8. Human articular chondrocytes express neutrophil collagenase. J Biol Chem 271: 11023–11026
87. Okada Y, Shinmei M, Tanaka O, Naka K, Kimura A, Nakanishi I et al. (1992) Localization of matrix metalloproteinase 3 (stromelysin) in osteoarthritic cartilage and synovium. Lab Invest 66: 680–690
88. Sirum KL, Brinckerhoff CE (1989) Cloning of the genes for human stromelysin and stromelysin 2: differential expression in rheumatoid synovial fibroblasts. Biochemistry 28: 8691–8698
89. Hembry RM, Bagga MR, Reynolds JJ, Hamblen DL (1995) Immunolocalisation studies on six matrix metalloproteinases and their inhibitors, TIMP-1 and TIMP-2, in synovia from patients with osteo- and rheumatoid arthritis. Ann Rheum Dis 54: 25–32
90. Nawrocki B, Polette M, Clavel C, Morrone A, Eschard JP, Etienne JC et al. (1994) Expression of stromelysin 3 and tissue inhibitors of matrix metallo-proteinases, TIMP-1 and TIMP-2, in rheumatoid arthritis. Pathol Res Pract 190: 690–696
91. Mohtai M, Smith RL, Schurman DJ, Tsuji Y, Torti FM, Hutchinson NI et al. (1993) Expression of 92-kD type IV collagenase/gelatinase (gelatinase B) in osteoarthritic cartilage and its induction in normal human articular cartilage by interleukin-1. J Clin Invest 92: 179–185
92. Buttner FH, Chubinskaya S, Margerie D, Huch K, Flechtenmacher J, Cole AA et al. (1997) Expression of membrane type 1 matrix metalloproteinase in human articular cartilage. Arthritis Rheum 40: 704–709
93. Ohuchi E, Imai K, Fujii Y, Sato H, Seiki M, Okada Y (1997) Membrane type 1 matrix metalloproteinase digests interstitial collagens and other extracellular matrix macromolecules. J Biol Chem 272: 2446–2451

94. Takino T, Sato H, Shinagawa A, Seiki M (1995) Identification of a second membrane-type metalloproteinase (MT-MMP-2) gene from a human placenta cDNA library. MT-MMPs form a unique membrane-type subclass in the MMP family. J Biol Chem 270: 23 013 – 23 020

95. Imai K, Ohuchi E, Aoki T, Nomura H, Fujii Y, Sato H et al. (1996) Membrane-type matrix metalloproteinase 1 is a gelatinolytic enzyme and is secreted in a complex with tissue inhibitor of metalloproteinases 2. Cancer Res 56 : 2707 – 2710

96. Martel-Pelletier J, McCollum R, Fujimoto N, Obata K, Cloutier JM, Pelletier JP (1994) Excess of metalloproteases over tissue inhibitor of metalloprotease may contribute to cartilage degradation in osteoarthritis and rheumatoid arthritis. Lab Invest 70 : 807 – 815

97. Apte SS, Mattei M-G, Olsen BR (1994) Cloning of the cDNA encoding human tissue inhibitor of metalloproteinases-3 (TIMP-3) and mapping of the TIMP3 gene to chromosome 22. Genomics 19 : 86 – 90

98. Dean DD, Martel-Pelletier J, Pelletier JP, Howell DS, Woessner JF Jr (1989) Evidence for metalloproteinase and metalloproteinase inhibitor imbalance in human osteoarthritic cartilage. J Clin Invest 84 : 678 – 685

99. Greene J, Wang M, Liu YE, Raymond LA, Rosen C, Shi YE (1996) Molecular cloning and characterization of human tissue inhibitor of metalloproteinase 4. J Biol Chem 271 : 30 375 – 30 380

100. Bigg HF, Shi YE, Liu YE, Steffensen B, Overall CM (1997) Specific, high affinity binding of tissue inhibitor of metalloproteinases-4 (TIMP-4) to the COOH-terminal hemopexin-like domain of human gelatinase A. TIMP-4 binds progelatinase A and the COOH-terminal domain in a similar manner to TIMP-2. J Biol Chem 272 : 15 496 – 15 500

101. Will H, Atkinson SJ, Butler GS, Smith B, Murphy G (1996) The soluble catalytic domain of membrane type 1 matrix metalloproteinase cleaves the propeptide of progelatinase A and initiates autoproteolytic activation. Regulation by TIMP-2 and TIMP-3. J Biol Chem 271 : 17 119 – 17 123

102. Pelletier JP, Mineau F, Faure MP, Martel-Pelletier J (1990) Imbalance between the mechanisms of activation and inhibition of metalloproteases in the early lesions of experimental osteoarthritis. Arthritis Rheum 33 : 1466 – 1476

103. Wolfe GC, MacNaul KL, Buechel FF, McDonnell J, Hoerrner LA, Lark MW et al. (1993) Differential in vivo expression of collagenase messenger RNA in synovium and cartilage: Quantitative comparison with stromelysin messenger RNA levels in human rheumatoid arthritis and osteoarthritis patients and in two animal models of acute inflammatory arthritis. Arthritis Rheum 36 : 1540 – 1547

104. Dean DD, Woessner JF Jr (1985) Extracts of human articular cartilage contain an inhibitor of tissue metalloproteinases. Prog Clin Biol Res 180 : 265 – 267

105. Lohmander LS, Hoerrner LA, Lark MW (1993) Metalloproteinases, tissue inhibitor and proteoglycan fragments in knee synovial fluid in human osteoarthritis. Arthritis Rheum 36 : 181 – 189

106. Clark IM, Powell LK, Ramsey S, Hazleman BL, Cawston TE (1993) The measurement of collagenase, tissue inhibitor of metalloproteinases (TIMP), and collagenase-TIMP complex in synovial fluids from patients with osteoarthritis and rheumatoid arthritis. Arthritis Rheum 36 : 372 – 379

107. Gomez DE, Alonso DF, Yoshiji H, Thorgeirsson UP (1997) Tissue inhibitors of metalloproteinases: structure, regulation and biological functions. Eur J Cell Biol 74 : 111 – 122

108. Leco KJ, Apte SS, Taniguchi GT, Hawkes SP, Khokha R, Schultz GA et al. (1997) Murine tissue inhibitor of metalloproteinases-4 (TIMP-4): cDNA isolation and expression in adult mouse tissues. FEBS Lett 401 : 213 – 217

109. Nagase H, Enghild JJ, Suzuki K, Salvesen G (1990) Stepwise activation mechanisms of the precursor of matrix metalloproteinase 3 (stromelysin) by proteinases and (4-aminophenyl) mercuric acetate. Biochemistry 29 : 5783 – 5789

110. Eeckhout Y, Vaes G (1977) Further studies on the activation of procollagenase, the latent precursor of bone collagenase. Effects of lysosomal cathepsin B, plasmin and kallikrein, and spontaneous activation. Biochem J 166 : 21 – 31

111. Martel-Pelletier J, Cloutier JM, Pelletier JP (1990) Cathepsin B and cysteine protease inhibitors in human OA: Effect of intra-articular steroid injections. J Orthop Res 8:336–344
112. Buttle DJ, Handley CJ, Ilic MZ, Saklatvala J, Murata M, Barrett AJ (1993) Inhibition of cartilage proteoglycan release by a specific inactivator of cathepsin B and an inhibitor of matrix metalloproteinases. Evidence for two converging pathways of chondrocyte-mediated proteoglycan degradation. Arthritis Rheum 36:1709–1717
113. Murphy G, Cockett MI, Stephens PE, Smith BJ, Docherty AJ (1987) Stromelysin is an activator of procollagenase. A study with natural and recombinant enzymes. Biochem J 248:265–268
114. Ogata Y, Enghild JJ, Nagase H (1992) Matrix metalloproteinase 3 (stromelysin) activates the precursor for the human matrix metalloproteinase 9. J Biol Chem 267:3581–3584
115. Knauper V, Lopez-Otin C, Smith B, Knight G, Murphy G (1996) Biochemical characterization of human collagenase-3. J Biol Chem 271:1544–1550
116. Knauper V, Will H, Lopez-Otin C, Smith B, Atkinson SJ, Stanton H et al. (1996) Cellular mechanisms for human procollagenase-3 (MMP-13) activation. Evidence that MT1-MMP (MMP-14) and gelatinase a (MMP-2) are able to generate active enzyme. J Biol Chem 271:17124–17131
117. Atkinson SJ, Crabbe T, Cowell S, Ward RV, Butler MJ, Sato H et al. (1995) Intermolecular autolytic cleavage can contribute to the activation of progelatinase A by cell membranes. J Biol Chem 270:30479–30485
118. Knauper V, Smith B, Lopez-Otin C, Murphy G (1997) Activation of progelatinase B (proMMP-9) by active collagenase-3 (MMP- 13). Eur J Biochem 248:369–373
119. d'Ortho MP, Will H, Atkinson S, Butler G, Messent A, Gavrilovic J et al. (1997) Membrane-type matrix metalloproteinases 1 and 2 exhibit broad-spectrum proteolytic capacities comparable to many matrix metalloproteinases. Eur J Biochem 250:751–757
120. Caron JP, Fernandes JC, Martel-Pelletier J, Tardif G, Mineau F, Geng C et al. (1996) Chondroprotective effect of intraarticular injections of interleukin-1 receptor antagonist in experimental osteoarthritis: suppression of collagenase-1 expression. Arthritis Rheum 39:1535–1544
121. van de Loo FA, Joosten LA, van Lent PL, Arntz OJ, van den Berg WB (1995) Role of interleukin-1, tumor necrosis factor alpha, and interleukin-6 in cartilage proteoglycan metabolism and destruction. Effect of in situ blocking in murine antigen- and zymosan-induced arthritis. Arthritis Rheum 38:164–172
122. Plows D, Probert L, Georgopoulos S, Alexopoulou L, Kollias G (1995) The role of tumour necrosis factor (TNF) in arthritis: studies in transgenic mice. Rheumatol Eur Suppl 2:51–54
123. Chikanza IC, Roux-Lombard P, Dayer JM, Panayi GS (1993) Tumour necrosis factor soluble receptors behave as acute phase reactants following surgery in patients with rheumatoid arthritis, chronic osteomyelitis and osteoarthritis. Clin Exp Immunol 92:19–22
124. Pelletier JP, Faure MP, Di Battista JA, Wilhelm S, Visco D, Martel-Pelletier J (1993) Coordinate synthesis of stromelysin, interleukin-1, and oncogene proteins in experimental osteoarthritis. An immunohistochemical study. Am J Pathol 142:95–105
125. Pelletier JP, Martel-Pelletier J (1989) Evidence for the involvement of interleukin 1 in human osteoarthritic cartilage degradation: protective effect of NSAID. J Rheumatol 16:19–27
126. Farahat MN, Yanni G, Poston R, Panayi GS (1993) Cytokine expression in synovial membranes of patients with rheumatoid arthritis and osteoarthritis. Ann Rheum Dis 52:870–875
127. Wood DD, Ihrie EJ, Dinarello CA, Cohen PL (1983) Isolation of an interleukin 1 like factor from human joint effusions. Arthritis Rheum 26:975–983
128. Martel-Pelletier J, Zafarullah M, Kodama S, Pelletier JP (1991) In vitro effects of interleukin 1 on the synthesis of metalloproteases, TIMP, plasminogen activators and inhibitors in human articular cartilage. J Rheumatol 18 (Suppl 27): 80–84

129. Mosley B, Urdal DL, Prickett KS, Larsen A, Cosman D, Conlon PJ et al. (1987) The inter-leukin-1 receptor binds the human interleukin-1 alpha precursor but not the interleukin-1 beta precursor. J Biol Chem 1262:2941–2944
130. Siders WM, Klimovitz JC, Mizel SB (1993) Characterization of the structural requirements and cell type specificity of IL-1α and IL-1ß secretion. J Biol Chem 268: 22170–22174
131. Pelletier JP, McCollum R, Cloutier JM, Martel-Pelletier J (1995) Synthesis of metallo-proteases and interleukin 6 (IL-6) in human osteoarthritic synovial membrane is an IL-1 mediated process. J Rheumatol 22:109–114
132. Black RA, Kronheim SR, Cantrell M, Deeley MC, March CJ, Prickett KS et al. (1988) Generation of biologically active interleukin-1 beta by proteolytic cleavage of the inactive precursor. J Biol Chem 263:9437–9442
133. Kronheim SR, Mumma A, Greenstreet T, Glackin PJ, Van Ness K, March CJ et al. (1992) Purification of interleukin-1 beta converting enzyme, the protease that cleaves the inter-leukin-1 beta precursor. Arch Biochem Biophys 296:698–703
134. Wilson KP, Black JA, Thomson JA, Kim EE, Griffith JP, Navia MA et al. (1994) Structure and mechanism of interleukin-1 beta converting enzyme. Nature 370:270–275
135. Gearing AJ, Beckett P, Christodoulou M, Churchill M, Clements J, Davidson AH et al. (1994) Processing of tumour necrosis factor-alpha precursor by metalloproteinases. Nature 370:555–557
136. Aggarwal BB, Kohr WJ, Hass PE, Moffat B, Spencer SA, Henzel WJ et al. (1985) Human tumor necrosis factor. Production, purification, and characterization. J Biol Chem 260:2345–2354
137. Black RA, Rauch CT, Kozlosky CJ, Peschon JJ, Slack JL, Wolfson MF et al. (1997) A metal-loproteinase disintegrin that releases tumour-necrosis factor-alpha from cells. Nature 385:729–733
138. Amin AR, Patel IR, Attur M, Patel R, Thakker G, Solomon K et al. (1997) A novel snake venom-like protease (SVP) from human arthritis-affected cartilage has properties of TNF-alpha convertase regulation in arthritis-affected cartilage. Arthritis Rheum (Suppl): S78 (Abstract)
139. Slack J, McMahan CJ, Waugh S, Schooley K, Spriggs MK, Sims JE et al. (1993) Indepen-dent binding of interleukin-1 alpha and interleukin-1 beta to type I and type II inter-leukin-1 receptors. J Biol Chem 268:2513–2524
140. Tartaglia LA, Goeddel DV (1992) Two TNF receptors. Immunol Today 13:151–153
141. Arend WP (1993) Interleukin-1 receptor antagonist. Adv Immunol 54:167–227
142. Martel-Pelletier J, McCollum R, Di Battista JA, Faure MP, Chin JA, Fournier S et al. (1992) The interleukin-1 receptor in normal and osteoarthritic human articular chondrocytes. Identification as the type I receptor and analysis of binding kinetics and biologic func-tion. Arthritis Rheum 35:530–540
143. Sadouk M, Pelletier JP, Tardif G, Kiansa K, Cloutier JM, Martel-Pelletier J (1995) Human synovial fibroblasts coexpress interleukin-1 receptor type I and type II mRNA: The increased level of the interleukin-1 receptor in osteoarthritic cells is related to an increased level of the type 1 receptor. Lab Invest 73:347–355
144. Alaaeddine N, Di Battista JA, Pelletier JP, Cloutier JM, Kiansa K, Dupuis M et al. (1997) Osteoarthritic synovial fibroblasts possess an increased level of tumor necrosis factor-receptor 55 (TNF-R55) that mediates biological activation by TNF-alpha. J Rheumatol 24:1985–1994
145. Westacott CI, Atkins RM, Dieppe PA, Elson CJ (1994) Tumour necrosis factor-alpha receptor expression on chondrocytes isolated from human articular cartilage. J Rheumatol 21:1710–1715
146. Loetscher H, Pan YCE, Lahm HW, Gentz R, Brockhaus M, Tabuchi H et al. (1990) Molec-ular cloning and expression of the human 55 kd tumor necrosis factor receptor. Cell 61:351–359
147. Hohmann HP, Remy R, Brockhaus M, van Loon AP (1989) Two different cell types have different major receptors for human tumor necrosis factor (TNF alpha). J Biol Chem 264:14927–14934

148. Scheurich P, Thoma B, Ucer U, Pfizenmaier K (1987) Immunoregulatory activity of recombinant human tumor necrosis factor (TNF)-alpha: induction of TNF receptors on human T cells and TNF-alpha-mediated enhancement of T cell responses. J Immunol 138:1786–1790

149. Guerne PA, Zuraw BL, Vaughan JH, Carson DA, Lotz M (1989) Synovium as a source of interleukin-6 in vitro: Contribution to local and systemic manifestations of arthritis. J Clin Invest 83:585–592

150. Nietfeld JJ, Wilbrink B, Helle M, van Roy JL, den Otter W, Swaak AJ et al. (1990) Interleukin-1-induced interleukin-6 is required for the inhibition of proteoglycan synthesis by interleukin-1 in human articular cartilage. Arthritis Rheum 33:1695–1701

151. Lotz M, Guerne PA (1991) Interleukin-6 induces the synthesis of tissue inhibitor of metalloproteinases-1/erythroid potentiating activity. J Biol Chem 266:2017–2020

152. Lotz M, Moats T, Villiger PM (1992) Leukemia inhibitory factor is expressed in cartilage and synovium and can contribute to the pathogenesis of arthritis. J Clin Invest 90:888–896

153. Hamilton JA, Waring PM, Filonzi EL (1993) Induction of leukemia inhibitory factor in human synovial fibroblasts by IL-1 and tumor necrosis factor-alpha. J Immunol 150:1496–1502

154. Campbell IK, Waring P, Novak U, Hamilton JA (1993) Production of leukemia inhibitory factor by human articular chondrocytes and cartilage in response to interleukin-1 and tumor necrosis factor alpha. Arthritis Rheum 36:790–794

155. Carroll GJ, Bell MC (1993) Leukaemia inhibitory factor stimulates proteoglycan resorption in porcine articular cartilage. Rheumatol Int 13:5–8

156. Yao Z, Painter SL, Fanslow WC, Ulrich D, Macduff BM, Spriggs MK et al. (1995) Human IL-17: a novel cytokine derived from T cells. J Immunol 155:5483–5486

157. Jovanovic D, Di Battista JA, Martel-Pelletier J, Jolicoeur FC, He Y, Zhang M et al. (1998) Interleukin-17 (IL-17) stimulates the production and expression of proinflammatory cytokines, IL-beta and TNF-alpha, by human macrophages. J Immunol 160:3513–3521

158. Attur MG, Patel RN, Abramson SB, Amin AR (1997) Interleukin-17 up-regulation of nitric oxide production in human osteoarthritis cartilage. Arthritis Rheum 140:1050–1053

159. Pelletier JP, Mineau F, Ranger P, Tardif G, Martel-Pelletier J (1996) The increased synthesis of inducible nitric oxide inhibits IL-1Ra synthesis by human articular chondrocytes: possible role in osteoarthritic cartilage degradation. Osteoarthritis Cartilage 4:77–84

160. Farrell AJ, Blake DR, Palmer RM, Moncada S (1992) Increased concentrations of nitrite in synovial fluid and serum samples suggest increased nitric oxide synthesis in rheumatic diseases. Ann Rheum Dis 51:1219–1222

161. McInnes IB, Leung BP, Field M, Wei XQ, Huang FP, Sturrock RD et al. (1996) Production of nitric oxide in the synovial membrane of rheumatoid and osteoarthritis patients. J Exp Med 184:1519–1524

162. Grabowski PS, Wright PK, Van't Hof RJ, Helfrich MH, Ohshima H, Ralston SH (1997) Immunolocalization of inducible nitric oxide synthase in synovium and cartilage in rheumatoid arthritis and osteoarthritis. Br J Rheumatol 36:651–655

163. Charles IG, Palmer RM, Hickery MS, Bayliss MT, Chubb AP, Hall VS et al. (1993) Cloning, characterization and expression of a cDNA encoding an inducible nitric oxide synthase from the human chondrocyte. Proc Natl Acad Sci USA 90:11419–11423

164. Pelletier JP, Jovanovic D, Fernandes JC, Manning PT, Connor JR, Currie MG et al. (1998) Selective inhibition of inducible nitric oxide synthase reduces in vivo the progression of experimental osteoarthritis. Arthritis Rheum (In Press)

165. Connor JR, Manning PT, Settle SL, Moore WM, Jerome GM, Webber RK et al. (1995) Suppression of adjuvant-induced arthritis by selective inhibition of inducible nitric oxide synthase. Eur J Pharmacol 273:15–24

166. Stefanovic-Racic M, Meyers K, Meschter C, Coffey JW, Hoffman RA, Evans CH (1994) N-monomethyl arginine, an inhibitor of nitric oxide synthase, suppresses the development of adjuvant arthritis in rats. Arthritis Rheum 37:1062–1069

167. Dinarello CA (1996) Biologic basis for interleukin-1 in disease. Blood 87:2095–2147

168. Joosten LA, Helsen MM, van de Loo FA, van den Berg WB (1996) Anticytokine treatment of established type II collagen-induced arthritis in DBA/1 mice. A comparative study using anti-TNF alpha, anti- IL-1 alpha/beta, and IL-1Ra. Arthritis Rheum 39 : 797 – 809

169. Bakker AC, Joosten LAB, Arntz OJ, Helsen MMA, Bendele AM, Van de Loo FAJ et al. (1997) Prevention of murine collagen-induced arthritis in the knee and ipsilateral paw by local expression of human interleukin-1 receptor antagonist protein in the knee. Arthritis Rheum 40 : 893 – 900

170. Campion GV, Lebsack ME, Lookabaugh J, Gordon G, Catalano M (1996) Dose-range and dose-frequency study of recombinant human interleukin-1 receptor antagonist in patients with rheumatoid arthritis. The IL-1Ra Arthritis Study Group. Arthritis Rheum 39 : 1092 – 1101

171. Giri JG, Newton RC, Horuk R (1990) Identification of soluble interleukin-1 binding protein in cell-free supernatants. Evidence for soluble interleukin-1 receptor. J Biol Chem 265 : 17 416 – 17 419

172. Lantz M, Gullberg U, Nilsson E, Olsson I (1990) Characterization in vitro of a human tumor necrosis factor-binding protein. A soluble form of a tumor necrosis factor receptor. J Clin Invest 86 : 1396 – 1342

173. Svenson M, Hansen MB, Heegaard P, Abell K, Bendtzen K (1993) Specific binding of interleukin-1(IL-1)-beta and IL-1 receptor antagonist (IL-1ra) to human serum. High-affinity binding of IL-1ra to soluble IL-1 receptor type I. Cytokine 5 : 427 – 435

174. Roux-Lombard P, Punzi L, Hasler F, Bas S, Todesco S, Gallati H et al. (1993) Soluble tumor necrosis factor receptors in human inflammatory synovial fluids. Arthritis Rheum 36 : 485 – 489

175. Cope AP, Aderka D, Doherty M, Engelmann H, Gibbons D, Jones AC et al. (1992) Increased levels of soluble tumor necrosis factor receptors in the sera and synovial fluid of patients with rheumatic diseases. Arthritis Rheum 35 : 1160 – 1169

176. Tartaglia LA, Weber RF, Figari IS, Reynolds C, Palladino MA Jr, Goeddel DV (1991) The two different receptors for tumor necrosis factor mediate distinct cellular responses. Proc Natl Acad Sci USA 88 : 9292 – 9296

177. Aderka D, Engelmann H, Maor Y, Brakebusch C, Wallach D (1992) Stabilization of the bioactivity of tumor necrosis factor by its soluble receptors. J Exp Med 175 : 323 – 329

178. Higuchi M, Aggarwal BB (1992) Inhibition of ligand binding and antiproliferative effects of tumor necrosis factor and lymphotoxin by soluble forms of recombinant P60 and P80 receptors. Biochem Biophys Res Commun 182 : 638 – 643

179. Peppel K, Crawford D, Beutler B (1991) A tumor necrosis factor (TNF) receptor-IgG heavy chain chimeric protein as a bivalent antagonist of TNF activity. J Exp Med 174 : 1483 – 1489

180. Tartaglia LA, Pennica D, Goeddel DV (1993) Ligand passing: the 75-kDa tumor necrosis factor (TNF) receptor recruits TNF for signaling by the 55-kDa TNF receptor. J Biol Chem 268 : 18 542 – 18 548

181. Hart PH, Vitti GF, Burgess DR, Whitty GA, Piccoli DS, Hamilton JA (1989) Potential antiinflammatory effects of interleukin 4: suppression of human monocyte tumor necrosis factor alpha, interleukin 1, and prostaglandin E2. Proc Natl Acad Sci USA 86 : 3803 – 3807

182. Lacraz S, Nicod L, Galve-de Rochemonteix B, Baumberger C, Dayer JM, Welgus HG (1992) Suppression of metalloproteinase biosynthesis in human alveolar macrophages by interleukin-4. J Clin Invest 90 : 382 – 388

183. Jenkins JK, Malyak M, Arend WP (1994) The effects of interleukin-10 on interleukin-1 receptor antagonist and interleukin-1beta production in human monocytes and neutrophils. Lymphokine Cytokine Res 13 : 47 – 54

184. de Waal Malefyt R, Figdor CE, Huijbens R, Mohan-Peterson S, Bennett B, Culpepper JA et al. (1993) Effects of IL-13 on the phenotype, cytokine production, and cytotoxic function of human monocytes. J Immunol 151 : 6370 – 6381

185. Jovanovic D, Pelletier JP, Alaaeddine N, Mineau F, Geng C, Ranger P et al. (1998) Effect of IL-13 on cytokines, cytokine receptors and inhibitors on human osteoarthritic synovium and synovial fibroblasts. Osteoarthritis Cartilage 6 : 40 – 49

186. Hart PH, Ahern MJ, Jones CA, Jones KL, Smith MD, Finlay-Jones JJ (1993) Synovial fluid macrophages and blood monocytes differ in their responses to IL-4. J Immunol 151 : 3370 – 3380

187. Donnelly RP, Crofford LJ, Freeman SL, Buras J, Remmers E, Wilder RL et al. (1993) Tissue-specific regulation of IL-6 production by IL-4. Differential effects of IL-4 on nuclear factor-κB activity in monocytes and fibroblasts. J Immunol 151 : 5603 – 5612

188. Hart PH, Ahern MJ, Smith MD, Finlay-Jones JJ (1995) Regulatory effects of IL-13 on synovial fluid macrophages and blood monocytes from patients with inflammatory arthritis. Clin Exp Immunol 99 : 331 – 337

189. Alaaeddine N, Di Battista JA, Pelletier JP, Kiansa K, Cloutier JM, Martel-Pelletier J (1998) Inhibition of TNF-alpha-induced PGE_2 production by the antiinflammatory cytokines IL-4, IL-10 and IL-13 in osteoarthritic (OA) synovial fibroblasts: distinct targeting in the signaling pathways. (Submitted)

190. Hunter T, Karin M (1992) The regulation of transcription by phosphorylation. Cell 70 : 375 – 387

191. Hunter T (1995) Protein kinases and phosphatases: the yin and yang of protein phosphorylation and signaling. Cell 80 : 225 – 236

192. Bonin PD, Chiou WJ, McGee JE, Singh JP (1990) Two signal transduction pathways mediate interleukin-1 receptor expression in Balb/c3T3 fibroblasts. J Biol Chem 265 : 18 643 – 18 649

193. Munoz E, Beutner U, Zubiaga A, Huber BT (1990) IL-1 activates two separate signal transduction pathways in T helper type II cells. J Immunol 144 : 964 – 969

194. Donati D, Baldari CT, Macchia G, Massone A, Telford JL, Parente L (1990) Induction of gene expression by IL-1 in NIH 3T3 cells. Possible requirement of protein kinase C activity and independence from arachidonic acid metabolism. J Immunol 145 : 4115 – 4120

195. Kolesnick R, Golde DW (1994) The sphingomyelin pathway in tumor necrosis factor and interleukin-1 signaling. Cell 77 : 325 – 328

196. Munoz E, Zubiaga A, Huang C, Huber BT (1992) Interleukin-1 induces protein tyrosine phosphorylation in T cells. Eur J Immunol 22 : 1391 – 1396

197. Geng Y, Valbracht J, Lotz M (1996) Selective activation of the mitogen-activated protein kinase subgroups c-Jun NH_2 terminal kinase and p38 by IL-1 and TNF in human articular chondrocytes. J Clin Invest 98 : 2425 – 2430

198. Beasley D, McGuiggin M (1994) Interleukin 1 activates soluble guanylate cyclase in human vascular smooth muscle cells through a novel nitric oxide-independent pathway. J Exp Med 179 : 71 – 80

199. Deng T, Karin M (1994) c-Fos transcriptional activity stimulated by H-Ras-activated protein kinase distinct from JNK and ERK. Nature 371 : 171 – 175

200. Conca W, Kaplan PB, Krane SM (1989) Increases in levels of procollagenase messenger RNA in cultured fibroblasts induced by human recombinant interleukin 1 beta or serum follow c-jun expression and are dependent on new protein synthesis. J Clin Invest 83 : 1753 – 1757

201. Schonthal A, Herrlich P, Rahmsdorf HJ, Ponta H (1988) Requirement for fos gene expression in the transcriptional activation of collagenase by other oncogenes and phorbol esters. Cell 54 : 325 – 334

202. Karin M (1995) The regulation of AP-1 activity by mitogen-activated protein kinases. J Biol Chem 270 : 16 483 – 16 486

203. Angel P, Imagawa M, Chiu R, Stein B, Imbra RJ, Rahmsdorf HJ et al. (1987) Phorbol ester-inducible genes contain a common *cis* element recognized by a TPA-modulated trans-acting factor. Cell 49 : 729 – 739

204. Kiley SC, Jaken S (1994) Protein kinase C: Interactions and consequences. Trends in Cell Biology 4 : 223 – 227

205. Lo YYC, Conquer JA, Grinstein S, Cruz TF (1998) Interleukin-1β induction of c-fos and collagenase expression in articular chondrocytes: Involvement of reactive oxygen species. J Cell Biochem 69 : 19 – 29

206. Geng Y, Lotz M (1995) Increased intracellular Ca2+ selectively suppresses IL-1-induced NO production by reducing iNOS mRNA stability. J Cell Biol 129 : 1651–1657
207. Luo L, Cruz TF, McCulloch C (1997) Interleukin 1-induced calcium signalling in chondrocytes requires focal adhesions. Biochem J 324 : 653–658
208. Rzymkiewicz DM, Tetsuka T, Daphna-Iken D, Srivastava S, Morrison AR (1996) Interleukin-1β activates protein kinase Cd in renal mesangial cells. Potential role in prostaglandin E₂ up-regulation. J Biol Chem 271 : 17 241–17 246
209. Miller C, Zhang M, Zhao J, Pelletier JP, Martel-Pelletier J, Di Battista JA (1998) Transcriptional induction of cyclooxygenase-2 gene by okadaic acid inhibition of phosphatase activity in human chondrocytes: Co-stimulation of AP-1 and CRE nuclear binding proteins. J Cell Biochem 69 : 392–413
210. Schutze S, Potthoff K, Machleidt T, Berkovic D, Wiegmann K, Kronke M (1992) TNF activates NF-kappa B by phosphatidylcholine-specific phospholipase C-induced "acidic" sphingomyelin breakdown. Cell 71 : 765–776
211. Baeuerle PA, Baltimore D (1988) I kappa B: a specific inhibitor of the NF-kappa B transcription factor. Science 242 : 540–546
212. Beg AA, Finco TS, Nantermet PV, Baldwin AS Jr (1993) Tumor necrosis factor and interleukin-1 lead to phosphorylation and loss of I kappa B-alpha: a mechanism for NF-kappa B activation. Mol Cell Biol 13 : 3301–3310
213. Henkel T, Machleidt T, Alkalay I, Kronke M, Ben-Neriah Y, Baeuerle PA (1993) Rapid proteolysis of I kappa B-alpha is necessary for activation of transcription factor NF-kappa B. Nature 365 : 182–185
214. DiDonato JA, Mercurio F, Karin M (1995) Phosphorylation of I kappa B-alpha precedes but is not sufficient for its dissociation from NF-kappa B. Mol Cell Biol 15 : 1302–1311
215. Mercurio F, Zhu H, Murray BW, Shevchenko A, Bennett BL, Li J et al. (1997) IKK-1 and IKK-2: cytokine-activated IkappaB kinases essential for NF-kappaB activation. Science 278 : 860–866
216. Palombella VJ, Rando OJ, Goldberg AL, Maniatis T (1994) The ubiquitin-proteasome pathway is required for processing the NF-kappa B1 precursor protein and the activation of NF-kappa B. Cell 78 : 773–785
217. Appleby SB, Ristimäki A, Neilson K, Narko K, Hla T (1994) Structure of the human cyclooxygenase-2 gene. Biochem J 302 : 723–727
218. Schutze S, Berkovic D, Tomsing O, Unger C, Kronke M (1991) Tumor necrosis factor induces rapid production of 1′2′diacylglycerol by a phosphatidylcholine-specific phospholipase C. J Exp Med 174 : 975–988
219. Hannun YA (1994) The sphingomyelin cycle and the second messenger function of ceramide. J Biol Chem 269 : 3125–3128
220. Schutze S, Nottrott S, Pfizenmaier K, Kronke M (1990) Tumor necrosis factor signal transduction. Cell-type-specific activation and translocation of protein kinase C. J Immunol 144 : 2604–2608
221. Karin M, Liu Zg, Zandi E (1997) AP-1 function and regulation. Curr Opin Cell Biol 9 : 240–246
222. Treisman R (1992) The serum response element. Trends Biochem Sci 17 : 423–426
223. Angel P, Hattori K, Smeal T, Karin M (1988) The jun proto-oncogene is positively autoregulated by its product, Jun/AP-1. Cell 55 : 875–885
224. Angel P, Karin M (1991) The role of Jun, Fos and the AP-1 complex in cell-proliferation and transformation. Biochim Biophys Acta 1072 : 129–157
225. Godfrey RW, Johnson WJ, Hoffstein ST (1987) Recombinant tumor necrosis factor and interleukin-1 both stimulate human synovial cell arachidonic acid release and phospholipid metabolism. Biochem Biophys Res Commun 142 : 235–241
226. Suffys P, Van Roy F, Fiers W (1988) Tumor necrosis factor and interleukin 1 activate phospholipase in rat chondrocytes. FEBS Lett 232 : 24–28
227. Pfeilschifter J, Lempart UG, Naumann A, Minne HW, Ziegler R (1989) Transforming growth factor beta increases insulin-like growth factor I (IGFI) secretion in osteoblast-like cells. Acta Endocrinol 120 (Suppl 1): 144–145

228. Clark MA, Chen MJ, Crooke ST, Bomalaski JS (1988) Tumour necrosis factor (cachectin) induces phospholipase A2 activity and synthesis of a phospholipase A2-activating protein in endothelial cells. Biochem J 250 : 125–132

229. Neale ML, Fiera RA, Matthews N (1988) Involvement of phospholipase A2 activation in tumour cell killing by tumour necrosis factor. Immunology 64 : 81–85

230. Lin LL, Wartmann M, Lin AY, Knopf JL, Seth A, Davis RJ (1993) cPLA2 is phosphorylated and activated by MAP kinase. Cell 72 : 269–278

231. Nemenoff RA, Winitz S, Qian NX, Van Putten V, Johnson GL, Heasley LE (1993) Phosphorylation and activation of a high molecular weight form of phospholipase A2 by p42 microtubule-associated protein 2 kinase and protein kinase C. J Biol Chem 268 : 1960–1964

232. Liu J, Mathias S, Yang Z, Kolesnick RN (1994) Renaturation and tumor necrosis factor-alpha stimulation of a 97-kDa ceramide-activated protein kinase. J Biol Chem 269 : 3047–3052

233. Vietor I, Schwenger P, Li W, Schlessinger J, Vilcek J (1993) Tumor necrosis factor-induced activation and increased tyrosine phosphorylation of mitogen-activated protein (MAP) kinase in human fibroblasts. J Biol Chem 268 : 18 994–18 999

234. Haliday EM, Ramesha CS, Ringold G (1991) TNF induces c-fos via a novel pathway requiring conversion of arachidonic acid to a lipoxygenase metabolite. EMBO J 10 : 109–115

235. Chang DJ, Ringold GM, Heller RA (1992) Cell killing and induction of manganous superoxide dismutase by tumor necrosis factor-alpha is mediated by lipoxygenase metabolites of arachidonic acid. Biochem Biophys Res Commun 188 : 538–546

236. Samuelsson B, Dahlen SE, Lindgren JA, Rouzer CA, Serhan CN (1987) Leukotrienes and lipoxins: structures, biosynthesis, and biological effects. Science 237 : 1171–1176

237. Meier B, Radeke HH, Selle S, Younes M, Sies H, Resch K et al. (1989) Human fibroblasts release reactive oxygen species in response to interleukin-1 or tumour necrosis factor-alpha. Biochem J 263 : 539–545

238. Zimmerman RJ, Chan A, Leadon SA (1989) Oxidative damage in murine tumor cells treated *in vitro* by recombinant human tumor necrosis factor. Cancer Res 49 : 1644–1648

239. Yamauchi N, Kuriyama H, Watanabe N, Neda H, Maeda M, Niitsu Y (1989) Intracellular hydroxyl radical production induced by recombinant human tumor necrosis factor and its implication in the killing of tumor cells *in vitro*. Cancer Res 49 : 1671–1675

240. Han J, Lee JD, Bibbs L, Ulevitch RJ (1994) A MAP kinase targeted by endotoxin and hyperosmolarity in mammalian cells. Science 265 : 808–811

241. Lin A, Minden A, Martinetto H, Claret FX, Lange-Carter C, Mercurio F et al. (1995) Identification of a dual specificity kinase that activates the Jun kinases and p38-Mpk2. Science 268 : 286–290

242. Rothe M, Wong SC, Henzel WJ, Goeddel DV (1994) A novel family of putative signal transducers associated with the cytoplasmic domain of the 75 kDa tumor necrosis factor receptor. Cell 78 : 681–692

4.5
Role of Growth Factors and Cartilage Repair

W. B. van den Berg, P. M. van der Kraan and H. M. van Beuningen

4.5.1
The Osteoarthritic Process

Osteoarthritis (OA) is characterized by focal lesions of the articular cartilage, and concomitant hypertrophic reactions in the bone compartment. The latter includes sclerosis in the subchondral bone and new bone formation at the joint margins, the so-called osteophytes. The overall picture resembles a failure in attempt at repair. It is still debated whether the initiating process in human OA originates from changes in the underlying bone, with the articular cartilage trying to cope with this condition, or that the initial failure is in the cartilage itself. Given the heterogeneous character of the ill defined condition of human OA it might well be that both options do apply. It is long recognized that OA may occur as a consequence of multiple causes, ranging from blunt joint trauma, biomechanical overloading and inborn or acquired joint incongruency, to genetic defects in matrix components, inappropriate matrix assembly, or an imbalance of synovial and cartilaginous homeostasis. Probably the joint has only a limited capacity to react to various insults and, in fact, the osteoarthritic lesion does reflect a common endpoint. However, it seems likely that the mediators involved in the process may be different in the initial stages of the various forms.

Features in the OA cartilage include enhanced proteolytic activity and imbalance with their natural inhibitors, as well as an overactive chondrocyte showing enhanced production of proteoglycans and collagen, combined with an impairment of the cell to orchestrate adequate assembly of the macromolecules into the cartilage matrix. This might be due to the observed changes in the subtypes of proteoglycans and collagens produced by the OA chondrocytes, often showing embryonic elements, or is caused by yet unidentified blockades in the lesional tissue, hampering proper remodeling and substitution.

4.5.1.1
The Hypertrophic Stage

As an illustration of complexity of the OA process, meniscal damage or ligament rupture both cause an abrupt shift in biomechanical loading of articular cartilage and bone, with potential lesions and cellular response in that tissue, but it will also generate an attempted repair reaction in the damaged tissues, be it in this case either cartilaginous or ligamentous in nature. It is first recognized in the anterior cruciate ligament transection model in dogs and confirmed in other models [1–3], that the early changes in the articular cartilage reflect a hypertrophic reaction, with enhanced synthesis of matrix and increase in matrix content. This is followed by a stage of increased matrix turnover, with net depletion of matrix components, and, finally, damage and loss of the collagen network. The hypertrophic stage clearly precedes the occurrence of the lesional stage, with its characteristic focal loss of cartilage. It seems likely that excessive production and/or activation of growth factors is a major event in this early phase. Whether this growth factor response is pathogenic on its own (on the long run), or reflects the attempted repair with ultimate failure, remains to be elucidated. Basic understanding of the role of growth factors in articular cartilage and interplay with other cartilage associated mediators will help to clarify this issue.

4.5.1.2
Late Stages of OA

In late stages of the OA process further activation of the synovial tissue is a likely event. Excessive release of matrix components or even wear particles from the damaged cartilage will trigger synovial macrophages and fibroblasts, resulting in generation of a broad range of "inflammatory" mediators, including TNF and IL-1. This synovial activation may even extend to an immune reaction, under conditions where the individual loses its tolerance against autoantigens from the cartilage (Fig. 1). Mediators found in OA and RA synovium, taken at late stages of the diseases, display considerable similarity, be it that in general the levels are higher in the RA synovium. Apart from direct effects of growth factors on articular cartilage, it is of utmost importance to understand the interplay between growth factors and "inflammatory" cytokines and to identify the critical balances which lead to characteristic OA or RA cartilage pathology.

4.5.2
Growth Factors and Articular Cartilage

Due to the overwhelming efforts in cloning technology there is a rapidly growing list of growth factors, which have been shown to affect articular chon-

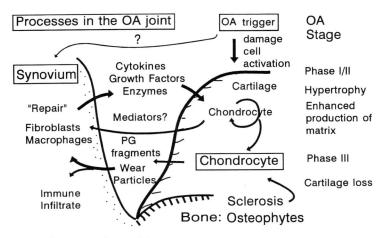

Fig. 1. Scheme of events in the OA joint

Table 1. Effect of various growth factors on cartilage

Growth Factor	Stimulation of cartilage proteoglycan synthesis	Effect chondrocyte phenotype/ differentiation	Present in OA joint
Insulin-like Growth Factors (IGF)	Refs 4–7	Refs 8–10	Refs 11[a], 12[b], 13[c], 14[abc]
Transforming Growth Factors (TGF-β)	Refs 22–24	Refs 8, 10, 27	Refs 28[c], 29[c], 30[a]
Bone- and Cartilage-derived Morphogenetic Proteins (BMP, CDMP)	Refs 35–38	Refs 39–41	Ref 37[a]

Refs, references.
[a] Cartilage.
[b] Synovial tissue.
[c] Synovial fluid.

drocytes. Table 1 shows a selection of well known and novel growth factors, implicated in cartilage damage and repair.

4.5.2.1
IGF

A first group of important growth factors to be mentioned is that of the IGFs. Insulin-like growth factors, as the name implies, are growth factors which are abundant in serum and share some properties with insulin. IGF-2 is an abundant factor in the embryonic stage, whereas IGF-1 is the dominant factor in adult life. Both IGF-1 and IGF-2 signal through the type I IGF receptor. The type II receptor is a mannose 6-phosphate receptor and its exact role in regulation of metabolism remains obscure. Although IGF-1 is more prominent, it can not be excluded that IGF-2 becomes of relevance under pathological conditions in adulthood, or at repair sites, often showing embryonic elements. IGF-1 is a potent stimulant of chondrocyte proteoglycan synthesis and markedly inhibits proteoglycan breakdown. In that sense, it is an important homeostatic factor for cartilage, the more so since it was found that IGF-1 is the main anabolic stimulus for chondrocyte proteoglycan synthesis present in serum and synovial fluid [5]. It also appears a crucial factor in culture systems of articular cartilage [4–7]. Since serum contains high levels of IGF-1, originating from the liver, it is commonly thought that the bulk of IGF-1 in synovial fluid is coming from the circulation. In addition, normal chondrocytes do make IGFs and recently, expression of both IGF-1 and IGF-2 message was demonstrated in synovium and cartilage of OA patients [11, 12]. In normal cartilage, IGF-1 is not mitogenic, but it has been claimed that IGF-1 stimulates proliferation in a damaged matrix, suggesting a further role in cartilage repair. The action of IGFs is under the control of a set of IGF-binding proteins, which can be produced by the chondrocyte [14]. The various binding proteins were shown to provide both carrier as well as

IGF-blocking activity. Cells isolated from OA cartilage make enhanced levels of IGF-bps, herein potentially limiting IGF action [15].

4.5.2.2
PDGF, FGF

A second category of growth factors displaying diverse activity at chondrocytes comprises PDGF, FGF and TGFβ. These factors can be produced by the chondrocyte but also in considerable quantities by activated synovial tissue. They are found in synovial lining cells as well as sublining cells, and levels are generally higher in RA as compared to OA synovium [16, 17]. PDGF was shown to contribute to matrix homeostasis, with no apparent mitogenic effect. Both enhanced synthesis as well as decreased proteoglycan degradation was noted [18]. In contrast, bFGF is capable of promoting either anabolic or catabolic processes, dependent on growth factor dose and condition of the cartilage [19].

4.5.2.3
TGFβ

TGFβ (transforming growth factor) is a factor of particular interest. It is the prototypic member of the large TGF superfamily, sharing functional and signaling homology with the more recently discovered BMPs (bone morphogenetic proteins). TGFβ is a highly pleiotropic factor, showing immunosuppressive activity as well as potent chemotactic activity and being a strong stimulus for fibroblast proliferation. It is rather unique amongst the growth factors in that it inhibits enzyme release from various cell types and enhances the production of enzyme inhibitors such as TIMP [20, 21]. This unique pattern is found in both synovial cells and chondrocytes. Linked to this behaviour, TGFβ is considered as an important feedback regulator of tissue damage, following inflammatory episodes. With regard to cartilage, it can markedly stimulate matrix production by activated chondrocytes [22–24], predominantly after preexposure to TGFβ. Normal cartilage is not sensitive. Moreover, it is demonstrated that TGFβ enhances aggrecan production, but also stimulates the production of the smaller proteoglycans, which are found in OA cartilage [25, 26]. The retarded responsiveness in normal cartilage/chondrocytes probably reflects a prerequisite TGFβ induced shift in receptor expression.

TGFβ can be produced by numerous cell types, including chondrocytes. It is released in a latent form, linked to latency associated peptide (LAP). Dissociation from LAP does occur by proteases, which are abundantly produced in inflamed tissues. Synovium and cartilage contain large amounts of latent TGFβ. Apart from production by activated tissue cells or infiltrating macrophages, these stores of latent TGFβ provide a major element in the TGFβ reactivity of a tissue after local insults. Significant levels of TGFβ are found in the synovial fluid as well as the synovia and cartilage of osteoarthritic processes [28–30]. Coexpression with TNF and IL-1 is seen at sites containing inflammatory infiltrates [31], whereas exclusive expression of TGFβ is noted in fibrotic areas.

4.5.2.4
Morphogenetic Proteins

The bone morphogenetic proteins (BMPs) are members of the TGFβ superfamily, and share the potential to stimulate chondrocytes. Although the name suggests that these factors are mainly involved in processes in the bone, some of the BMPs (BMP-2, BMP-7 and BMP-9) also display a strong stimulation of chondrocyte proteoglycan synthesis. The BMPs use BMP-specific receptors on the cell surface and generate different down stream proteins as compared to TGFβ [32, 33]. Like TGFβ, most of the BMPs members signal through heteromeric complexes of type II and type I serine/threonine kinase receptors. Within these complexes receptor II transphosphorylates and activates receptor I, which then transmits the signal to a down stream family of signal transduction molecules, the Smads [33]. Smads are rapidly phosporylated after signaling and it becomes clear that Smad1, 5 and 8 are phosphorylated in response to BMP, whereas Smad2 and 3 are essential in the TGFβ pathway. Thereafter, these Smads associate with Smad4, which is now considered as an obligate element in signaling of the whole TGFβ superfamily. This may explain some of the overlapping functions of the various members, but it also provides the intriguing condition that TGFβ and BMP pathways can inhibit each other by competing for common components. Recently, another class of Smad proteins has been identified, represented by Smad 6 and 7. These Smads act as negative regulators of TGFβ and BMP signaling [34]. Further description of the fine tuning of this regulation goes beyond the scope of the present paper, but it is becoming clear that genetic diversity in Smads may be linked to pathology, for instance tumor growth, and that these molecules may offer therapeutic targets in the regulation of various cell functions, including those of chondrocytes.

The potential of BMPs to stimulate cartilage proteoglycan synthesis has long been recognized [35, 36, 38], but its application in cartilage repair has been questioned with regard to the risk of further dedifferentiation of chondrocytes and eventual calcification and bone formation. Recent studies with chondrocytes, in which a truncated type II BMP receptor was introduced, revealed that BMP-2 signaling through this receptor is required for maintenance of the differentiated phenotype, control of proliferation and hypertrophy [41]. Recent studies with chondrocytes of young calves [42] suggested that BMP-2 maintained the chondrocyte phenotype in long term culture (4 weeks), not inducing a hypertrophic chondrocyte and identical data were obtained with BMP-9 (personal comm). Moreover, in studies with mature articular chondrocytes in alginate it was shown that BMP-7 (identical to Osteogenic Protein, OP-1) stimulates mature human articular chondrocytes, with continued expression of the chondrocyte phenotype. It was claimed that BMP-7 is a more potent stimulator of synthesis of cartilage-specific macromolecules, as compared to TGFβ [43].

4.5.2.4.1
In Vivo Effects of BMPs

We have injected BMP-2 and BMP-9 into the knee joint of normal mice and found that these morphogenetic growth factors markedly stimulate chon-

Fig. 2.
Differential kinetics of
TGFβ and BMP-2 effect on
chondrocyte proteoglycan
synthesis

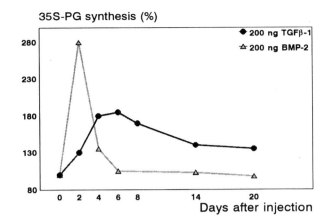

drocyte proteoglycan synthesis (up to 300%), which is far above the levels reached with TGFβ [38]. However, the stimulatory effect is transient, with a return to normal in a few days, whereas TGFβ provides more prolonged stimulation (Fig. 2). The latter is probably linked to TGFβ autoinduction and sensibilization of the chondrocyte to TGFβ stimulation.

4.5.2.4.2
CDMPs

Cartilage-derived morphogenetic proteins (CDMPs 1 and 2) are recently discovered members of the TGFβ superfamily, which are essential for the formation of cartilaginous tissue during early limb development [44]. A null mutation in the CDMP-1 gene was characterized by chondrodysplasia [45]. It is hoped that these CDMPs provide growth factors with a more selective cartilage directed profile. Although TGFβ and BMPs can stimulate chondrocytes they have major effects on multiple cell types and considerable side effects will seriously hamper their application in cartilage repair. CDMP-1 and -2 were detected in healthy and OA cartilage and shown to be able to promote cartilage matrix recovery after enzymatic depletion, with maintenance of normal phenotype [37].

4.5.2.5
Synergy of Growth Factors

Although the various growth factors have been dicussed with regard to their distinct activities, it should be mentioned that considerable synergy may occur. Moreover, the one growth factor can often induce itself as well as other growth factors, creating a highly regulated interplay. For example, in cartilage repair of traumatic defects it is well recognized that FGF together with other growth factors provides much better tissue engeneering. Although FGF on its own is hardly stimulatory to matrix production, its mitogenic and transforming

activity adds to chondrogenic potential [46, 47]. In addition, IGF-1 together with
TGFβ creates a much greater potential to induce a proper chondrocyte phenotype in *in vitro* culture systems [48, 49]. Intriguingly, TGFβ was shown to inter-
fer with the production of IGF-1 as well as IGF binding proteins and to dephos-
phorylate the IGF-1 receptor, with apparent upregulation of IGF binding. We
also noted no separate effect, but marked synergy with IGF-1 for a number of
growth factors in activation of chondrocyte proteoglycan synthesis in intact
murine cartilage [50]. However, the apparent IGF nonresponsiveness observed
in arthritic cartilage could still not be overruled with the application of growth
factor cocktails [50].

4.5.3
Balance with Destructive Cytokines

Absolute levels of growth factors in the joints of RA and OA patients can be
indicative of their role. However, the pattern of cartilage destruction and attempted repair is quite different in RA and OA, yet enhanced levels of growth
factors are found in both conditions. This suggests that other, yet unidentified
factors are of pivotal importance, or that other aspects determine the particular response, such as defined receptor expression patterns on chondrocytes,
shedded soluble receptors, binding proteins, or different counterbalance with
destructive cytokines.

Cytokines can be broadly catagorized in three major subclasses: destructive
cytokines, regulatory cytokines, and anabolic growth factors (Fig. 3). As a prime
example of a destructive cytokine, IL-1 induces enhanced protease release, and
inhibits chondrocyte proteoglycan and collagen synthesis. Regulatory mediators
such as IL-4 and IL-10 inhibit IL-1 production, enhance the production of IL-1ra
and furthermore reduce the levels of iNOS (inducible NO synthase) in chondrocytes. In this, IL-4 provides at least three levels of potential counterbalancing of
IL-1 action: reducing production levels, but also enhancing scavenge of IL-1 with
IL-1ra, as well as decreasing the IL-1 effect by reduction of NO, a pivotal secundary
mediator in IL-1 mediated inhibition of chondrocyte proteoglycan synthesis.

Fig. 3.
Interplay between
cytokines and growth
factors in cartilage

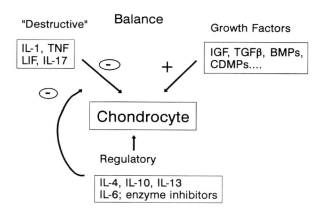

Moreover, enzymatic breakdown is reduced with IL-4 [51]. Optimal therapeutic effect *in vivo* is achieved with the combination of IL-4 and IL-10 [52, 53].

Factors from the anabolic category, such as IGF-1 and TGFβ, do not really interfere with IL-1 production or action, but in fact display opposing activity: stimulation of proteoglycan and collagen synthesis, and suppression of protease action, the latter by inhibition of release of enzymes and/or upregulation of enzyme inhibitors. This plain counteraction further underlines the relevance of mediator balances. Prime examples of the categories are depicted in Fig 3.

4.5.3.1
Subclasses of Destructive Cytokines

Apart from IL-1, the cytokines TNFα, LIF (leukemia inhibitory factor) and IL-17 are listed in the destructive catagory. Although these mediators share activities in common with IL-1, it is clear that IL-1 is by far the most potent destructive cytokine [54, 55]. Direct intraarticular injection of IL-1 caused proteoglycan synthesis inhibition, whereas TNF has to be dosed 1000-fold higher to get a modest effect. Elegant studies in TNF transgenic mice revealed that TNF overexpression leads to chronic arthritis, yet treatment with antibodies to the IL-1 receptor fully abolished the destructive process [56]. Intriguingly, TNF levels were still high in these animals, excluding a direct cartilage destructive effect in vivo. The only role attributed to TNF in this respect is an IL-1 inducing potential and a capacity to cause synergistic destructive activity, together with IL-1. Within the process of OA, TNF levels are relatively low as compared to RA. However, TNF receptor expression on OA chondrocytes appeared to be enhanced [57]. Moreover, a new Tace-like activity was recently described in OA chondrocytes, contributing in regulation of TNF [58].

IL-17 is a novel cytokine, displaying IL-1 like activity. It was demonstrated that its action on chondrocytes, with marked NO production, was independent of induction of IL-1 and it was claimed in other studies that the major effect was chondrocyte mediated cartilage breakdown. We have used human recombinant IL-17 *in vitro* and *in vivo* in the mouse and in our hands the suppression of chondrocyte proteoglycan synthesis was evident, although IL-17 appeared less potent as compared to IL-1. The claimed effect of marked cartilage degradation was not identified in our studies. IL-17 is considered a factor released from activated T memory cells. Although OA chondrocytes are sensitive to IL-17 [59], a major role in the OA cartilage destruction is unlikely. A final factor to be discussed is LIF. This mediator can induce IL-1, but shows cartilage destructive activity, independent of IL-1 [60]. Suppression of chondrocyte proteoglycan synthesis appeared independent of NO production [61], providing an additional pathway of cartilage pathology. Its potential role in the OA process remains to be elucidated.

4.5.4
Counteraction of IL-1

Growth factors may display a complex interaction with IL-1. As an example, pre-exposure of chondrocytes to FGF enhances the subsequent protease release after IL-1 exposure, probably linked to enhanced IL-1 receptor expression [62]. PDGF also stimulates IL-1 dependent protease release, yet reduces IL-1 mediated inhibition of proteoglycan synthesis [63]. This suggests that certain growth factors can enhance cartilage repair, but simultaneously promote cartilage breakdown. Other growth factors such as IGF-1 and TGFβ stimulate synthesis and reduce IL-1 mediated breakdown, both activities consistent with repair. This counteraction is still operational after preexposure to IL-1, implying that IL-1 does not induce a state of growth factor nonresponsiveness, in general [64]. Intriguingly, kinetics of IL-1 and TGFβ effects may differ and the potential of TGFβ to inhibit breakdown is attenuated by its slow effect on TIMP mRNA levels [65]. On the other hand, studies in TGFβ knock-out mice revealed increased iNOS and NO levels in the absence of TGFβ [66]. Since the suppressive IL-1 effect on chondrocyte proteoglycan synthesis is strongly NO dependent [67], this might explain why we observe a much stronger counteraction by TGFβ on IL-1 induced proteoglycan synthesis inhibition as compared with proteoglycan breakdown, in vivo.

4.5.4.1
Growth Factors In Vivo

We have analysed the process of IL-1/growth factor counteraction in vivo, using direct injection into the murine knee joint. Intriguingly, it was found that TGFβ profoundly counteracted IL-1 mediated proteoglycan synthesis suppression in the articular cartilage, whereas BMP-2 was unable to do so (Fig. 4): its stimulatory potential was fully overruled by IL-1, even at high BMP-2 concentrations [68, 69]. This is the more remarkable since the absolute level of BMP-2 stimulation of chondrocyte proteoglycan synthesis was much higher as compared to that of TGFβ, in the absence of IL-1. It is as yet unclear why BMP-2 can not counteract IL-1, but the BMP-2 nonresponsiveness might be related to down regulation of BMP-2 receptors or a blockade of intracellular pathways, potentially linked to iNOS. Apart from effects on synthesis, TGFβ also had a

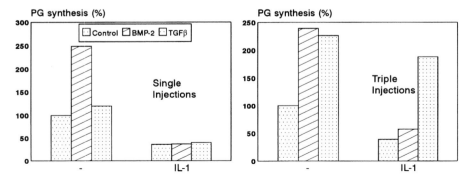

Fig. 4. Cartilage proteoglycan synthesis at day 2 after the last of single and triple injections of TGFβ or BMP. Left bars in the absence of IL-1; right bars in the presence of IL-1

marked impact on the IL-1 induced cartilage proteoglycan depletion. It is conceivable that, dependent on relative concentration of IL-1 and TGFβ, the net effect on cartilage would be either a reduced or an enhanced proteoglycan content.

Remarkably, IL-1/TGFβ counteraction was evident in the articular cartilage, but such a balance was not noted in the nearby chondrophyte formation at the joint margins. The latter process is a prominent action of TGFβ on chondrogenic cells in the periosteum, resulting in development of chondroblasts and deposition of proteoglycans [24, 38]. Apparently, these chondroblasts are not sensitive to IL-1, at least not in the sense of normal chondrocytes with the typical pattern of suppressed synthesis.

4.5.4.2
Repair in Inflammation

Subsequent to the studies in a plain IL-1 driven process, we analysed the potential counteraction of TGFβ and BMP-2 in a full-blown arthritic process, induced by intraarticular injection of Zymosan (yeast particles). In line with the above data, TGFβ markedly counteracted the inflammation mediated cartilage proteoglycan depletion, which is a largely IL-1 dependent event, whereas BMP-2 was fully unable to show significant counteraction (Fig. 5). Repeated local administration of TGFβ in the knee joint clearly stimulated chondrocyte proteoglycan synthesis, restored PG content of the depleted cartilage, but had no suppressive effect on the inflammatory process [70].

Of note, TGFβ promoted outgrowth of chondrophytes as an unwanted side effect. BMP-2 also promoted chondrophytes, but at different sites of the joint margins, mainly reflecting outgrowth from epiphyseal growth plate cartilage [38].

4.5.5
Involvement of Growth Factors in OA Cartilage

To obtain some insight in key factors in OA cartilage pathology, it is imperative to identify the critical changes in the articular cartilage and to try to fit these patterns with actions of particular mediators or combinations of mediators. Under normal conditions, cartilage maintains its homeostasis by a regulated balance of synthesis and degradative events. In theory, cartilage pathology may arise from local overproduction of destructive mediators or a shortage of controling mediators, including inhibitors and anabolic growth factors. Moreover, a shift in responsiveness of the chondrocyte to these mediators may contribute to loss of homeostasis. There is no doubt that the OA chondrocyte displays an altered phenotype, which remains present after at least a number of passages in culture. It is yet unclear whether this state reflects cause or outcome of the OA process.

An intriguing observation in human OA cartilage is the enhanced sensitivity of the chondrocytes to undergo stimulation of proteoglycan synthesis by TGFβ. Normal cartilage does not show enhanced proteoglycan synthesis upon first

Fig. 5.
No apparent suppression of
inflammation, but markedly
enhanced levels of proteoglycans in the articular
cartilage by coinjection of
TGFβ. **A:** control; **B:** TGFβ

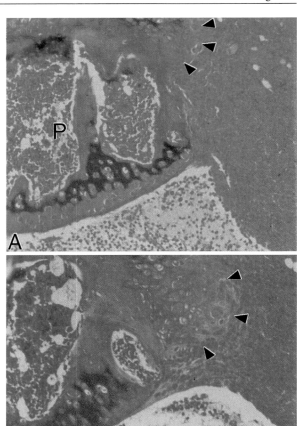

exposure to TGFβ. Only after a number of days in culture, in particular in the
presence of TGFβ, the chondrocytes start to show this profile, probably under
the influence of a TGFβ induced shift in phenotype [22, 71, 72]. The fact that OA
chondrocytes already show this pattern suggests previous exposure to TGFβ
and critical involvement of this factor in the disease process. Further indication
of a role of TGFβ in OA is provided by the marked and prolonged upregulation of chondrocyte proteoglycan synthesis and induction of osteophytes in
the murine knee joint, upon repeated local injection of TGFβ [24]. Osteophytes
are characteristic OA features and it was shown that repeated local injection with another growth factor, IGF-1, does not induce these hallmarks, nor
the enhanced PG synthesis, whereas BMP-2 induces only a transient rise in
PG synthesis and different types of chondrophytes and osteophytes (Fig. 6,
[38]).

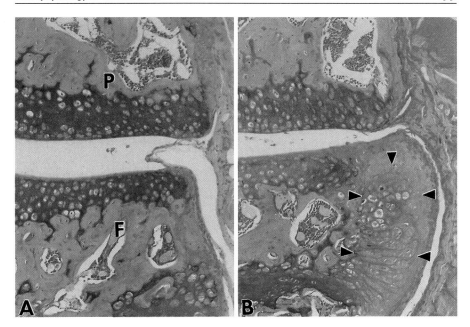

Fig. 6. Pattern of outgrowth of chondrogenic tissue after injection of saline (A) or BMP-2 (B)

4.5.5.1
Models of OA

When the pattern of chondrocyte proteoglycan synthesis is evaluated in experimental models of OA, it is a consistent finding that proteoglycan content and synthesis is enhanced [1–3] in early OA, in sharp contrast to the suppressed proteoglycan synthesis seen in inflammatory models (Fig. 7). The latter profile is proven to be IL-1 dependent [54, 67].

Given the discussion above on growth factor/cytokine counteraction, the pattern in the OA models is compatible with enhanced activity of anabolic growth factors, or a combination of high levels of growth factors, overruling suppressive cytokines such as IL-1. BMP-2 is not a likely mediator of this process and TGFβ seems more obvious. Although IGF-1 can stimulate cartilage proteoglycan synthesis *in vitro*, we could not find further enhancement of cartilage proteoglycan synthesis *in vivo*, upon local IGF-1 administrations, probably indicating that endogenous levels are already optimal. At later stages, when signs of focal OA cartilage destruction become evident, suppression of synthesis is noted, which might be compatible with more dominant IL-1 action or an ultimate failure of anabolic growth factors, lacking to keep up the counteraction.

Analysis of growth factor expression in spontaneous OA in STR/ORT mice demonstrates both enhanced levels of TGFβ mRNA as well as IL-1 in lesional cartilage [30], potentially in line with enhanced TGFβ levels. It should be noted

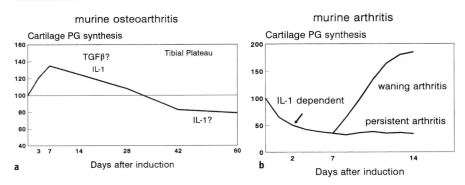

Fig. 7a–b. Cartilage proteoglycan synthesis in various stages of experimental OA (a) and joint inflammation (b)

that TGFβ activation from latent stores is also a major element in tissue repair processes and production levels need not necessarily be upregulated to a large extent. A complicating factor in understanding of the role of TGFβ is provided by the recent studies on the type II TGFβ receptor expression in an ACL OA model in the rabbit [73]. Shortly after OA induction a reduced level was found, indicative of insufficient TGFβ signaling. Intriguingly, TGFβ type II receptor knock-out mice display signs of spontaneous OA, also suggesting that impaired TGFβ signaling causes failure in cartilage repair and ultimate OA cartilage pathology [74].

Given the strong impact of TGFβ on chondrocyte proteoglycan synthesis, it is acceptable that both overproduction of TGFβ as well as impaired signaling of TGFβ may cause cartilage pathology. Deficient anabolic stimulation would reflect a continued threat to the cartilage, provided that microtrauma are formed in the cartilage on a regular base, even under normal loading conditions, needing continued and adequate repair. On the other hand, the profile of hypertrophy and enhanced proteoglycan synthesis in early OA is not compatible with lack of anabolic growth factor signaling and makes overstimulation a more likely event to occur.

4.5.5.2
Is TGFβ Pathogenic?

Remarkably, prolonged exposure to enhanced levels of TGFβ does result in OA-like cartilage pathology in C57Bl mice. Apart from the characteristic osteophytes, the femoral cartilage of the murine knee joint shows typical loss of proteoglycans close to the tidemark, as well as irregular spacing, at sites where lesions develop in spontaneous murine OA in this mouse strain with aging (Fig. 8). These observations were obtained after repeated intraarticular injection of recombinant TGFβ.

Recently, we backed up this data by showing similar OA-like cartilage pathology in this area after a single injection of an adenoviral gene construct, yielding

Fig. 8A–C.
Lesions in the tibial plateau after repeated TGFβ injection (**B**), in comparison with normal tissue (**A**) and lesions observed in experimental OA (**C**). The deep lesions after TGFβ suggest the initiation of tearing processes, seen in murine OA

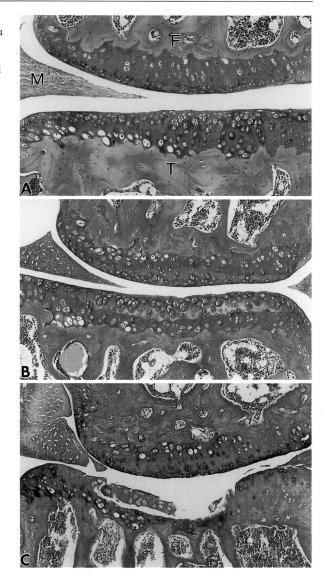

sustained levels of active TGFβ instead of the repeated peak levels after consecutive injections of recombinant TGFβ. The sustained TGFβ production with the gene construct comes more close to the *in vivo* situation and it is comforting to note that the earlier findings of characteristic OA pathology could be confirmed.

In trying to understand how excessive TGFβ might cause cartilage pathology, it should be noted that TGFβ exposure induces a characteristic chondrocyte phenotype, with a shift in subclasses of proteoglycans made, and the risk of

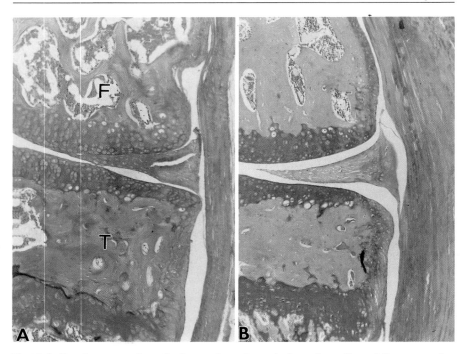

Fig. 9A, B. Development of cartilaginous tissue in and along the collateral ligament, after repeated TGFβ injection. **A:** normal; **B:** TGFβ

impaired matrix assembly. We recently showed that both IGF-1 and TGFβ enhanced the proteoglycan synthesis in chondrocytes cultured in Alginate, but that TGFβ induced a shift in the compartmentalization of PGs, deposited closely around the chondrocyte or further away from the cell [75]. Moreover, it was reported that TGFβ enhanced the level of the novel collagenase MMP-13 (collagenase-3) in activated chondrocytes, in sharp contrast to the general expectation that TGFβ reduces destructive protease release, in general [76]. It remains to be seen whether TGFβ induced MMP-13 plays a role in the OA cartilage pathology. Finally, TGFβ not only induces an initial increase in levels of cartilage proteoglycans, but also promotes deposition of proteoglycans in ligament and tendon structures, herein inducing enhanced stiffnes in these structures, with loss of joint flexibility and impairment of proper joint movement (Fig. 9).

Intriguingly, similar lesions are noted in spontaneous OA in aging mice. Moreover, expression of TGFβ and BMP has been noted in ectopic proteoglycan deposition in ligament structures [77, 78].

4.5.5.3
Pathways in OA

It remains to be seen whether some or all of these aspects contribute to growth factor induced OA pathology and studies with specific TGF blockers have to be

Fig. 10.
Scheme of events in OA

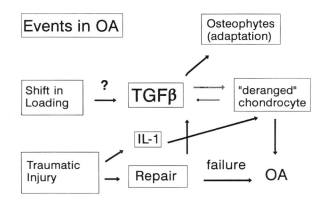

awaited before final conclusions can be drawn [79]. Meanwhile, it is tempting to draw up a scheme of putative events in the OA process (Fig. 10), with elements of excessive growth factor involvement, reflecting the dark side of tissue repair. The latter is a well accepted phenomenon in pathologic tissue fibrosis in kidney and liver disease as well as excessive scarring in wound healing [80]. Accepted causes of OA such as ligament rupture or shift in load bearing give rise to excessive TGFβ activation. Ongoing attempted repair of damaged ligaments is the prototype of tissue repair and subsequent release of TGFβ, whereas biomechanical overload also results in TGFβ generation. *In vitro* loading of chondrocytes enhances TGFβ production, whereas impairment of chondrocyte proteoglycan synthesis after immobilization can be overruled by TGFβ supplementation [81]. This TGFβ induces osteophytes at the joint margins, as an adaptive process to cope with the changed loading conditions. In addition to TGFβ induction of an altered chondrocyte phenotype, IL-1 produced during the tissue damage and modest inflammatory repair reaction might contribute to the deranged phenotype.

It has been shown that after prolonged exposure to IL-1, the production of cartilage specific collagen types such as type II and type IX is reduced, whereas an increase is noted in type I and III collagen [82]. This shift may contribute to inadequate matrix repair. In addition, recent studies with IL-1ra in the canine OA model demonstrated some protection (see chapter Pelletier in this book) and we also noted some suppression of OA pathology in a mouse model, when induced in an IL-1β knockout or an iNOS knockout, both compatible with a contribution of IL-1 to the cartilage destruction.

4.5.5.4
OA Chondrocytes

Apart from excessive TGFβ, in the context of minor IL-1 levels, OA pathology may be promoted by inadequate functioning of other anabolic growth factors. There is no evidence that IGF levels are limiting in synovial fluid of OA patients. However, in experimental joint inflammation, IGF nonresponsiveness is noted in chondrocytes, compatible with the low level of proteoglycan synthesis and production of aberrant, small proteoglycans. The latter could be mimicked in normal cartilage, upon culture in the absence of IGF [83, 84]. A distinct variant of improper IGF signaling seems to be present in OA cartilage. The chondrocytes make enhanced levels of IGF binding proteins, potentially limiting the homeostatic action of IGF-1 [15]. The seemingly contradictory enhancement of overall proteoglycan synthesis should then be viewed in the light of concomitant overstimulation with other growth factors, such as TGFβ. If IGF nonresponsiveness is the primary causative element in the OA chondrocytes, the lack of response might be overcome with excessive levels of IGF-1, then warranting therapeutic approaches with IGF. Of interest, steroids display actions similar to IGF, and low doses may be applied instead of IGF, to bypass problems related to disturbed IGF signaling [85].

4.5.6
Final Remarks

Since the OA condition seems to reflect a failure in attempted repair, it was long considered that plain application of growth factors might be of benefit. However, if the underlying process still activates destructive cytokines, degradative enzymes or even excessive amounts of pathogenic growth factors, it seems a waste of time to add excessive amounts of the dominant growth factor in normal homeostasis, IGF-1, without controling the pathogenic events. Whether anti-IL-1, combined with anti-protease should provide a fruitful complementary therapy remains to be seen. A serious complication in therapy is the deranged phenotype of the OA chondrocyte, including disturbed receptor expression and/or signaling. If it is intrinsic, even the complementary treatments might be unsuccessful. If the deranged phenotype is a reflection of prolonged exposure to excessive levels of destructive mediators, combination therapies seem a logic extension. Apart from the usage of IGF, it should be considered to use novel factors. Further characterization of the members of the rapidly growing list of morphogenetic proteins in bone and cartilage might provide novel options. A largely neglected area is the interplay between factors from underlying bone and the adjacent cartilage. There is no doubt that homeostasis is markedly disturbed in the bone of an OA joint and further understanding of cross regulation between these compartments is warranted [86, 87]. Finally, osteophytes are a hallmark of the OA process, but it is still not understood whether they are good or bad for the further progression of OA cartilage lesions. In experimental OA models osteophytes are always seen, generally preceding the occurrence of cartilage erosions [88]. They develop out of chondrophytes [38], reflecting an enormous potential of the joint to generate new cartilage. Understanding of the final differentiation of the cells in this ectopic area and the successive mediators and receptor expression involved in maturation might provide new clues to improve cartilage repair at other sites in the OA joint.

References

1. Adams ME, Brandt KD (1991) Hypertrophic repair of canine articular cartilage in osteo-arthritis after anterior cruciate ligament transection. J Rheumatol 18: 428–435
2. Van der Kraan PM, Vitters EL, van Beuningen HM, van den Berg WB (1992) Proteoglycan synthesis and osteophyte formation in "metabolically"and "mechanically" induced murine degenerative joint disease: An in-vivo autoradiographic study. Int J Exp Pathol 73: 335–350
3. Gaffen JD, Cleave SJ, Crossman MV, Bayliss MT, Mason RM (1995) Articular cartilage proteoglycans in osteoarthritic STR/Ort mice. Osteoarthritis Cartilage 3: 95–104
4. Tyler JA (1989) Insulin-like growth factor-1 can decrease degradation and promote synthesis of proteoglycan in cartilage exposed to cytokines. Biochem J 260: 543–548
5. Schalkwijk J, Joosten LAB, van den Berg WB, van Wijk JJ, van de Putte LBA (1989) Insulin-like growth factor stimulation of chondrocyte proteoglycan synthesis by human synovial fluid. Arthritis Rheum 32: 66–71
6. Tesch GH, Handley CJ, Cornell HJ, Herington AC (1992) Effects of free and bound insulin-like growth factors on proteoglycan metabolism in articular cartilage explants. J Orthop Res 10: 14–22
7. Van Beuningen HM, Arntz OJ, van den Berg WB (1993) Insulin-like growth factor stimu-lation of articular chondrocyte proteoglycan synthesis. Availability and responses at dif-ferent ages. Br J Rheum Dis 32: 1037–1043
8. Böhme K, Winterhalter KH, Bruckner P (1995) Terminal differentiation of chondrocytes in culture is a spontaneous process and is arrested by TGF-ß2 and basic fibroblast growth factor in synergy. Exp Cell Res 216: 191–198
9. Wroblewski J, Edwall-Arvidsson C (1995) Inhibitory effects of basic fibroblast growth factor on chondrocyte differentiation. J Bone Miner Res 10: 735–742
10. Ballock RT, Heydemann A, Wakefield LM, Flanders KC, Roberts AB, Sporn MB (1993) TGF-β1 prevents hypertrophy of epiphyseal chondrocytes: Regulation of gene expres-sion for cartilage matrix proteins and metalloproteinases. Dev Biol 158: 414–429
11. Middleton JF, Tyler JA (1992) Upregulation of insulin-like growth factor-1 gene expression in the lesions of osteoarthritic human articular cartilage. Ann Rheum Dis 51: 440–447
12. Keyszer GM, Heer AH, Kriegsmann J, Geiler T, Keysser C, Gay RE, Gay S (1995) Detection of insulin-like growth factor-1 and -2 in synovial tissue specimens of patients with rheuma-toid arthritis and osteoarthritis by *in situ* hybridization. J Rheumatol 22: 275–281
13. Denko CW, Boja B, Moskowitz RW (1996) Growth factors, insulin-like growth factor-1 and growth hormone, in synovial fluid and serum of patients with rheumatic disorders. Osteoarthritis Cartilage 4: 245–249
14. Martel-Pelletier J, Di Battista JA, Lajeunesse D, Pelletier JP (1998) IGF/IGFBP axis in cartilage and bone in osteoarthritis pathogenesis. Inflamm Res 47: 90–100
15. Doré S, Pelletier JP, Di Battista JA, Tardif G, Brazeau P, Martel-Pelletier JM (1994) Human osteoarthritic chondrocytes possess an increased number of insulin-like growth factor-1 binding sites but are unresponsive to its stimulation. Arthritis Rheum 37: 253–263
16. Nakashima M, Eguchi K, Aoyagi T, Yamashita I, Ida H, Sakai M et al. (1994) Expression of basic fibroblast growth factor in synovial tissues from patients with rheumatoid arthri-tis. Detection by immunohistochemical staining and *in situ* hybridization. Ann Rheum Dis, 53: 45–50
17. Remmers EF, Sano H, Lafyatis R, Case JP, Kumkumian GK, Hla T et al. (1991) Production of plateled derived growth factor β chain (PDGF-B/c-sis) mRNA and immunoreactive PDGF-β-like polypeptide by rheumatoid synovium: coexpression with heparin binding acidic fibroblast growth factor. J Rheumatol 18: 7–13
18. Schafer SJ, Luyten FP, Yanagishita M, Reddi AH (1993) Proteoglycan metabolism is age related and modulated by isoforms of plateled-derived growth factor in bovine articular cartilage explant cultures. Archiv Biochem Biophys 302: 431–438
19. Sah RL, Chen AC, Grodzinsky AJ, Trippel SB (1994) Differential effects of bFGF and IGF-1 on matrix metabolism in calf and adult bovine cartilage explants. Archiv Biochem Bio-phys 308: 137–147

20. Gunther M, Haubeck HD, van de Leur E, Blaser J, Bender S, Gutgemann I, Fischer DC, Tschesche H, Greiling H, Heinrich PC, Graeve L (1994) TGF-β1 regulates tissue inhibitor of metalloproteinases-1 expression in differentiated human articular chondrocytes. Arthritis Rheum 37 : 395 – 405

21. Wright JK, Cawston TE, Hazleman BI (1991) TGF-β stimulates the production of the tissue inhibitor of metalloproteinases (TIMP) by human synovial and skin fibroblasts. Biochem Biophys Acta 1094 : 207 – 210

22. Van der Kraan PM, Vitters EL, van den Berg WB (1992) Differential effect of transforming growth factor β on freshly isolated and cultured articular chondrocytes. J Rheumatol, 19 : 140 – 145

23. Morales TI (1994) TGF-β and insulin-like growth factor-1 restore proteoglycan metabolism of bovine articular cartilage after depletion by retinoic acid. Archiv Biochem Biophys 315 : 190 – 198

24. Van Beuningen HM, van der Kraan PM, Arntz OJ, van den Berg WB (1994) Transforming growth factor-ß1 stimulates articular chondrocyte proteoglycan synthesis and induces osteophyte formation in the murine knee joint. Lab Invest 71 : 279 – 290

25. Roughley PJ, Melching LI, Recklies AD (1994) Changes in the expression of decorin and biglycan in human articular cartilage with age and regulation by TGFβ. Matrix Biol 14 : 51 – 59

26. CS-Szabo G, Roughley PJ, Plaas AHK, Glant TT (1995) Large and small proteoglycans of osteoarthritic and rheumatoid articular cartilage. Arthritis Rheum 38 : 660 – 668

27. Wu LNY, Genge BR, Ishikawa Y, Wuthier RE (1992) Modulation of cultured chicken growth plate chondrocytes by TGF-β1 and basic fibroblast growth factor. J Cell Biochem 49 : 181 – 198

28. Fava R, Olsen N, Keski-Oja J, Moses H, Pingus T (1989) Active and latent forms of TGFβ activity in synovial effusions. J Exp Med 169 : 291 – 296

29. Schlaak JF, Meyer zum Buschenfelde KH, Marker-Hermann E (1996) Different cytokine profiles in the synovial fluid of patients with osteoarthritis, rheumatoid arthritis and seronegative spondylarthropathies. Clin Exp Rheumatol 14 : 155 – 162

30. Chambers MG, Bayliss MT, Mason RM (1997) Chondrocyte cytokine and growth factor expression in murine osteoarthritis. Osteoarthritis Cartilage 5 : 301 – 308

31. Chu CQ, Field M, Abney E, Zheng RQH, Allard S, Feldmann M et al. (1991) TGF-β1 in rheumatoid synovial membrane and cartilage/pannus junction. Clin Exp Immunol, 86 : 380 – 386

32. Yamashita H, Ten Dijke P, Heldin CH, Miyazono K (1996) Bone morphogenetic protein receptors. Bone 19 : 569 – 574

33. Attisano L, Wrana JL (1998) Mads and Smads in TGFβ signaling. Curr Opin Cell Biol, 10 : 188 – 194

34. Hayashi H, Abdollah S, Qiu Y, Cai J, Xu YY, Grinnell BW, Richardson MA, Topper JN, Grimbone JMA, Wrana JL, Falb D (1997) The MAD-related protein Smad7 associates with the TGFβ receptor and functions as an antagonist of TGFβ signaling. Cell 89 : 1165 – 1173

35. Luyten FP, Yu YM, Yanagishita M, Vukicevic S, Hammonds RG, Reddi AH (1992) Natural bovine osteogenic and recombinant human bone morphogenetic protein-2B are equipotent in the maintenance of proteoglycans in bovine articular cartilage explant cultures. J Biol Chem 267 : 3691 – 3695

36. Lietman SA, Yanagishita M, Sampath TK, Reddi AH (1997) Stimulation of proteoglycan synthesis in explants of porcine articular cartilage by recombinant osteogenic protein-1 (bone morphogenetic protein-7). J Bone Joint Surg, 79 A: 1132 – 1137

37. Erlacher L, NG CK, Ullrich R, Krieger S, Luyten FP (1998) Presence of cartilage-derived morphogenetic proteins in articular cartilage and enhancement of matrix replacement in vitro. Arthritis Rheum 41 : 263 – 273

38. Van Beuningen HM, Glansbeek HL, van der Kraan PM, van den Berg WB (1998) Differential effects of local application of BMP-2 or TGF-β1 on both articular cartilage composition and osteophyte formation. Osteoarthritis Cartilage 6 : 306 – 317

39. Chen P, Vukicevic S, Sampath TK, Luyten FP (1995) Osteogenic protein-1 promotes growth and maturation of chick sternal chondrocytes in serum-free cultures. J Cell Sciences 108 : 105 – 114

40. Hiraki Y, Inoue H, Shigeno C, Sanma Y, Bentz H, Rosen DM, Asada A, Suzuki F (1991) Bone morphogenetic proteins (BMP-2 and BMP-3) promote growth and expression of the differentiated phenotype of rabbit chondrocytes and osteoblastic MC3T3-E1 cells *in vitro*. J Bone Miner Res 6 : 1373 – 1385

41. Enomoto-Iwamoto M, Iwamoto M, Mukudai Y, Kawakami Y, Nohno T, Higuchi Y, Takemoto S, Ohuchi H, Noji S, Kurisu K (1998) Bone morphogenetic protein signaling is required for maintenance of differentiated phenotype, control of proliferation, and hypertrophy in chondrocytes. J Cell Biol 140 : 409 – 418

42. Sailor LZ, Hewick RM, Morris EA (1996) Recombinant human bone morphogenetic protein-2 maintains the articular chondrocyte phenotype in long-term culture. J Orthop Res 14 : 937 – 945

43. Flechtenmacher J, Huch K, Thonar EJMA, Mollenhauer JA, Davies SR, Schmid TM, Puhl W, Sampath TK, Aydelotte MB, Kuettner KE (1996) Recombinant human osteogenic protein 1 is a potent stimulator of the synthesis of cartilage proteoglycans and collagens by human articular chondrocytes. Arthritis Rheum 39 : 1896 – 1904

44. Luyten FP (1997) Molecules in focus. Cartilage-derived morphogenetic protein-1. Int J Biochem Cell Biol 29 : 1241 – 1244

45. Thomas JT, Lin K, Nandedkar M, Camargo M, Cervenka J, Luyten FP (1996) A human chondrodysplasia due to a mutation in a TGF-β superfamily member. Nat Genet 12 : 315 – 317

46. Frenz DA, Liu W, Williams JD, Hatcher V, Galinovic-Schwartz V, Flanders KC, van de Water TR (1994) Induction of chondrogenesis: requirement for synergistic interaction of basic fibroblast growth factor and TGF-β. Developm 120 : 415 – 424

47. Otsuka Y, Mizuta H, Takagi K, Iyama KI, Yoshitake Y, Nishikawa K, Suzuki F, Hiraki Y (1997) Requirement of fibroblast growth factor signaling for regeneration of epiphyseal morphology in rabbit full-thickness defects of articular cartilage. Develop Growth Differ 39 : 143 – 156

48. Tsukazaki T, Usa T, Matsumoto T, Enomoto H, Ohtsuru A, Namba H, Iwasaki K, Yamashita S (1994) Effect of TGF-β on the insulin-like growth factor-I autocrine/paracrine axis in cultured rat articular chondrocytes. Exp Cell Res 215 : 9 – 16

49. Yaeger PC, Masi TL, Buck de Ortiz JL, Binette F, Tubo R, McPherson JM (1997) Synergistic action of TGF-ß and IGF-1 induces expression of type II collagen and aggrecan genes in adult human articular chondrocytes. Exp Cell Res 237 : 318 – 325

50. Verschure PJ, Joosten LAB, van der Kraan PM, van den Berg WB (1994) Responsiveness of articular cartilage from normal and inflamed mouse knee joints to various growth factors. Ann Rheum Dis 53 : 455 – 460

51. Nemoto O, Yamada H, Kikuchi T, Shimmei M, Obata K, Sato H, Seiki M (1997) Suppression of matrix metalloproteinase-3 synthesis by IL-4 in human articular chondrocytes. J Rheumatol 24 : 1774 – 1779

52. Joosten LAB, Lubberts E, Durez P, Helsen MMA, Jacobs MJM, Goldman M, van den Berg WB (1997) Role of IL-4 and IL-10 in murine collagen-induced arthritis: Protective effect of IL-4 and IL-10 treatment on cartilage destruction. Arthritis Rheum 40 : 249 – 260

53. Lubberts E, Joosten LAB, Helsen MMA, van den Berg WB (1998) Regulatory role of IL-10 in joint inflammation and cartilage destruction in murine SCW arthritis. More therapeutic benefit with IL-4/IL-10 combination therapy than with IL-10 treatment alone. Cytokine 10 : 361 – 369

54. Van de Loo AAJ, Joosten LAB, van Lent PLEM, Arntz OJ, van den Berg WB (1995) Role of Interleukin-1, Tumor Necrosis Factor-1 and Interleukin-6 in cartilage proteoglycan metabolism and destruction. Effect of *in situ* cytokine blocking in murine antigen- and zymosan-induced arthritis. Arthritis Rheum 38 : 164 – 172

55. Van Meurs JBJ, van Lent PLEM, Singer II, Bayne EK, van de Loo FAJ, van den Berg WB (1998) IL-1ra prevents expression of the metalloproteinase-generated neoepitope VDIPEN in antigen-induced arthritis. Arthritis Rheum 41 : 647 – 656

56. Probert L, Plows D, Kontogeorgos G, Kollias G (1995) The type I IL-1 receptor acts in series with TNF to induce arthritis in TNF-transgenic mice. Eur J Immunol 25:1794–1797

57. Webb GR, Westacott CI, Elson CJ (1997) Chondrocyte tumor necrosis factor receptors and focal loss of cartilage in osteoarthritis. Osteoarthritis Cartilage 5:427–437

58. Patel IR, Attur MG, Patel RN, Stuchin SA, Abagyan RA, Abramson SB, Amin AR (1998) TNF-α convertase enzyme from human arthritis-affected cartilage: Isolation of cDNA by differential display, expression of the active enzyme, and regulation of TNF-α. J Immunol, 160:4570–4579

59. Attur MG, Patel RN, Abramson SB, Amin AR (1997) IL-17 up-regulation of nitric oxide production in human osteoarthritis cartilage. Arthritis Rheum 40:1050–1053

60. Bell MC, Carroll GJ (1995) Leukemia inhibitory factor (LIF) suppresses proteoglycan synthesis in porcine and caprine cartilage explants. Cytokine 7:137–141

61. Van de Loo FAJ, Arntz OJ, van den Berg (1997) Effect of IL-1 and leukemia inhibitory factor on chondrocyte metabolism in articular cartilage from normal and IL-6-deficient mice: Role of nitric oxide and IL-6 in the suppression of proteoglycan synthesis. Cytokine, 9:453–462

62. Chandrasekhar S, Harvey AK (1989) Induction of IL-1 receptors on chondrocytes by fibroblast growth factor: A possible mechanism for modulation of IL-1 activity. J Cell Physiol 138:236–246

63. Smith RJ, Justen JM, Sam IM, Rohloff NA, Ruppel PI, Brunden MN et al. (1991) Platelet-derived growth factor potentiates cellular responses of articular chondrocytes to IL-1. Arthritis Rheum 34:697–706

64. Verschure PJ, Joosten LAB, van de Loo FAJ, van den Berg WB (1995) IL-1 has no direct role in the IGF-1 nonresponsive state during experimentally induced arthritis in murine knee joints. Ann Rheum Dis 54:976–982

65. Lum ZP, Hakala BE, Mort JS, Recklies AD (1996): Modulation of the catabolic effects of IL-1β on human articular chondrocytes by TGF-β. J Cell Physiol 166:351–359

66. Vodovotz Y, Geiser AG, Chesler L, Letterion JJ, Cambell A, Lucia MS, Sporn MB, Roberts AB (1996) Spontaneously increased production of nitric oxide and aberrant expression of the inducible nitric oxide synthase in vivo in the TGFβ1 null mouse. J Exp Med 183:2337–2342

67. Van de Loo FAJ, Arntz OJ, van Enckevort FHJ, van Lent PLEM, van den Berg WB (1998) Reduced cartilage proteoglycan loss during zymosan-induced gonarthritis in NOS2-deficient mice and in anti-IL-1-treated wild-type mice with unabated joint inflammation. Arthritis Rheum 41:634–646

68. Van Beuningen HM, van der Kraan PM, Arntz OJ, van den Berg WB (1994) In vivo protection against interleukin-1-induced articular cartilage damage by transforming growth factor-β1: age related differences. Ann Rheum Dis 53:593–600

69. Glansbeek HL, van Beuningen HM, Vitters EL, Morris EA, van der Kraan PM, van den Berg WB (1997) Bone morphogenetic protein-2 stimulates articular cartilage proteoglycan synthesis in vivo but does not counteract IL-1 effects on proteoglycan synthesis and content. Arthritis Rheum 40:1020–1028

70. Glansbeek HL, van Beuningen HM, Vitters EL, van der Kraan PM, van den Berg WB (1998) Stimulation of articular cartilage repair in established arthritis by local administration of TGFβ into murine knee joints. Lab Invest 78:133–142

71. Lafeber FPJG, van der Kraan PM, Huber-Bruning O, van den Berg WB, Bijlsma JWJ (1993) Osteoarthritic human cartilage is more sensitive to transforming growth factor β than is normal cartilage. Br J Rheumatol 32:281–286

72. Lafeber FPJG, van Roy HLAM, van der Kraan PM, van den Berg WB, Bijlsma JWJ (1997) TGFß predominantly stimulates phenotypically changed chondrocytes in osteoarthritic human cartilage. J Rheumatol 24:536–542

73. Boumediene K, Conrozier T, Mathieu P, Richard M, Marcelli C, Vignon E, Pujol JP (1998) Decrease of cartilage TGF-β receptor II expression in the rabbit experimental osteoarthritis – potential role in cartilage breakdown. Osteoarthritis Cartilage 6:146–149

74. Serra R, Johnson M, Filvaroff EH, LaBorde J, Sheehan DM, Derynck R, Moses HL (1997) Expression of a truncated, kinase-defective TGF-β type II receptor in mouse skeletal tissue promotes terminal chondrocyte differentiation and osteoarthritis. J Cell Biol 139:541–552

75. Van Osch GJVM, van den Berg WB, Hunziker EB, Häuselmann HJ (1998) Differential effects of IGF-1 and TGFβ-2 on the assembly of proteoglycans in pericellular and territorial matrix by cultured bovine articular chondrocytes. Osteoarthritis Cartilage 6:187–195

76. Moldovan F, Pelletier JP, Hambor J, Cloutier JM, Martel-Pelletier J (1997) Collagenase-3 (matrix metalloprotease 13) is preferentially localized in the deep layer of human arthritic cartilage *in situ. In vitro* mimicking effect by TGFβ. Arthritis Rheum 40:1653–1661

77. Kawaguchi H, Kurokawa T, Hoshino Y, Kawahara H, Ogata E, Matsumoto T (1992) Immunohistochemical demonstration of bone morphogenetic protein-2 and TGF-β in the ossification of the posterior longitudinal ligament of the cervical spine. Spine, 17: S33-S36

78. Hoshi K, Amizuka N, Kurokawa T, Ozawa H (1997) Ultrastructure and immunolocalization of TGF-ß in chondrification of murine ligamenous fibroblasts and endochondral calcification induced by recombinant human bone morphogentic protein-2. Acta Histochem Cytochem 30:371–379

79. Glansbeek HL, van Beuningen HM, Vitters EL, van der Kraan PM, van den Berg WB (1998) Expression of recombinant human soluble type II TGFβ in Pichia pastoris and Escherichia coli: Two powerful systems to express a potent inhibitor of TGFβ1. Protein Expression Purification 12:201–207

80. Border WA, Ruoslahti E (1992) TGF-β in disease. The dark side of tissue repair. J Clin Invest 90:1–7

81. Zerath E, Holy X, Mouillon JM, Farbos B, Machwate M, Andre C, Renault S, Marie PJ (1997) TGF-β2 prevents the impaired chondrocyte proliferation induced by unloading in growth plates of young rats. Life Sciences 24:2397–2406

82. Goldring MB, Birkhead J, Sandell IJ, Kimura T, Krane SM (1988) IL-1 suppresses expression of cartilage-specific types II and IX collagen and increases type I and III collagens in human chondrocytes. J Clin Invest 82:2026–2037

83. Verschure PJ, van Marle J, Joosten LAB, van den Berg WB (1995) Chondrocyte IGF-1 receptor expression and responsiveness to IGF-1 stimulation in mouse articular cartilage during various phases of experimentally-induced arthritis. Ann Rheum Dis 54:645–653

84. Verschure PJ, van Marle J, Joosten LAB, van den Berg WB (1996) Histochemical analysis of IGF-1 binding sites in mouse normal and experimentally induced arthritic articular cartilage. Histochem J 28:13–23

85. Verschure PJ, van der Kraan PM, Vitters EL, van den Berg WB (1994) Stimulation of proteoglycan synthesis by Triamcinolone acetonide and insulin-like growth factor-1 in normal and arthritic murine articular cartilage. J Rheumatol 21:920–926

86. Dequeker J, Mohan R, Finkelman RD, Aerssens J, Baylink DJ (1993) Generalized osteoarthritis associated with increased insulin-like growth factor types I and II and TGF-β in cortical bone from the iliac crest. Possible mechanism of increased bone density and protection against osteoporosis. Arthritis Rheum 36:1702–1708

87. Westacott CI, Webb GR, Warnock MG, Sims JV, Elson CJ (1997) Alteration of cartilage metabolism by cells from osteoarthritic bone. Arthritis Rheum 40:1282–1291

88. Van Osch GJVM, van der Kraan PM, Blankevoort L, Huiskes R, van den Berg WB (1996) Relation of ligament damage with site specific cartilage loss and osteophyte formation in collagenase induced osteoarthritis in mice. J Rheumatol 23:1227–1232

4.6
Role of Crystal Deposition in the Osteoarthritic Joint

G. M. McCarthy

The presence of intra-articular calcium-containing crystals such as basic calcium phosphate (BCP) (hydroxyapatite, octacalcium phosphate, tricalcium phosphate) and calcium pyrophosphate dihydrate (CPPD) is strongly linked to osteoarthritis. The basis of cartilage damage by crystals has been the subject of numerous investigations. The crystals are thought to either initiate the degenerative process or to amplify ongoing degeneration. However, controversies persist concerning the relationship between calcium-containing crystals and cartilage degeneration despite ample data in support of their role [1].

4.6.1
Clinical Associations of Calcium-Containing Crystals

Prototypic of other arthritides associated with calcium-containing crystal deposition is a distinctive type of destructive arthropathy described by McCarty et al. in 1981 ("Milwaukee Shoulder Syndrome", MSS) [2], by Neer et al. in 1983 ("cuff tear arthropathy") [3] and by Dieppe et al. in 1984 ("apatite associated destructive arthritis") [4]. The gross anatomical features of MSS are often bilateral and include disappearance of the superior part of the fibrous rotator cuff and intra-articular portion of the tendon of the long-head of biceps; glenohumeral degenerative changes with loss of articular cartilage, marginal osteophytes, bony remodeling of both the humeral head and the glenoid fascia; upward subluxation of the humeral head with eburnation of the superior aspect as it forms a pseudoarthrosis with the coracoacromial vault and medial clavicle; synovial hypertrophy with frequent formation of pedunculated loose bodies and separation of the acromion into two parts along the plane of the original epiphysis. Frequently, large, non-inflammatory joint effusions are associated.

The etiologic role of basic calcium phosphate (BCP) crystals in MSS was first observed by McCarty et al. Synovial fluid studies of patients with MSS showed microaggregates of BCP crystals and particulate collagens with few leukocytes [5]. Synovial biopsies from patients with MSS showed increased numbers of villi, focal synovial lining hyperplasia and chondromatosis associated with intra- and extracellular BCP crystal deposits [6]. Since BCP crystals are identified from all affected joints, it was postulated that BCP crystals play an active role in the pathogenesis of MSS.

Several other patterns of arthritis have been associated with BCP crystals including primary osteoarthritis, an erosive polyarthritis and an acute inflammatory arthritis. Articular BCP crystal deposition also occurs as a consequence of several other conditions and may be termed secondary BCP arthropathies or periarthropathies (Table 1) [7].

BCP crystals are common in osteoarthritic (OA) knee effusions, often associated with synovial proliferation and severe degenerative arthritis. Several studies have suggested that the incidence of BCP crystals in synovial fluid from pa-

Table 1. Basic calcium crystal-associated joint disease

Calcific periarthritis
  Unifocal
  "Hydroxyapatite pseudopodagra"
  Multifocal
  Familial

Calcific tendonitis and bursitis

Intra-articular BCP arthropathies
  Acute (gout-like) attacks
  Milwaukee shoulder/knee syndrome
  (Idiopathic destructive arthritis; cuff tear arthropathy)
  Erosive polyarticular disease
  Mixed crystal deposition disease (BCP and CPPD)

Secondary BCP crystal arthropathies/periarthropathies
  Chronic renal failure
  Hypercalcemia states
  Calcinosis
  Neurological injury/paralysis
  Following local corticosteroid injection
  Miscellaneous

Tumoral calcinosis
  Hyperphosphatemic
  Nonhyperphosphatemic

---

tients with knee OA is between 30–60% [8, 9]. Indeed, it has been suggested that many OA joint fluids contain CPPD or BCP crystals that are too small or too few in number to be identified by conventional techniques [10]. The presence of BCP crystals correlates strongly with radiographic evidence of cartilaginous degeneration [11] and is associated with larger joint effusions when compared with joint fluid from OA knees without crystals [12]. Leukocyte levels in synovial fluid from osteoarthritic joints are no different whether or not crystals are present [9].

A polyarticular erosive form of arthritis associated with BCP crystals has also been described. Pain and swelling were most prominent in the wrists, metacarpophalangeal joints and proximal interphalangeal joints. Massive articular calcification was observed radiographically and joint damage was progressive [13]. Peri-articular BCP arthropathies include calcific periarthritis, tendonitis and bursitis [7]. For the most part, these appear to be related to isolated local dystrophic calcifications the etiology of which remain obscure and in general, these calcifications appear to be asymptomatic. In some individuals, however, dramatic inflammatory episodes may occur with severe pain, swelling and erythema resembling gout.

CPPD crystal deposition has been associated with the acute inflammatory arthritis of "pseudogout". It is also associated with chronic "pyrophosphate arthropathy" which is clinically distinguished from primary OA by its pattern of affected joints, greater severity and prominent inflammatory component. Inflammatory features may be sufficiently severe to cause confusion with rheumatoid disease [14]. A study of factors affecting radiographic progression of knee osteoarthritis showed that CPPD crystal deposition predicted poor clinical and radiographic outcome [15]. In a community-based study of an elderly population, OA was associated with chondrocalcinosis, particularly in the lateral tibiofemoral compartment of the knee and in the first three metacarpophalangeal joints [16].

BCP crystals are frequently observed together with CPPD and under these circumstances have been referred to as "mixed crystal deposition disease". In pathological joint effusions, the mixture is as common as the presence of either crystal alone [17].

4.6.2
Calcium-Containing Crystal Location and Identification

Basic calcium phosphate (BCP) crystals consist of partially carbonate substituted hydroxyapatite, octacalcium phosphate and rarely tricalcium phosphate [18]. Pathological calcifications in a wide variety of human tissues are composed of BCP crystals. They have long been known to deposit in periarticular locations in conditions such as calcific periarthritis and tendonitis. More recently, BCP crystals have also been found in intra-articular locations including synovial fluid, synovium and hyaline cartilage [19]. They are ultramicroscopic in size and therefore can be seen as individual particles only by transmission electron microscopy (TEM). These crystals have a remarkable tendency to clump as spheroidal microaggregates, which vary from about 1 to 50 μm in diameter. These clumps may be seen by light microscopy or by scanning electron microscope (SEM) where they look like snowballs. They are invariably associated with particulate collagens in synovial fluid [20].

Deposition of BCP cuboid crystals has been reported in OA and elderly normal femoral head articular cartilage and also in normal femoral head articular cartilage from a range of joint sites across a broad patient age spectrum [21]. Their crystalline composition is magnesium-substituted tricalcium phosphate (magnesium whitlockite) as suggested morphologically and as determined by scanning electron microscopy and X-ray diffraction [22]. An active role of these crystals in the propagation of cartilage degeneration has been suggested but remains to be confirmed [23].

Calcium pyrophosphate dihydrate (CPPD; $Ca_2P_2O_7.2H_2O$) crystals are relatively specific for articular tissue although periarticular deposits of CPPD have been reported in tendons, dura mater, ligamenta flava and the olecranon bursa, as well as in isolated "tophi"[14].

BCP crystals obtained from joint fluid have been carefully identified by scanning and transmission electron microscopy, X-ray energy dispersive analysis, direct chemical analysis for calcium and phosphate, X-ray diffraction by the powder method and Fourier transform infrared spectroscopy [20]. Alizarin red S staining of synovial fluid pellets has been suggested as a screening technique for BCP crystals [24]. This method is sensitive to 0.005 μg of hydroxyapatite (HA) standard per millilitre, but it is not specific for calcium phosphates and may provide many false positive results. A semiquantitative technique using the binding of (^{14}C) ethane-1-hydroxyl-1, 1-diphosphonate (EHDP) to BCP crystals has proved useful as a screening test and is sensitive to about 2 µg of HA standard [25]. Diphosphonates are analogues of inorganic pyrophosphate (PP_i) that adsorb to the surface of calcium phosphate crystals but not to MSU, CPPD, cartilage fragments, particulate collagens, or to any other known particulate in joint fluid. Such adsorption is not inhibited to any significant extent by PPi at the levels found in synovial fluid. Synovial fluid pellets that bound EHDP were examined routinely by scanning electron microscopy (SEM). Microspheroidal aggregates approximately 1 to 19 µm in diameter were generally found and were further characterized by x-ray energy dispersive analysis. The molar calcium/phosphorus was virtually identical to that of a HA standard [5].

Using TEM, magnesium whitlockite crystals have been frequently observed scattered amongst intramatrical lipidic debris, particularly pericellularly, in areas of cell necrosis and amongst close-packed tangential fibers between the articular surface and initial superficial zone chondrocytes of articular cartilage [23].

CPPD crystals can be identified by polarized light microscopy when they appear as anisotropic (nonrefractile) or weakly positively birefringent rhomboidal crystals. Most patients whose joint fluid contains CPPD crystals will have radiographic evidence of calcified fibrocartilage and/or of hyaline articular cartilage although some will appear radiographically normal [14].

4.6.3
Current Concepts of the Role of Calcium-Containing Crystals in the Pathophysiology of Osteoarthritis

Concurrence of articular calcium-containing crystal deposition and degenerative joint disease is well established and ample data support their role in cartilage degeneration.

Clinically, the joint degeneration of calcium-containing crystal deposition differs from the joint degeneration of primary osteoarthritis (OA) [14]. If crystals were simply an epiphenomenon of cartilage degeneration, we would expect to see CPPD or BCP crystals in the joints most commonly affected by primary OA. Instead, crystal deposition disease frequently involves shoulders, wrists and elbows, sites rarely affected by primary OA. Not only is the distribution of joint involvement distinct, but the severity of joint degeneration is magnified in the presence of calcium-containing crystals. Some investigators speculate that articular crystals cause cartilage degeneration directly whereas others hypothesize that clinically undetectable cartilage metabolic or structural aberrations are primary and these aberrations cause defects in matrix or chondrocyte metabolism that favor both crystal formation and degeneration. Thus, degeneration and crystal formation would be viewed as parallel events of common derivation [26]. An intermediate view is that a primary metabolic abnormality leads to degeneration but that secondary crystal deposits accelerate deterioration, the "amplification loop" hypothesis [27].

The exact basis of cartilage damage by calcium-containing crystals remains somewhat speculative. In theory, crystals in cartilage could directly injure chondrocytes. However, in pathological specimens crystals are rarely seen in imme-

Fig. 1.
Proposed pathogenic
mechanism of calcium-
containing crystal-induced
cartilage degeneration.
BCP, basic calcium phos-
phate; CPPD, calcium
pyrophosphate dihydrate;
MMP, matrix metallo-
protease

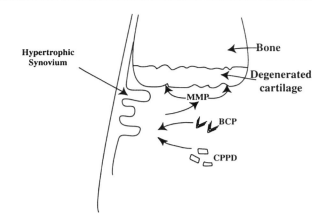

diate contact with chondrocytes and even less frequently found engulfed by chondrocytes [28]. It is more likely that cartilage damage results when synovial lining cells ingest crystals and then release matrix-degrading enzymes or secrete cytokines that stimulate chondrocytes to release matrix-degrading enzymes (Fig. 1). This concept is further supported by data from a study of the role of CPPD crystal-induced synovitis in the development of accelerated OA in CPPD deposition disease [29]. A lapine model of OA, induced by partial lateral meniscectomy and section of the fibular collateral and sesamoid ligaments, was used in the study. In meniscectomized right knees, following repeated (weekly) injections of CPPD crystals (either 1 or 10 mg), there was more severe OA at 8 weeks compared with noninjected contralateral meniscectomized left knees. The intensity of associated synovial inflammation correlated with intra-articular CPPD administration and dosage. Although the doses administered were considerably higher than concentrations found *in vivo*, the data support a worsening effect of chronic CPPD crystal-induced synovitis on experimental OA and suggest a role for CPPD crystal-induced inflammation in the progression of OA lesions in clinical CPPD crystal deposition disease.

4.6.4
In Vitro Studies

Potential mechanisms by which calcium-containing crystals may promote articular damage have been explored and will be presented below. These include their mitogenic properties, their ability to induce metalloproteases and their ability to stimulate prostaglandin synthesis.

4.6.4.1
Mitogenic Effect of Calcium-Containing Crystals

Synovial lining proliferation of varying degrees is common in crystal-associated arthritis and the crystals themselves are at least partly responsible for proliferation [6]. Increased cell numbers in the synovial lining enhance the capacity for secretion of cytokines, which may promote chondrolysis and cause secretion of proteolytic enzymes. BCP crystals in concentrations found in pathologic human joint fluids stimulated mitogenesis in quiescent cultured human skin fibroblasts, canine synovial fibroblasts and mouse 3T3 cells in a concentration-dependent manner [30, 31]. Growth stimulation also occurred with CPPD, calcium urate, calcium sulfate, calcium carbonate and calcium diphosphonate crystals [30, 32]. Both onset and peak (^{3}H)-thymidine incorporation induced by these crystals was delayed 2–3 hours compared to cells stimulated with serum. This lag time may in part represent time required for phagocytosis and intracellular dissolution of crystals. Addition of control particles of similar size such as diamond dust or latex beads did not stimulate mitogenesis. Monosodium urate monohydrate (MSU) crystals were weakly mitogenic and much less so than calcium urate, suggesting that the calcium content of crystals is important for mitogenesis. Synthetic BCP was as mitogenic as BCP obtained from a patient with calcinosis, indicating that the crystal and not a contaminant was responsible [30]. The mitogenic effect of the calcium-containing crystals was not the result of increased ambient medium calcium concentration from crystal dissolution, since conditioned medium from cells which had been exposed to and which had dissolved BCP crystals did not stimulate (^{3}H)-thymidine incorporation by fibroblasts [32].

The mechanism of BCP crystal-induced mitogenesis has been explored. Firstly, it was hypothesized that the abnormal proliferation of synovial cells may be at least in part, due to endocytosis and intracellular dissolution of crystals producing an increased cytoplasmic calcium concentration which activates a calcium-dependent pathway leading to mitogenesis. This concept was supported by the following evidence. Direct cell-crystal contact is required for crystal-induced mitogenesis since cultures exposed to crystals were growth-stimulated but in cultures inverted to prevent cell-crystal contact, no growth stimulation occured [33]. To study the requirement for crystal phagocytosis following cell-crystal interaction, cells were exposed to ^{45}Ca-labeled BCP and (^{3}H)-thymidine. Cells containing ^{45}Ca-labeled BCP were separated by gradient centrifugation and found to have incorporated significantly more (^{3}H)-thymidine than those without BCP [34]. In cultured macrophages, inhibition of crystal endocytosis with cytochalasin B inhibited crystal dissolution, further supporting the requirement of phagocytosis [35]. Calcium-containing crystals are acid soluble. Following phagocytosis, intracellular crystal dissolution likely occurs in the acid medium of the phagolysosomes. Chloroquine, ammonium chloride and bafilomycin A$_1$, all lysosomotrophic agents which raise lysosomal pH, significantly inhibit intracellular crystal dissolution and (^{3}H)-thymidine uptake in a dose-dependent manner in fibroblasts exposed to BCP crystals [36].

The intracellular calcium response to basic calcium phosphate crystals in fibroblasts has subsequently been determined using the photoactive dye, fura-2 [37]. Addition of media containing BCP crystals to fibroblasts in monolayer culture caused an immediate 10-fold increase in intracellular calcium which returned to baseline within 8 minutes. This increase was derived mostly from extracellular calcium as it was not seen when BCP were added in calcium-free media. A second rise of intracellular calcium started at 60 minutes, continued to increase up to at least 3 hours and was derived from intracellular dissolution of phagocytosed crystals.

Current evidence suggests, therefore, that phagocytosis followed by intracellular crystal dissolution occurs when BCP crystals and fibroblasts come into contact with each other and that this process contributes to BCP crystal-induced mitogenesis.

Secondly, it was noted that BCP crystals also stimulate mitogenesis by a process similar to platelet-derived growth factor (PDGF). PDGF is a peptide growth factor which renders quiescent fibroblasts and many other anchorage-dependent cell lines "competent" to respond to 'progression' growth factors such as insulin-like growth factor-1 (IGF-1), which are required for progression through the cell cycle. BCP crystals could substitute for PDGF as a competence growth factor and, like PDGF, acted synergistically with IGF-1 or plasma. Furthermore, blocking antibodies against IGF-1 diminished the mitogenic response of 3T3 cells to BCP [38]. Some differences have been observed between the biochemical and cellular mechanisms of action of PDGF and BCP crystals. Mitchell et al. demonstrated that BCP crystal induced mitogenesis in Balb/c-3T3 fibroblasts involves a rapid membrane associated event which requires the presence of the serine/threonine protein kinase C (PKC), one of the major mediators of signals generated upon external stimulation of cells by hormones, neurotransmitters and growth factors. Down regulation of PKC activity in Balb/c-3T3 cells inhibited BCP crystal-mediated induction of the proto-oncogenes c-*fos* and c-*myc* but had no effect on that stimulated by PDGF [39].

It was therefore recognized that the increased intracellular calcium concentration that occurs as phagocytosed crystals dissolve is only one signal for mitogenesis. When growth factors such as PDGF bind to their membrane receptors, phospholipase C (a phosphodiesterase) is stimulated to hydrolyze phosphatidylinositol 4,5-bisphosphate (PIP_2) to the intracellular messengers, inosital triphosphate (IP_3) and diacylglycerol (DAG) [40]. IP_3 releases calcium from the endoplasmic reticulum, modulating the activities of calcium-dependent and calcium/calmodulin-dependent enzymes such as protein kinases and proteases [41].

DAG, the other hydrolysis product of PIP_2, is a potent activator of PKC [42]. Rothenberg and Cheung reported elevated phospholipase C degradation of inosital phospholipid in rabbit synovial cells in response to BCP crystal stimulation [43]. BCP crystals significantly increased inosital-1-phosphate in (^3H)-inosital-labeled cells within 1 minute, and levels were maximum at 1 hour. Increased amounts of inositol mono-, bis-, and trisphosphates were all measured after crystal ingestion supporting the concept that BCP crystals enhance phospholipase C activity in synovial fibroblasts.

Since BCP crystals increased phospholipase C activity, resultant increased DAG accumulation and finally increased PKC activity was expected. Accordingly, the role of PKC in BCP-induced mitogenesis was examined. The effects of BCP crystals and PDGF on DNA synthesis were compared in Balb/c-3T3 fibroblasts. In some cultures, PKC was depleted by incubation of the cells with a high concentration of tumor-promoting phorbol diester (TPA), an analogue of DAG. Chronic TPA stimulation down-regulates PKC, in contrast to acute treatment which activates PKC. Stimulation of DNA synthesis by BCP was inhibited after downregulation of PKC implying an important role for PKC in BCP-induced mitogenesis. As noted above, no effect on PDGF-stimulated DNA synthesis was observed under the same conditions [39]. Subsequently, it has been confirmed that the mitogenic response to BCP crystals is associated with PKC activation in human fibroblasts [44]. In contrast, BCP crystals do not activate phosphatidylinositol 3-kinase or tyrosine kinases confirming that cell activation by BCP crystals is selective in mechanism [44].

A class of genes known as proto-oncogenes play an important role in controlling cell proliferation. Fos and myc proteins, both products of the proto-oncogenes c-*fos* and c-*myc*, are localized to the cell nucleus and bind to specific DNA sequences [45, 46]. Stimulation of 3T3 fibroblasts with either BCP crystals or PDGF results in the expression of c-*fos* within minutes, reaching maximal expression approximately 30 minutes after stimulation. Induction of c-*myc* transcription by BCP or PDGF occurs within 1 hour and is maximal at about 3 hours after stimulation. Such stimulated cells maintain elevated transcription of c-*myc* for at least 5 hours [47]. The expression of c-*fos* and c-*myc* is increased in response to BCP crystal stimulation in a manner similar to the increase produced by PDGF. However, in PKC down-regulated cells both TPA and BCP crystal stimulation of c-*fos* and c-*myc* are markedly inhibited, whereas in contrast, the induction of these transcripts by PDGF is unaffected.

Members of the mitogen activated protein kinases (MAPK) family are key regulators of a variety of intracellular signal transduction cascades. One subclass of this family, the p42/p44 MAPKs, is believed to regulate cell proliferation by a mechanism that includes the activation of proto-oncogenes c-*fos* and c-*jun*. BCP and CPPD crystals both activate a protein kinase signal transduction pathway involving p42 and p44 MAPKs suggesting that this pathway may contribute to calcium-containing crystal-induced mitogenesis [48].

Finally, the transcription factor nuclear factor κB (NF-κB) appears to contribute to BCP crystal-induced mitogenesis. NF-κB, first described as a regulator of the immunoglobulin kappa (Ig κ) light-chain gene, is an inducible transcription factor critical to many signal transduction pathways because it regulates the expression of a wide variety of important genes. Induction of NF-κB ordinarily involves release from cytoplasmic inhibitory proteins, collectively referred to as IκB. NF-κB induction is followed by translocation of the active transcription factor complex into the nucleus. BCP crystals induce NF-κB in Balb-c/3T3 fibroblasts and human foreskin fibroblasts (HFF) [44].

Many stimuli other than BCP crystals activate NF-κB. These include cytokines and activators of PKC such as the phorbol ester TPA [49]. Several signal-transduction pathways may be involved but all of these stimuli act by means of protein kinases that phosphorylate (and thus degrade) IκB. It was originally proposed that IκB might serve as a substrate for kinases such as PKC and protein kinase A, based on *in vitro* studies [50, 51]. Recently, however, a high molecular mass IκB kinase (IKK) complex has been identified [52]. These kinases specifically phosphorylate critical serine residues of IκB. Activation of NF-κB by TNF- and IL-1 requires the successive action of NF-κB-inducing kinase (NIK) and IκB kinase [53]. The molecular mechanisms by which NIK becomes activated are not yet understood. Although BCP crystals activate both PKC and NF-κB, it is not known to what extent these two events are linked. Since the critical modification for IKK activation appears to be phosphorylation, it is possible that PKC plays a role in BCP crystal-induction of NF-κB by inducing phosphorylation and activation of IKK [54]. In support of this concept, the PKC inhibitor staurosporine inhibited both BCP crystal-induced mitogenesis and NF-κB [44]. Alternatively, it is possible that staurosporine inhibits IKK since, although it is a potent inhibitor of PKC, it also inhibits PKA and other protein kinases [55].

The mechanism of BCP crystal-induced mitogenesis in fibroblasts, therefore, has been shown to involve at least two distinct, but necessary, processes. The first is a fast, membrane-associated event resulting in PKC and MAPK activation, NF-κB induction and proto-oncogene induction. The second event is a slower intracellular dissolution of the crystals which raises intracellular calcium leading to the activation of a number of calcium-dependent processes stimulating mitogenesis. Figure 2 depicts our current concept of the biologic effects of calcium-containing crystals.

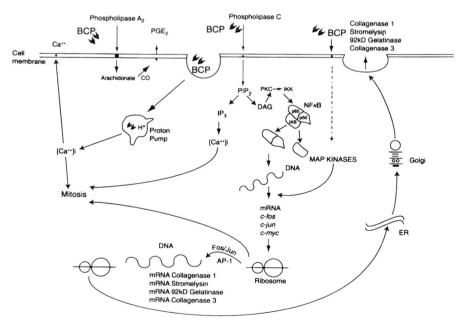

Fig. 2. Some biological effects of calcium-containing crystals. BCP, basic calcium phosphate; CO, cyclo-oxygenase; ER, endoplasmic reticulum; PKC, protein kinase C; DAG, diacylglycerol; PIP$_2$, phosphatidylinositol 4,5-bisphosphate; IP$_3$, inositol 1,4,5-triphosphate; NF-κB, nuclear factor κB; MAPK, mitogen-activated protein kinase; IKK, IκB kinase

4.6.4.2
Matrix Metalloprotease Induction by Calcium-Containing Crystals

Current data suggests that the mediators of tissue damage from calcium-containing crystals include the matrix metalloproteases (MMP) collagenase-1 (MMP-1), stromelysin (transin, MMP-3), 92 kD gelatinase (gelatinase B/MMP-9) and collagenase-3 (MMP-13). The MMP family share a number of chief characteristics. The enzymes cleave one or more components of the extracellular matrix. Activity is inhibited by tissue inhibitor of metalloproteinases (TIMP). The proteinases are secreted in zymogen form which can be activated by proteinases or by organomercurials. The catalytic mechanism depends on zinc at the active site. The cDNA sequences of the MMP family all show homology to that of collagenase [56].

Collagenase is a critical regulator of extracellular matrix remodeling because of it's unique ability to degrade the native collagen fibril [56]. Stromelysin degrades type 4 collagen and many other components of extracellular matrix including proteoglycan and laminin [57]. 92 kD gelatinase accelerates the breakdown of matrix components such as gelatin, collagens type IV, V and XI and elastin [58]. Collagenase-3 is expressed in human osteoarthritic cartilage and degrades type II collagen more efficiently than collagenase-1 [59].

The massive lysis of intra-articular collagenous structures which typifies MSS strongly suggests collagen matrix-degrading metalloprotease activity. Furthermore, collagenase and neutral protease activity was demonstrated in the synovial fluid from the shoulder joints of some, but not all, patients with MSS [5]. The neutral protease activity was likely due to stromelysin but the presence of gelatinase was not evaluated. Similarly, Lohmander et al. measured concentrations of stromelysin and collagenase-1 in a variety of joint disorders including OA and calcium pyrophosphate arthropathy. ELISA's were performed using monoclonal and polyclonal antibodies. Both proteins were detected in disease groups 15 – 45 times that of the control groups. The highest concentrations of both enzymes were found in pyrophosphate arthropathy [60].

On account of the association between synovial fluid BCP crystals and joint destruction, a hypothesis was formulated in which BCP crystals and possibly particulate collagens are endocytosed by synovial-lining cells. These cells are then stimulated to proliferate and secrete proteases. This hypothesis was tested in vitro by adding natural or synthetic BCP, CPPD and other crystals to cultured human or canine synovium cells. Neutral protease and collagenase activity was augmented in a dose-related fashion approximately 5 to 8 times over control cultures incubated without crystals [61].

We recently expanded studies of metalloprotease induction and secretion using HFF proliferating in response to BCP crystals. We demonstrated the coordinate induction of collagenase-1, stromelysin and 92 kD gelatinase messenger RNA (mRNA) accumulation in BCP crystal-stimulated cultures. This was followed by secretion of collagenase-1, stromelysin and 92 kD gelatinase protein into conditioned media, identified by Western blot using specific antibodies. Activity of each enzyme was also confirmed [62, 63]. BCP crystals also caused collagenase-1 and collagenase-3 mRNA accumulation in adult porcine articular chondrocytes [64, 65]. This was followed by secretion of collagenase-1 (un-published observation) and collagenase-3 protein into conditioned media.

Since intracellular crystal dissolution is important in BCP crystal-induced mitogenesis, we evaluated the role of crystal dissolution in BCP crystal-induced MMP production. Raising lysosomal pH with bafilomycin A_1 to inhibit intracel-lular BCP crystal dissolution attenuated the proliferative response of human fibroblasts to BCP crystals but did not inhibit MMP synthesis and secretion [36].

It has been shown that the collagenase promoter contains a *cis* element term-ed the TPA response element (TRE) which is involved in increased transcrip-tion in response to tumor necrosis factor alpha (TNFα) [66] and phorbol esters [67]. Increased transcription modulated through the TRE depends on the tran-scription factor, activator protein-1 (AP-1) a heterodimer composed of the pro-tein products of c-*fos* and c-*jun*, both primary response genes, which interact to stimulate transcription of AP-1 responsive genes [67]. Synthesis of fos is essen-tial for phorbol (TPA) induction of collagenase and also for the cells response to IL-1, TNFα and serum factors [56]. Thus, inhibitors of protein synthesis such as cycloheximide would be expected to interfere with this mechanism of tran-scriptional activation. Cycloheximide blocks the response to IL-1β and TNFα which suggests that the response is dependent on the synthesis of fos and jun. Both c-*fos* and c-*jun* messenger RNA (mRNA) levels are increased by TNFα [66]. Similarly, cycloheximide blocks BCP crystal induction of collagenase-1, stromelysin and 92-kD gelatinase mRNA in human fibroblasts and also colla-genase-3 mRNA in adult porcine articular chondrocytes [62, 63, 65]. BCP crystals induce c-*fos* and c-*jun* mRNA and activate the transcription factor AP-1 in human fibroblasts [44].

The clinical features of OA suggest a prominent contribution of matrix me-talloproteases. In the presence of calcium-containing crystals, joint degenera-tion is exaggerated. Current data suggests that the clinical manifestations of cal-cium-containing crystal deposition disease result, in part, from the direct stimulation of MMP production by fibroblasts and chondrocytes upon contact with the crystals.

4.6.4.3
Stimulation of Prostaglandin Synthesis by Calcium-Containing Crystals

In addition to the stimulation of growth stimulation and enzyme secretion, cal-cium-containing crystals caused the release of prostaglandins from cultured mammalian cells, especially PGE_2 [61, 68, 69]. All PGE_2 release occurred in the first hours after cells were exposed to crystals. Rothenberg confirmed and ex-tended this work. He demonstrated that phosphatidyl choline and phosphatidyl ethanolamine are the major sources of arachidonic acid for PGE_2 synthesis con-firming that the phospholipase A_2/cyclooxygenase pathway is the predominant route for PGE_2 production. BCP crystals appeared to stimulate synthesis of both phospholipase A_2 and cyclooxygenase [70].

Although PGE compounds are local mediators of inflammation, evidence from both *in vitro* and *in vivo* experiments indicates that they can suppress diverse effector systems of inflammation. Both PGE_1 and PGE_2 also increase concentrations of cyclic AMP in human synovial cells in culture and suppress synovial cell proliferation [71, 72]. Since radioimmunoassays do not usually distinguish between PGE_1 and PGE_2 [73]. PGE_1 may also have been released in response to BCP crystals. Whether the augmented PGE production induced by these crystals significantly down-regulates their other biologic effects is an important question and may be one mechanism accounting for the clinical observation of accelerated articular damage in the presence of the cyclooxygenase inhibitor indomethacin [74].

We studied the effects of PGE_2, PGE_1 and its analogue, the drug misoprostol on the mitogenic response of human fibroblasts to BCP crystals. All three agents inhibited the mitogenic response to BCP crystals in a concentration-dependent manner. PGE_1 and misoprostol were more potent. PGE_1 and misoprostol, but not PGE_2, inhibited collagenase mRNA accumulation in response to BCP crystals [75, 76].

Various classes of PG increase intracellular cAMP levels and increased cAMP levels inhibit mitogenesis in certain cell types. We explored the mechanism of inhibition of BCP crystal-mediated cell activation by PGE. We showed that PGE_1 is a more potent inducer of intracellular cAMP than PGE_2 and that PGE_1 inhibits BCP crystal induced mitogenesis and MMP production through the cyclic AMP signal transduction pathway [76]. It is possible that the augmented PGE production induced by BCP crystals downregulates their other biological effects (mitogenesis and MMP production) by a feedback mechanism.

4.6.5
Calcium-Containing Crystal Induced Inflammation

The chronic destructive arthropathies or osteoarthritis associated with CPPD or BCP crystals are probably much more important medically than are the dramatic acute inflammatory syndromes associated with neutrophilic phagocytosis [7, 14]. Firstly, they are more common. Secondly, chronic joint destruction is irreversible whereas acute inflammatory events can be readily treated. Furthermore, repeated, isolated inflammatory events are usually required over long periods of time before permanent joint damage ensues. The presence of calcium-containing crystals in osteoarthritic synovial fluids (SF) is common; however, associated episodes of acute inflammation with leukocytosis appear relatively uncommon clinically in OA and MMS. The phlogistic potential of crystals may be somewhat modified by intra-synovial inhibitory factors. Terkeltaub et al. have demonstrated the ability of serum and plasma to markedly suppress neutrophil responsiveness to BCP crystals [77]. Factors causing such inhibition appeared to be crystal-bound proteins. Of the crystal-bound plasma proteins studied, α_2-HS glycoprotein (AHSG) appeared to be the most potent and specific inhibitor of neutrophil responsiveness to BCP crystals. AHSG is a liver-derived serum protein known to be greatly concentrated relative to other serum proteins in bone and mineralizing tissues [78]. AHSG was present in non-inflammatory synovial fluids and could be detected on native synovial fluid BCP crystals [77]. The authors concluded that AHSG could modulate the inflammatory potential of BCP crystals *in vivo*. When the inflammatory potential of BCP crystals was evaluated using the rat air pouch model, variations in fluid volumes and white cell counts occured according to specific surface area of the various crystal types tested and their calcium:phosphorus ratios [79]. The authors postulate that BCP heterogeneity may be one explanation for their variable tolerance in human joints.

4.6.6
Role of Cytokines

Recently, there has been progress in understanding the mechanism of cartilage breakdown in osteoarthritis [80]. The initial cleavage of cartilage matrix molecules is extracellular and is mediated primarily by proteases [56]. The major proteases involved appear to be collagenase and stromelysin. Chondrocytes are capable of exhaustive degradation of their extracellular matrix [81]. Interleukin-1 (IL-1), produced by synovial cells, polymorphs and chondrocytes, has been suggested as the most potent stimulator of cartilage degradation [81]. IL-1 stimulates increases in proteinase transcription, synthesis and secretion by chondrocytes and synoviocytes while inhibiting matrix synthesis [80]. Although it is possible that matrix degradation in calcium-containing crystal arthropathies is cytokine mediated, neither BCP nor CPPD crystals induced IL-1 production *in vitro*, unlike monosodium urate crystals [82]. Current data strongly supports direct stimulation of MMP production by fibroblasts and chondrocytes upon contact with calcium-containing crystals.

4.6.7
Implications for Treatment

There are no available drugs to inhibit deposition nor effect reabsorption of the crystals [75]. This contrasts with gout where accumulation of urate crystals can be eliminated with hypouricemic therapy [83]. Both normal and abnormal joint tissues generate extracellular inorganic pyrophosphate (PPi). CPPD crystal deposition is driven by a local abnormality of excess articular PPi production [84]. Hyaline articular and fibrocartilage, tendon and ligament in organ culture release PPi into the ambient medium [85]. Basal PPi release is stimulated twofold or more by transforming growth factor β (TGFβ) and this increase is inhibited by probenecid, insulin-like growth factor or inhibitors of protein synthesis [86]. Pharmacological control of excess local PPi levels might prevent CPPD crystal deposition much as control of excess urate prevents monosodium urate deposition in gout.

  Recently phosphocitrate, a potent inhibitor of hydroxyapatite crystal formation and a relatively non-toxic compound, was shown to inhibit the mitogenic effect of BCP crystals in a concentration dependent manner. This inhibition appeared to be specific since the same concentrations of phosphocitrate had no impact on basal, PDGF-induced or serum-induced (^{3}H)-thymidine incorporation [87]. Phosphocitrate also blocked BCP crystal-induced proto-oncogene and collagenase transcription [88]. Its mechanism of action is being explored at present and recently it was shown to inhibit calcium-containing crystal induction of MAPK. This compound may ultimately prove useful in protecting articular tissues from the harmful biologic effects of calcium-containing crystals such as CPPD or BCP [48].

Others have shown that PGE_1 can have anti-inflammatory and tissue protective action [73]. Misoprostol, a PGE_1 analogue, is already approved for use in humans to prevent gastrointestinal damage induced by non-steroidal inflammatory drugs [89]. We have demonstrated the ability of these E-series prostaglandins to interfere with the biological effects of BCP crystals [75, 76]. These characteristics may also be of therapeutic importance in the future.

Calcium-containing crystal deposition diseases and their role in the cartilage damage which characterizes osteoarthritis remains incompletely understood. Their importance in terms of morbidity will likely amplify as the aged population increases. Further studies of the mechanisms important for crystal deposition and for their biological effects are essential to rational prevention or reversal of the consequences of calcium-containing crystal deposition.

References

1. Schumacher HR (1995) Synovial inflammation, crystals, and osteoarthritis. J Rheumatol, 22 [Suppl 43]:101–103
2. McCarty DJ, Halverson PB, Carrera G., Brewe, BJ, Kozin FK (1981) Milwaukee shoulder: association of microspheroids containing hydroxyapatite crystals, active collagenase, and neutral protease with rotator cuff defects, i. Clinical aspects. Arthritis Rheum, 4: 464–473
3. Neer CS, Craig EV, Fakuda H (1983) Cuff-tear arthropathy. J Bone Joint Surg, 65 A:1232–1244
4. Dieppe PA, Doherty M, Macfarlane DG, Hutton CW, Bradfield JW, Watt I (1984) Apatite associated destructive arthritis. Br J Rheumatol, 23:84–91
5. Halverson PB, Cheung HS, McCarty DJ, Garancis J, Mandel N (1981) Milwaukee shoulder: association of microspheroids containing hydroxyapatite crystals, active collagenase, and neutral protease with rotator cuff defects. ii. Synovial fluid studies. Arthritis Rheum, 24: 474–483
6. Garancis JC, Cheung HS, Halverson PB, McCarty DJ (1981) Milwaukee shoulder: Association of microspheroids containing hydroxyapatite crystals, active collagenase and neutral protease with rotator cuff defects.iii. Morphologic and biochemical studies of an excised synovium showing chondromatosis. Arthritis Rheum, 24:484–491
7. Halverson PB, McCarty DJ (1997) Basic calcium phosphate (apatite, octacalcium phosphate, tricalcium phosphate) crystal deposition diseases; calcinosis, in Arthritis and allied conditions. A textbook of rheumatology. Koopman WJ (ed) Williams and Wilkins: Baltimore, MD p 2127–2146
8. Gibilisco PA, Schumacher HR, Hollander JL, Soper KA (1985) Synovial fluid crystals in osteoarthritis. Arthritis Rheum, 28:511–515
9. Dieppe PA, Crocker PR, Corke CF, Doyle DV, Willoughby DA (1972) Synovial fluid crystals. Q J Med, 192:533–553
10. Swan A, Chapman B, Heap P, Seward H, Dieppe P (1994) Submicroscopic crystals in osteoarthritic synovial fluids. Ann Rheum Dis, 53:467–470
11. Halverson PB, McCarty DJ (1986) Patterns of radiographic abnormalities associated with basic calcium phosphate and calcium pyrophosphate crystal deposition in the knee. Ann Rheum Dis, 45:603–605
12. Carroll GJ, Stuart RA, Armstrong JA, Breidahl PD, Laing BA (1991) Hydroxyapatite crystals are a frequent finding in osteoarthritic synovial fluid, but are not related to increased concentrations of keratan sulfate or interleukin-1β. J Rheumatol, 18:861–866

13. Schumacher HR, Miller JL, Ludivico C, Jessar RA (1981) Erosive arthritis associated with apatite crystal deposition. Arthritis Rheum, 24:31–37
14. Ryan L, McCarty D (1997) Calcium pyrophosphate crystal deposition disease, pseudogout and articular chondrocalcinosis, in Arthritis and Allied Conditions, Koopman W (ed) Williams and Wilkins: Baltimore, MD. p.2103–2125
15. Ledingham J, Regan M, Jones A, Doherty M (1995) Factors affecting radiographic progression of knee osteoarthritis. Ann Rheum Dis, 54:53–58
16. Sanmarti R, Kanterewicz E, Pladevall M, Panella D, Brugues Tarradellas J, Munoz Gomez J (1996) Analysis of the association between chondrocalcinosis and osteoarthritis: a community based study. Ann Rheum Dis, 5:30–33
17. Dieppe P, Doyle D, Huskisson E, Willoughby D, Crocker P (1978) Mixed crystal deposition and osteoarthritis. Br Med J, 1:150
18. McCarty DJ, Lehr JR, Halverson PB (1983) Crystal populations in human synovial fluid. Identification of apatite, octacalcium phosphate and tricalcium phosphate. Arthritis Rheum, 26:247–251
19. Halverson P, McCarty D (1988) Clinical aspects of basic calcium phosphate crystal deposition. Rheum Dis North Am, 14:427–439
20. McCarty D (1988) Crystal identification in human synovial fluids. Rheum Dis Clin North Am, 14:253–267
21. Scotchford CA, Ali SY (1995) Magnesium whitlockite deposition in articular cartilage: a study of 80 specimens from 70 patients. Ann Rheum Dis, 54:339–344
22. Scotchford C, Vickers M, Ali S (1995) The isolation and characterization of magnesium whitlockite crystals from human articular cartilage. Osteoarthritis Cartilage, 3:79–94
23. Scotchford C, Ali S (1997) Association of magnesium whitlockite crystals with lipid components of the extracellular matrix in human articular cartilage. Osteoarthritis Cartilage 5:107–119
24. Paul H, Reginato AJ, Schumacher HR (1983) Alizarin red S staining as a screening test to detect calcium compounds in synovial fluid. Arthritis Rheum, 6:191–200
25. Halverson P, McCarty DJ (1979) Identification of hydroxyapatite crystals in synovial fluid. Arthritis Rheum, 22:389–395
26. Bjelle A (1981) Familial pyrophosphate arthropathy occurence and crystal identification. Scand J Rheumatol, 24:464–473
27. Doherty M, Watt I, Dieppe P (1982) Localised chondrocalcinosis in postmenisectomy knees. Lancet, 1:1207–1210
28. Schumacher H (1988) Pathology of crystal deposition diseases. Rheum Dis Clin North Am, 14:269–288
29. Fam AG, Morava-Protzner I, Purcell C, Young BD, Bunting PS, Lewis AJ (1995) Acceleration of experimental lapine osteoarthritis by calcium pyrophosphate microcrystalline synovitis. Arthritis Rheum, 38:201–210
30. Cheung HS, Story MT, McCarty DJ (1984) Mitogenic effects of hydroxyapatite and calcium pyrophosphate dihydrate crystals on cultured mammalian cells. Arthritis Rheum, 27:668–674
31. Barnes D, Colowick S (1977) Stimulation of sugar uptake and thymidine incorporation in mouse 3T3 cells by calcium phosphate and other extracellular particles. Proc Natl Acad Sci USA, 74:5593–5597
32. Cheung HS, McCarty DJ (1985) Mitogenesis induced by calcium-containing crystals: role of intracellular dissolution. Exp Cell Res, 157:63–70
33. Bowen-Pope D, Rubin H (1983) Growth stimulatory precipitate of Ca^{++} and pyrophosphate. J Cell Physiol, 17:51–61
34. Borkowf A, Cheung HS, McCarty DJ (1987) Endocytosis is required for the mitogenic effect of basic calcium phosphate crystals. Calcif Tiss Int, 40:173–176
35. Owens J, Cheung H, McCarty D (1986) Endocytosis precedes dissolution of basic calcium phosphate crystals by murine macrophages. Calcif Tiss Int, 36:645–650
36. McCarthy GM, Cheung HS, Abel SM, Ryan LM (1998) Basic calcium phosphate crystal-induced collagenase production:role of intracellular crystal dissolution. Osteoarthritis Cartilage, 6:205–213

37. Halverson P, Greene A, Cheung H (1998) Intracellular calcium responses to basic calcium phosphate crystals in fibroblasts. Osteoarthritis Cartilage, 6:324–329
38. Cheung HS, Van Wyk JJ, Russell WE, McCarty DJ (1986) Mitogenic activity of hydroxyapatite: Requirement for somatomedin. C J Cell Physiol, 128:143–148
39. Mitchell PG, Pledger W, Cheung HS (1989) Molecular mechanism of basic calcium phosphate crystal-induced mitogenesis. Role of protein kinase C. J Biol Chem, 264:14071–14077
40. Berridge M (1987) Inosital phosphate and diacylglycerol: two interacting second messengers. Annu Rev Biochem, 56:159–194
41. Rasmussen H (1986) The calcium messenger system. Part II. N Engl J Med, 314:1164–1170
42. Kikkawa U, Nishizuka Y (1986) The role of protein kinase C in transmembrane signalling. Annu Rev Cell Biol, 2:149–178
43. Rothenberg R, Cheung H (1988) Rabbit synoviocyte inositol phosphate metabolism is stimulated by hydroxyapatite crystals. Am J Physiol, 254:C554–C559
44. McCarthy GM, Augustine JA, Baldwin AS, Christopherson PA, Cheung HS, Westfall PR, Scheinman RI (1987) Molecular mechanism of basic calcium phosphate crystal-induced activation of human fibroblasts. Role of nuclear factor kB, activator protein 1 and protein kinase c. J Biol Chem, In press
45. Cochran B, Zullo J, Verma I, Stiles C(1984) Expression of *c-fos* and of a fos-related gene is stimulated by PDGF. Science, 226:1080–1082
46. Kelly K, Cochran B, Stiles C, Leder P (1983) Cell-specific regulation of the *c-myc* gene by lymphocyte mitogens and platelet-derived growth factor. Cell, 35:603–610
47. Cheung HS, Mitchell P, Pledger WJ (1989) Induction of expression of *c-fos* and *c-myc* proto-oncogenes by basic calcium phosphate crystals: effect of beta-interferon. Cancer Res, 49:134–138
48. Nair D, Misra RP, Sallis JD, and Cheung HS (1997) Phosphocitrate inhibits a basic calcium phosphate and calcium pyrophosphate dihydrate crystal-induced mitogen-activated protein kinase cascade signal transduction pathway. J Biol Chem, 272:18920–18925
49. Barnes P, Karin M (1997) Nuclear factor-κB-a pivotal transcription factor in chronic inflammatory diseases. N Engl J Med, 336:1066–1071
50. Baeuerle PA, Baltimore D (1988) IκB: a specific inhibitor of the NF-κB transcription factor. Science, 242:540–546
51. Shirakawa F, Mizel SB (1989) In vitro activation and nuclear translocation of NF-κB catalyzed by cyclic AMP-dependent protein kinase and protein kinase C. Mol Cell Biol, 9: 2424–2430
52. Mercurio F et al (1997) IKK-1 and IKK-2: cytokine-activated IκB kinases essential for NF-κB activation. Science, 278:860–866
53. Woronicz JD, Gao X, Cao Z, Rothe M, Goeddel DV (1997) IκB kinase-*b*: NF-κB activation and complex formation with IκB kinase-*a* and NIK. Science, 278:866–869
54. DiDonato JA. Hayakawa M, Rothwarf DM, Zandi E, Karin M (1997) A cytokine-responsive IκB kinase that activates the transcription factor NF-κB. Nature, 388:548–554
55. Tamaoki T (1991) Use and specificity of staurosporine, UCN-01 and calphostin C as protein kinase inhibitors. Methods Enzymol, 201:340–347
56. Woessner JF (1991) Matrix metalloproteinases and their inhibitors in connective tissue remodeling. FASEB J, 5:2145–2154
57. Fini M, Karmilowicz, Ruby P, Belman A, Borges K, Brinckerhoff C (1987) Cloning of a complimentary DNA for rabbit proactivator. A metalloproteinase that activates synovial cell collagenase shares homology with stromelysin and transin and is co-ordinately regulated with collagenase. Arthritis Rheum, 30:1254–1264
58. Mohtai M, Lane Smith R, Schurman DJ, Tsuji T, Torti FM, Hutchinson NI, Stetler-Stevenson WG, Goldberg GI (1993) Expression of 92-kD type IV collagenase/gelatinase (gelatinase B) in osteoarthritic cartilage and its induction in normal human articular cartilage by interleukin-1. J Clin Invest, 92:179–185
59. Mitchell P, Magna H, Reeves L, Lopresti-Morrow L, Yocum S, Rosner P, Geoghegan K, Hambor J (1996) Cloning, expression, and type II collagenolytic activity of matrix metalloproteinase-13 from human osteoarthritic cartilage. J Clin Invest, 97:761–768

60. Lohmander LS, Hoerrner LA, Lark MW (1993) Metalloproteinases, tissue inhibitor, and knee proteoglycan fragments in knee synovial fluid in human osteoarthritis. Arthritis Rheum, 36:181–189

61. Cheung H, Halverson, McCarty D (1981) Release of collagenase, neutral protease, and prostaglandins from cultured mammalian synovial cells by hydroxyapatite and calcium pyrophosphate dihydrate crystals. Arthritis Rheum, 24:1338–1344

62. McCarthy GM, Mitchell PG, Struve JS, Cheung HS (1992) Basic calcium phosphate crystals cause co-ordinate induction and secretion of collagenase and stromelysin. J Cell Physiol, 153:140–146

63. McCarthy G, Macius A, Christopherson P, Ryan L, Pourmotabbed T (1998) Basic calcium phosphate crystals induce synthesis and secretion of 92-kD gelatinase (matrix metalloproteinase 9/gelatinase B) in human fibroblasts. Ann Rheum Dis, 57:56–60

64. Mitchell PG, Struve JA, McCarthy GM, Cheung HS (1992) Basic calcium phosphate crystals stimulate cell proliferation and collagenase message accumulation in cultured adult articular chondrocytes. Arthritis Rheum, 35:343–350

65. McCarthy G, Christopherson P, Mitchell P (1997) Basic calcium phosphate crystals and tumor necrosis factor α induce matrix metalloprotease 13 (collagenase-3) in adult porcine articular chondrocytes. Arthritis Rheum, 40:S127

66. Brenner D, O'Hara M, Angel P, Chojkier M, Karin M (1989) Prolonged activation of *jun* and collagenase genes by tumor necrosis factor α. Nature, 337:661–663

67. Angel P, Baumann I, Stein B, Delius H, Rahmsdorf H, Herrich P (1987) 12-O-tetradecanoyl-phorbol-13-acetate induction of the human collagenase gene is mediated by an inducible enhancer element located in the 5′-flanking region. Mol Cell Biol, 7:2256–2266

68. Dayer J-M, Evequoz V, Zavadil-Grob C, Grynpas MD, Cheng P-T, Schnyder, Trechsel U, Fleisch H (1987) Effect of synthetic calcium pyrophosphate and hydroxyapatite crystals on the interaction of human blood mononuclear cells with chondrocytes, synovial cels and fibroblasts. Arthritis Rheum, 30:1372–1381

69. McCarty D, Cheung H (1985) Prostaglandin (PG) E2 generation by cultured canine synovial fibroblasts exposed to microcrystals containing calcium. Ann Rheum Dis, 4:316–320

70. Rothenberg R (1987) Modulation of prostaglandin E2 synthesis in rabbit synoviocytes. Arthritis Rheum, 30:266–274

71. Baker D, Krakauer K, Tate G, Laposata M, Zurier R (1988) Suppression of human synovial cell proliferation by dihomo-g-linoleic acid. Arthritis Rheum, 2:1273–1281

72. Newcombe D, Ciosek C, Ishikawa Y, Fahey J (1974) Human synoviocytes: activation and desensitization by prostaglandins and L-epinephrine. Proc Natl Acad Sci USA, 72:3124–3128

73. Zurier R (1990) Prostaglandin E1: Is it useful? J Rheumatol, 17:1439–1441

74. Rashad S, Hemingway A, Rainsford K, Revell P, Low F, Walker F (1989) Effect of non-steroidal anti-inflammatory drugs on the course of osteoarthritis. Lancet, ii:519–521

75. McCarthy GM, Mitchell PG, Cheung HS (1993) Misoprostol, a prostaglandin E1 analogue, inhibits basic calcium phosphate crystal-induced mitogenesis and collagenase accumulation in human fibroblasts. Calcif Tissue Int, 53:434–437

76. McCarthy G, Cheung H (1994) The role of cyclic-3′,5′-adenosine monophosphate in prostaglandin-mediated inhibition of basic calcium phosphate crystal-induced mitogenesis and collagenase induction in cultured human fibroblasts. Biochim Biophys Acta, 1226:97–104

77. Terkeltaub R, Santoro D, Mandel G, Mandel N (1988) Serum and plasma inhibit neutrophil stimulation by hydroxyapatite crystals. Evidence that serum a2-HS glycoprotein is a potent and specific crystal-bound inhibitor. Arthritis Rheum, 31:1081–1089

78. Triffit J (1978) Plasma disappearance of rabbit a2-HS glycoprotein and its uptake by bone tissue. Calcif Tiss Res, 26:155–161

79. Prudhommeaux F et al (1996) Variation in the inflammatory properties of basic calcium phosphate crystals according to crystal type. Arthritis Rheum, 39:1319–1326

80. Hamerman D (1989) The biology of osteoarthritis. N Engl J Med, 320:1322–1330

81. Poole A (1990) Enzmatic degradation: cartilage destruction, in Cartilage changes in osteoarthritis, K. Brandt (ed) Indiana University School of Medicine: Indianapolis, IN
82. Malawista S, Duff G, Atkins E, Cheung H, McCarty D (1985) Crystal-induced endogenous pyrogen production. Arthritis Rheum, 28:1039 –1046
83. McCarthy G, Barthelemy C, Veum J, Wortmann R (1991) Influence of anti-hyperuricemic therapy on the clinical and radiographic progression of gout. Arthritis Rheum, 34: 1489 –1494
84. Ryan L, McCarty D (1995) Understanding inorganic pyrophosphate metabolism: toward prevention of calcium pyrophosphate dihydrate crystal deposition. Ann Rheum Dis, 54: 939 – 941
85. Rosenthal A, McCarty B, Cheung H, Ryan L (1993) A comparison of the effect of transforming growth factor B1 on pyrophosphate elaboration from various articular tissues. Arthritis Rheum, 36:539 – 542
86. Rosenthal A, Ryan L (1990) Probenecid inhibits transforming growth factor B1-induced pyrophosphate elaboration by chondrocytes. J Rheumatol, 21:896 – 900
87. Cheung H, Sallis J, Mitchell P, Struve (1990) Inhibition of basic calcium phosphate crystal-induced mitogenesis by phosphocitrate. Biochem Biophys Res Commun, 171:20 – 25
88. Cheung H, Sallis J, Struve J (1996) Specific inhibition of basic calcium phosphate and calcium pyrophosphate crystal-induction of metalloproteinase synthesis by phosphocitrate. Biochim Biophys Acta, 1315:105 – 111
89. Walt R (1992) Misoprostol for the treatment of peptic ulcer and anti-inflammatory drug-induced gastroduodenal ulceration. N Engl J Med, 327:1575 – 1580

CHAPTER 5

Diagnosis and Monitoring of Osteoarthritis

5.1
Direct Visualization of the Cartilage

X. AYRAL and M. DOUGADOS

To date, therapy for osteoarthritis (OA) has been directed at improving symptoms, primarily pain. Research is now exploring agents that may alter the course of OA. These potential disease modifying drugs for OA (DMOADs) are being designed to prevent, delay or even reverse OA changes in the joint. Research into DMOADS requires standardized and reproducible outcome measurements that evaluate changes in the joint. Since many of the potential DMOADS are directed at altering the breakdown of articular cartilage, a measurement of the quantity, integrity and/or quality of articular cartilage would prove of value [1].

Arthroscopy provides a direct, inclusive magnified view of the six articular surfaces of the knee. Direct visualization through the arthroscope is more sensitive than the plain radiograph or magnetic resonance imaging (MRI) in detecting cartilage lesions [2]. Indeed, arthroscopy is so sensitive and specific in the evaluation of cartilage, it has prompted some to view arthroscopy as the "Gold Standard" for assessment of articular cartilage, whereby other methods will be judged [3]. Direct visualization permits evaluation of the synovium [4]. This is particularly significant in the anterior compartment of the knee where OA abnormalities are often patchy in distribution [5]. Direct visualization of the tissues by arthroscopy allows for macroscopic quantification of synovitis [6] and for guided biopsy of such focal synovial abnormalities.

Over the last few decades, arthroscopy has been established to be of value for diagnosis and surgical intervention in numerous disorders of the knee. There is an evolving methodology that utilizes knee arthroscopy in clinical research utilizing baseline and follow-up arthroscopy to monitor the course of knee OA. For this purpose, arthroscopy is used for diagnostic purposes, and since it is mostly directed at evaluation of cartilage, it is often named "chondroscopy." [7] Sequential arthroscopies permit an evaluation of the natural history of OA. In clinical research, the natural history in one cohort of patients could easily be compared to an intervention in another cohort of patients [7].

Issues that have interfered with the development of arthroscopy for clinical research include the following:

- The invasive nature of arthroscopy
- The lack of a validated, standardized scoring system of chondropathy
- The lack of standardized guidelines for videorecording the articular cartilage surfaces during arthroscopy

5.1.1
Can Arthroscopy Be Simplified?

5.1.1.1
Local Anesthesia

Therapeutic arthroscopy is often performed under general or spinal anesthesia. The procedure requires a preoperative and operative anesthetist consultation with as much as 2 days of hospitalization. Postoperative thigh rehabilitation is often necessary due to the potential deleterious effect of the tourniquet on nerve and muscle recovery [8]. Explorative arthroscopy conducted for research purposes can be simplified by the use of local anesthesia administered subcutaneously and intraarticularly. Lidocaine or marcaine can provide skin and synovial anesthesia. With the use of local anesthesia, the procedure is almost always performed on an outpatient basis in an ambulatory surgery center.

Arthroscopy under local anesthesia is safe, reliable and relatively inexpensive and is an alternative to arthroscopy under general or spinal anesthesia [9]. Eriksson *et al.* compared arthroscopy under local, spinal and general anesthesia [9]. Patient satisfaction under local or spinal anesthesia was similar (77 % of satisfied patients) but not as good as general anesthesia (97% of satisfied patients). Blackburn *et al.* compared arthroscopy under local anesthesia to magnetic resonance imaging (MRI) of the knee [2]. Both were well tolerated by their 16 patients. When asked about which procedure they preferred, 8 patients preferred arthroscopy, 2 preferred MRI, and 6 felt the two procedures were equally tolerable.

In a prospective study including 84 patients undergoing chondroscopy under local anesthesia [7], tolerance was evaluated as "good" (62 percent) or "very good" (28 percent) by 90 percent of the patients. There was no pain in 25 percent with some pain during or immediately following the procedure in 75 percent. In relation to the ambulatory surgery, post arthroscopy daily activities were hampered in 79 percent of the patients (for up to one day in 44 percent, up to two days in 55 percent, and up to one week in 79 percent). One month after chondroscopy, 82 percent of the patients felt improved.

As a guide to tolerability of anesthesia, in a clinical trial 36/39 (95 percent) patients accepted a second chondroscopy after one year of follow-up [10]. The lack of follow-up in the remaining 3 patients was not related to the technique [10].

McGinty and Matza compared the diagnostic accuracy of arthroscopy performed under local or general anesthesia with postarthroscopy visualization by arthrotomy [11]. Under this system, arthroscopy was slightly more accurate under local anesthesia (95 percent) than general anesthesia (91 percent). It appears that the benefits of local anesthesia are not outweighed by a loss in accuracy. Nevertheless, performance of arthroscopy under local anesthesia requires specific training, even for experienced arthroscopists.

5.1.1.2
Small Glass Lens Arthroscope

Knee arthroscopy is often performed with a 4.0 mm glass lens arthroscope requiring a 5.5 mm trochar. Chondroscopy is intended to obtain information on the status of the articular surfaces. In some patients with contracted ligaments or residual muscle tension (because of local anesthesia), the posterior part of femorotibial compartments may not be accessible with a standard 4.0 mm scope. The 2.7 mm arthroscope has a similar field of view as the 4.0 mm arthroscope and most often permits the inspection of all compartments. Continuous knee irrigation provided by the 2.7 mm arthroscope is adequate to clear the joint of blood and debris allowing a clear field for visualization [7]. Technically, the 25 or 30 degree angle provides a wide field and a better view. Smaller diameter (1.8 mm, ~ 16-gauge) fiberoptic arthroscopes (sometimes called "needlescopes") can be inserted into the joint by needle puncture rather than stab incision but, among other disadvantages, they provide a smaller field of view, a dimmer and grainier picture due to fiberoptic transmission and lower irrigation, tend to bend and fracture fiberoptics and are often only straight viewing [12]. The images obtained by the needlescope appear to be insufficient for clinical research on cartilage and synovial lesions as they tend to underestimate cartilage and synovial abnormalities. Compared to standard arthroscopy, the sensitivity for detecting abnormalities of needlescope arthroscopy is 89 percent for cartilage and 71 percent for synovial abnormalities [12].

5.1.1.3
Tourniquet

An inflated thigh tourniquet is routinely used under general or spinal anesthesia for therapeutic arthroscopy to minimize bleeding but it cannot be tolerated under local anesthesia. Bleeding during chondroscopy is a potential problem for visualization rather than patient safety. Chondroscopy includes enough joint irrigation so that bleeding is most often not of concern. However, some arthroscopists include epinephrine in the local anesthesia to reduce bleeding. Rapid absorption of the epinephrine could cause a transient adverse clinical event, but is avoided by verifying the absence of vascular puncture when performing local anesthesia.

5.1.1.4
Joint Lavage

In a prospective, open, uncontrolled study, 82 percent of the patients felt improved one month after chondroscopy [7]. It is believed the lavage performed during the procedure (usually 1 liter of normal saline) prompted clinical improvement of joint symptoms. This beneficial effect of joint lavage has been reported in controlled studies [13–15] and might partially counterbalance the invasivity of the technic. This beneficial effect of arthroscopy needs to be considered when evaluating the benefits of any potential DMOAD.

5.1.2
How to Score Chondropathy?

Some degree of quantification of the severity of chondropathy is needed to monitor the lesions over time. This can provide the basis for comparing treatment in groups of patients. Articular cartilage lesions can be defined by three baseline parameters: depth, size and location. Over the years, several arthroscopic classification systems have been devised in an attempt to describe and categorize the articular cartilage damage [16–21].

5.1.2.1
Previous Classifications (Table 1)

Some systems take only into account the depth of the lesions (Beguin [16], Insall [17]) and give qualitative information on the surface appearance of articular cartilage. They do not provide a quantitative approach to cartilage lesions.

Some systems (Outerbridge [18], Hungerford and Ficat [19], Bentley [20], Casscels [21]) combine the depth and the size of the most severe chondropathy of the articular surface under a single descriptive category but present obvious discrepancies.

The Outerbridge classification system [18] subdivides cartilage lesions: Grade I: softening and swelling of the cartilage without fissuring (true chondromalacia); Grade II: fragmentation and fissuring with a diameter of 1/2 inch or less; Grade III: fragmentation and fissuring with a diameter of greater than 1/2 inch; Grade IV: erosion of cartilage with exposure of subchondral bone. Grade II and Grade III have identical depth and their size is estimated while the size of grade I and IV is not described. This system has been used for classifying patients in a cross-sectional study [3] but appears inadequate for accurate outcome measurements of chondropathy in longitudinal studies as the size of grades I and IV is not evaluated and the size of grades II and III is not a continuous variable.

Hungerford and Ficat subdivide cartilage lesions in closed and open chondromalacia [19]. Closed chondromalacia (grade I) represents true chondromalacia (softening-swelling) and open chondromalacia (grade II) represents open (fissurated) chondropathy. The size of a grade I lesions, according to Ficat and Hungerford, begins as 1 cm^2 in an area which extends progressively in all directions. This description leads to confusion as to the total extent of involvement of the surface area of any grade I lesion. Grade II includes three different depths of chondropathy: superficial and deep fissures and exposure of subchondral bone with no reference to the size. This system cannot lead to an accurate quantitative approach of articular cartilage breakdown.

Table 1. Review of previous classification symptoms of articular cartilage

Author	Surface description of articular cartilage	Diameter	Location
Outerbridge[a]	I – softening and swelling II – Fragmentation and fissuring III – Fragmentation and fissuring IV – Erosion of cartilage down to bone	I. None II. <1/2" III. >1/2" IV. None	Start most frequently on medial facet of patella; later extends to lateral facet "mirror" lesion on intercondylar area of femoral condyles; upper border medial femoral condyle
Hungerford and Ficat[a]	I – Closed chondromalacia. Simple softening (small blister) macroscopically, surface is intact, varying degrees of severity from simple softening to "pitting edema", loss of elasticity	I. 1 cm^2 and then extends progressively in all directions	Lateral facet – 2° excessive lateral pressure
	II – Open chondromalacia a. Fissures – single or multiple, relatively superficial or extending down to subchondral bone b. Ulceration – localized loss of cartilage substance, exposes dense subchondral bone. When extensive, bone has polished appearance (eburnated)	II. None	Medial facet – 2° incongruence and combination of compression and shearing forces
	Chondrosclerosis – abnormally hard, not depressible	Not localized but involves entire contact zone	
	Tuft formation – multiple deep fronds of cartilage separated from one another by deep clefts which extend to subchondral bone		Centered on crest separating medial and odd facets
	Superficial surface changes - surface fibrillation; longitudinal striations present in the axis of movement of the joint		
Bentley[a]	I – Fibrillation or fissuring II – Fibrillation or fissuring III – Fibrillation or fissuring IV – Fibrillation with or without exposure of subchondral bone	I. <0.5 cm II. 0.5–1.0 cm III. 1.0–2.0 cm IV. >2.0 cm	Most common at junction of medial and odd facets of patella

Table 1 (Continued)

Author	Surface description of articular cartilage	Diameter	Location
Casscells[a]	I – Superficial area of erosion II – Deeper layers of cartilage involved III – Cartilage is completely eroded and bone is exposed IV – Articular cartilage completely destroyed	I. ≤1 cm II. 1–2 cm III. 2–4 cm IV. "wide area"	Patella and anterior femoral surfaces
Insall[a]	I – Swelling and softening of cartilage (closed chondromalacia) II – Deep fissures extending to subchondral bone III – Fibrillation IV – Erosive changes and exposures of subchondral bone (osteoarthrosis)	None	I–IV: midpoint of patellar crest with extension equally onto medial and lateral patellar facets. IV: also involves opposite or mirror surface of femur Upper and lower 1/3 nearly always spared (patella); femur never severe
Beguin/Locker	I – Softening – swelling II – Superficial fissures III – Deep fissures, down to bone IV – Exposure of subchondral bone	None	None

[a] Reproduced from reference 22 with the kind permission of the publishers : The American Journal of Sports Medicine.

In the classification proposed by Bentley and Dowd [20], grade I, II and III have identical appearance (fibrillation or fissuring), and the distinction between the grades is based on the diameter of the involvement (Table 1). No mention is made of true chondromalacia. Grade IV describes two different depths of chondropathy: fibrillation with or without exposure of subchondral bone, with a fixed size of more than 2.0 cm. Which grade would be assigned to an exposure of subchondral bone less than 2.0 cm in size ?

Casscels et al . assigned a specific size-range diameter in centimeters to a particular depth of lesion, with the prerequisite that the less the depth, the smaller the size [21] (Table 1). Which grade would be assigned to superficial lesions covering the entire articular surface?

The above systems lack consistency in providing information on depth, size and location of cartilaginous lesions. Guidelines for a system suggest the following are needed:

– All the different articular cartilage lesions of a given articular surface must be evaluated, and not only the most severe chondropathy in order to score the overall articular cartilage breakdown.
– Depth and size of each cartilage lesion must be rated separately.
– The evaluation of depth must distinguish chondromalacia, superficial fissures, deep fissures, and exposure of subchondral bone.
– The evaluation of size must be as accurate as possible to allow detection of change with time.

Location of chondropathy is a qualitative variable involving two types of information: (1) the articular surface of the knee that is affected by the chondral lesion, (2) the part of this articular surface that is affected by the chondral lesion. A system for scoring chondropathy can be applied globally to the joint or specifically to each of the three compartments of the knee, that is, patello-femoral, medial tibiofemoral, lateral tibiofemoral. Nevertheless, without quantitative joint mapping, the description of the location of chondropathy on a given articular surface remains qualitative.

5.1.2.2
Newer Classifications

5.1.2.2.1
Noyes and Stabler

In 1989, Noyes and Stabler proposed a system for grading articular cartilage lesions at arthroscopy (22). They separate the description of the surface appearance, the depth of involvement, and the diameter and location of the lesions (Table 2). They distinguish three surface grades : articular surface intact (grade 1), articular surface damaged, open lesion (grade 2), and bone exposed (grade 3). Each grade is divided into subtypes A or B, depending upon the depth of involvement. Grade 1 implies chondromalacia. Type 1A corresponds to a moderate degree of softening of the articular cartilage; type 1B corresponds to an extensive softening resulting in swelling of the articular surface. A grade 2 lesion is characterized by any disruption of the articular surface without visua-

Table 2. Classification of articular cartilage lesions (Noyes and Stabler)

Surface description	Extent of involvement	Diameter (mm)	Location	Degree of knee flexion
1. Cartilage surface intact	A. Definite softening with some resilience remaining	< 10 ≤ 15 ≤ 20 ≤ 25 > 25	Patella A. Proximal 1/3 　Middle 1/3 　Distal 1/3 B. Odd facet 　Middle facet 　Lateral facet	Degree of knee flexion where the lesion is in weight-bearing contact (e.g., 20°–45°)
	B. Extensive softening with loss of resilience (deformation)		Trochlea	
			Medial femoral condyle	
2. Cartilage surface damaged: cracks, fissures, fibrillation, or fragmentation	A. < 1/2 thickness B. ≥ 1/2 thickness		a. Anterior 1/3 b. Middle 1/3 c. Posterior 1/3	
			Lateral femoral condyle a. Anterior 1/3	
3. Bone exposed	A. Bone surface intact		b. Middle 1/3 c. Posterior 1/3	
	B. Bone surface cavitation		Medial tibial condyle a. Anterior 1/3 b. Middle 1/3 c. Posterior 1/3	
			Lateral tibial condyle a. Anterior 1/3 b. Middle 1/3 c. Posterior 1/3	

Reproduced from [22] with the kind permission of the publishers: The American Journal of Sports Medicine.

lized exposure of bone. A type 2A lesion is less than one-half thickness (superficial fissures); type 2B is more than one-half thickness (deep fissures, down to bone). Grade 3 indicates any surface with exposed bone. Type 3A indicates that the normal bony contour remains; type 3B indicates cavitation or erosion of bone surface. Lesions are reported on a knee diagram and the diameter of each lesion is estimated by the examiner in millimeters using a graduated probing hook. Depending on the diameter and depth of the lesion, a point scaling system is used to calculate the score of chondropathy for each compartment and finally to calculate an overall joint score.

This system is the first attempt to score chondropathy. We offer this critique:

- In this system, all the chondral lesions are represented on the knee diagram as a full circle with a unique diameter defined by the graduated hook. This is a semi-objective estimate of size because most cartilage lesions are not circular, but rather oval or irregularly shaped. Moreover, degenerative cartilage lesions often have the appearance of escarrotic skin lesions with the deepest breakdown located at the middle central point and surrounded by more superficial cartilage lesions. A diameter cannot be attributed to this "surrounding lesion" which is crown-shaped.
- In this system, any lesion less than 10 mm in diameter is not considered clinically significant and therefore no points are subtracted. This induces a lack of sensitivity. In monitoring the outcome of DMOAD, all lesions, even the smallest, must be described.
- The point scaling system proposed to score simultaneously depth and diameter of chondral lesions is arbitrary. It is not based on statistical methodology, nor on clinical assessment and ponderation of the severity of the lesions.
- This system has not been validated.

5.1.2.2.2
Global Assessment and SFA Systems

Two methods for scoring chondropathy have been more recently proposed [7, 23, 24].

The first method is a subjective approach based on the investigator's overall assessment of chondropathy reported on a set of 100 mm Visual Analogue Scales (VAS) in which "0" indicates the absence of chondropathy and "100" the most severe chondropathy [7]. One VAS is used for each articular surface of the knee: patella, trochlea, medial femoral condyle, lateral femoral condyle, medial tibial plateau and lateral tibial plateau. A VAS score is calculated for each of the 3 compartments of the knee and is obtained by averaging the VAS scores from the two corresponding articular surfaces of the compartment.

The second method is a more objective and analytic approach which includes an articular diagram of the knee with grading for location, depth and size of all the different cartilaginous lesions (Table 3) [23, 24].

Location

Areas defined included the patella, trochlea, medial femoral condyle, medial tibial plateau, lateral femoral condyle and the lateral tibial plateau.

Depth

The system is based on the classification of chondropathy proposed by French arthroscopists Beguin and Locker [16] (Fig. 1):

Grade 0   Normal cartilage.

Grade I   Chondromalacia including softening with or without swelling; it can be assimilated to grade 1, type A and B, of Noyes and Stabler.

Grade II   Cartilage demonstrates superficial fissures, either single or multiple, giving a "velvet-like" appearance to the surface; grade II also includes

Fig. 1 a, b. Depth of articular cartilage lesions according to the classification proposed by Beguin and Locker (16). **a** Diagram of grades. Grade 0, normal articular cartilage; Grade I, softening with or without swelling; Grade II, superficial fissures; Grade III, deep fissures, down to bone; Grade IV, exposure of subchondral bone. **b** Examples of grades (chondroscopy – 2.7 mm arthroscope – local anesthesia). Reading from left to right: Grade 0, normal medial femorotibial compartment; Grade I, swelling of the lateral femoral condyle; Grade II, "velvet-like" aspect of the patella; Grade III, "crab-meat-like" aspect of the patella; Grade III, deep ulceration of the medial femoral condyle; Grade IV, exposure of subchondral bone of the medial femoral condyle

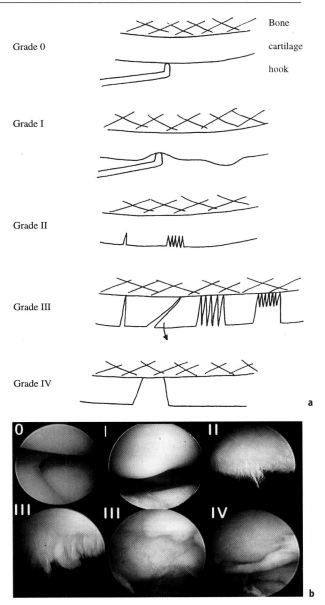

superficial erosion. Fissures and erosions do not reach subchondral bone and can be assimilated to the grade 2 A of Noyes and Stabler in which lesions are less than one-half thickness.

Grade III There are deep fissures of the cartilage surface, down to subchondral bone, which is not directly visualized but may be touched with an arthroscopy probe; grade III lesions may take different aspects: a "shark's mouth-like" aspect or a detached chondral flap due to a single deep fissure, a "crab-meat-like" aspect due to multiple deep tears; grade III also includes deep ulceration of the cartilage creating a crater which remains covered by a thin layer of cartilage. Grade III can be assimilated to the grade 2B of Noyes and Stabler in which lesions are more than one-half thickness.

Grade IV There is exposure of subchondral bone with intact bone surface or with cavitation. It can be assimilated to grade 3, type A and B, of Noyes and Stabler.

The different grades are summarized in Figure 1. In knee OA, cartilage breakdown often shows a combination of different grades, the most severe grade being surrounded by milder lesions (Table 3).

Size

The size and shape of each grade of chondropathy is recorded on a knee diagram (Table 3) by the arthroscopist. This step is crucial for evaluation. Then, the size is evaluated as a percentage of the articular surface. The percentage can be calculated by computer using numerization of the drawing on the knee diagram or calculated directly from the diagram by a trained investigator. Unless fully trained, the investigator has a tendency to overestimate the size of the lesions. A practical way to calculate the size of each chondropathy covering a given articular surface is to determine the number of times this area could be traced within the whole (100%) articular surface on the diagram. Dividing 100% by the resulting number indicates the size of chondropathy in percent. As an example, if tracing a given chondropathy four times on the diagram of the femoral condyle fills the diagram, the size of this given chondropathy is 25% of the femoral condyle (obtained by dividing 100%, the whole articular surface of the femoral condyle, by 4). Examples of different sizes of chondropathy are exposed in Figure 2.

Location, depth and size of the different chondropathies are reported on a special form (Table 3). This form lists 8 different quantitative variables, that is, sizes of chondropathy from grade I to grade IV for each compartment. The comparison of chondropathy severity between patients and/or between arthroscopies performed at different times in the same patient require the integration of these different quantitative variables in a single score of chondropathy. For this purpose, the French Society of Arthroscopy (Société Française d'Arthroscopie: SFA) carried out a prospective and multicenter study with 14 arthroscopists, selected on the basis of their experience in arthroscopy and considered in this study as "standard of reference". Seven hundred and fifty-five subjects who had undergone arthroscopy of the knee were enrolled in this study. Criteria for assessment of severity of chondropathy were as follows: 1) investigator's overall assessment, using a 100-mm-long Visual Analogue Scale (VAS); and 2) depth, size and location of cartilage lesions recorded on a diagram. For the establishment of chondropathy scoring, multivariate analyses were carried out using logistic multiple regression in which

Table 3. Calculation of SFA score and SFA grade from one example of articular cartilage lesions visualized by arthroscopy and recorded on knee diagram and case record form

Knee diagram (right knee)

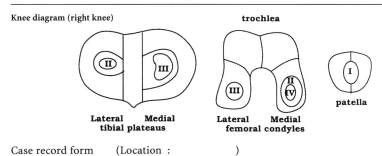

Case record form   (Location :   )

Grade	Medial compartment			Lateral compartment			Femoropatellar compartment		
	Femur	Tibia	Mean value	Femur	Tibia	Mean value	Patella	Trochlea	Mean value
0	60	65	62.5	80	75	77.5	80	100	90
I	0	0	0	0	0	0	20	0	10
II	30	0	15	0	25	12.5	0	0	0
III	0	35	17.5	20	0	10	0	0	0
IV	10	0	5	0	0	0	0	0	0

Each value given represents the size of the corresponding grade expressed in percentage of the corresponding whole articular surface. Each column totals 100%.
0, normal; I, softening-swelling; II, superficial fissures; III, deep fissures; IV, exposure of sub-chondral bone.

SFA score = size (%) of grade I lesions × 0.14 + size (%) of grade II lesions × 0.34 + size (%) of grade III lesions ×0.65 + size (%) of grade IV lesions ×1.00
- Medial score: 15 × 0.34+17.5 × 0.65 + 5 × 1.00 = *21.475*
- Lateral score: 12.5 × 0.34 + 10 × 0.65 = *10.75*
- Femoropatellar score: 10 × 0.14 = *1.4*

SFA grade (for definition, see Table 4)
- Medial grade = *IV*
- Lateral grade = *III*
- Femoropatellar grade = *I*

the investigator's overall assessment of chondropathy using the VAS comprised the dependent variables and the depth and size of the lesion were the independent variables. Multivariate parametric and nonparametric analyses were performed on two-thirds of the patients and resulted in two systems of assessing chondropathy: the SFA scoring system [23, 24] and the SFA grading system [23]. After the SFA systems were established, their validity was evaluated and confirmed on the remaining one-third of the patients by correlating the SFA score and SFA grade with the investigator's overall assessment using the VAS.

Size	10 %	25 %	30 %	40 %	50 %
Knee diagram (right knee)	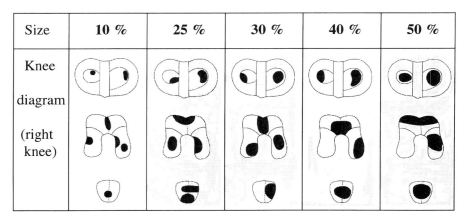				

Fig. 2. Size of articular cartilage lesions. Each *solid black area* represents the percentage of cartilar damage of each articular surface

The SFA score is a continuous variable graded between "0" and "100". The score is obtained for each compartment as follows:

SFA score = A + B + C + D

where

- A = size (percent) of grade I lesions × 0.14
- B = size (percent) of grade II lesions × 0.34
- C = size (percent) of grade III lesions × 0.65
- D = size (percent) of grade IV lesions × 1.00
- Size (percent) = average percent of surface for the medial femoral condyle and medial tibial plateau (medial tibiofemoral compartment), lateral femoral condyle and lateral tibial plateau (lateral tibiofemoral compartment) or trochlea and patella (patellofemoral compartment).

The coefficients of severity of chondropathy (0.14, 0.34, 0.65, 1.00) were obtained by parametric multivariate analysis [24].

The SFA grade is a semi-quantitative variable. The above numbers [size (percent) of grade I to IV lesions] are placed in a formula to provide a summary grade (or category of chondropathy severity of the compartment) for each of the knee compartments (Table 4). The formula for each compartment was obtained by nonparametric multivariate analysis using a tree structured regression [23]. There are 6 categories for the patellofemoral compartment (0 to V) and 5 categories for the medial and lateral tibiofemoral compartments (0 to IV). One example of the SFA score and the SFA grade is calculated in Table 3.

5.1.2.2.3
ACR System

In 1995, a committee of the American College of Rheumatology (ACR) proposed a scoring system for cartilage [25]. This system takes into account depth, size

Table 4. French Society of Arthroscopy (SFA) system for grading chondropathy at knee arthroscopy. Adapted from [23]

Category	Grade[a] 0 (%[b])	Grade III (%)	Grade IV (%)
Medial tibiofemoral compartment			
0	100		
I	≥ 80 < 100		0
II	< 80	< 15	0
III	< 80	≥ 15	0
	or ≥ 65		≥ 1
IV	< 65		≥ 1
Lateral tibiofemoral compartment			
0	100		
I	≥ 85 < 100	< 10	< 10
II	< 85	< 10	< 10
III		≥ 10	< 10
IV			≥ 10
Patellofemoral compartment			
0	100		
I	≥ 85 < 100	< 10	< 2.5
II	< 85	< 10	< 2.5
III		≥ 10	< 2.5
IV			≥ 2.5 < 25
V			≥ 25

[a] Grade derived from cartilage surface changes (Beguin and Locker classification), see text and Table 3.

[b] Percentage derived from extent of surface involved with the grade changes; see text and Table 3.

and location of chondral lesions. The lesions are recorded on a knee diagram. Depth of each lesion is assessed by the grades proposed by Noyes and Stabler. The size of each lesion is evaluated in percentage. An arbitrary point scaling system is applied to obtain an overall score, called damage score. The reliability of the damage score has been evaluated [25]. Videotapes of 10 arthroscopies were each viewed on two separate occasions by three rheumatologist-arthroscopists in blinded fashion. Damage score demonstrated significant intraobserver reliability (r = 0.90, 0.90, 0.80; p < 0.01 for each) and interobserver reliability (r = 0.82, 0.80, 0.70; p < 0.05 for each).

5.1.3
The Validation of Arthroscopic Quantification of Chondropathy By Using VAS Score and SFA Scoring and Grading Systems

The main characteristics of an outcome measure, that is, simplicity, reliability, validity, clinical relevance, sensitivity to change and discriminant capacity have been evaluated for these 2 scoring systems.

5.1.3.1
Simplicity

Arthroscopy will always be an invasive procedure because of the incision required, but can be rendered less complex by the use of local anesthesia, performance on an outpatient basis, elimination of the tourniquet and use of a small glass lens arthroscope (cf chapter 5.1.1).

5.1.3.2
Reliability

Intraobserver reliability of chondropathy measurement using either VAS score of chondropathy, or SFA score and SFA grade is good [7, 26] and better than interobserver reliability [7] (reliability coefficient, 0.928 and 0.989 for intraobserver reliability of the arthroscopic quantification of chondropathy by using SFA score and VAS score, respectively ; reliability coefficient, 0.529 and 0.936 for interobserver reliability by using SFA score and VAS score, respectively [26]). Thus, it appears that arthroscopy videotapes from a clinical study should be reviewed by a single trained investigator. For multicenter studies, training sessions will be needed to improve interobserver evaluations of depth and size of the cartilage lesions [27].

5.1.3.3
Validity

Intrinsic validity was evaluated by calculating the correlations between the different arthroscopy scales (VAS score and SFA systems). A strong correlation was found between these different systems, as the evaluation of cartilage status by the SFA scoring system accounts for 84, 81 and 83 percent of the variability of the overall assessment (VAS score) of the medial, lateral and femoro-patellar compartment ($r = 0.92, 0.90, 0.91$, respectively), and the evaluation by the SFA grading system accounts for 75, 77 and 78 percent of the variability of the overall assessment for these compartments ($r = 0.87, 0.88, 0.88$, respectively) [26]. Nevertheless, the three methods of quantifying chondropathy (VAS score, SFA score and SFA grade) appear to be of complementary interest and are used together at this time in clinical trials in osteoarthritis. The VAS score and the SFA score are more appropriate to detect minimal changes in severity of chondropathy over time as they represent a continuous variable. SFA grade permits to classify a population of osteoarthritis patients into homogenous categories of chondropathy severity and to investigate specifically subgroups of osteoarthritic patients. Although a highly significant correlation exists between the VAS and the SFA score, there are some discrepancies between these two technics; the SFA score usually shows a lower value then the VAS score [26]. This is likely due to the fact that evaluating objectively the extent of chondropathy in percent lowers the final SFA score; a single deep fissure represents impressive chondropathy (high subjective VAS score) but a very small surface (low objective SFA score). Moreover, the investigator might be influenced by the location of chondropathy on the articular surface (weight-bearing areas or not) when recording his subjective overall assessment of the severity of chondropathy on the 100 mm visual analogue scale.

Extrinsic validity was evaluated by calculating the correlations between the arthroscopic quantification of chondropathy and radiological joint space narrowing on weight-bearing X-rays [7, 26]. Arthroscopic and roentgenographic evaluations of chondropathy are closely correlated. There was a strong correlation between: 1) the overall assessment of chondropathy (VAS) and radiological medial joint space narrowing evaluated in percentage ($r = 0.646, p < 0.0001$) [7]; 2) the SFA score and joint space narrowing of the medial and lateral femorotibial compartments evaluated in millimeters ($r = -0.59, p < 0.01$ and $r = -0.39, p < 0.01$, respectively) [26]; 3) the SFA grade and joint space narrowing of the medial and lateral femorotibial compartments evaluated in millimeters ($r = -0.48, p < 0.01$ and $r = -0.31, p < 0.01$, respectively) [26]. Nevertheless, arthroscopy appears to be more sensitive than plain radiographs. Mild cartilage lesions but also severe and deep cartilage erosions may remain undetected, even on weight bearing radiographs [3, 7, 26]. In 33 patients fulfilling ACR criteria for OA with joint space narrowing of the medial compartment of less than 25 percent on weight-bearing X-rays, chondropathy was found at arthroscopy in 30 patients, with a mean VAS score of 21 mm, ranging from 2 mm to 82 mm and above 10 mm in 24 patients [7].

5.1.3.4
Clinical Relevance

The clinical relevance was evaluated in a cross sectional study of the severity of chondropathy at arthroscopy [26]. This was correlated with the clinical characteristics of the patients, including demographic data, baseline characteristics and clinical activity of OA. They found a statistically significant correlation ($p < 0.05$) between articular cartilage damage: 1) of the three compartments (medial, lateral, femoro-patellar) of the knee and patient age; and 2) of the medial compartment and the body mass index. At variance, no statistically significant correlation was found between articular cartilage damage of the knee and clinical activity (pain, Lequesne's index, AIMS2). Conversely, a longitudinal study performed with a one year arthroscopy follow-up in 41 patients showed that changes in the severity of cartilage lesions correlated with changes in functional disability (Lequesne's index : $r = 0.34, p = 0.03$) and quality of life (AIMS2 : $r = 0.35, p = 0.04$) [26].

5.1.3.5
Sensitivity to Change

Chondroscopy demonstrated statistically significant worsening in knee OA cartilage lesions between two arthroscopic evaluations performed one year apart in 41 patients [26]. The mean VAS score of the medial compartment moved from 45 ± 28 at entry to 55 ± 31 after one year ($p = 0.0002$) and the SFA score from 31 ± 21 to 37 ± 24 ($p = 0.0003$). Significant worsening was also reported in a one

year trial of 26 patients with post-traumatic patella chondromalacia [28].
Sensitivity to change might be explained by the precision of the technique and
enrollment of patients with active OA of the knee. These patients had prior
failure of analgesics, NSAIDs, physical exercises and intra-articular glucocorticoid injection leading to joint lavage. It should be noted that several longitudinal arthroscopic studies that demonstrated cartilage abnormalities noted
reversible changes in occasional patients [26, 28, 29].

5.1.3.6
Discriminant Capacity

A preliminary study of repeated hyaluronic acid injections suggested that chondroscopy may be capable of identifying chondromodulating agents [10].

5.1.4
Guidelines for Videorecording Articular Cartilage Surfaces at Knee Arthroscopy

Arthroscopies conducted for clinical or research purposes are most often recorded on videotape. The arthroscopist needs to prepare on the videorecording by making sure the appropriate equipment is available and functional.
For clinical trials, centralized reading and grading of arthroscopies may be
needed.

5.1.4.1
Clarity of the Image

Clarity of the videorecording can be improved by:

- Using a local intra-articular anesthesia with epinephrine to reduce bleeding
- Performing abundant articular lavage before starting to record in order to
  remove debris and cellular material
- Continuously focusing the camera
- Maximizing light intensity by providing enough light for visualization but
  avoiding overexposure ("flash") of the articular cartilage
- Removing any condensation on the camera or scope

5.1.4.2
Complete Exploration

The aim of arthroscopy is to explore the entire six articular surfaces of the knee
joint. Areas of normal cartilage should receive as much attention as areas of
damage, in order that the reader can assess what percentage of the total
cartilage is damaged. The arthroscopist can briefly assess any cartilage lesion,
but should not focus on specific lesions before making a general examination
by sweeping along the whole articular surface from medial to lateral edge and
inversely, and from back to front in order to allow the reader to assess the size
of any lesion. The exploration of each articular surface should be performed

twice and slowly to ensure that no area is missed. The femoral condyles should be explored from 20° to 90° of knee flexion, whilst maintaining valgus or varus pressure, to allow the inspection of their posterior surfaces.

5.1.5
Conclusion

Arthroscopy, performed under local anesthesia, is a relevant outcome measure of OA in clinical research. Arthroscopy could potentially lead to reducing the duration and number of patients in clinical trials on DMOADs in OA.

References

1. M Brandt K, Bellamy N, Moskowitz R, Menkes CJ, Pelletier JP et al. (1994) Guidelines for testing slow acting drugs in OA. J Rheumatol Supplement 41 : 65–71
2. Blackburn PM, Kramer J, Marcelis S, Pathria MN, Trudell D, Haghighi P et al. (1994) Arthroscopic evaluation of knee articular cartilage: a comparison with plain radiographs and magnetic resonance imaging. J Rheumatol 21 : 675–679
3. Fife RS, Brandt KD, Braunstein EM, Katz BP, Shelbourne KD, Kalinski LA et al. (1991) Relationship between arthroscopic evidence of cartilage damage and radiographic evaluation of joint space narrowing in early OA of the knee. Arthritis Rheum 34 : 377–382
4. Kurosaka M, Ohno O, Hirohata K (1991) Arthroscopy evaluation of synovitis in the knee joints. Arthroscopy 7 : 162–170
5. Lindblad S, Hedfors E (1987) Arthroscopic and immunohistologic characterization of knee joint synovitis in OA. Arthritis Rheum 30 : 1081–1088
6. Ayral X, Mayoux-Benhamou A, Dougados M (1996) Proposed scoring system for assessing synovial membrane abnormalities at arthroscopy in knee osteoarthritis. Br J Rheumatol 35 (Suppl 3), 14–17
7. Ayral X, Dougados M, Listrat V, Bonvarlet JP, Simonnet J, Poiraudeau S et al. (1993) Chondroscopy: A new method for scoring chondropathy. Sem Arthritis and Rheum 22 : 289–297
8. Dobner J, Nitz A (1982) Postmeniscectomy tourniquet palsy and functional sequelae. Am J Sports Med 10 : 211–14
9. Eriksson E, Haggmark T, Saartok T, Sebik A, Ortengren B (1986) Knee arthroscopy with local anesthesia in ambulatory patients. Orthopedics 9 : 186–188
10. Listrat V, Ayral X, Paternello F, Bonvarlet JP, Simonnet J, Amor B et al. (1997) Arthroscopic evaluation of potential structure modifying activity of hyaluronan (Hyalgan®) in osteoarthritis of the knee. Osteoarthritis Cartilage 5 : 153–160
11. Mc Ginty JB, Matza RA (1978) Arthroscopy of the knee. J Bone Jt Surg 60-A, 787–789
12. Ike RW, Rourke KS (1993) Detection of intra-articular abnormalities in OA of the knee. A pilot study comparing needle arthroscopy with standard arthroscopy. Arthritis Rheum 36 : 1353–1363
13. Livesley PJ, Doherty M, Needhoff M, Moulton A (1991) Arthroscopic lavage of osteoarthritic knees. J Bone Jt Surg 73-B, 922–926
14. Ike RW, Arnold WJ, Rothschild E, Shaw HL (1992) The Tidal Irrigation Cooperating Group. Tidal irrigation versus conservative medical management in patients with OA of the knee: a prospective randomized study. J Rheumatol 19 : 772–779
15. Chang RW, Falconer J, Stulberg SD, Arnold WJ, Manheim LM, Dyer AR (1993) A randomized, controlled trial of arthroscopic surgery versus closed-needle joint lavage for patients with OA of the knee. Arthritis Rheum 36 : 289–296
16. Beguin J, Locker B (1983) Chondropathie rotulienne. In 2ème journée d'arthroscopie du genou, No. 1, pp 89–90 (Lyon)

17. Insall JN (1984) Disorders of the patellae. In Surgery of the Knee. Churchill Livingston, New York pp 191–260
18. Outerbridge RE (1961) The etiology of chondromalacia patellae. J Bone Jt Surg 43-B, 752–57
19. Ficat RP, Philippe J, Hungerford DS (1979) Chondromalacia patellae: a system of classification. Clin Orthop Rel Res 144: 55–62
20. Bentley G, Dowd G (1984) Current concepts of etiology and treatment of chondromalacia patellae. Clin Orthop Rel Res 189: 209–228
21. Casscels SW (1978) Gross pathological changes in the knee joint of the aged individual: a study of 300 cases. Clin Orthop Rel Res 132: 225–235
22. Noyes FR, Stabler CL (1989) A system for grading articular cartilage lesions at arthroscopy. Am J Sports Med 17: 505–513
23. Dougados M, Ayral X, Listrat V, Gueguen A, Bahuaud J, Beaufils P, et al. (1994) The SFA system for assessing articular cartilage lesions at arthroscopy of the knee. Arthroscopy 10: 69–77
24. Ayral X, Listrat V, Gueguen A, Bahuaud J, Beaufils P, Beguin J et al. (1994) Simplified arthroscopy scoring system for chondropathy of the knee (revised SFA score). Revue du Rhumatisme (English Edition) 31: 89–90
25. Klashman D, Ike R, Moreland L, Skovron ML, Kalunian K (1995) Validation of an OA data report form for knee arthroscopy. Arthritis Rheum 38 (9 suppl), S 178, Abstract 154
26. Ayral X, Dougados M, Listrat V, Gueguen A, Bonvarlet JP, Simonnet J, Amor B (1996) Arthroscopic evaluation of chondropathy in osteoarthritis of the knee. J Rheumatol 23: 698–706
27. Ayral X, Gueguen A, Ike RW, Bonvarlet JP, Frizziero L, Kalunian K et al. (1998) Interobserver reliability of the arthroscopic quantification of chondropathy of the knee. Osteoarthritis and Cartilage 6: 160–166
28. Raatikainen T, Vaananen K, Tamelander G (1990) Effect of glycosaminoglycan polysulfate on chondromalacia patella. A placebo controlled 1 year study. Acta Orthopaedica Scandinavica 61: 443–448
29. Fujisawa Y, Masuhara K, Shiomi S (1979) The effects of high tibial osteotomy on OA of the knee. An arthroscopic study of 54 knee joints. Orthop Clin North Am 10: 585–608

5.2
Radiographic Imaging of Osteoarthritis

C. Buckland-Wright

5.2.1
Introduction

Radiography is the easiest way to identify the anatomical changes in joint structure that confirm the existence of osteoarthritis (OA), with joint space narrowing, corresponding to cartilage loss [1, 2]; subchondral sclerosis and osteophyte formation, the joint's bony response to the increased mechanical load consequent upon cartilage degeneration and loss [3]. The ease of radiography in detecting these characteristic features, together with the ready availability and ease of interpretation of radiographs, has led to its use as the principal method for imaging OA joints.

The emphasis, by many authors, on loss of articular cartilage thickness, assessed indirectly on the radiograph as a narrowing of the interbone distance, underscores its significance as a principal component within the disease process. Nevertheless, it is essential to remember that OA is a condition affecting an organ, the synovial joint, and not just a particular tissue. Articular cartilage is intimately related to the underlying bone [4], together they act as a functional unit. Thus changes in one of the tissue layers will inevitably involve alterations in the other. Diagnostic radiology should assess the changes not only in articular cartilage but in particular those in the juxta and peri-articular bone which precede those in cartilage detectable as joint space narrowing.

Today, it is recognised that effective treatment of the condition is dependent upon early diagnosis, so joint anatomy is not irreparably altered and that there is sufficient cartilage tissue to respond to therapy [5]. For diagnosis of early osteoarthritis to be effective we need to know which of the radio-anatomic features, in each of the major joints, is a reliable indicator of the onset and progression of the disease. This chapter reviews which of these features of OA in the hand, knee and hip.

Additionally, diagnostic radiography is influenced by the sensitivity of the imaging system, which determines its ability to detect small anatomical changes characteristic of the disease process. The sensitivity is a function of the image quality which comprises both tissue contrast and spatial resolution, characteristic of the x-ray system (see Table 1 in [6]). These parameters are, in turn, affected by the perspective or plane in which the anatomical features are imaged. This is defined by the radiographic view of the joint, which must be constant both within as well as between patient examinations. This chapter addresses these aspects of radiography in OA by answering the following questions:

1) What procedures in standard radiography limit reliable diagnostic assessment of OA joints?
2) What procedures are necessary to ensure good quality control in radiography, so as to enhance radiographic diagnosis in OA?
3) Which radioanatomical features are the most reliable criteria for diagnosis and for assessing progression in OA of the hand, knee and hip?
4) How many patients are required to detect a therapeutic effect in knee OA?

5.2.2
What Procedures in Standard Radiography Limit Reliable Diagnostic Assessment of OA Joints?

The lack of any proper standardisation in radiographic methods is well illustrated by the variety of procedures that have been used to examine the knee. Ahlback [7] recommended that standard radiography of this joint in patients should be taken standing since he found that when the patient was x-rayed lying down, the knee cartilage was not loaded and the joint space width appeared artificially wide, giving a false impression of the state of the patients knee. When the patient is standing on a fully extended straight knee, this was still not ideal as a number of investigators [8–11] showed that a flexed knee revealed greater joint space loss than in the straight knee view.

Apart from the position of the joint, there are several steps in the production of a standard radiograph that make it difficult to ensure quality control [12]:

- The clinician making the request may not indicate precisely what is required (many OA knees are still obtained with the subject lying down).
- The radiology technician performing the examination may have his or her own idiosyncratic methods of positioning patients, especially when faced with someone who has difficulty standing or walking.
- The person assessing the radiographic features may be unaware of what has gone on beforehand.

This variability in the number of personnel, the radiographic procedure and the process of evaluation lead to errors in assessment of the dimensions of features recorded in the radiographs [12]. This is demonstrated by the findings in the following studies.

Longitudinal studies [13, 14] of the radiographic changes seen following the administration of non-steroidal anti-inflammatory drugs (NSAIDs) to patients with OA of the knee showed no radiographic progression after 2 years and only minimal changes between treatment groups. The absence of significant changes in these investigations was observed in other longitudinal studies of the knee [15, 16]. The inability to detect significant radiographic changes in joint anatomy lead to the following statements:

- "Two years was too short a time to detect significant changes in knee structure using conventional radiographic methods" [13].
- "Anatomical changes in many OA joints remain relatively stable over many years" [16].

It also led to the proposal that more sensitive techniques, such as microfocal radiography, should be evaluated [13, 17].

5.2.3
What Procedures are Necessary to Ensure Good Quality Control in Radiography, so as to Enhance Radiographic Diagnosis in OA?

Protocols for precise radio-anatomical positioning of joints are essential if disease related changes in joint anatomy are to be reliably assessed from sequential radiographic examinations. It can not be emphasised strongly enough that their use is essential to maintain quality control in a procedure which involves several isolated steps with respect both to the number of personnel involved and the technical procedure. Indeed, worthwhile radiographic assessment for both diagnosis and for therapeutic trials require protocols defining the precise position of the joint, standard criteria for x-ray beam alignment, allowance for inherent radiographic magnification and precise definition of anatomical boundaries for measurements of radiographic features [12]. The following principles form the basis for such protocols:

1. The radio-anatomical position of a joint must occupy a plane in which the central ray of the x-ray beam will pass between the margins of the joint space so that both margins and the space are optimally defined in a position consistent with the functional loading of that joint (Figs. 1, 2, 4, and 6).

2. Standardisation of the radio-anatomical position should ensure:
   - that the radiographic features to be evaluated can be assessed accurately and reproducibly in the same plane and on successive occasions
   - that the dimensions obtained for the radiographic feature are accurately recorded in the image and are neither an underestimate nor overestimate of its actual size.

The rationale for the radio-anatomical position for the hand, knee and hip is outlined in the following sections. The protocols for standard radiography of these joints are described elsewhere [18].

5.2.3.1
Dorsi-palmar Radiography of the Wrist and Hand

In hand OA, joint space width is evaluated in joints from which cartilage loss may be uneven. Spreading the fingers will alter joint alignment or radiography of both hands in ulnar deviation, can lead to an incorrect assessment of joint space narrowing. Fingers held together and in line with the axis of the wrist and fore-arm (Fig. 1) when laid flat on the x-ray film holder will be under the combined action of both the flexor and extensor groups of the finger muscles. Thus, each joint will be under muscular load along its own axis, providing a reproducible method for evaluating the joint space.

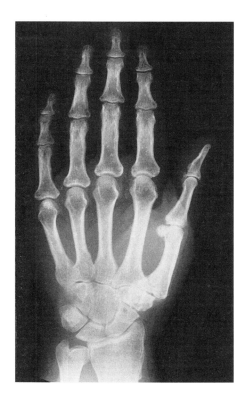

Fig. 1. Standard dorsi-palmar radiograph of a wrist and hand with the fingers held in line with the axis of the wrist and forearm

Fig. 2. a Diagram of the leg in the standing semi-flexed position and its position relative to the x-ray tube on the right and the film cassette placed in front of the image intensifier tube to the left. In this position the tibial plateau is horizontal, parallel to the central x-ray beam (*broken line*) and perpendicular to the x-ray film. **b** Standard anteroposterior radiograph of an OA knee in the standing semi-flexed position with the x-ray beam centred on the joint space. The tibial spines are centrally located relative to the femoral notch and the anterior and posterior margins of the medial compartment (*right*) are superimposed

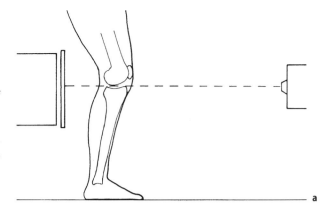

a

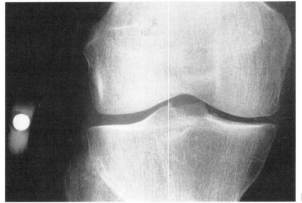

b

5.2.3.2
Knee Radiography

The knee is one of the most difficult joints to examine well radiographically because of its structural complexity and wide range of movement. In addition, there is now an awareness that OA may affect different compartments of the joint and may be focally distributed even within compartments [19–21]. Recent epidemiological and clinical studies have highlighted the importance of examining the patellofemoral joint in evaluating OA of the knee [20, 22, 23]. Indeed, as these authors have shown, patellofemoral or combined patellofemoral and medial tibiofemoral compartment disease is found in approximately 50% of all OA knee patients. Therefore, separate protocols describing the radio-anatomical positioning for the tibiofemoral and patellofemoral compartments have been described [18, 24].

5.2.3.3
Anteroposterior Radiography of the Tibiofemoral Compartment

The Osteoarthritis Research Society Clinical Trials guidelines [25] described two different protocols for radiography of the OA knee, the Standing Fully Extended View [26 – 28] and the Standing Semi-Flexed View [11, 18, 19, 24, 29, 30].

5.2.3.3.1
The Similarities

The two protocols for knee radiography described in the guidelines, are both based on similar principles, initially proposed by Buckland-Wright [12] and Buckland-Wright et al [19]:

– each knee is to be radiographed separately
– the central ray of the x-ray beam must be centred upon the middle of the joint, defined by the joint space
– the x-ray beam must be aligned with the medial compartment so that it is parallel with the tibial plateau [26 – 28], and so as to ensure that the anterior and posterior lips of the medial tibial plateau are superimposed (Fig. 2) [12, 19]
– the tibial spines must appear centrally placed relative to the femoral notch
– the radio-anatomic position of the joint is visualised with the aid of fluoroscopy; and
– following the first exposure, the outline of the foot is drawn on a sheet of paper placed there beforehand, to facilitate joint positioning at subsequent examinations.

Such procedures are undertaken so as to ensure that the dimensions of the joint space are reliably recorded on the radiographic film and are not distorted by variations either in the angle of projection of the x-ray beam or the positioning of the joint within and between patients.

5.2.3.3.2
The Differences

The techniques differ with respect to two important features. These are the manner in which the joint is positioned and the way in which the image magnification is controlled.

Standing Fully Extended View

This view is based upon an existing methodology, originally described by Ahlback [7] and subsequently adopted by the WHO/AAOS workshop [31]. In this position the knee is 'locked' into a straight leg stance. The femoral condyles role forward onto the anterior edge of the tibial plateau so that the weight of the body is transmitted across the joint, anterior to the attachment of the collateral and cruciate ligaments (Fig. 3). With the knee in extension, the body's weight passes down at the anterior region of the joint and is counter-balanced by the tension in the collateral and cruciate ligaments. A source of error can arise from the observation that articular cartilage is often spared at the anterior margin of the tibia, even when it has been almost completely lost from the central articular region of the tibial plateau (Fig. 3). Thus joint space width measurements in the medial compartment of knees in the straight leg stance provides a false image of the extent of cartilage preservation in the central articular region of the joint.

Standing Semi-Flexed View

In this view, using fluoroscopy, each knee is flexed until the medial compartment tibial plateau is horizontal relative to the floor of the room and parallel to the central ray of the x-ray beam. Each knee is radiographed separately as the required degree of flexion usually varies between the left and right knees of the same patient and among individuals. This variation is due to differences in the angle of inclination of the tibial plateau. In the semi-flexed position, the femoral condyle occupies a postero-central position on the articular surface of the tibia (Fig. 3). This position co-insides with the site of principal load across the joint during its normal function [32]. It is also the site at which arthroscopy has

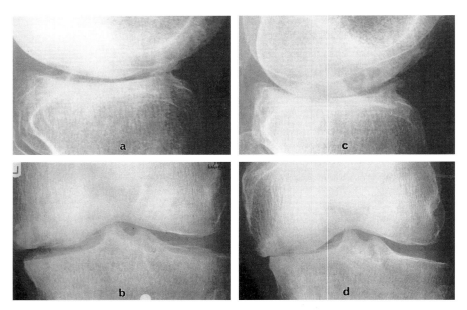

Fig. 3a–d. Weight bearing standard radiographs of a knee with advanced OA. The lateral view of the knee in the extended position **a** shows the femoral condyle forward on the anterior region of the tibia, a space is visible between the tibia and femur, seen also in the antero-posterior view of the knee in extension **b**. The lateral view of the same joint radiographed in the semi-flexed position **c** shows the tibia occupying a postero-central region of the tibial plateau. No joint space is visible in this or the antero-posterior view **d**. The space visible in the extended view of the knee does not correspond to articular cartilage thickness at the central region of the tibio-femoral joint, but to a "gap" produced by the femoral condyle rolling forward onto the tibial eminence seen in **a**

revealed highest prevalence of articular cartilage destruction [10]. Thus joint space width measurements in the medial compartment of the knees in the semi-flexed position provides a reliable assessment of the extent of cartilage preservation in the central articular region of the joint.

Radiographic Magnification

Correction for the effect of radiographic magnification is required where measurements are undertaken of joint space width and other radiographic features. The standing extended view requires the knees to be placed as close as possible to the x-ray film-cassette so as to minimise the degree of radiographic magnification. Nevertheless, the distance between the centre of the joint and the film varies between patients, for example, due either to obesity or the restriction of joint movement as a result of pain or osteophytosis [11, 12]. In this view, the radiographic magnification was found to range from $\times 1.09$ to $\times 1.35$, resulting in a significant effect upon the accuracy and precision of joint space width measurements [11]. Whereas, in the standing semi-flexed view, since the distance of the knee from the film-cassette will vary with each joint radiographed, a metal ball of known size (5 mm) is placed over the head of the fibula (Fig. 2). The image of this ball is used to correct for radiographic magnification [2, 11]. In therapeutic trials, failure to correct for the effect of radiographic magnification has a significant adverse effect upon the power calculations leading to an increase in the number of patients required for a therapeutic study [5, 33].

Recommendations

The standing semi-flexed view plus correction for the effect of radiographic magnification is recommended where measurements are to be undertaken of the radiographic features. Computerised automated methods for measuring joint space width have been developed and validated for use in standard and high definition macroradiographs [11, 30].

5.2.3.4
Axial Radiography of the Patellofemoral Compartment

Currently two different radiographic views are used in the assessment of patello-femoral OA, the medio-lateral and axial or skyline view of the joint. In a detailed evaluation of the two views Jones et al. [34] and Cicuttini et al. [35] found that the axial or skyline view was more readily and reproducibly achieved than the lateral view, permitting more precise localisation of the changes in the lateral and medial facets of the joint (Fig. 4).

Examination of the patellofemoral joint in the axial or skyline view can be obtained using Ahlback's method [7], with the patient standing and the knee flexed to 30° from the vertical (Fig. 5). In this position the joint is under functional load, ensuring that the articular surfaces are in close apposition, providing a more reliable assessment of cartilage thickness than when the patient is radiographed in the supine position [24]. In the latter position, the muscles around the knee are relaxed and the patella is no longer held in a position under functional load and as a result the patella may be subluxed.

Fig. 4. Axial, or skyline radiograph of a right patellofemoral compartment with the knee in the standing semi-flexed view. The patellar articular margins used in joint space width measurements are identified by the *arrows*

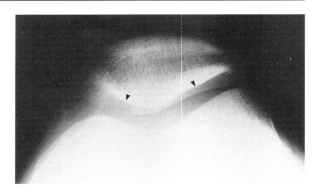

Fig. 5. General view showing the position of the patient and associated equipment for a skyline view of the patello-femoral compartment. The *broken line* indicates the alignment of the central ray of the x-ray beam

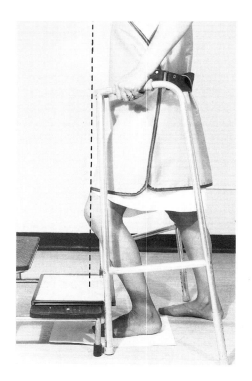

5.2.3.5
Anteroposterior Radiography of the Hip

Three factors affect the precision of joint space width assessment in the hip, patient position, limb rotation and the direction of the centre of the x-ray beam.

Recent radiographic studies [36, 37], comparing OA hips of the same individuals after examination in both the supine and erect position have shown that when the joint space is narrower than 2.5 mm, the measured interbone distance was significantly smaller when the patient was standing than it was when the subject was lying down [38].

Evaluation of the effect of limb rotation at the hip joint in cadavers showed that with medial rotation the minimum joint space was smaller than in the neutral position, i. e. when the foot is straight [24]. The effect of medial rotation results in tightening of the powerful lateral rotator muscles of the hip joint, driving the femoral head medially into the acetabulum.

We have found [30] that displacement of the x-ray tube away from the centre of the joint can significantly alter the measurement of joint space width. This has recently been confirmed by Conrozier and his colleagues [38] who found a benefit in centering the beam over the hip joint rather than at the supra-pubic position, for detecting subtle changes in hip joint space.

5.2.3.5.1
Recommendations

In those joints in which the status of the articular cartilage is to be assessed, the hip should be radiographed with the patient standing and the feet internally rotated to ensure the femoral head is closely applied to the articular surface of the acetabulum. The central ray of the x-ray beam must be aligned with the centre of the femoral head for accurate and precise measurements (Fig. 6). These recommendations are the basis of the published protocol [18].

Fig. 6. Standard antero-posterior weight bearing radiograph of an OA hip taken with a 10° internal rotation of the foot

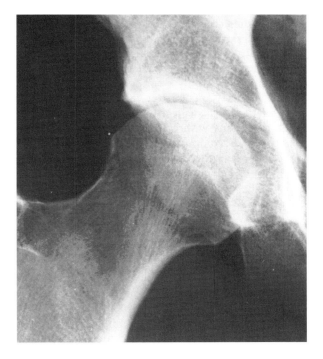

5.2.4
Which Radioanatomical Features are the Most Reliable for Diagnosis and for Assessing Progression in OA of the Hand, Knee and Hip?

Should all features be assessed in all joints and be given equal importance? The evidence to date suggests that this is not a useful approach because radiographic features of OA are variable, not only between joints, such as hip, hand and knee [39] but also within areas of a single joint, such as the tibiofemoral and patellofemoral compartments of the knee [20]. For each joint or compartment, a set of criteria need to be developed for diagnosis and for evaluating outcome [20, 39]. Quantitative methods are required to determine the extend and progression of the disease [24].

5.2.4.1
Methods for Quantifying the Extent and Progression in OA

Semi-quantitative grading systems based on global score of the radiographic features [40], although widely used to assess disease progression, suffer from two limitations which are based on the following assumptions:

- The change in any one radiographic feature is linear and constant during the course of disease progression.
- The relationship between the different radiographic features is constant.

Consequently, recent workers [41–44] have turned to scoring individual radiographic features of OA. Although this approach requires confirmation by future studies, these methods remain susceptible to fairly high levels of inter-observer variation.

Alternatively, direct measurement of the radiographic features is undertaken, usually of the interbone distance. Measurement of radiographic features is dependent not only upon image quality but also upon the measurement procedure [12, 45]. The latter varies among investigators; some do not describe their methods [13, 46], others use a ruler [47] or callipers [1, 48] and/or a magnifying lens with a fitted graticule [49]. Measurement reproducibility is greatest with computerised techniques using digitally stored radiographic images [30, 50], where inter- and intra-observer variability is virtually eliminated [30]. A more detailed review of the methods of measurement and the sites at which to take measurements of the different radiographic features is described elsewhere [24].

5.2.4.2
Dorsi-palmar View of the Hand

5.2.4.2.1
Semi-quantitative Assessment

Kallman et al. [51] and Altman et al. [52] in their methods for scoring individual radiographic features in OA, include osteophytes, joint space narrowing and

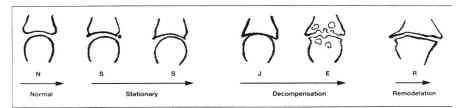

Fig. 7. Diagram of the radiographic changes used to score radiographic progression in the fingers of patients with hand osteoarthritis (with permission from Verbruggen and Veys 1995)

periarticular subchondral erosions as the most important features to assess in the distal and proximal interphalangeal joints as well as the first carpometacarpal joint. Additional features of interest include periarticular subchondral sclerosis and joint malalignment without subluxation.

The four point grading scale allocated to these features by Altman et al. [52] underestimates the complexity of the anatomical changes observed and described by Verbruggen and Veys [53]. They identified five distinct phases of disease progression (Fig. 7). The nonaffected joint (N), the stationary osteoarthritic joint (S) based on the presence of osteophytes and/or joint space narrowing and/or subchondral sclerosis. Most of the joints at this stage remained in the S-phase for 2 to 3 years. This was followed by obliteration of the joint space (J-phase) which also lasted between 2 to 3 years. The J-phase preceded or coincided with the appearance of subchondral cysts eroding the entire subchondral plate (erosive or E-phase). The erosive episodes subsiding spontaneously to be followed a repair and remodelling (R-phase). This last phase led to the regeneration of a subchondral plate covered by cartilaginous tissue, with the formation of large osteophytes producing a nodular appearance to the affected finger joints. Verbruggen and Veys [53] found that this method permit rapid assessment of OA progression.

5.2.4.2.2
Quantitative assessment

Measurement of the extent and progression of OA features recorded in high definition macroradiographs [54–56] in a group of patients found quite different and distinct patterns of progression affecting the bony features of osteophytosis and subchondral sclerosis compared with those of joint space width.

Radiographic detection of the existence of OA in hand joints at an initial or baseline examination, was confirmed by the presence of bony features, with osteophytosis being the most sensitive of these since it was more readily detected in radiographs. In evaluating disease progression osteophytosis alone, as measured by an increase in their number and size was the most the sensitive parameter confirming the criteria first established by Kellgren and Lawrence [40] and later by others [39, 51].

Fig. 8. Distribution of the percentage incidence of osteophyte formation at the juxta-articular margins and capsular attachments at the joints of the wrist and hand in patients with hand osteo-arthritis

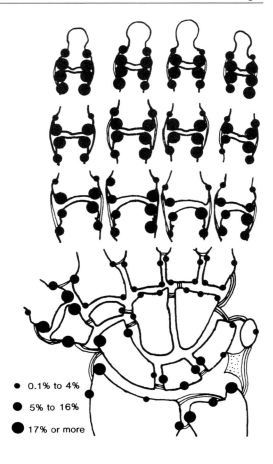

- 0.1% to 4%
- 5% to 16%
- 17% or more

Osteophytes were present not only in the digits but also in the wrist. In the latter, they were much larger at the first carpometacarpal joint [55]. Osteophyte number and size were found to be greatest at the joint margins, in the dominant hand, at the joints of the second and third compared to the fourth and fifth phalanges, in the joints of the third phalangeal ray and at the second distal interphalangeal joint respectively (Fig. 8) [55]. Subchondral cortical sclerosis showed a similar bony response [56]. These sites of increased bone formation correspond to those at which the largest forces occur in the hand, viz. in the dominant side, the finger tripod used in precision grip, power grip and pulp pinch grip respectively [55, 56].

Radiographic detection of cartilage destruction and loss from measurements of joint space narrowing is a sensitive method of assessing disease progression in hand OA, confirming the findings of previous reports [39, 51]. However, the sensitivity of joint space width measurements in detecting the presence of OA at an initial examination is poor and unreliable, since over half the patients at entry into this study had normal joint space width measurements compared to the non-arthritic reference group. Our studies in OA [54, 56] indicate that although the earliest changes may occur in cartilage, radiographic detection of the destruction and loss of this tissue is a late phenomenon of the disease. Joint space loss was symmetrical in both hands. Its change showed that, over a period of time, narrowing progressed proximally from the distal interphalangeal to proximal interphalangeal, metacarpophalangeal and wrist joints [56]. The findings, when taken in context of the role of mechanical factors in bony changes described above, suggest that genetic or other constitutional factors determine the onset of cartilage changes in OA [56].

5.2.4.3
Knee: Anteroposterior View of the Tibiofemoral Joint

5.2.4.3.1
Semi-quantitative Assessment

The most important radiographic features in the knee are joint space narrowing, marginal osteophytes and subchondral sclerosis [52]. Spiking of the tibial spines although unreliable as a single independent feature [57], has been found to be of value in assessing progression [39]. As discussed above, joint space width assessment in the straight leg stance of the knee is not reliable since it does not provide an assessment of the extent of cartilage preservation in the central articular region of the joint. Thus, in straight leg radiographs greater emphasis must be placed on the bony features for assessing disease status.

5.2.4.3.2
Quantitative Assessment

Determination of the degree of narrowing and loss of the articular cartilage is reliably undertaken with the knee in either the semi-flexed position [6] or in the 'tunnel' or 'schuss' position [19, 58] where the knee is flexed to an angle of 130° between the shafts of the tibia and femur. Joint space width measurements in the medial compartment of the knees in these flexed positions provides a reliable assessment of the extent of cartilage preservation in the central articular region of the joint. In an assessment of the standing semi-flexed and tunnel views it was found that the combination of these two views detected narrowing of the interbone distance more frequently than either view alone, but that the standing semi-flexed view alone failed to detect narrowing in 22% of OA knees [19]. The mechanism responsible for this difference in articular cartilage thickness between views is not clear. Nevertheless, these findings indicate that in medial diseased compartment cartilage loss occurs in the central articular region of the tibial plateau, seen in the semi-flexed view, and additionally, over the popliteal surface of the femoral condyle as detected in the tunnel view. Lateral compared with medial compartment disease is less common [59] with joint space width measurements on the lateral side being less precise [11].

In knees with medial compartment disease osteophytes are not confined to the diseased compartment. Indeed, marginal osteophytes appear either in the medial or lateral compartment and at the respective tibial spines. We have measured the size of osteophytes in both compartments and found that on average osteophytes are larger in the medial diseased compartment than in the lateral and that their size correlates with the degree of joint space loss in the medial compartment. Interestingly, the size of osteophytes in the lateral compartment of the same knees also correlates with the degree of joint space loss in the medial compartment [19]. Osteophyte formation is thus an expression of the disease in the tibio-femoral joint rather than of either the medial or lateral compartment. In this study, as in OA of the hand [54], osteophytes and subchondral sclerosis were found to be well developed in as many as 40 % of the OA knees with minimal or no joint space narrowing. Indicating that in OA bony changes develop ahead of articular cartilage destruction measured as a reduction in the interbone distance [19].

5.2.4.4
Knee: Axial View of the Patellofemoral Joint

5.2.4.4.1
Semi-quantitative Assessment

The most important features in this joint are the same as those for the tibiofemoral compartment, with the addition that subluxation can play a more important role. Longitudinal studies are required to evaluate the sensitivity of the different features using either semi-quantitative scoring or methods of direct measurement.

5.2.4.5
Anteroposterior View of the Hip

5.2.4.5.1
Semi-quantitative Assessment

Although, the radiographic features considered the most important for global assessment were joint space narrowing and subchondral sclerosis [39], the current emphasis is on scoring separately the following individual features for assessing change: joint space narrowing, subchondral bony lucencies, marginal osteophytes and subchondral bony sclerosis [52]. Subclassification of the disease has been according to the pattern of migration of the femoral head within the acetabulum [3, 60, 61].

In a radiographic analysis of OA hip patients attending hospital, Ledingham and her colleagues [62] found that the differences in radiographic progression, according to the pattern of femoral head migration, was in keeping with previous studies [63–65]. There was a higher occurrence of overall radiographic change and change in individual features occurred in hips with superior migration and a lower occurrence in those with medial or axial migration. The superolateral pattern, in particular, showed an increased frequency of change in all radiographic features which may, in part, relate to the greater mechanical stresses associated with this pattern of migration [62]. Women were also found to have increased frequency of radiographic change in both overall and individual radiographic features and confirmed that they develop a more severe form of hip osteoarthritis than men [62]. A worse prognosis was also detected in those patients with atrophic or limited bone response [61, 62], characterised by poor osteophyte and subchondral sclerosis formation.

5.2.4.6
Recommendations for Early Detection in OA Joints

The earliest radiographic features to appear in OA joints are the changes to bone, with osteophytes being more important in the hand and knee, and subchondral sclerosis in the hip. These features are detected in the radiographs ahead of articular cartilage destruction measured as joint space narrowing. However, the latter is of greater value in the assessment of progression than osteophytes.

5.2.5
How Many Patients are Required to Detect a Therapeutic Effect in Knee OA?

Guidelines for the design and conduct of clinical trials in patients with OA have been prepared by the Task Force of the Osteoarthritis Research Society [5]. They incorporated the recommendations of earlier committees WHO/ILAR [1], WHO and AAOS [66], GREES [67] and OMERACT III [68] where the outcome, for a disease modifying drug (DMOAD), should assess the effect of a drug on joint structure. The primary outcome measure for knee should be minimum joint space width since this is more sensitive than global scoring [5, 69]. The overriding conclusion of the guidelines was that for the reliable assessment of progression in OA, it was absolutely essential for reproducible radiographs to be obtained.

5.2.5.1
Effect of Protocols Upon Measurement Accuracy and Precision

The effect of protocols for standardisation of radiographic and mensural procedures upon the accuracy and precision of computerised measurement of minimum joint space width in the tibiofemoral compartment of the knee was assessed in the standing semi-flexed view for both standard and macroradiography of the knee. These findings were compared with the manual measurement of minimum joint space width in the standing extended view of the knee, without correction for radiographic magnification [11]. Twenty five patients with knee OA had standard and microfocal radiographs taken of the knee in both views twice on the same day and again two weeks later. For each of the procedural comparisons identified in Fig. 9, reproducibility was calculated as the standard deviation in the four similar measurements for each knee, and accuracy as the mean absolute error with respect to the mean macroradiographic measurement.

Although a more detailed explanation for the findings is presented elsewhere [11], the results show that for measurement of medial compartment joint space width, computerised was more accurate than manual; correction for radio-

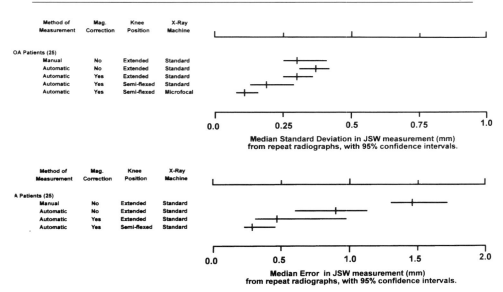

Fig. 9. Relative precision (*top*) and accuracy (*bottom*) of knee joint space width measurements under varying radiographic and mensural procedures described in the text. The bars give the median values with 95% confidence intervals for precision and accuracy of joint space width measurements under each of the procedural conditions listed to the left. Original values published in [11]. No value is given for the accuracy of joint space width measurements using microfocal radiography, since we had previously shown that this measurement reliably and accurately measured articular cartilage thickness in the medial tibio-femoral compartment [2]

graphic magnification improved precision and accuracy; measurements in the semi-flexed view were more precise and accurate than those in the standing extended knee position; and macroradiography increased measurement precision over that which could be achieved by standard radiography.

5.2.5.2
Quantifying Outcome

The advantages of the use of high definition macroradiography upon the precision of joint space width measurement in OA knees is shown in Fig. 9, where it is significantly more precise than that obtained from standard radiographs of knees in the same radiographic view. The difference between standard and microfocal radiography can be assessed by reference to two important questions for studies aimed at determining disease progression or monitoring the effect of therapy:

– What is the minimum interval change required in joint space width measurement?
– What is the minimum time interval required to detect a significant change in joint space width?

5.2.5.2.1
Minimum Interval Change in Joint Space Width Measurement

The minimum interval change as defined by Cummings and Black [70] is the change in any parameter that can be measured with 95% confidence with a particular technique. Based on the results of the assessment of accuracy and reproducibility of joint space width measurements [11] the minimum interval change in the medial compartment joint space width was between 9% and 15% in standard radiography and between 4% and 9% for microfocal radiography. The minimum interval change required was smaller in those knees with early OA [11].

5.2.5.2.2
Minimum Time Interval to Detect a Significant Change in Joint Space Width Measurement

Using the published figures for the annual rate of joint space narrowing in knees with definite OA of 0.20 mm/year [24, 33] and those for accuracy and precision of joint space width measurements [11], we determined that the time it would take to measure a significant change in joint space width, with a 95% confidence interval, would be 23 months for standard plain film compared with 13 months using microfocal radiography of OA knees [6].

5.2.5.3
Power Calculations

Using the mean and standard deviation of the annual rate of joint space narrowing it is possible to determine the number of knees that would be required to detect a significant change in joint space width in patients receiving drug treatment versus a placebo. For studies using standard or microfocal radiographic examination of patients with early knee OA, i.e. those most likely to respond to treatment [5, 71, 72], the criteria for selecting the study knee is based upon the following:

1) The knee must have a medial tibio-femoral compartment joint space width > 2 mm (where both knees in a patient have a joint space width > 2 mm, the knee with the smaller joint space is selected).
2) Osteophytosis and subchondral sclerosis should be visible.
3) The joint must have had pain for at least 15 days in one month.

For a double-blind study of 2 years duration, comparing an active agent against placebo, in which patient groups are of equal size with medial or bi-compartmental involvement, the total number of knees required to detect a significant difference in minimum joint space width, using standard or microfocal radiography of the joint in the standing semi-flexed position, is shown in Table 1.

For an agent with a therapeutic effect which, in comparison to the placebo, resulted in a 30% protection against joint space loss over 2 years, a study using microfocal radiography would require 111 knees in each group to detect such an effect with 90% power and a statistical significance of p = 0.05, using com-

Table 1. Required number of knees for therapeutic studies, of 2 years duration, for patients with early OA (joint space width >2 mm), using computer measurement of minimum joint space width (JSW) from standard[a] and macro-radiographs[b] of joints in the standing semi-flexed position. The agent's therapeutic effect (the difference in joint space narrowing compared to that in the placebo group) is expressed as a percentage of the placebo group joint space narrowing. For each percentage effect the total number of knees has been determined, using the formula for calculating sample size [73], for the different power levels and a significance P = 0.05

Power level	Therapeutic effect		
	30%	50%	80%
Standard radiography			
95%	460	164	66
90%	372	134	52
80%	278	100	40
Macroradiography			
95%	274	100	40
90%	222	80	32
80%	166	60	24

Mean annual rate of joint space narrowing = 0.183 mm/year.
[a] with associated standard deviation for joint space width measurement using standard radiography = 0.249 mm.
[b] with associated standard deviation for joint space width measurement using macroradiography = 0.196 mm.

puterised measurement of joint space width. Whereas, 186 knees are required in each group using the same techniques and standard radiography [24]. Currently these figures represent our "best guess", and provide more an indication of the reduction in sample size afforded by the protocols for microfocal compared to standard radiography.

5.2.5.4
Recommendations

High definition macroradiography will detect disease progression and the response to treatment, as measured by change in joint space width in knee OA, within a shorter period and with a fewer patients than when using standard radiography.

References

1. Lequesne M, Brandt K, Bellamy R, Moskowitz R, Menkes CJ, Pelletier J-P (1994) Guidelines for testing slow acting drugs in OA. Proceedings Vth Joint WHO and ILAR Task Force Meeting. J Rheumatol 21 [Suppl 41]:65–73
2. Buckland-Wright JC, Macfarlane DG, Lynch JA, Jasani MK, Bradshaw CR (1995a) Joint space width measures cartilage thickness in osteoarthritis of the knee: high resolution plain film and double contrast macroradiographic investigation. Ann Rheum Dis 54:263–268

3. Resnick D, Niwayama G (1995): Degenerative disease of extraspinal locations. In: Resnick D, Niwayama G (eds) Diagnosis of Bone and Joint Disorders. 2nd edn. Saunders, Philadelphia pp 1365–1479

4. Sokoloff L (1987) Loading and motion in relation to ageing and degeneration of joints: implications for prevention and treatment of osteoarthritis. In: Helminen HJ, Kiviranta I, Saamanen A-M, Tammi M, Paukkonen K, Jurvelin J (eds) Joint loading, biology and health of articular structures. Bristol, Wright, pp 412–424

5. Altman R, Brandt K, Hochberg M and Moskowitz R (1996) Design and conduct of clinical trials in patients with osteoarthritis: recommendations from the task force of the osteoarthritis research society. Osteoarthritis Cartilage 4:217–243

6. Buckland-Wright JC (1997) Current status of imaging procedures in the diagnosis, prognosis and monitoring of osteoarthritis. In: Bellamy N (ed) Osteoarthritis. Baillière's Clin Rheumatol 11:727–748

7. Ahlback S (1968) Osteoarthritis of the knee: a radiographic investigation. Acta Radiol 277 [Suppl]:7–72

8. Resnick D, Vint V (1980) The "tunnel" view in assessment of cartilage loss in osteoarthritis of the knee. Radiology 137:547–548

9. Rosenberg TD, Paulos LE, Parker RD, Coward DB, Scott SM (1988) The forty-five-degree posteroanterior flexion weight-bearing radiograph of the knee. J Bone Joint Surg 70 A: 1479–1483

10. Messieh SS, Fowler PJ, Munro T (1990) Anteroposterior radiographs of the osteoarthritic knee. J Bone Joint Surg 72B:639–640

11. Buckland-Wright JC, Macfarlane DG, Williams SA, Ward RJ (1995b) Accuracy and precision of joint space width measurements in standard and macro-radiographs of osteoarthritic knees. Ann Rheum Dis 54:872–880

12. Buckland-Wright JC (1994) Quantitative radiography of osteoarthritis. Ann Rheum Dis 53:268–275

13. Dieppe P, Cushnaghan J, Jasani MK, McCrae F, Watt I (1993) A two year, placebo-controlled trial of non-steroidal anti-inflammatory therapy in osteoarthritis of the knee joint. Br J Rheumatol 32:595–600

14. Williams HJ, Ward JR, Egger MJ, Neuner R, Brooks RH, Clegg DO, Field EH, Skosey JL, Alarcon GS, Wilkens RF, et al. (1993) Comparison of naproxen and acetaminophen in a two-year study of treatment of osteoarthritis of the knee. Arthritis Rheum 36:1196–1206

15. Massardo L, Watt I, Cushnaghan J, Dieppe P (1989) Osteoarthritis of the knee joint: an eight year prospective study. Ann Rheum Dis 48:893–897

16. Spector TD, Dacre JE, Harris PA, Huskisson EC (1992) Radiological progression of osteoarthritis: an 11 year follow up study of the knee. Ann Rheum Dis 51:1107–1110

17. Peyron JG (1991) Clinical features of osteoarthritis, diffuse idiopathic skeletal hyperostosis, and hypermobility syndromes. Curr Opin Rheumatol 3:653–661

18. Buckland-Wright JC (1998a) Protocols for radiography. In: Brandt K, Lohmander S and Doherty M (eds) Textbook of Osteoarthritis. Oxford University Press, Oxford, pp 578–580

19. Buckland-Wright JC, Macfarlane DG, Jasani MK, Lynch JA (1994) Quantitative microfocal radiographic assessment of osteoarthritis of the knee from weight bearing tunnel and semi-flexed standing views. J Rheumatol 21:1734–1741

20. Dieppe P, Kirwan J (1994) The localization of osteoarthritis. Br J Rheumatol 33:201–203

21. Felson DT, Radin EL (1994) What causes knee osteoarthritis: are different compartments susceptible to different risk factors? J Rheumatol 21:181–183

22. McAlindon TE, Snow S, Cooper C, Dieppe PA (1992) Radiographic patterns of the knee joint in the community: the importance of the patello-femoral joint. Ann Rheum Dis 51: 844–849

23. McAlindon TE, Cooper C, Kirwan J, Dieppe PA (1992) Knee pain and disability in the community. Br J Rheumatol 31:189–192

24. Buckland-Wright JC (1995) Protocols for precise radio-anatomical positioning of the tibiofemoral and patellofemoral compartments of the knee. Osteoarthritis Cartilage 3 [Suppl A]:71–80

25. Buckland-Wright JC, Scott WW and Peterfy (1996) Radiographic imaging techniques. Appendix III to design and conduct of clinical trials in patients with osteoarthritis. Osteoarthritis Cartilage 4:238–240
26. Ravaud P, Auleley G, Chastang C et al. (1996a) Knee joint space width measurement: an experimental study of the influence of radiographic procedure and joint positioning. Br J Rheumatol 35:761–766
27. Ravaud P, Chastang C, Auleley G et al. (1996b) Assessment of joint space width in patients with osteoarthritis of the knee: a comparison of four measuring instruments. J Rheumatol 23:1749–1755
28. Ravaud P, Graudeau B, Auleley G et al. (1996c) Radiographic assessment of knee osteoarthritis: reproducibility and sensitivity to change. J Rheumatol 23:1756–1764
29. Buckland-Wright JC (1998b) Quantitation of radiographic changes. In: Brandt K, Lohmander S and Doherty M (eds) Textbook of Osteoarthritis. Oxford University Press, Oxford, pp 459–472
30. Lynch JA, Buckland-Wright JC, Macfarlane DG (1993) Precision of joint space width measurement in knee osteoarthritis from digital image analysis of high definition macroradiographs. Osteoarthritis Cartilage 1:209–218
31. Dieppe PA, Brandt K, Lohmander S, Felson D (1995) Detecting and measuring modification in osteoarthritis: the need for standardized methodology. J Rheumatol 22:201–203
32. Maquet P (1976) Biomechanics of the knee. Springer-Verlag, Berlin
33. Mazzuca SA, Brandt KD, Katz BP (1997) Is conventional radiography suitable for evaluation of a disease-modifying drug in patients with knee osteoarthritis? Osteoarthritis Cartilage 5:217–226
34. Jones AC, Ledingham J, McAlindon T, Regan M, Hart D, MacMillan PJ, Doherty M (1993) Radiographic assessment of patellofemoral osteoarthritis. Ann Rheum Dis 52:655–658
35. Cicuttini FM, Baker J, Hart DJ, Spector TD (1996) Choosing the best method for radiological assessment of patellofemoral osteoarthritis. Ann Rheum Dis 55:134–136
36. Conrozier T, Tron AM, Mathieu P, Vignon E, Lequesne M (1993) Measurement of x-ray hip joint space in the weight bearing and non weight bearing position. Rev Rhum Engl Ed 60:582
37. Lequesne M (1995) Quantitative measurements of joint space during progression of osteoarthritis: "chondrometry". In: Kuettner KE, Goldberg V (eds) Osteoarthritic Disorders. American Academy of Orthopaedic Surgeons, Rosemont pp 427–444
38. Conrozier T, Lequesne MG, Tron AM, Mathieu P, Berdah L, Vignon E (1997) The effects of position on the radiographic joint space in osteoarthritis of the hip. Osteoarthritis Cartilage 5:17–22
39. Altman R, Fries JF, Block DA, Carstens J, Cooke TD, Genant H, Gofton P, Groth H, McShane DJ, Murphy WA, Sharp JT, Spitz P, Williams CA, Wolf F (1987) Radiological assessment of progression in osteoarthritis. Arthritis Rheum 30:1214–1225
40. Kellgren JH, Lawrence JS (1957) Radiological assessment of osteoarthrosis. Ann Rheum Dis 16:494–501
41. Croft P, Cooper C, Wickham C, Coggon D (1990) Defining osteoarthritis of the hip for epidemiological studies. Am J Epidemiol 132:514–522
42. Lane NE, Nevitt MC, Genant HK, Hochberg MC (1993) Reliability of new indices of radiographic osteoarthritis of the hand and hip and lumbar disc degeneration. J Rheumatol 20:1911–1918
43. Spector TD, Hart DJ, Byrne J, Harris PA, Dacre JE, Doyle DV (1993) Definition of osteoarthritis of the knee for epidemiological studies. Ann Rheum Dis 52:790–794
44. Hart D, Spector T, Egger P, Coggon D, Cooper C (1994) Defining osteoarthritis of the hand for epidemiological studies: the Chingford study. Ann Reum Dis 53:220–223
45. Dieppe PA (1995) Recommended methodology for assessing the progression of osteoarthritis of the hip and knee joints. Osteoarthritis Cartilage 3:73–77
46. Dougados M, Gueguen A, Nguyen M, Thiesce A, Listrat V, Jacob L, Nakashe JP, Gabriel KR, Lequesne M, Amor B (1992) Longitudinal radiologic evaluation of osteoarthritis of the knee. J Rheumatol 19:378–384

47. Jonsson K, Buckwalter K, Helvie M, Niklason L, Martel W (1992) Precision of hyaline cartilage thickness measurements. Acta Radiol 33:234–239
48. Lequesne M, Winkler P, Rodriguez P, Rahlfs VW (1992) Joint space narrowing in primary osteoarthritis of the hip. Results of a three year controlled trial. Arthritis Rheum 35 [Suppl 9]:S135
49. Laoussadi S, Menkes CJ (1991) Amélioration de la précision de la mesure visuelle de la hauteur de l'interligne articulaire du genou et de la hanche à l'aide d'une loupe graduée. Revue du Rhumatisme et des Maladies Osteoarticulaires 58:678
50. Dacre JE, Coppock JS, Herbert KE, Perrett D, Huskisson EC (1989) Development of a new radiographic scoring system using digital image analysis. Ann Rheum Dis 48:194–200
51. Kallman DA, Wigley FM, Scott WW, Hochberg MC, Tobin JD (1989) New radiographic grading scales for osteoarthritis of the hand. Arthritis Rheum 32:1584–1591
52. Altman RD, Hochberg M, Murphy WA, Wolfe F, Lequesne M (1995) Atlas of individual radiographic features in osteoarthritis. Osteoarthritis Cartilage 3[Suppl A]:3–70
53. Verbruggen G, Veys EM (1995) Numerical scoring systems for the progression of osteoarthritis of the finger joints. Rev Rheum Engl Ed 62:27S–32S
54. Buckland-Wright JC, Macfarlane DG, Lynch JA, Clark B (1990) Quantitative microfocal radiographic assessment of progression in osteoarthritis of the hand. Arthritis Rheum 33:57–65
55. Buckland-Wright JC, Macfarlane DG, Lynch JA (1991) Osteophytes in the arthritic hand: their incidence, size, distribution and progression. Ann Rheum Dis 50:627–630
56. Buckland-Wright JC, Macfarlane DG, Lynch JA (1992) Relationship between joint space width and subchondral sclerosis in the osteoarthritic hand: a quantitative microfocal study. J Rheumatol 19:788–795
57. Donnelly S, Hart DJ, Doyle DV, Spector TD (1996) Spiking of the tibial tubercles – a radiological feature of osteoarthritis? Ann Rheum Dis 55:105–108
58. Piperno M, Hellio M-P, Conrozier T, Bochu M, Mathieu P, Vignon E (1998) Quantitative evaluation of joint space width in femorotibial osteoarthritis: comparison of three radiographic views. Osteoarthritis Cartilage 6: in press
59. Thomas RH, Resnick D, Alazraki NP, Daniel D, Greenfield R (1975) Compartmental evaluation of osteoarthritis of the knee. Radiology 116:585–594
60. Gofton JP (1971) Studies in osteoarthritis of the hip: part 1. Classification. Can Med Assoc J 104:679–683
61. Solomon L (1976) Patterns of osteoarthritis of the hip. J Bone Joint Surg 58B:176–183
62. Ledingham J, Dawson S, Preston B, Milligan G, Doherty M (1993) Radiographic progression of hospital referred osteoarthritis of the hip. Ann Rheum Dis 52:263–267
63. Cameron HU, Macnab I (1975) Observations on osteoarthritis of the hip joint. Clin Orthop 108:31–40
64. Danielsson LG (1964) Incidence and prognosis of coxarthrosis. Acta Orthop Scand 66:1–114
65. Perry G, Smith MJG, Whiteside CG (1972) Spontaneous recovery of the joint space in degenerative hip disease. Ann Rheum Dis 31:440–448
66. Kuettner K, Goldberg V (eds) (1995) Osteoarthritic disorders. American Academy of Orthopaedic Surgeons, Rosemont
67. Group for the Respect of Ethics and Excellence in Science (GREES osteoarthritis section) (1996) Recommendations for the registration of drugs used in the treatment of osteoarthritis. Ann Rheum Dis 55:552–557
68. Bellamy N, Kirwan J, Boers M, et al. (1996) Recommendations for a core set of outcome measures for future phase III clinical trials in knee, hip, and hand osteoarthritis: consensus development at OMERACT III. J Rheumatol 24:799–802
69. Hochberg MC (1996) Quantitative radiography in osteoarthritis, c: analysis. In: Bird HA and Dougados M (eds) Imaging techniques part I: traditional methods. Baillière's Clin Rheumatol 10:421–428
70. Cummings SR, Black D (1986) Should perimenopausal women be screened for osteoporosis? Ann Intern Med 104:817–823

71. Buckland-Wright JC, Macfarlane DG, Lynch JA, Jasani MK (1995c) Quantitative micro-focal radiography detects changes in OA knee joint space width in patients in placebo-controlled trial of NSAID therapy. J Rheumatol 22:937–943
72. Fife RS, Brandt KD, Braunstein EM, Katz BP, Shelbourne KD, Kalasinski LA, Ryan S (1991) Relationship between arthroscopic evidence of cartilage damage and radiographic evidence of joint space narrowing in early osteoarthritis of the knee. Arthritis Rheum 34:377–382
73. Bourke GJ, Daly LE, McGiluray J. Interpretation and uses of Medical Statistics. Blackwell, Oxford

5.3
Magnetic Resonance Imaging in Osteoarthritis

Y. Jiang, C. G. Peterfy, J. J. Zhao, D. L. White, J. A. Lynch and H. K. Genant

5.3.1
Introduction

Magnetic Resonance Imaging (MRI) is a complex technology which has advanced rapidly since its introduction to medical science in the early 1970s, and which has revolutionized medical imaging in general. A non-invasive technique with no ionizing radiation, MRI depicts anatomy with true multi-planar versatility and provides three dimensional (3-D) images in arbitrary orientations, though it is relatively expensive and time consuming. Because earlier MRI technique had limited spatial resolution and poor contrast between cartilage and adjacent structures, the use of MRI in osteoarthritis has been comparatively slow to develop. Many of these earlier difficulties have been overcome by progressive improvements in MRI hardware, e.g., gradient strength and performance and coil design, and to the development of more efficient pulse sequences and cartilage-selective techniques [1–3]. Generally, patients tolerate this technique well, allowing repeated serial examinations, and offering the opportunity to register serially acquired images, and to monitor changes over time. Clinical MRI systems at most major hospitals in the world can perform sophisticated examinations making multi-institutional and even multinational investigations feasible [4, 5]. MRI will undoubtedly play an increasingly important role in the development of our understanding of osteoarthritis as well as in our efforts to combat the disease.

Morphological changes in osteoarthritis can be measured by direct inspection of the joint with arthroscopy, or through noninvasive imaging techniques. The inability to evaluate articular cartilage and other important articular tissues non-invasively has been a major problem in the study and treatment of osteoarthritis. Unlike x-ray based imaging modalities such as radiography or CT that provide information mainly on osseous changes [6–9], MRI is capable of visualizing simultaneously all components of the joint (Fig. 1), in addition to potentially quantifying compositional and functional parameters of articular tissues relevant to osteoarthritis. This capability for whole-organ evaluation of the joint is

Fig. 1. Three-dimensional display of the knee MRI shows the articular cartilage in yellow and joint fluid in blue, as viewed from a posteromedial vantage point

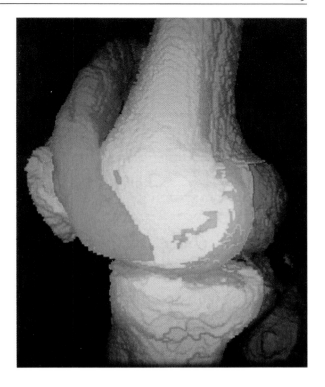

particularly cogent to the current view of osteoarthritis as a disease of organ failure, analogous to heart failure. Unlike other imaging techniques for which the image greyscale is generally linked to only one or two tissue characteristics (e. g., physical density and atomic number for radiography and CT, acoustic impedance mismatch for ultrasonography, and differential uptake of radiotracer for scintigraphy), MRI owes its great range of different tissue contrast to as many as six tissue characteristics (proton density, T_1 relaxation, T_2 and T_2^* relaxation, proton diffusion and bulk flow, magnetization transfer, magnetic susceptibility). The degree to which each of these factors influences the MRI depends on the pulse sequence and the imaging parameters used. This adds to the complexity of MRI. Considerable technical expertise is necessary to properly utilize this sophisticated modality and to interpret its images.

5.3.2
Technical Considerations

5.3.2.1
Basic Principles of MRI

MRI is based on the natural magnetization produced by hydrogen nuclei (protons) or "spins" as they spin or precess about their axes, and on the application of high magnetic fields, transmission of radiofrequency (rf) waves and detection of rf signals from protons. The most abundant sources of hydrogen protons in the body are water (H_2O) and fat ($-CH_2-$), and it is from these two substances that MRI derives virtually all of its signal. When the protons are placed within the very high magnetic field (B_0) in the bore of an MR imager magnet, they show a net tendency to align their nuclear magnetic moments along this magnetic field (longitudinal magnetization), much like a compass needle aligns with the magnetic field of the earth. The precession frequency (resonant frequency or Larmor frequency) of the protons is directly proportional to the field strength of the magnet, which may vary from 0.1 tesla to 2.0 tesla for clinical MR imaging scanners. Exposure of these protons to a second field rf pulse that is rotating and perpendicular to the original static field of the magnet and tuned to the resonant frequency of the protons (90° rf pulse) resonates and realigns the protons transversely (transverse magnetization) with this new field. This rotation of one magnetic field (the proton fields) against another (the main magnetic field) induces an alternating electrical current in receiver wires in an imaging coil near the patient. This current is fed to a computer for analysis to generate the MR image by Fourier transformation. The magnitude of this current and, therefore, the signal intensity on an MRI depend on regional variations in the amount of hydrogen protons in a sample, micromagnetic influences exerted on these protons by other substances in the sample, and the type and timing of the radio-frequency pulses used during imaging. The multiplicity of factors gives an unparalleled range of tissue contrast on MRI.

5.3.2.1.1
T1 Relaxation

Once the rf pulse is turned off, the protons relax, gradually tipping back to their original longitudinal alignment with the static field of the MRI magnet. This process of recovering longitudinal magnetization is called spin-lattice or T1 relaxation. Some substances, such as fat, show very rapid T1 relaxation, while others, such as water, show slow recovery of T1 relaxation. Under conditions of rapid rf pulsing (typically, a sequence of 192 to 512 rf pulses is used to generate MRI), slow-T1 substances, such as water, are not given sufficient time to recover between the pulses, and therefore exhibit low signal intensity, while fast-T1 substances, such as fat, show high signal intensity. Short-TR (repetition time, e.g., 500 msec) sequences therefore generate contrast (relative signal intensity difference) among tissues on the basis of differences in T1 and are accordingly referred to as T1 weighted. "Paramagnetic" substances, such as methemoglobin found in subacute hematomas, and gadolinium (Gd)-containing MRI contrast media (e.g., Gd-DTPA), increase T1 recovery in adjacent water protons and thereby increase their signal intensity on short-TR (T1-weighted) images. If, alternatively, a long TR (e.g., 2000 msec) is used, permitting both fat and water to almost completely recover, both substances generate high signal intensity.

5.3.2.1.2
T2 Relaxation

T2 relaxation refers to the loss of transverse magnetization, and therefore signal, as individual protons fall out of phase with each other. Since the resonant frequency of individual protons is dependent on the field strength of their immediate magnetic environment, microheterogeneities in the field resulting from effects of neighboring proton fields on each other will cause internuclear differences in precession frequency leading to loss of phase coherence among adjacent protons. Loss of phase coherence of the individual magnetic moments decreases the magnitude of the mean net magnetization vector, and therefore the MRI signal observed.

MRI signal can be sampled at different times by generating "echoes" with either a 180° "rephasing" rf pulse (spin echo technique) or a sudden reversal of the polarity of the magnetic gradient used for spatial encoding (gradient echo). The later this echo is acquired, i. e., the longer the echo time (TE), the greater the degree of dephasing that will have occurred, and thus the smaller the amplitude of the echo. Accordingly, free water, which shows slow T2 relaxation, retains relatively high signal intensity on spin-echo MRI acquired with long (>80 msec) TE, while fat and bound water appear dark on the same long-TE images.

5.3.2.1.3
Magnetic Susceptibility Effects and T2* Relaxation

Warping of the magnetic field at interfaces between substances that have very different magnetic susceptibilities (the degree to which a substance magnetizes when exposed to a magnetic field) also dephases local protons. Magnetic-susceptibility effects occur between trabecular bone and marrow tissue, at the boundary between articular cartilage and subchondral bone, and in tissues containing hemosiderin deposits from chronic hemorrhage, heavy calcification or metal, e. g., following surgery. Signal loss resulting from the combination of fixed magnetic heterogeneities (magnetic susceptibility effects) and internuclear interactions (T2 relaxation) is referred to as T2* relaxation, which is usually considerably shorter than T2. Signal lost to fixed magnetic heterogeneities, but not that lost to T2 relaxation, can be recovered by rephasing the protons with a 180° rf pulse (spin echo). Long echo time (TE) sequences thus generate contrast among tissues on the basis of T2, and when combined with a long TR to minimize the effects of T1 on contrast, are referred to as T2-weighted. The spin-echo technique corrects for fixed magnetic heterogeneities and therefore can generate true T2-weighted images, while the gradient-echo technique, which is faster than spin echo but does not correct for magnetic susceptibility effects, produces so-called T2*-weighted images which are highly vulnerable to magnetic susceptibility effects, such as those caused by metallic prostheses. The signal intensity of fat in the marrow space, which has a heterogeneous magnetic field, is lower than that of fat in adipose tissue when imaged with gradient-echo technique, while fat in both compartments appears the same with spin echo imaging. Magnetic susceptibility effects are more severe on high field strength magnets.

Since T_1, T_2 and T_2^* relaxation occur simultaneously in any tissue during MR imaging, tissues are discriminated on MRI by manipulating imaging parameters, such as TR, TE and flip angle, and by the use of contrast agents.

Both T_1-weighting (short TR) and T_2-weighting (long TE) involve discarding MR signal. If these effects are eliminated, signal intensity reflects only the proton density. Accordingly, long-TR/short-TE images are often referred to as proton-density-weighted. However, even the shortest finite TE attainable is too long to completely escape T_2 relaxation, and extremely long TRs (> 2500 msec) are not practical for imaging *in vivo*. Therefore, even so called proton-density-weighted images contain some T_1 and T_2 contrast.

The MRI spatial resolution is determined by the dimensions of voxels, or the individual volume elements. All signals within a single voxel are averaged. Therefore, if an interface with high signal intensity on one side and low signal intensity on the other side passes through the middle of a voxel, the interface is depicted as an intermediate signal intensity band the width of the voxel. This effect is known as partial-volume averaging. Voxel size is determined by multiplying slice thickness by the pixels (picture elements), the size of the in-plane subdivisions of the image. Pixel size, in turn, is determined by dividing the field of view (FOV) by the image matrix. The smaller the voxel, the greater the spatial resolution. However, as voxel size decreases, so does signal-to-noise ratio (S/N). Accordingly, high-resolution imaging requires sufficient S/N to support the spatial resolution. S/N can be increased by shortening TE (less T_2 decay), increasing TR (more T_1 recovery), imaging at higher field strength (greater longitudinal magnetization) or utilizing specialized coils which reduce noise (small surface coil, quadrature coil, phased array of small coils). Specialized sequences, such as three-dimensional (3-D) gradient echo also provide greater S/N.

5.3.2.2
Imaging Sequences

5.3.2.2.1
Spin Echo

Spin echo, a commonly used sequence for most clinical MRI applications (Figs. 2–4), uses a 180° rf pulse to rephase the protons following the original 90° excitation pulse. It has the advantage of correcting for fixed magnetic heterogeneities and minimizing susceptibility effects.

T_1-weighted spin echo images attempt to separate different tissues on the basis of inherent differences in T_1 relaxation by employing short TR. T_2 decay is minimized on these images by using short TE. Substances that show high signal intensity on T_1-weighted images include fat, methemoglobin in subacute hematomas, and substances exposed to Gd-containing contrast agents. Most other substances appear dark on T_1-weighted images. The T_2-weighted spin-echo technique attempts to discriminate tissues on the basis of inherent differences in T_2 relaxation by using long TE. Tissues that show high signal intensity on T_2-weighted images contain significant amounts of free water.

Fig. 2. Osteoarthritis in the knee. Coronal gradient spine-echo T1 weighted image shows large marginal osteophytes of the femoral condyles and the tibial plateaus

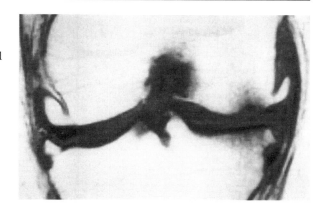

Fig. 3 A, B. Coronal spin-echo T1 weighted (**A**) and gradient-echo T 2* weighted (**B**) images show advanced changes of osteoarthritis of the glenohumeral joint, with joint space narrowing, osteophyte formation, loss of articular cartilage, and subchondral cystic changes

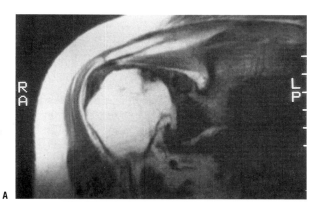

A

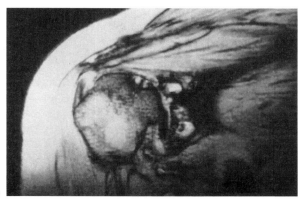

B

Fig. 4A–C. Osteoarthritis in the ankle. Coronal (**A**) and sagittal (**B**) spin-echo T1 weighted, and sagittal gradient-echo T2* weighted (**C**) images of the ankle show joint space narrowing, osteophyte formation, loss of articular cartilage, and cystic changes in the sub-chondral bone

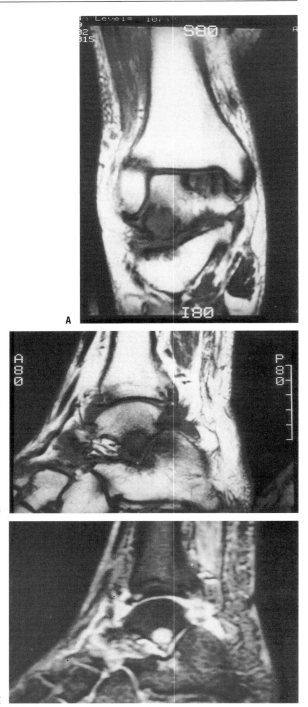

T2-weighted imaging, however, requires relatively long imaging times because of the long TR, and offers poor S/N because of signal decay due to T2 relaxation. Proton-density-weighted images collect an earlier echo (short TE) while waiting for the late-echo (long-TE) in the sequence, as the short-TE images have greater S/N and provide better anatomical detail, but depict both free water and fat with high signal intensity and provide poor image contrast between fat and water. Abnormalities such as trauma, infection or neoplasia arising in adipose or the fatty marrow may not be apparent on proton-density-weighted images.

5.3.2.2.2
Gradient Echo

Gradient-echo technique employs partial flip-angles ($< 90°$) and collects echoes by gradient reversal rather than $180°$ rf pulses. It is faster than spin echo. The rapid speed permits 3-D acquisition which allows thinner slice thicknesses and improves S/N.

5.3.2.2.3
Fast Spin Echo

This recently introduced technique is capable of generating heavily T2-weighted spin echo images with high spatial resolution in only a fraction of the time required for conventional spin echo imaging. It is particularly useful for imaging the articular cartilage. However, fat tends to remain high in signal intensity even on relatively long-TE fast spin-echo images and may obscure abnormalities in fatty tissue. This often necessitates the use of fat suppression (Fig. 5).

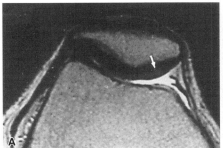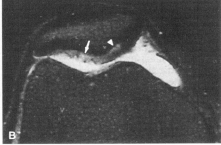

Fig. 5A, B. Patterns of signal alteration in articular cartilage. A Axial T2-weighted fast spin echo image of the patella (TR 2500, TE 102, 8 echo train) shows a focus of increased signal intensity just beneath the bulging but otherwise intact articular surface (*arrow*). B Axial T2 weighted fast spin echo image of the patella (same parameters as A) obtained with fat suppression shows transmural signal increase and surface fraying in the cartilage over the lateral facet (*arrow*) as well as deep linear signal paralleling the subchondral surface of the medial facet (*arrowhead*). The deep signal pattern may reflect early basal delamination of the cartilage from mechanical failure, an abnormality that may not be apparent on arthroscopy

5.3.2.2.4
Fat Suppression

The most widely used technique for suppressing signal from fat on MRI is called frequency-selective saturation. Protons in fat precess at different frequency than those in water because of their different microenvironment, a phenomenon known as chemical shift. By applying a narrow bandwidth rf saturating pulse tuned to the frequency of fat at the beginning of the sequence, the magnetization of fat protons can be selectively suppressed or saturated with no significant effect on protons in water. This technique, also called chemical-shift selective (CHESS) fat suppression, applied to a T 2-weighted fast spin echo sequence generates images in which fat has a low signal intensity while free water in fatty tissue has a high signal intensity (Figs. 5, 6). Subtle T1 contrast, e. g., between articular cartilage and synovial fluid, is usually overshadowed on T1-weighted images by the far greater difference in signal intensity between fat and most other tissues. By selectively suppressing the signal intensity of fat, it is possible to expand the scale of image intensities across smaller differences in T1, augmenting residual T1 contrast. Fat saturation can also be used to increase contrast between fat and other substances on T1-weighted images, such as high signal intensity methemoglobin and gadolinium (Gd)-containing contrast material, which also show rapid T1 relaxation.

5.3.2.2.5
Magnetization Transfer

A similar technique can be used to suppress the signal of water indirectly through a mechanism called magnetization transfer. Magnetization transfer

Fig. 6. Fat-suppressed T1-weighted 3-D gradient-echo image of the knee from a normal volunteer offers superb morphological delineation of articular cartilage

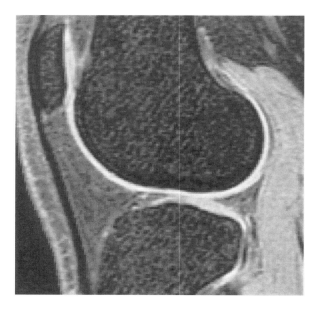

reflects the thermodynamic equilibrium between freely mobile protons in tissue water, and protons constrained by macromolecules within the same tissue. Since the macromolecular protons are relatively immobile, they exhibit an extremely short T_2 relaxation time (<1 msec) and do not contribute directly to the MR signal on conventional MRI. Selective loss of longitudinal magnetization from this pool, invoked by a number of different techniques [10], causes a transfer of magnetization from the MR-visible pool of mobile water protons to the MR-invisible macromolecular pool in order to maintain equilibrium. This manifests as a loss of signal intensity from the tissue depending on the tissue-specific rate constant for this equilibrium reaction and the relative proportions of water and macromolecular protons in the tissue. Collagen is a particularly good macromolecular substrate for this reaction [11]. Cartilage [12], hyperplastic synovium [13] and muscle also exhibit pronounced magnetization-transfer effect [3, 11, 14]. Fat and joint fluid, on the other hand, do not show any substantial magnetization transfer and thus do not loose signal intensity under conditions in which macromolecular protons are selectively saturated. These tissue-dependent differences in susceptibility to magnetization transfer can be exploited to generate additional image contrast among articular structures [12, 14]. In addition, it may be possible to quantify specific macromolecular constituents of different tissues by measuring the magnetization-transfer effect. In cartilage, for example, collagen is the dominant macromolecule involved, with only minor contributions, if any, made by proteoglycans and other constituents [11]. Magnetization-transfer techniques are therefore useful for imaging the articular cartilage (Figs. 7, 8).

5.3.3
MRI of Articular Cartilage

5.3.3.1
Histological, Biochemical, and MRI Features of Normal Articular Cartilage

The MRI appearance of articular cartilage reflects its complex histological and biochemical composition (Figs. 6, 8, 9) [15–17]. It is a relatively fibrous tissue with marked three-dimensional anisotropy. It can be conceptualized as two phases: a fluid phase composed of water and ions, and a solid one consisting of aggregated proteoglycans and other glycoproteins, fibrous collagen, and chondrocytes [17]. The deepest layer of cartilage (constituting approximately 5% of the total thickness) is calcified and serves to anchor an extensive network of collagen fibrils radiating from the subjacent calcified layer towards the surface in large dense bundles connected by numerous smaller cross ties or bridging fibrils. This deep noncalcified layer is known as the radial zone. More superficially, in the upper radial zone, the individual collagen fibrils become thinner and band together in a more regular and tight parallel array with fewer cross ties [18]. Superficial to this layer, the transitional zone contains more randomly organized collagen fibrils with numerous obliquely oriented fibrils to resist the shearing forces that arise in this region [17]. The most superficial zone at the articular surface is a thin layer of densely packed, tangentially arranged collagen fibrils known as the superficial tangential zone, which resist tensile

Fig. 7 A, B. Magnetization-transfer subtraction technique for depicting articular cartilage. Sagittal images of an amputated knee after intraarticular injection of 55 ml saline to simulate a joint effusion. **A** Conventional T2*-weighted, thin-partitioned sagittal 3-D gradient echo (TR 60, TE 7, flip angle 20°) shows poor contrast between cartilage (*c*) and joint fluid (*e*). **B** Addition of pulsed magnetization transfer to the same imaging sequence markedly decreased signal intensity in cartilage (*c*) but has significantly less effect on effusion (*e*), bone (*b*), or adipose tissue (*f*). This combined high cartilage fluid contrast with sufficient spatial resolution to allow delineation of small surface defects in the cartilage (*long arrow*) in addition to more generalized area of cartilage thinning (*arrowheads*). Contrast at the cartilage-bone interface, however, was decreased

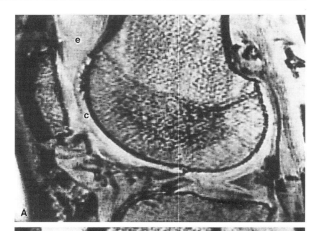

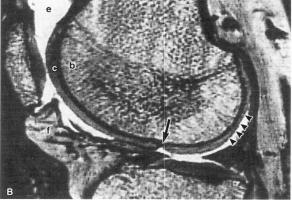

forces during compressive loading and form a water-impermeable barrier to interstitial fluid loss during compression [17]. The fine network of collagen fibrils in cartilage is further organized into parallel leaves or lamina that radiate vertically from the calcified zone [16]. Superficially, these lamina become thinner and arch over to form tightly packed horizontal leaves at the articular surface, though the fibrils of the superficial tangential zone are not necessarily continuous with those of the deeper layers [19].

Trapped within this complex fibrous meshwork are numerous aggregated (compressed) proteoglycan molecules [17]. Hydrophilic proteoglycan molecules maintain a high water content and therefore a high proton density in cartilage, since negatively charged SO_3^- and COO^- moieties in the glycosaminoglycans (GAG) of the proteoglycans repel each other, and attract counter ions (usually Na^+) that in turn draw water osmotically into the cartilage. The combination of electrostatic repulsion between adjacent GAGs and Donnan osmotic pressure produces a swelling pressure that keeps the articular cartilage inflated and the collagen fibrils under tension. The balance between this swelling pressure and

Fig. 8A, B. Osteoarthritis in the patellofemoral joint. Axial gradient-echo T2* weighted images (A) on which articular cartilage can not be appreciated, while magnetization transfer subtraction image (B) clearly demonstrates articular cartilage. Both images reveal osteophyte formation at the joint margins, and increased amount of a joint effusion

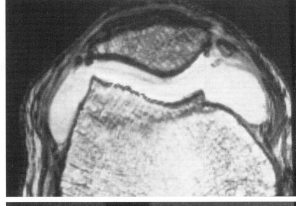

A

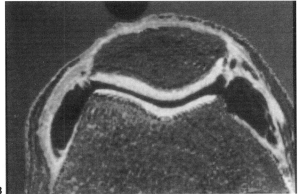

B

the uniform resistance provided by the collagen network determines the degree of compression of the proteoglycan molecules, the number of negative charges exposed, and therefore the level of hydration of the articular cartilage. Water content is greatest at the articular surface and decreases slightly towards the subchondral bone [17, 20, 21]. Proteoglycan concentration, on the other hand, increases in the deep layers of cartilage [21, 22]; though these deep proteoglycans appear to be more highly aggregated [23].

Cartilage water resides primarily in the interfibrilar space due to the high osmotic pressure. Since the superficial tangential zone of cartilage is impermeable to water, compression of the cartilage causes interstitial water to flow horizontally through the porous solid matrix, proteoglycans and collagen. Resistance to this flow of water is extremely high due to the presence of chondroitin sulfate, and water is thus forced to bear the majority of the compressive load [17]. This fluid pressurization mechanism is the basis for the compressive stiffness of cartilage and its load bearing capacity.

This high proton density constitutes the potential for generating MR signal in cartilage. However, equally important as the amount of water protons is their state. Constraint or "binding" of otherwise mobile protons primarily by col-

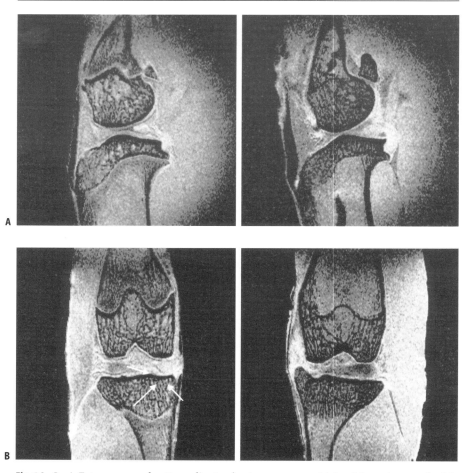

Fig. 9A–B. **A** Fat-suppressed 3-D gradient-echo images were obtained from knees of adult rabbits, using a Helmholtz coil and a 2-Tesla system (GE/Bruker), imaged in sagittal plane (TR 110/TE 3.5 ms; NEX 2; fat-sat; voxel dimensions 137 μm X 137 μm in-plane X 312 μm thick). The acquisition time was 1 h. Sagittal slice through the medial chondyle show normal structure of cartilage, menisci, subchondral bone and trabecular bone network in normal control (*left*); decreased cartilage thickness, osteosclerosis and osteophytes at 3-month post bilateral partial medial meniscectomy. **B** Coronal slices near the anterior edge of the tibial plateau through the medial chondyle show normal structure of cartilage and subchondral bone and trabecular bone network in normal control (*left*), subchondral osteosclerosis and a large conspicuous osteophyte on the medial margin of the tibial plateau of a meniscectomized knee (*right*).

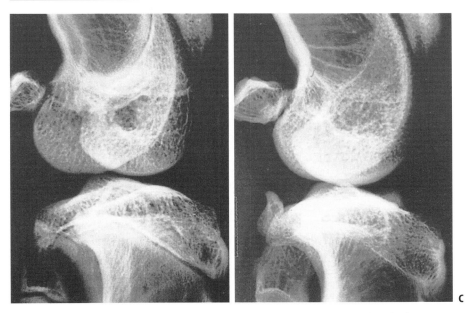

C

Fig. 9C. Radiographs show normal structure of subchondral bone and trabecular bone network in a normal knee of a control rabbit (*left*), increased thickness and density of the subchondral bone and osteosclerosis of a menisectomized rabbit (*right*)

lagen promotes T2 relaxation and speeds up the rate of signal loss. The content and distribution of hydrophilic proteoglycan molecules and the anisotropic organization of collagen fibrils influence not only the amount of water, i.e., proton density, in cartilage but also the state or the relaxation properties, i.e., T2, of this water, giving cartilage a characteristic "zonal" or laminate appearance on MRI [21, 24–26]. On very short TE images (<5 msec) higher resolution images of cartilage typically show a bi-laminar appearance with a low signal superficial lamina corresponding to the superficial tangential cone and the remainder of the cartilage (Gold et al).

Also, some of the zones may not be visible under certain conditions. The thin, low signal-intensity bands in the superficial tangential zone (the first zone), and upper radial zone (the third zone) can be obscured by partial-volume averaging in curved and obliquely sectioned portions of the cartilage [18]. Because of the linear parallel arrangement of collagen in the radial zone, when the fibrils are oriented at 55° relative to the static magnetic field, angular anisotropy of T2 relaxation or magic-angle phenomenon can result in increased signal intensity in the normally low signal-intensity lamina [18, 27]. The superficial tangential zone also shows angular anisotropy of T2, though the orientation of these fibrils varies from site to site on the articular surface [4]. Also, this zone will not be visible when viewed against a dark background, e.g., joint fluid on fat-suppressed, T1-weighted gradient echo images.

On intermediate TE images (5–40 msec) cartilage shows a trilaminar appearance: a low-signal superficial lamina; an intermediate-signal transitional and upper radial lamina; and a low-signal deep lamina composed of the remainder of the upper radial, deep radial and deep calcified zones [4, 28]. With very heavy T 2-weighting, signal also drops out of the transitional lamina, and cartilage becomes homogeneously low in signal intensity. When low spatial resolution is employed additional lamina may sometimes appear on short TE images. These are due to truncation artifacts from the high contrast at the cartilage/fluid interface [18], and can be avoided by increasing the matrix size.

5.3.3.2
Compositional Changes in Cartilage in Osteoarthritis

In early osteoarthritis, there is a net degradation of collagen in the superficial layers of cartilage, resulting in surface fibrillation and increased permeability to water [29]. As proteoglycans are lost, the remaining compressed proteoglycans are allowed to swell and thus expose more negatively-charged GAGs to attract cations and water [17, 30–35]. However, proteoglycan loss decreases the frictional drag on interstitial water flow and thus undermines the fluid pressurization mechanism and compressive stiffness of cartilage. This has the effect of transferring more of the load to the already weakened solid matrix [17]. This renders the swollen, edematous cartilage more susceptible to mechanical injury. Ultimately the cartilage either repairs itself or breaks down and sloughs off.

Acute mechanical trauma and compressive loading can develop transverse shear forces and cause horizontal cracks in the deep calcified layer of cartilage [36] and separation of the cartilage from subchondral bone [33]. Basal splitting or delamination of the cartilage in this manner may be a mechanism of cartilage degeneration [36–38] not only in normal cartilage exposed to excessive mechanical loading, but also in osteoarthritis, in which joint laxity and shifting contact points during normal activity may overload areas of abnormally weakened cartilage.

Increases in cartilage water content increase the proton density of cartilage, and removal of the intrinsic T 2-shortening effects of the proteoglycan-collagen matrix on water unmasks more of the water signal [39], which increase the signal intensity (Fig. 5) in areas of matrix damage on conventional MRI sequences. This is early chondromalacia, the earliest sign of cartilage injury, and may be seen before any loss of thickness has occurred. There may be mild swelling of the cartilage during this stage. As the compositional and biomechanical properties of articular cartilage continue to deteriorate, substance loss begins to occur. This may be focal or diffuse, restricted to superficial fraying and fibrillation, or involve partial to full thickness of cartilage. In some cases, focal swelling or "blistering" of the cartilage may be seen without disruption of the articular surface [19]. Consistent with this, foci of high signal intensity are often seen in the cartilage of osteoarthritis patients on T 2-weighted images, and have been shown to correspond to arthroscopically demonstrable abnormalities [40, 41]. Patterns of abnormal cartilage signal include superficial, transmural and deep linear changes. The latter may reflect deep degenerative changes initiated by basal delamination of the cartilage at the calcified layer or tide mark [33, 36, 37], Early changes confined to the deep layers of cartilage, may not be detectable by inspection of the articular surface alone during arthroscopy; although, focal separation in the deep layers of cartilage may ultimately lead to attrition of the overlying cartilage, occasionally with in growth of the subchondral bone to form a central osteophyte.

In addition to subjective examinations using specialized techniques, it is possible to obtain quantitative information about the composition of articular cartilage. For example, the fractional water content and the diffusion coefficient of water in cartilage can be accurately measured with noninvasive MRI techniques [42, 43]. Both of these parameters increase with damage to the proteoglycan and collagen matrix in cartilage disease. The concentration of mobile protons (water content) in cartilage decreases from the articular surface to the subchondral bone, which is consistent with direct measurements using other techniques [20]. Proteoglycan content can also be probed by cationic MR contrast agents, such as manganese (Mn^{++}), in much the same way that the cationic dye, toludine blue, is used to stain cartilage proteoglycans on histological preparations [44], or by imaging sodium instead of hydrogen [45]. Manganese shortens T1 relaxation and therefore increases the signal intensity of cartilage on T1-weighted images in proportion to the negative charge density, i.e., GAG content of the tissue. Fujioka, et. al [46] have shown decreased Mn^{++} enhancement in osteoarthritic cartilage.

It is also possible to quantify T2 changes using widely available techniques [28, 47]. By combining the data from images of the same cartilage acquired with several different TE's, it is possible to estimate the T2 of the cartilage by fitting an exponential curve to the observed signal intensity values for each pixel. The T2 can be estimated in this way for a specific region of interest in the cartilage, or depicted in image mode as a map of the entire cartilage in which the signal intensity of each pixel corresponds to the T2 at that site [28]. However, this approach, while widely available and relatively easy to use tends to underestimate T2, partly because of increased diffusion-related effects with increasing TE [48]. Underestimation of T2 is greatest in chondromalacic cartilage, where water diffusion is increased. Unless special techniques are employed, the potential increase in T2 measurable with this technique in chondromalacic cartilage will be slightly suppressed by diffusion-related effects. Nevertheless, large changes of T2 might still be demonstrable.

MRI thus shows considerable promise for detecting and monitoring very early compositional changes in degenerating articular cartilage.

5.3.3.3
Morphological Changes in Cartilage

Evaluation of morphological changes in cartilage is dependent on high spatial resolution and high contrast at the articular surface and the cartilage bone interface. This is best achieved with a fat-suppressed, T1 weighted 3-D gradient-echo technique [4] which has been shown to accurately detect focal defects as verified by arthroscopy and direct inspection of cadaveric specimens. A virtually identical contrast pattern can be achieved with magnetization-transfer subtraction images that depict the articular cartilage as an isolated band of high signal intensity sharply contrasted against the adjacent low signal intensity joint fluid, intraarticular adipose tissue and subchondral bone marrow, but this method is twice as slow since subtraction is required, less widely available than fat-suppressed T1-weighted imaging [3, 13]. Subtraction of images acquired with and without the magnetization-transfer pulse produce a map of the tissue distribution of magnetization transfer in the joint.

In addition to subjective evaluation of focal defects, surface irregularities, and generalized thinning of articular cartilage on a slice-by-slice basis (Figs. 2–5, 9–11), a variety of morphological parameters, such as the thickness, volume, geometry and surface topography of cartilage can be quantified using 3-D MRI data. By summing the voxels contained with in the 3-D reconstructed image of the cartilage, the exact volume of these complexly shaped structures can be determined [84]. Moreover, unlike cartilage thickness measurements made from individual sections, values for total cartilage volume are relatively unaffected by minor variations in the plane of section and are less demanding in terms of spatial resolution. Total volume is therefore a more robust parameter for serial measurements in patients with arthritis. In a study of whole amputated knees and patellar specimens obtained from total knee arthroplasty, the volume of articular cartilage over the femur, tibia and patella determined by MRI correlated well with the corresponding volumes determined by scraping the cartilage off the bones and measuring their displacement of water in graduated cylinders [3]. This technique may therefore be useful for monitoring changes in cartilage volume over time in patients with arthritis. Currently, measuring cartilage volume in this way demands considerable human input. Accurate segmentation of the articular cartilage, especially in patients with

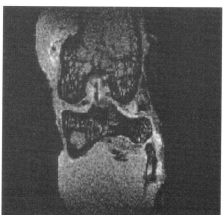 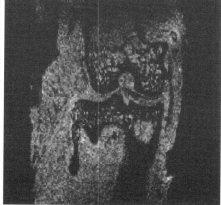

Fig. 10. Coronal sections near the posterior part of the tibial plateau through the medial chondyle show normal structure of cartilage and subchondral bone and trabecular bone network in the control knee (*left*); decreased cartilage thickness and subchondral osteosclerosis in the other knee (*right*) with anterior cruciate ligament tear of a same rabbit

Fig. 11. Fat-suppressed T1-weighted 3-D gradient-echo image of the knee from a patient with osteoarthritis shows osteophytes in the patellar, the distal femur, and the proximal tibia, and decreased cartilage thickness

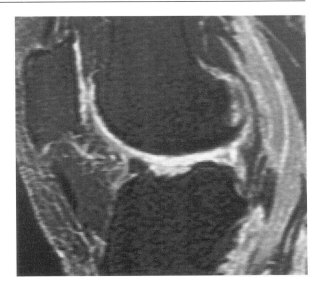

osteoarthritis, requires special expertise and perceptual skills on the part of the reader. Although many techniques available today are at least semi-automated, an experienced eye is still necessary to confirm and, often, to edit manually the primary segmentation to assure accuracy. Improvements in the degree of automation of this process would be extremely useful.

Total volume measurements offer little spatial information about the distribution of changes and are relatively insensitive to focal loss. Theoretically, a loss of cartilage in one region could be balanced by an equivalent increase in volume elsewhere in the joint, and thereby elude detection by this method. By subdividing 3-D reconstructions of the articular cartilage into several smaller regions [49] it is possible to evaluate the volume at specific sites, such as the weight-bearing surfaces of the femorotibial joints. However, the precision of such measurements decreases as the subdivisions are made smaller. Ultimately, extremely high spatial resolution is necessary to maintain precision. If sufficient resolution can be achieved within a reasonable imaging time, the prospect of mapping the cartilage thickness in vivo becomes feasible (Fig. 12) [50, 51]. Cartilage thickness maps may render insight into the importance of the location of cartilage lesions to the progression of osteoarthritis. Unlike total cartilage volume measurements, which are relatively unaffected by minor variations in limb orientation between serial examinations [3], monitoring cartilage thickness over time requires some method of precisely registering (i.e., realigning) and reslicing serially acquired images.

Image registration techniques that rely on matching anatomical structures or surfaces, or externally placed markers [52, 53] are limited by the image resolution because the criteria used to specify the landmarks are defined only to the nearest voxel. Pixel-intensity correlation techniques [54, 55], however, are capable of matching images to within a fraction of a voxel [56]. Therefore, with adequate

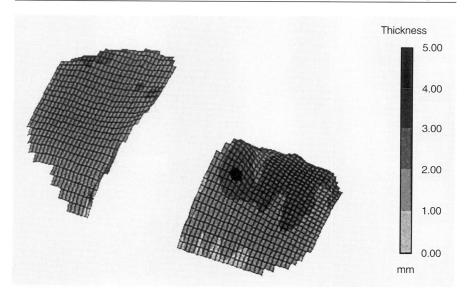

Fig. 12. Cartilage thickness map of the tibial cartilages in a human knee *in vivo*. B-spline geometric models of the tibial cartilages were generated using the same method as for *in situ* contact area mapping by MR imaging. Regional cartilage thickness (perpendicular to the cartilage-bone interface) is depicted in intervals of 1 mm

attention to spatial resolution and precise image registration [85], it should be feasible to monitor regional changes in cartilage thickness in individual patients over time using MRI; although, this has yet to be demonstrated directly.

5.3.4
MRI of Bone and Bone Marrow in Osteoarthritis and Related Conditions

Calcification and cortical and trabecular bone does not generate any detectable signal because of its relative lack of constituent hydrogen protons, and are depicted as curvilinear signal voids on MRI. They are silhouetted by the intermediate and high signal intensity tissues lining them, such as marrow and adipose. Bone abnormalities (Figs. 2–4, 9–11) associated with osteoarthritis include osteophytosis, subchondral bone sclerosis, subchondral cyst formation, and marrow edema. Because of its multiplanar tomographic capabilities, MRI is more sensitive than either projectional radiography (Fig. 9) or computed tomography (CT) for demonstrating most of these kind of changes [57]. Osteophytes also, are better delineated with MRI than by conventional radiography – particularly central osteophytes, which are especially difficult to identify radiographically [58]. Central osteophytes may develop for different reasons than marginal osteophytes and thus have different implications to the disease. Bone sclerosis is also visible on MRI and presents a low signal intensity on all pulse sequences due to the presence of dense calcification and fibrosis. MRI is also capable of delineating sites of enthesitis and periostitis. High resolution MRI is an additional MR-based technique for studying trabecular microarchitecture [59, 60]. It may be possible to monitor trabecular changes in the subchondral bone, in order to determine their importance in the development and progression of osteoarthritis (Figs. 9, 10).

MRI is uniquely capable of imaging the bone marrow, and is currently the most sensitive, though not the most specific, technique for detecting osteonecrosis, osteomyelitis, infiltrating primary or secondary neoplasia, and trauma, especially bone contusion and undisplaced fracture [61]. Conditions arising in this compartment generally remain occult on radiographs until the cortical and trabecular bones themselves are affected. In each of these cases, increased free water, which appears low in signal intensity on T_1-weighted images and high in signal intensity on T_2-weighted images, shows high contrast with the normal marrow fat, which has high signal intensity on T_1-weighted images and low signal intensity on T_2-weighted images. An exception is T_2-weighted fast spin echo, which depicts both fat and water with relatively high signal intensity and requires fat suppression to generate contrast between these marrow constituents. Gradient echo techniques, at least at high field strengths, are generally insensitive to marrow pathology because of magnetic susceptibility effects in cancellous bone. Areas of subchondral marrow edema are often seen in joints with progressive osteoarthritis [37]. Usually, these areas of focal bone marrow edema in osteoarthritis develop at sites of articular cartilage loss or chondromalacia [62]. Histologically, these areas typically show fibrovascular infiltration. They may be due to mechanical injury to the subchondral bone caused by shifting articular contact points at sites of biomechanically failing cartilage and/or loss of joint stability, or presumably from pulsion of synovial fluid through the defect into uncovered subchondral bone. Occasionally, epiphyseal marrow edema is seen some distance from the articular surface or at enthyses. To what extent these marrow changes contribute to local pain and disability or are predictive of disease progression remains unclear.

5.3.5
MRI of Synovium and Joint Fluid

Normal synovium is generally too thin to visualize on conventional MRI, and can be difficult to discriminate from the adjacent joint fluid or articular cartilage. Some degree of synovial thickening can be found in a majority of osteoarthritic joints [63]. Whether this synovitis contributes directly to articular cartilage loss in osteoarthritis, or simply arises in reaction to the breakdown of cartilage by other causes remains uncertain [64]. However, synovitis may be important to the symptoms and disability of osteoarthritis, and may pose different treatment requirements than those directed only towards cartilage protection.

In many cases, the only sign of synovitis is the presence of a joint effusion. However, the amount of synovial fluid that normally resides in diarthroidial joints varies considerably throughout the body. The ankle in particular may contain a relatively large amount of synovial fluid under normal conditions [65].

The appropriate threshold for defining a quantity of joint fluid as abnormal is still unknown. Using 3-D reconstruction methods, it is possible to quantify the amount of free fluid in a joint by MRI [66]. This may be useful for monitoring treatment response in patients with arthritis or for studying the normal role of synovial fluid in joint physiology *in vivo*.

The signal behavior of nonhemorrhagic joint fluid is dominated by free water and with slow T_1 recovery and slow T_2 decay, and so shows intensely high signal on T_2-weighted images. Hemorrhagic effusions may contain methemoglobin, which has a very short T_1 and shows high signal intensity on T_1-weighted images, and/or deoxyhemoglobin, which shows rapid T_2 relaxation and thus appears low in signal intensity on T_2-weighted images. In chronic recurrent hemarthrosis, hemosiderin accumulation in the synovium may lower signal intensity on both T_1- and T_2-weighted images. Hemorrhage often develops in popliteal cysts as they dissect between the gastrocnemius and soleus muscles of the calf. Leakage of synovial fluid from ruptured Baker's cysts may produce a feathery pattern of free water signal or Gd-DTPA enhancement along the fascial planes between the muscles behind the knee [67].

Inflamed, edematous synovium usually exhibits slow T_2 relaxation reflecting its high interstitial water content. It may be difficult to discriminate thickened synovial tissue from adjacent joint fluid or cartilage. Hemosiderin deposition or chronic fibrosis can lower the signal intensity of hyperplastic synovial tissue on long-TE images (T_2-weighted) and occasionally even short-TE images (T_1-weighted, proton-density-weighted, all gradient-echo sequences). Most synovial tissue exhibits a slightly shorter T_1 than does joint fluid, but under normal circumstances the contrast on T_1-weighted images is relatively poor.

Gadolinium, a heavy metal, exerts a paramagnetic effect on nearby water protons causing them to relax more rapidly by T_1. Water-containing tissues exposed to chelates of Gd (e.g., Gd-DTPA) show increased signal intensity on T_1-weighted images in proportion to the tissue concentration of this contrast material. Intravenously administered Gd-DTPA is rapidly distributed to vascular tissues such as inflamed synovium. Gd-DTPA, a relatively small molecule, diffuses rapidly out of even normal capillaries and leaks into the adjacent joint fluid over time [13, 68, 69]. Immediately after a bolus intravenous injection of Gd-DTPA, the synovial lining of a joint may appear discrete and intensely enhanced. Contrast between the high-signal intensity synovium and any adjacent high signal intensity adipose tissue can be augmented by fat suppression. Soon after, the zone of enhancement begins to thicken as the Gd-DTPA diffuses centripetally through the adjacent joint fluid, which may result in over estimation of the amount of synovial hyperplasia. The rate at which these two compartments equilibrate their signal intensities depends on a number of factors, including the rate of blood flow to the synovium, the volume of the synovial tissue, the total volume of the joint effusion, and the degree of mechanical mixing of the joint fluid. In an immobilized large joint, such as the knee, a sizable effusion may take as long as an hour to equilibrate with the synovial tissue, while in intensely inflamed or very small joints, such as the metacarpophalangeal joints, this equilibration can be extremely rapid (<5 min) [70]. Additionally, 10–15 min of active mobilization after injection can diffusely enhance the joint cavity and produce an arthrographic effect, or indirect MR arthrography, in even large joints [71]. Once in the joint fluid, electrostatic forces inhibit diffusion of this anionic agent into the negatively charged articular cartilage, and the articular cartilage is therefore delineated on T1-weighted images, though it may diffuse into diseased cartilage that is deficient in negatively charged proteoglycans [72].

In addition to quantifying the amount and distribution of inflamed synovium and joint fluid in arthritic joints, it is possible to objectively grade the severity of the synovitis by monitoring the rate of synovial enhancement with Gd-containing contrast over time using rapid, sequential T1-weighted MRI in one or several joints [69, 73 – 75]. A rapid synovial enhancement rate and high maximal enhancement following bolus injection of Gd-DTPA correlate with severe inflammation and hyperplasia, while sluggish enhancement corresponds to chronic fibrotic synovium. Though it is difficult to control for subtle differences in the pharmacokinetics of the Gd-DTPA between examinations, the slope and maxima of synovial enhancement – time curves correlate with the histological severity of the synovitis [75, 76], and can be shown to decrease markedly following therapy. In contrast, synovial enhancement rates did not correlate with the degree of synovial fibrosis or the degree of multiplication of the synovial lining.

5.3.6
MRI of Other Articular Components

The supporting articular structures, e.g., ligaments, menisci, local tendons, and glenoid labrum are important in maintaining the static and dynamic stability, efficient mechanical loading distribution, and functional integrity of the joints. Loss of these functions promotes biomechanical wear and ultimately joint failure. This is evident from the high incidence of osteoarthritis following meniscectomy [77–79], cruciate ligament tears, and rotator cuff tears [80]. These structure are composed primarily of collagen, which provides tensile strength but also constrains and dephases water protons. T2 relaxation is typically so rapid (<1 msec) [27] that most of the signal decays before it can be sampled by even the shortest TEs attainable with conventional MR systems (~5 msec), and generally appear low in signal intensity on all pulse sequences, silhouetted by high signal intensity substances, such as adipose fat or synovial fluid.

Intact ligaments appear as dark bands that can be traced to their insertions (Fig. 6). Discontinuity is intuitively a direct sign of ligamentous disruption. However, this may be mimicked by obliquity of the plane of section through an intact ligament. Special planes may be necessary to delineate certain ligaments. The anterior cruciate ligament in the knee is best seen on oblique sagittal images with the knee in neutral position, or on direct sagittal images with the leg in slight abduction, while the inferior glenohumeral ligament, a principal static stabilizer of the shoulder in abduction, is difficult to visualize unless the shoulder is positioned in abduction and external rotation [81]. With multiplanar reformatting, very thorough analysis of ligamentous integrity is possible regardless of the original plane of image acquisition.

The menisci consist of fibrocartilage and contain abundant collagen fibers spatially arranged to withstand the tensile stresses during weight bearing. Fiber orientation is predominantly circumferential, particularly in the peripheral half of the meniscus, which accounts for the propensity of tears to run longitudinally, as they follow the split lines between the collagen fibers rather than traversing fibers. When there is focal loss of collagen, as with myxoid or eosinophilic degeneration which is usually also accompanied by increased local water content, this $T2$-shortening effect is diminished and water signal is unmasked and manifests as globular or linear areas of intermediate signal intensity within the meniscus on short-TE images (i.e. $T1$-weighted or proton-density-weighted spin-echo or any gradient-echo sequence) that tend to fade away at longer TEs. These signal abnormalities are not tears and do not, in distinction, violate the articular surfaces of the meniscus. Meniscal tears can be associated with gross deformity of the meniscal surface, but most often are only apparent as linear intermediate signal intensity extending to an otherwise smooth articular surface on the short-TE images. Occasionally, a sufficient amount of joint fluid tracks into a meniscal tear to be visualized on $T2$-weighted images, but in most instances, undisplaced tears of the menisci cannot be seen on long-TE images. Short-TE images are thus highly sensitive (>90%) but somewhat nonspecific for meniscal tears, whereas long-TE images are insensitive, though highly specific when present.

MRI is sensitive to the full spectrum of tendon pathology, and has been shown to identify tendonitis and rupture with greater accuracy than clinical examination [82]. Normal tendons show smooth margins and homogeneously low signal intensity on long-TE ($T2$-weighted) MRI. Tendon rupture can be partial or complete, and is depicted by varying degrees of tendon discontinuity on MRI or high intratendinous signal intensity on $T2$-weighted MRI. In tenosynovitis, fluid can be seen within the tendon sheath, but the tendon itself appears normal. Tendonitis usually results in enlargement and irregularity of the tendon, but the most reliable sign is increased signal intensity within the tendon on $T2$-weighted images. Tendon rupture may result from mechanical fraying of tendons passing over jagged osteophytes and sharp-edged erosions, or from direct tenosynovial invasion of the tendon [83]. Tendon avulsion at sites of enthesitis may also occur. The most common tendons to rupture are the extensors in the wrist and hand, the rotator cuff tendons of the shoulder and the tibilais posterior tendon in the ankle. Tendonitis and rupture of the rotator cuff and long head of the biceps are among the most common causes of pain and disability in the shoulder. Complete rotator cuff tear results in superior subluxation of the humeral head and often leads to osteoarthritis. Tendon repair or tendon transfer is therefore indicated in cases of rupture, not only to restore function, but to prevent the rupture of additional tendons. Even with the appropriate surgery, patients are often left with some residual functional deficit. Prophylactic tenosynovectomy is often performed in patients with persistent tenosynovitis in an effort to reduce the risk of tendon rupture. A majority of these patients already show tenosynovial invasion of the tendon at the time of elective surgery [83].

Muscles contain somewhat less collagen and therefore exhibit intermediate signal intensity on both $T1$- and $T2$-weighted images. Muscular inflammation is occasionally seen in association with inflammatory arthritis, appearing as increased signal intensity on T 2-weighted MRI, both because of elevated water content with interstitial edema and T 2 prolongation associated with the loss of collagen. Conversely, postinflammatory fibrosis tends to lower signal intensity on T 2-weighted images, while fatty atrophy marbles muscles with high signal intensity fat on T 1-weighted images. Typically, muscle involvement shows a focal distribution.

5.3.7
Summary

MRI can noninvasively delineate all the articular constituents simultaneously and is also capable of probing compositional and functional parameters of disease in these tissues. Potentially, MRI can identify very early changes associated with cartilage degeneration when clinical symptoms may be minimal or absent. Early detection of patients who are at risk for developing progressive disease may allow appropriate treatment to be initiated earlier, when there may be a greater chance of favorable outcome. Furthermore, MRI can provide objective and quantitative measures of subtle morphological and compositional variations in different articular tissues over time, and therefore may offer more reliable and reproducible measures of disease progression and treatment response in patients with osteoarthritis than are currently available by other methods. This will facilitate the assessment of new therapies for osteoarthritis, and may allow faster clinical studies, with fewer patients, and potentially less cost. Further work is necessary to thoroughly validate and optimize some of these extremely promising measures so that they can be employed as powerful means for exploring the pathophysiology of osteoarthritis and potential new therapies.

References

1. Recht MP, Kramer J, Marcelis S, Pathria M, Trudell D, Haghighi P, Sartoris DJ, Resnick D (1993) Abnormalities of articular cartilage in the knee: analysis of available MR techniques. Radiology 187:473–478
2. Peterfy CG, van Dijke CF, Lu Y, Nguyen A, Connick T, Kneeland B, Tirman PFJ, Lang P, Dent S, Genant HK (1995) Quantification of articular cartilage in the metacarpophalangeal joints of the hand: accuracy and precision of 3-D MR imaging. AJR 165:371–375
3. Peterfy CG, van Dijke CF, Janzen DL, Glüer C, Namba R, Majumdar S, Lang P, Genant HK (1994b) Quantification of articular cartilage in the knee by pulsed saturation transfer and fat-suppressed MRI: optimization and validation. Radiology 192:485–491
4. Peterfy CG, Genant HK (1996) Emerging applications of magnetic resonance imaging for evaluating the articular cartilage. Radiol Clin N Am 34:195–213
5. Dieppe P, Altman RD, Buckwalter JA, Felson DT, Hascall V, Lohmander LS, Peterfy CG, Roos H, Kuetner KE (1995) Standardization of methods used to assess the progression of osteoarthritis of the hip or knee joints. In: Keutner KE, Goldberg VM (eds) Osteoarthritic Disorders. American Academy of Orthopedic Surgeons, Rosemont, pp 481–496
6. Genant HK (1983) Methods of assessing radiographic change in rheumatoid arthritis. Am J Med 30:35–47
7. Genant HK, Doi K, Mall JC (1975) Optical versus radiographic magnification for fine detail skeletal radiography. Invest Radiol 10:160–172

8. Buckland-Wright JC, Macfarlane DG, Lynch JA, Jasani MK, Bradshaw CR (1995) Joint space width measures cartilage thickness in osteoarthritis of the knee: high resolution plain film and double contrast macroradiographic investigation. Ann Rhem Dis 54:263–268

9. Buckland-Wright JC, Macfarlane DG, Jasani MK, Lynch JA (1994) Quantitative microfocal radiographic assessment of osteoarthritis of the knee from weight bearing tunnel and semi-flexed standing views. J Rheum 21:1734–1741

10. Hajnal JV, Baudouin CJ, Oatridge A, Young IR, Bydder GM (1992) Design and implementation of magnetization transfer pulse sequences for clinical use. J Comput Assist Tomogr 16:7–18

11. Kim DK, Ceckler TL, Hascall VC, Calabro A, Balaban RS (1993) Analysis of water-macromolecule proton magnetization transfer in articular cartilage. Magn Reson Med 29:211–215

12. Woolf SD, Chesnick S, Frank JA, Lim KO, Balaban RS (1991) Magnetization transfer contrast: MR imaging of the knee. Radiology 179:623–628

13. Peterfy CG, Majumdar S, Lang P, van Dijke CF, Sack K, Genant H (1994a) MR imaging of the arthritic knee: improved discrimination of cartilage, synovium and effusion with pulsed saturation transfer and fat-suppressed T1-weighted sequences. Radiology 191:413–419

14. Hall LD, Tyler JA (1995) Can quantitative magnetic resonance imaging detect and monitor the progression of early osteoarthritis? In: Kuetner KE, Goldberg VM (eds) Osteoarthritic Disorders. American Academy of Orthopedic Surgeons, Rosemont, pp 67–84

15. Hunziker E (1992) Articular cartilage structure in humans and experimental animals. In: Kuetner et al. (eds) Articular Cartilage and Osteoarthritis. Raven, New York, pp 183–199

16. Jeffery AK, Blunn GW, Archer CW, Bentley G (1991) Three-dimensional collagen architecture in bovine articular cartilage. J Bone Joint Surg 73B:795–801

17. Mow VC, Ratcliffe A, Poole AR (1992) Cartilage and diarthroidial joints as paradigms for hierarchical materials and structures. Biomaterials 13:67–97

18. Rubenstein JD, Kim JK, Morava-Protzner I, Stanchev PL, Henkelamn RM (1993) Effects of collagen orientation on MR imaging characteristics of bovine cartilage. Radiology 188:219–226

19. Hwang WS, Li B, Jin LH, Ngo K, Schachar NS, Hughes NF (1992) Collagen fibril structure of normal, aging, and osteoarthritic cartilage. J Pathol 167:425–433

20. Volpi M, Katz EP (1991) On the adaptive structures of the collagen fibrils of bone and cartilage. J Biomech 24:67–77

21. Paul PK, Jasani MK, Sebok D, Rakhit A, Dunton AW, Douglas FL (1993) Variation in MR signal intensity across normal human knee cartilage. JMRI 3:569–574

22. Meachim G, Stockwell RA (1979) The matrix. In: Freeman MAR (ed) Adult articular cartilage. Pitman Medical, London, p 28

23. Oegema TR, Bradford DS, Cooper KM (1979) Aggregated proteoglycan synthesis in organ cultures of human nucleus pulposus. J Biol Chem 254:1579–1583

24. Modl JM, Sether LA, Haughton VM, Kneeland JB (1991) Articular cartilage: correlation of histologic zones with signal intensity at MR imaging. Radiology 181:853–855

25. Cole PR, Jasani MK, Wood B, Freemont AJ, Morris GA (1990) High resolution, high field magnetic resonance imaging of joints: unexpected features in proton images of cartilage. Br J Radiol 63:907–909

26. Fry ME, Jacoby RK, Hutton CW, Ellis RE, Pittard S, Vennart W (1991) High-resolution magnetic resonance imaging of the interphalangeal joints of the hand. Skeletal Radiol 20:273–277

27. Fullerton G, Cameron I, Ord V (1985) Orientation of tendons in the magnetic field and its effect on T2 relaxation times. Radiology 155:433–435

28. Dardizinski B, Mosher T, Li S, Van Slyke M, Smith M (1997) Spatial variation of T2 in human articular cartilage. Radiology 205:546–550

29. Dodge GR, Poole AR (1989) Immunohistochemical detection and immunochemical analysis of type II collagen degradation in human normal, rheumatoid and osteoarthritic articular cartilages and in explants of bovine articular cartilage cultured with interleukin-1. J Clin Invest 83:647–661

30. Buckwalter J, Rosenberg L, Hunziker E (1990) Articular cartilage: composition, structure, response to injury, and methods of facilitating repairs. In: Ewing J (ed) Articular Cartilage and Knee Joint Function. Raven, New York, pp 19–54

31. Mow V, Fithian D, Kelly M (1990) Fundamentals of articular cartilage and meniscus biomechanics. In: Ewing J (ed) Articular Cartilage and Knee Joint Function. Raven, New York, pp 1–18

32. Mankin HJ, Thrasher AZ (1975) Water content and binding in normal and osteoarthritic human cartilage. J Bone Joint Surg 57A:76–79

33. Armstrong CG, Mow VC (1982) Variations in the intrinsic mechanical properties of human cartilage with age, degeneration and water content. J Bone Joint Surg 64A: 88–94

34. Maroudas A, Venn M (1977) Chemical composition and swelling of normal and osteoarthritic cartilage. II. Swelling. Ann Rheum Dis 36:399–406

35. Lehner KB, Rechl HP, Gmeinwieser JK, Heuck AF, Lukas HP, Kohl HP (1989) Structure, function, degeneration of bovine hyaline cartilage: assessment with MR imaging *in vitro*. Radiology 170:495–499

36. Vener MJ, Thompson RCJ, Lewis JL, Oegema TR (1992) Subchondral damage after acute transarticular loading: an *in vitro* model of joint injury. J Orthop Res 10:759–769

37. Vellet AD, Marks P, Fowler P, Mururo T (1991) Occult posttraumatic lesions of the knee, prevalence, classification, and short-term sequelae evaluated with MR imaging. Radiology 178:271–276

38. Shahriaree H (1985) Chondromalacia. Contemp Orthop 11:27–39

39. König H, Sauter R, Deimling M, Vogt M (1987) Cartilage disorders: a comparison of spin-echo, CHESS, and FLASH sequence MR images. Radiology 164:753–758

40. Broderick LS, Turner DA, Renfrew DL, Schnitzer TJ, Huff JP, Harris C (1994) Severity of articular cartilage abnormality in patients with osteoarthritis: evaluation with fast spin-echo MR vs arthroscopy. AJR 162:99–103

41. Rose PM, Demlow TA, Szumowski J, Quinn SF (1994) Chondromalacia patellae: fat-suppressed MR imaging. Radiology 193:437–440

42. Xia Y, Farquhar T, Burton-Wuster N, Ray E, Jelinski LW (1994) Diffusion and relaxation mapping of cartilage-bone plugs and excised disks using microscopic magnetic resonance imaging. Magn Reson Med 31:273–282

43. Burstein D, Gray ML, Hartman AL, Gipe R, Foy BD (1993) Diffusion of small solutes in cartilage as measured by nuclear magnetic resonance (NMR) spectroscopy and imaging. J Orthop Res 11:465–478

44. Kusaka Y, Grunder W, Rumpel H, Dannhauer K-H, Gersone K (1992) MR microimaging of articular cartilage and contrast enhancement by manganese ions. Magn Reson Med 24:137–148

45. Lesperance LM, Gray ML, Burstein D (1992) Determination of fixed charge density in cartilage using nuclear magnetic resonance. J Orthop Res 10:1–13

46. Fujioka M, Kusaka Y, Morita Y, Hirasawa Y, Gersonde K (1994) Contrast-enhanced MR imaging of articular cartilage: a new sensitive method for diagnosis of cartilage degeneration. 40th Annual Meeting, Orthopedic Research Society, New Orleans

47. Roberts TPL, Roberts HC, Peterfy CG, White D, Jiang Y, Zhao J, Genant HK (1998) Magnetization transfer modulation of observed T2 changes in injured human cartilage. Proceeding of the International Society for Magnetic Resonance in Medicine, vol 1, 6th Scientific Meeting and Exhibition, Sydney, Australia, p 39

48. Xia Y, Farquhar T, Burton-Wurster N, Lust G (1997) Origin of cartilage laminae in MRI. JMRI 7:887–894

49. Pilch L, Stewart C, Gordon D, Inman R, Parsons K, Pataki I, Stevens J (1994) Assessment of cartilage volume in the femorotibial joint with magnetic resonance imaging and 3-D computer reconstruction. J Rheum 21:2307–2321

50. Eckstein F, Sitteck H, Gavazzenia A, Milz S, Putz R, Reiser M (1995) Assessment of articular cartilage volume and thickness with magnetic resonance imaging (MRI). (abstract) Trans Orthop Res Soc 20:194

51. Ateshian GA, Kwak SD, Soslowsky LJ, Mow VC (1994) A stereophotogrammetric method for determining in situ contact areas in diarthroidial joints, and a comparison with other methods. J Biomech 27:111–124
52. Pelizzari C, Chen GTY, Spelbring DR, Weichselbaum RR, Chen C (1989) Accurate three-dimensional registration of CT, PET and/or MR images of the brain. J Comput Assist Tomogr 13:20–26
53. Kessler ML, Pitluck S, Petti PL, Castro JR (1991) Integration of multimodality imaging data for radiotherapy treatment planning. Int J Radiation Oncol Biol Phys 21:1653–1667
54. Woods RP, Mazziotta JC, Cherry SR (1993) MRI-PET registration with automated algorithm. J Comput Assist Tomogr 17:536–546
55. Woods RP, Cherry SR, Mazziotta JC (1992) Rapid automated algorithm for aligning and reslicing PET images. J Comput Assist Tomogr 16:620–633
56. Hajnal JV, Saeed N, Saor EJ, Oatridge A, Young IR, Bydder GM (1995) A registration and interpolation procedure for subvoxel matching of serially acquired MR images. J Comput Assist Tomogr 19:289–296
57. Chan WP, Lang P, Chieng PU, Davison PA, Huang SC, Genant HK (1991) Three-dimensional imaging of the musculoskeletal system: an overview. J Formosan Med Assoc 90:713–722
58. Abrahim-Zadeh R, Yu JS, Resnick D (1994) Central (interior) osteophytes of the distal femur: imaging and pathological findings. Invest Radiol 29:1001–1005
59. Genant HK, Engelke K, Fuerst T, Gluer CC, Grampp S, Harris ST, Jergas M, Lang T (1996) Noninvasive assessment of bone mineral and structure – state of the art. J Bone Min 11:707–730
60. White D, Schmidlin O, Jiang Y, Zhao J, Majumdar S, Genant H, Sebastian A, Morris RC Jr (1997) MRI of trabecular bone in an ovarectomized rat model of osteoporosis. Proceeding of the International Society for Magnetic Resonance in Medicine, vol 2, 5th Scientific Meeting and Exhibition, Vancouver, Canada, p 1021
61. Resnick D (1995) Internal derangements of joints. In: Resnick D (ed) Diagnosis of Bone and Joint Disorders. Saunders, Philadelphia, pp 3063–3069
62. McAlindon TEM, I Watt, McCrea F, Goddard P, Dieppe PA (1991) Magnetic resonance imaging in osteoarthritis of the knee: correlation with radiogaphic and scintigraphic findings. Ann Rheum Dis 50:14–20
63. Fernandez-Madrid F, Karvonen RL, Teitge RA, Miller PR, An T, Negendank WG (1995) Synovial thickening detected by MR imaging in osteoarthritis of the knee confirmed by biopsy as synovitis. Magn Reson Imaging 13:177–183
64. Brandt KD (1995) Insights into the natural history of osteoarthritis and the potential for pharmacologic modification of the disease afforded by study of the cruciate-deficient dog. In: Keutner KE, Goldberg VM (eds) Osteoarthritic Disorders. American Academy of Orthopedic Surgeons, Rosemont, pp 419–426
65. Schweitzer ME, van Leersum M, Ehrlich SS, Wapner K (1994) Fluid in normal and abnormal ankle joints: amount and distribution as seen on MR images. AJR 162:11–114
66. Heuck AF, Steiger P, Stoller DW, Glüer CC, Genant HK (1989) Quantification of knee joint fluid volume by MR imaging and CT using three-dimensional data processing. J Comput Assist Tomogr 13:287–293
67. Eich GF, Hallé F, Hodler J, Seger R, Willi UV (1994) Juvenile chronic arthritis: imaging of the knees and hips before and after intraarticular steroid injection. Pediatr Radiol 24:558–563
68. Winalski CS, Aliabadi P, Wright RJ, Shortkroff S, Sledge CB, Weissman BN (1993) Enhancement of joint fluid with intravenously administered gadopentetate dimeglumine: technique, rationale, and implications. Radiology 187:185–197
69. Drapé J-L, Thelen P, Gay-Depassier P, Silbermann O, Benacerraf R (1993) Intraarticular diffusion of Gd-DOTA after intravenous injection in the knee: MR imaging evaluation. Radiology 188:227–234
70. Smith H-J, Larheim TA, Aspestrand F (1992) Rheumatic and nonrheumatic disease in the temporomandibular joint: gadolinium-enhanced MR imaging. Radiology 185:229–234

71. Vahlensieck M, Peterfy CG, Wischer T, Sommer T, Lang P, Schlippert U, Genant HK, Schild HH (1996) Indirect MR arthrography: optimization and clinical applications. Radiology 200:249–254
72. Bashir A, Gray ML, Burstein D (1996) Gd-DTPA as a measure of cartilage degradation. Book of Abstracts: Society of Magnetic Resonance 1995. Berkeley, Society of Magnetic Resonance: 207
73. König H, Sieper J, Wolf KJ (1990) Rheumatoid arthritis: evaluation of hypervascular and fibrous pannus with dynamic MR imaging enhanced with Gd-DTPA. Radiology 176:473–477
74. Yamato M, Tamai K, Yamaguchi T, Ohno W (1993) MRI of the knee in rheumatoid arthritis: Gd-DTPA perfusion dynamics. J Comput Assist Tomogr 17: 781–785
75. Tamai K, Yamato M, Yamaguchi T, Ohno W (1994) Dynamic magnetic resonance imaging for the evaluation of synovitis in patients with rheumatoid arthritis. Arthritis Rheum 37:1151–1157
76. Stiskal MA, Neuhold A, Szolar DH, Saeed M, Czerny C, Leeb B, Smolen J, Czembirek H (1995) Rheumatoid arthritis of the craniocervical region by MR imaging: detection and characterization. AJR 165:585–592
77. Lynch MA, Henning CE, Glick KRJ (1983) Knee joint surface changes: long-term follow-up meniscus tear treatment in stable anterior cruciate ligament reconstructions. Clin Orthop 172:148–153
78. White D, Jiang Y, Zhao J, Genant HK, Peterfy CG (1998) MRI of meniscectomy-induced osteoarthritis. Proceeding of the International Society for Magnetic Resonance in Medicine, vol 2, 6th Scientific Meeting and Exhibition, Sydney, Australia, p 1094
79. Jiang Y, White D, Zhao J, Peterfy C, Genant HK (1997) Meniscectomy-induced osteoarthritis model in rabbits: MRI and radiographic assessments. Arthritis Rheum 40:S89
80. Jiang Y, Zhao J, Ouyang X, Flynn M, van Holsbeeck M, Genant HK (1996) Decreased trabecular bone volume but osteosclerotic surface changes in the greater tuberosity in rotator cuff tears. Radiology 201:388
81. Tirman PFJ, Bost FW, Garvin GJ, Peterfy CG, Mall JC, Steinbach LS, Feller JF, Crues JV III (1994) Posterosuperior glenoid impingement: MRI and MR arthrographic findings with arthroscopic correlation. Radiology 193:431–436
82. Rubens DJ, Blebea JS, Totterman SMS, Hooper MM (1993) Rheumatoid arthritis: evaluation of wrist extensor tendons with clinical examination versus MR imaging – a preliminary report. Radiology 187:831–838
83. Williamson SC, Feldon P (1995) Extensor tendon ruptures in rheumatoid arthritis. Hand Clin 11:449–459
84. Peterfy CG, White DL, Zhao J, VanDijke CF, Genant HK (1998) Longitudinal measurement of knee articular cartilage volume in osteoarthritis. Arthritis Rheum 41:S361
85. Zhao J, Lynch JA, Peterfy CG, White DL, Jiang Y, Genant HK (1998) Evaluation of articular cartilage volume quantification following registration of MR Images in the knee. Arthritis Rheum 41:S144

5.4
The Role of Molecular Markers to Monitor Breakdown and Repair

L. S. LOHMANDER

5.4.1
Introduction

The functional deterioration and failure of joint cartilage in osteoarthritis results from changes in its cells and matrix. Significant changes occur in both synthesis, degradation and structure of matrix molecules of cartilage and other joint tissues during the different phases of development of OA.

Biochemical markers reflect these dynamic changes in the joint tissues and may serve as a window on the pathological processes in the joint. The markers are most likely to be useful to elucidate degradation mechanisms, to predict prognosis and to monitor response to treatment. Markers are currently being used in research for these purposes.

Osteoarthritis is thus a disease characterized by dynamic, measurable changes in the turnover of joint cartilage constituents. Further investigations in this area will likely lead to a better understanding of the mechanisms and regulation of these processes and will help make osteoarthritis a treatable disease.

Osteoarthritis (OA) is associated with a loss of the balance between synthesis and degradation of the macromolecules needed to provide articular cartilage with its biomechanical and functional properties. At the same time,

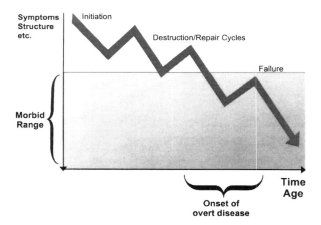

Fig. 1. Osteoarthritis might be seen as slowly progressing from an asymptomatic, pre-clinical phase into a symptomatic, morbid, clinical phase. During disease development, phases of destruction and repair alternate. In the pre-clinical phase, metabolic joint changes might be detected by molecular markers, structural changes by arthroscopy, MRI and later plain radiographs. In the symptomatic clinical phase, metabolic, structural and functional changes gradually increase. For many individuals, osteoarthritis development may never reach the symptomatic, morbid phase

changes occur in the structure and metabolism of the synovium, subchondral bone and other tissues of the joint. These processes result in the destruction of joint cartilage with concomitant structural and functional changes in other joint tissues. This causes changes in the function of the affected joints. In some patients these changes, often after an extended asymptomatic period, lead to pain, disability and handicap. It is this final end-stage of a long process that corresponds to the overt disease we call osteoarthritis (Fig. 1).

Current therapy of OA is largely symptomatic, and aims to decrease pain and improve function with analgesics, non-steroidal anti-inflammatory drugs or joint replacement. However, novel pharmaceutical interventions are now being investigated, based on an improved understanding of the critical processes involved in joint destruction [1], which may have the ability to decrease the rate of joint destruction in OA. The ability to reproducibly and sensitively monitor disease progression and outcome for both joint and patient in OA intervention trials is critical to development of such new disease-modifying treatment strategies. The growing realization of the major socioeconomic impact caused by OA provides further stimulus to this development (Consensus Document: The Bone and Joint Decade 2000–2010, [2]).

For clinical trials or for longitudinal follow-up studies, OA can be assessed by:

a) Patient-centered measures of joint pain and disability
b) Measurements of structural changes in the affected joints
c) Measurements of the disease process

Well documented examples of (a) are scoring systems such the "Index for Severity of Knee or Hip Disease" and the "WOMAC Osteoarthritis Index" [3–5]. Structural (anatomical) changes associated with OA (b) can be measured by plain radiographs, magnetic resonance imaging, arthroscopy or ultrasound [6–10]. The osteoarthritic disease process (c) can be monitored by bone scintigraphy, by metabolic markers, and possibly in the future by magnetic resonance imaging [8, 11–13].

Algofunctional scores, plain radiographs, magnetic resonance imaging and arthroscopy are now in use to assess OA in clinical trials. For a discussion of current issues in the design of symptom- and disease-modifying clinical trials in OA, the reader is referred to recent reviews [14–16].

Imaging of joints by plain x-ray examination is the current "gold-standard" to detect changes in joint structure in clinical trials of disease-modifying drugs in OA. Even with improved and standardized techniques for patient positioning and image measurements, plain x-ray examination remains an indirect measure of cartilage destruction, a "surrogate marker". Magnetic resonance imaging is finding an increased use as a measure to assess joint changes in OA, and the technology is in rapid development. Among other advantages over plain x-ray examination, it can monitor changes in volume of cartilage and other soft joint tissues, as well as bone structure. However, until methods to monitor joint cartilage quality or composition by magnetic resonance imaging appear, the technique suffers from the same weakness as x-ray examination: it provides only an indirect measure of the disease process, and documents the consequences of the process rather than the process itself.

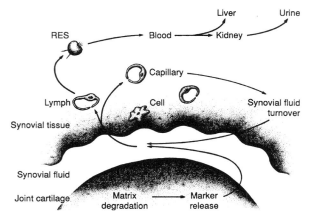

Fig. 2. Molecular fragments generated by degradation of cartilage matrix, or released from synovial tissue or bone into the joint fluid compartment are cleared by bulk flow through the synovial tissue matrix into the lymphatic vessels (Levick et al. 1992). Some fragments are eliminated or further degraded in the regional lymph nodes. Many and possibly most products of cartilage matrix metabolism are taken up and degraded in the liver. Some specific types of fragments, such as collagen cross-links, are not metabolized, but found in urine. Modified from [17]

Critical pathological processes associated with OA occur in the joint carti-lage, but also in the subchondral bone, synovium and other soft joint tissues. Because our ability to sample and monitor these tissues is limited, body fluid compartments such as joint fluid, blood and urine may serve as windows on these pathological processes in the joint (Fig. 2).

The metabolic alterations in joint tissues associated with OA (and other joint diseases) involves changes in both the degradation and synthesis of matrix molecules, which are then often released as fragments to joint fluid, blood and urine where they may be detected. Such molecular "markers" of e.g. cartilage matrix turnover could be used to prognosticate and monitor joint diseases such as rheumatoid arthritis and OA, and to identify disease mechanisms on the molecular level. Other potential markers of the OA disease process are as-sociated with the increased production and release to body fluids of enzymes or cytokines. For overviews and further references on molecular markers of OA and other joint diseases, several reviews are available [12, 13, 17–20]. This chapter to a large extent is based on these recent reviews, and attempts to briefly summarize the current status of research on markers which are directly associated with turnover of joint tissue matrix molecules, such as matrix molecule fragments and proteases potentially associated with their generation.

5.4.2
The Relationship Between Markers and Joint Tissue Synthesis and Degradation

A basic rationale for the concept of OA markers is that such markers reflect some aspects of the metabolic processes of joint tissues. However, the relationship between marker concentration in a body fluid compartment such as joint fluid, blood or urine with turnover processes in the joint tissues is complex.

For example, the concentration of a marker of cartilage matrix degradation in joint fluid may depend not only on the rate of degradation of cartilage matrix, but also on other factors such as the rate of elimination, or clearance, of the molecular fragment in question from the joint fluid compartment [21–23] and the amount of cartilage matrix remaining in the joint [24] (Figs. 2 and 3). Since clearance from the joint fluid compartment is increased by inflammation [21,25], differences in the rates of release of markers from joint cartilage into joint fluid between control joints and diseased inflamed joints may be underestimated. An estimate of the degradation rate of a cartilage matrix molecule in arthritis, based solely on the joint fluid concentration of its fragments, may thus actually lead to an underestimation of its metabolic rate.

In spite of these confounding factors, marker concentrations in joint fluid in general seem to correlate with the expected metabolic rate of joint cartilage matrix molecules [12]. As an example, the changes with time after joint injury and in development of osteoarthritis in synovial fluid concentrations of fragments of aggrecan, 846 epitope, cartilage oligomeric matrix protein (COMP) and collagen II C-propeptide [26–29] are consistent with the changes in meta-

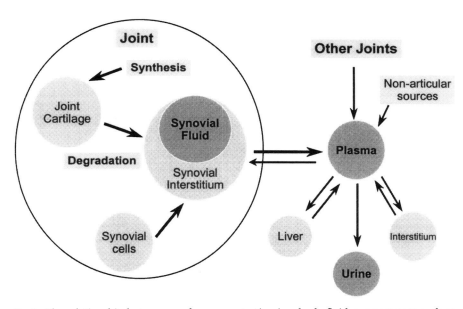

Fig. 3. The relationship between marker concentration in a body fluid compartment such as joint fluid, blood or urine with metabolic processes in the joint tissues is complex. The concentration of a marker of cartilage matrix degradation in joint fluid depends not only on the rate of degradation of cartilage matrix, but also on other factors such as the clearance of the molecular fragment in question from the joint fluid compartment (increased by inflammation) and the amount of cartilage matrix remaining in the joint. Marker concentrations in serum are, in addition, influenced by e.g. liver function. Modified from [23]

bolic rate observed for aggrecan, COMP and type II collagen in animal models *in vivo* and in human osteoarthritic cartilage *in vitro* [30 – 33].

The identification of the specific source of the molecular fragment can be a problem with regard to both the metabolic process and the tissue. An increased rate of release of molecular fragments may be present both as a result of a net increase in degradation (resulting in net loss from tissue), or as a result of an increased rate of degradation in the presence of an increased rate of new synthesis and replenishment (resulting in a steady state with regard to tissue concentration of the molecule). We therefore need markers with specificity for degradative and synthetic events, respectively. An example of the former is aggrecan fragments, and of the latter, collagen II C-propeptide.

Even with a molecular marker being associated with degradative events, the specific process source may need to be considered. For example, the fragments identified could result from the degradation of a newly synthesized matrix molecule which has not yet been incorporated into a functional matrix, a molecule recently incorporated into cell-associated matrix, or a resident matrix molecule which has a critical functional part of the mature matrix. The consequences on cartilage matrix integrity and function may well be different. In general, markers are not specific to these processes. This problem is also related to the largely unresolved question of the specific cartilage matrix compartment source (pericellular, territorial matrix or interterritorial matrix) of a molecular marker present in joint fluid, blood or urine. *In vitro* experimentation suggests that the metabolic rates of these cartilage matrix compartments may differ significantly [34]. Assay of some low-abundance epitopes associated with chondroitin sulfate sulfation patterns may help identify populations of newly synthesized aggrecan molecules [29, 35 – 38].

It may be suggested that fragments appearing in joint fluid of matrix molecules normally resident in cartilage are generated by metabolism of cartilage matrix. This assumption is not necessarily true. It relies, in turn, on the assumption that the molecule in question is significantly more abundant in cartilage than in any other joint tissue, or that its metabolic rate in cartilage is higher than in other joint tissues. While it is true that joint cartilage contains a far greater total mass of aggrecan compared to, e. g. the meniscus (Dahlberg et al. 1992), the total mass of COMP in the menisci of the knee may approach that in the joint cartilage of the knee [39]. Both chondrocytes and synovial cells produce stromelysin-1 [40], but the cell number in synovial tissue may be higher than in cartilage, suggesting that a significant proportion of the stromelysin-1 detected in joint fluid originates in the synovium. The specific source of the molecule or molecular fragment identified in joint fluid may thus not always be entirely evident, and is likely often more complex than originally proposed.

The question of the tissue source of markers of cartilage metabolism is highly relevant for markers assayed in serum or urine samples. Joint cartilage represents less than 10 % of body hyaline cartilage. Sources of the marker other than cartilage will also have to be considered. Moreover, in monoarticular disease, any markers released from the single affected joint are mixed with markers released from normal joints. It seems reasonable to suggest that determinations of cartilage markers in serum or urine may be of use in poly-articular or systemic disease, but are less likely to be useful in monoarticular disease.

Extra-articular factors which affect the clearance of the marker from the serum or urine compartment have to be considered. Physical activity may change the concentrations of some markers in both synovial fluid and serum [41]. The lymph nodes and the liver are responsible for the elimination of a great part of the molecular fragments released from cartilage and other connective tissues. Any change in the function of these organ systems will thus affect the clearance of cartilage markers from serum (Figs. 2 and 3). For example, the serum concentration of hyaluronan is greatly affected by changes in liver function [42].

A brief list of putative biochemical markers of cartilage, bone or synovial metabolism in joint fluid, serum and urine in OA is given in Table 1.

Table 1. Molecular markers of joint tissue metabolism in synovial fluid or serum in human osteoarthritis

Marker[a]	Process[b]	OA markers in synovial fluid[c,d] (references)	OA markers in serum[c,d] (references)
Cartilage			
Aggrecan			
Core protein fragments	Degradation of aggrecan	⇑ (Lohmander [67], Lohmander [26])	
Core protein epitopes (cleavage site specific neoepitopes)	Degradation of aggrecan	⇑ (Sandy [59], Lohmander [60], Lark [61[e]])	
Keratan sulfate epitopes	Degradation of aggrecan	⇑ (Campion [68], Belcher [49])	⇑ ⇔ ⇓ (Thonar [43], Campion [68], Mehraban [69], Spector [44], Poole [35], Lohmander and Thonar [46])
Chondroitin sulfate epitopes (846, 3B3, 7D4, etc.)	Synthesis/degradation of aggrecan	⇑ (Poole [35], Hazell [70], Slater [71], Lohmander [29], Plaas [37[e]], Plaas [38[e]])	⇑ (Poole [35])
Chondroitin sulfate ratio 6 S/4 S	Synthesis/degradation of aggrecan	⇓ (Shinmei [72])	
Small proteoglycans	Degradation of small proteoglycans	⇑[e] (Witsch-Prehm [73])	

Table 1 (continued)

Marker[a]	Process[b]	OA markers in synovial fluid[c,d] (references)	OA markers in serum[c,d] (references)
Cartilage matrix proteins			
Cartilage oligomeric matrix protein (COMP)	Degradation of COMP	⇑ (Saxne and Heinegård [74], Lohmander [27], Peterson [47])	⇑ (Sharif [52])
Cartilage collagens			
Type II collagen C-propeptide	Synthesis of type II collagen	⇑ (Shinmei [75], Lohmander [28], Yoshihara [58])	
Type II collagen α chain fragments	Degradation of type II collagen	⇑[e] (Hollander [76], Billinghurst [77], Atley [78])	
Matrix metalloprotein-ases and inhibitors	Synthesis and secretion	⇑ From synovium or joint cartilage?	⇑ ⇔ tissue source? (see below)
Meniscus			
Cartilage oligomeric matrix protein	Degradation of COMP	⇑ From joint cartilage, synovium or meniscus?	
Small proteoglycans	Degradation of small proteoglycans		
Synovium			
Hyaluronan	Synthesis of hyaluronan		⇑ (Goldberg [79], Hedin [80], Sharif [51])
Matrix metalloproteinases and inhibitors			
Stromelysin (MMP-3)	Synthesis and secretion of MMP-3	⇑ (Lohmander [26])	⇑ ⇔ (Zucker [57], Manicourt [56], Yoshihara [58])
Interstitial collagenase (MMP-1)	Synthesis and secretion of MMP-1	⇑ (Lohmander [26], Clark [55])	⇔ (Manicourt [56])
Tissue inhibitors of metallo-proteinases (TIMP)	Synthesis and secretion of TIMPs	⇑ (Lohmander [26], Manicourt [56])	⇔ (Yoshihara [58])
Type III collagen N-propeptide	Synthesis/degradation of type III collagen	⇑ (Sharif [81])	⇑ (Sharif [81])
Bone			
Bone sialoprotein (BSP)	Synthesis/degradation of BSP	⇑ ⇔ (Lohmander [82])	⇑[f] (Lohmander [82])

Table 1 (continued)

Marker[a]	Process[b]	OA markers in synovial fluid[c,d] (references)	OA markers in serum[c,d] (references)
Osteocalcin	Synthesis of osteocalcin	⇑ ⇔ (Sharif [83])	⇔ (Campion [68])
3-hydro-xypyridinium cross-links[g]	Degradation of bone collagens		

⇑ ⇔ ⇓: Increased, unchanged or decreased concentrations, respectively, compared with healthy controls.

[a] Markers have been assigned a predominant tissue source with regard to marker occurrence in joint fluid and serum.

[b] As discussed in this chapter (see Figs. 2 and 3) some individual marker levels may change both as a result of changes in synthesis and in degradation.

[c] A predominant increase or decrease, respectively, is assigned on the basis of representative publications on "active", not end-stage OA.

[d] Some recent and representative literature references are given, this is not a comprehensive review of the literature.

[e] In human OA cartilage.

[f] After acute knee injury.

[g] Results published only for urine, showing increased excretion [84, 85].

5.4.3
Uses of Molecular Markers

The demands on a marker will differ, depending on if it is to be used as a diagnostic test, a prognostic test or an evaluative test. For example, the diagnostic test focuses on the ability to detect differences between affected and non-affected individuals, expressed in terms of sensitivity and specificity of the test, or positive and negative predictive values. The prognostic test attempts to identify the individuals within a cohort which are the most likely to show a rapid disease progression. The evaluative test, finally, focuses on the ability of the marker to monitor change over time in the individual patient, often expressed as sensitivity to change or effect size. Additional uses of markers may also be contemplated, such as the ability of a marker to predict response to a treatment, such as a specific inhibitor of the collagenase responsible for cartilage collagen breakdown, or the protease responsible for cartilage aggrecan breakdown. Here, the presence or absence of degradation products of these matrix molecules in certain conditions would provide a rationale for targeting a specific protease for inhibition.

It has been suggested that markers may serve as diagnostic tests, helping to distinguish joints with OA from unaffected joints or other joint diseases. The concentration of keratan sulfate in serum was originally suggested to serve as a diagnostic test for generalized OA [43]. Subsequent experience has, however, failed to fulfill this promise [35, 44], although this serum marker may yet serve to reflect cartilage proteoglycan degradation in specific situations [45]. A considerable overlap exists between affected and non-affected individuals, and serum concentrations are influenced by age and gender [46]. Other studies have shown differences in knee joint fluid concentrations of aggrecan fragments, COMP fragments, and matrix metalloproteinases and their inhibitors between knee-healthy reference groups, rheumatoid arthritis, reactive arthritis and OA [26, 27, 47, 48]. While these investigations show significant differences in mean concentration values (or ratios between different markers) between the study groups with only moderate overlap, interpretation is confounded by the fact that comparisons between groups are cross-sectional and retrospective. Of further concern in these cross-sectional studies is the requirement for careful patient characterization, since sub-grouping may influence the results significantly [49]. The predictive power of the test to discriminate between groups is rarely discussed. Results from reports such as these will require confirmation in prospective studies.

Molecular markers might also be used for evaluating disease severity or staging, rather than the presence or absence of disease. In OA, disease severity is currently measured by, e.g. Kellgren and Lawrence grade of radiological changes, by the amount of cartilage loss on arthroscopy or by the patient's degree of pain and functional impairment. Several reports have suggested that assay of molecular markers of cartilage metabolism may provide complementary information on joint disease stage [24, 50]. While further experience in this area is needed, molecular markers have the potential to provide unique information on joint cartilage quality not currently available by other modalities of staging.

Biochemical assays of molecular markers developed to evaluate OA have also been promoted as *prognostic markers,* to predict the later worsening of OA. For example, it was shown that levels of serum hyaluronan (but not serum keratan sulfate) in patients with knee OA at study entry predicted subsequent progression of knee OA at the 5-year follow-up [51]. In the same study population, an increase in serum COMP during the first year after study entry, was associated with radiographic progression of the knee OA at 5-year follow-up [52]. Studies on groups of patients with rheumatoid arthritis have indicated that serum levels of COMP and the chondroitin sulfate epitope 846 are associated with rapid disease progression in that condition [53]. These reports describe results obtained on patient groups of limited size, and often do not specify the strength of the relationship between marker levels and disease progression. However, they suggest that further progress in the area of prognostic markers is likely with prospective, longitudinal studies on larger patient cohorts.

Of note here is a report of low-level increases in serum C-reactive protein in early osteoarthritis of the knee, and that levels of this protein predict progression of knee OA [54]. Likely, this increase reflects tissue-damaging processes within the joints, and may further be related to the increased levels of serum hyaluronan shown to predict knee OA progression [51]. Possibly, the synovium is responsible for a significant proportion of the increased serum hyaluronan, indicating a low-level synovitis. The presence of such a low-level synovitis may also be consistent with the increased concentrations of the matrix metalloproteinase stromelysin in synovial fluid and serum observed in OA and after joint injury [26, 55 – 58].

Markers that reflect the ongoing repair and degradative processes occurring within a joint, might be regarded as prognostic markers. As discussed, concentrations in joint fluid of molecular markers for both degradation and synthesis are consistent with the changes in metabolic rate observed for these molecules in animal models *in vivo* and in human osteoarthritic cartilage *in vitro*.

Markers may also be used to identify degradation mechanisms and to predict response to therapy. Structure analysis of the matrix molecule fragments released from or remaining in the cartilage matrix may yield important information on the character of the metabolic process or protease responsible for tissue destruction. Results with aggrecan fragments may serve as an example. The structures of the fragments released into joint fluid, and of those remaining in the matrix, are consistent with two separate proteolytic activities in cartilage matrix in OA [59 – 61]. One of these proteases generates fragments consistent with the action of a "classic" matrix metalloprotease such as stromelysin, while the other as yet unidentified protease generates fragments consistent with the action of a putative protease, "aggrecanase". Similar and ongoing structure analysis of fragments of cartilage collagens and matrix proteins may yield information the role of different proteases in different phases of disease development, critical for our understanding of cartilage metabolism in health and disease [18]. This information may in turn be used to predict responsiveness to treatment specific for a proteolytic activity such as a collagenase or "aggrecanase". The usefulness of this concept relies on the demonstration of disease mechanisms with at least a relative specificity for a condition or disease stage, and on the availability of agents specific for these processes.

Molecular markers have also been suggested as being useful to monitor response to therapy in OA, to be used as sensitive surrogate outcome measures in clinical trials of new disease-modifying treatments. Within this area, the possible ability of markers to provide "proof-of-principle" in early-stage clinical testing of new agents to inhibit cartilage breakdown, is of particular interest. Advances in our understanding of disease mechanisms, assisted by structure analysis of molecular fragments released from human joint cartilage, as outlined in the preceding paragraph, will be critical for progress. However, with the current absence of disease-modifying treatments in OA, the role of molecular markers in this area remains somewhat speculative. Experience from the treatment of rheumatoid patients is so far limited, but suggests that cartilage molecular markers are indeed responsive to treatment [48, 62 – 65]. Randomized, controlled clinical trials of new disease-modifying treatments of OA will represent important opportunities to validate OA markers as outcome measures.

Given that markers reflect the dynamic state of cartilage metabolism, it appears most likely that markers will be used to evaluate changes in disease: as prognostic tools to identify those at high risk of rapid progression, to identify the responders, and to assess the degree of response.

For all suggested uses of markers, but perhaps in particular for markers used to monitor treatment response, we shall require knowledge of the variability both over time in the individual and between individuals in representative and stable cohorts of appropriate size. Such data can be used to calculate the needed number of patients and the required response to treatment in a clinical trial setting. Similarly, we will need marker data for age- and gender-matched groups of joint-healthy and arthritic individuals at different stages of disease development. On the basis of such data, sensitivity, specificity and predictive power for diagnostic tests may be calculated. Only few such data have yet been published.

A recent report, however, presented assay results on samples of synovial fluid, serum, and urine obtained on 8 different occasions during one year from 52 patients with incipient knee osteoarthritis [66]. Both between-patient and within-patient coefficients of variation varied for markers in different body fluid compartments, with the lowest variability for serum keratan sulfate and the highest for synovial fluid markers (Fig. 4). For synovial fluid, aggrecan fragments showed the least variability, and matrix metalloproteinases the highest. One patient with septic arthritis showed a 5-fold peak increase in joint fluid aggrecan fragment concentrations, while the concentration of matrix metalloproteinase-3 increased 100-fold, and that for matrix metalloproteinase-1 more than 500-fold.

It was notable that the sensitivity to change differed between markers in the same body fluid compartment, reflecting a differing degree of responsiveness to pathologic processes between the cells and tissues primarily responsible for the

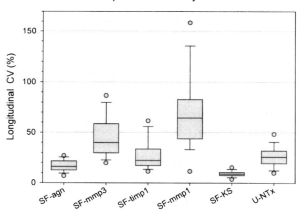

Fig. 4. Within-patient variability of markers. Variability expressed as Coefficient of Variation (CV) (SD/mean × 100). Box plots contain 25th to 75th percentiles within box, line in box is median. *Whiskers* represent 10th and 90th percentiles, *symbols* 5th and 95th percentiles. Synovial fluid markers: Aggrecan fragments (*SF-agn*), matrix metalloproteinase-3 (*SF-mmp3*), matrix metalloproteinase-1 (*SF-mmp1*). Serum marker: keratan sulfate (*SF-KS*). Urine marker: type I collagen N-telopeptide crosslink (*U-NTx*). (Data from [66])

production and release of these markers. An example is provided by the great differences in variability between aggrecan fragments, MMP-1 and MMP-3 in joint fluid. While aggrecan fragment concentrations reflect degradation and synthesis of joint cartilage aggrecan, MMP concentrations probably mirror synthesis, secretion and release of MMP's from both synovium and cartilage, which apparently may be more responsive to pathogenic stimuli. Even though the baseline variability for MMP-3 concentration was greater than for aggrecan fragments, the responsiveness to change was some 4-fold greater for MMP-3 than for aggrecan fragments. However, we still have little or no information with regard to diagnostic specificity for these or any other markers in OA.

The lower degree of variability of marker concentrations within patients, as compared to between patients, emphasizes the importance of knowledge of, and comparison with, baseline concentrations in clinical trials which propose to use joint markers as outcome measures. MMP-3 concentrations in synovial fluid may serve as an illustration of the use of data such as those presented here. If a decrease from a baseline concentration of 22 nM of MMP-3 to a concentration of 17 nM is taken as a relevant change (approximately 0.5 standard deviations), then some 30 patients per treatment arm would be sufficient to show this change with a power of 80 %. This example does not imply, however, that such a change would necessarily relate to a change in the osteoarthritic disease process, or be clinically relevant.

This review has presented data which support the notion that biochemical markers reflect the dynamic changes in the joint tissues that take place in OA, and may serve as a window on pathological processes in the joint. Osteoarthritis is a disease characterized by dynamic, measurable changes in the turnover of joint cartilage constituents. Further investigations in this area will help make osteoarthritis a treatable disease.

References

1. Vincenti MP, Clark IM, Brinckerhoff CE (1994) Using inhibitors of metalloproteinases to treat arthritis. Easier said than done? Arthritis Rheum 37:1115–1126
2. Consensus document (1998) The Bone and Joint Decade 2000–2010 for prevention and treatment of musculo-skeletal disorders. Acta Orthop Scand 69:67–86
3. Lequèsne MG, Mery C, Samson M, Gerard P (1987) Indexes of severity for osteoarthritis of the hip and knee. Validation – Value in comparison with other assessment tests. Scand J Rheumatol [Suppl] 65:85–89
4. Bellamy N, Buchanan WW, Goldsmith CH, Campbell J, Stitt LW (1988) Validation study of WOMAC: a health status instrument for measuring clinically important patient relevant outcomes to antirheumatic drug therapy in patients with osteoarthritis of the hip or knee. J Rheumatol 15:1833–1840
5. Rivest C, Liang M (1998). Evaluating outcome in osteoarthritis for research and clinical practise. In: Brandt KD, Doherty M, Lohmander LS (eds) Osteoarthritis. Oxford University Press, Oxford, pp 403–414
6. Hodgson RJ, Barry MA, Carpenter TA, Hall L, Hazleman B L, Tyler JA (1995) Magnetic resonance imaging protocol optimization for evaluation of hyaline cartilage in the distal interphalangeal joint of fingers. Invest Radiol 30:522–531
7. Buckland-Wright JC (1998) Quantitation of radiographic changes. In: Brandt KD, Doherty M, Lohmander LS (eds) Osteoarthritis. Oxford University Press, Oxford, pp 459–472

8. Peterfy CG (1998) Magnetic resonance imaging. In: Brandt KD, Doherty M, Lohmander LS (eds) Osteoarthritis. Oxford University Press, Oxford, pp 473–494

9. Ayral X, Altman RD (1998) Arthroscopic evaluation of knee articular cartilage. In: Brandt KD, Doherty M, Lohmander LS (eds) Osteoarthritis. Oxford University Press, Oxford, pp 494–505

10. Myers S (1998) Ultrasonography. In: Brandt KD, Doherty M, Lohmander LS (eds) Osteoarthritis. Oxford University Press, Oxford pp 512–518

11. Schauwecker DS (1998) Bone scintigraphy. In: Brandt KD, Doherty M, Lohmander LS (eds) Osteoarthritis. Oxford University Press, Oxford, p 506–511

12. Lohmander LS (1994) Articular Cartilage and Osteoarthrosis – The role of molecular markers to monitor breakdown, repair and disease. J Anat 184:477–492

13. Lohmander LS, Felson DT (1998) Defining and validating the clinical role of molecular markers in osteoarthritis. In: Brandt KD, Doherty M, Lohmander LS (eds) Osteoarthritis. Oxford University Press, Oxford, pp 519–530

14. Dieppe P, Altman R, Buckwalter J, Felson D, Hascall V, Kuettner K, Lohmander LS, Peterfy C, Roos H (1995) Standardisation of methods used to assess the progression of osteoarthritis of hip and knee. In: Kuettner K, Goldberg V (eds) Osteoarthritic Disorders. American Academy of Orthopedic Surgeons, Rosemont, pp 481–496

15. Altman R, Brandt K, Hochberg M, Moskowitz R, Bellamy N, Bloch DA, Buckwalter J, Dougados M, Ehrlich M, Lequèsne M, Lohmander LS, Murphy WA, Rosario-Jansen T, Schwartz B, Trippel S (1996) Design and conduct of clinical trials in patients with osteoarthritis: Recommendations from a task force of the Osteoarthritis Research Society. Osteoarthritis Cartilage 4:217–243

16. Bellamy N (1998) Design of clinical trials for evaluation of disease-modifying osteoarthritis drugs (DMOADS) and of new agents for symptomatic treatment of osteoarthritis. In: Brandt KD, Doherty M, Lohmander LS (eds) Osteoarthritis. Oxford University Press, Oxford, pp 531–542

17. Lohmander LS (1991) Markers of cartilage metabolism in arthrosis. A review. Acta Orthop Scand 62:623–632

18. Poole AR (1994) Immunochemical markers of joint inflammation, skeletal damage and repair; where are we now? Ann Rheum Dis 53:3–5

19. Saxne T, Heinegård D (1995) Matrix proteins: potentials as body fluid markers of changes in the metabolism of cartilage and bone in arthritis. J Rheumatol 22 [Suppl 43]:71–74

20. Lohmander LS, Saxne T, Heinegård D (eds) (1995) Molecular markers of joint and skeletal diseases. Acta Orthop Scand 66 [Suppl 266]:1–212

21. Wallis WJ, Simkin PA, Nelp WB (1987) Protein traffic in human synovial effusions. Arthritis Rheum 30:57–63

22. Levick JR (1992) Synovial fluid. Determinants of volume turnover and material concentration. In: Kuettner KE, Schleyerbach R, Peyron JG, Hascall VC (eds) Articular cartilage and osteoarthritis. Raven, New York, pp 529–541

23. Simkin PA, Bassett JE (1995) Cartilage matrix molecules in serum and synovial fluid. Current Opin Rheumatol 7:346–351

24. Dahlberg L, Ryd L, Heinegård D, Lohmander LS (1992) Proteoglycan fragments in joint fluid – influence of arthrosis and inflammation. Acta Orthop Scand 63:417–423

25. Myers SL, O'Connor BL, Brandt KD (1996) Accelerated clearance of albumin from the osteoarthritic knee: implications for interpretation of concentrations of "cartilage markers" in synovial fluid. J Rheumatol 23:1744–1748

26. Lohmander LS, Hoerrner LA, Lark MW (1993a) Metalloproteinases, tissue inhibitor and proteoglycan fragments in knee synovial fluid in human osteoarthritis. Arthritis Rheum 36:181–189

27. Lohmander LS, Saxne T, Heinegård D (1994) Release of cartilage oligomeric matrix protein (COMP) into joint fluid after injury and in osteoarthrosis. Ann Rheum Dis 53:8–13

28. Lohmander LS, Yoshihara Y, Roos H, Kobayashi T, Yamada H, Shinmei M (1996a) Procollagen II C-propeptide in joint fluid. Changes in concentrations with age, time after joint injury and osteoarthritis. J Rheumatol 23:1765–1769

29. Lohmander LS, Ionescu M, Jugessur H, Poole AR (1998a) Changes in joint cartilage aggrecan metabolism after knee injury and in osteoarthritis. Arthritis Rheum, in press

30. Eyre DR, McDevitt CA, Billingham ME, Muir H (1980) Biosynthesis of collagen and other matrix proteins by articular cartilage in experimental osteoarthritis. Biochem J 188:823–837

31. Carney SL, Billingham MEJ, Muir H, Sandy JD (1984) Demonstration of increased proteoglycan turnover in cartilage explants from dogs with experimental osteoarthritis. J Orthop Res 2:201–206

32. Aigner T, Stöss H, Weseloh G, Zeiler G, von der Mark K (1992) Activation of collagen type II expression in osteoarthritic and rheumatoid cartilage. Virchows Archiv B Cell Pathol 62:337–345

33. Heinegård D, Bayliss M, Lorenzo P (1998) Biochemistry and metabolism of normal and osteoarthritic cartilage. In: Brandt KD, Doherty M, Lohmander LS (eds) Osteoarthritis. Oxford University Press, Oxford, pp 74–84

34. Mok SS, Masuda K, Häuselmann HJ, Aydelotte MB, Thonar EJ-MA (1994) Aggrecan synthesized by mature bovine chondrocytes suspended in alginate. Identification of two distinct metabolic matrix pools. J Biol Chem 269:33021–33027

35. Poole AR, Ionescu M, Swan A, Dieppe PA (1994) Changes in cartilage metabolism in arthritis are reflected by altered serum and synovial fluid levels of the cartilage proteoglycan aggrecan -implications for pathogenesis. J Clin Invest 94:25–33

36. Visco DM, Johnstone B, Hill MA, Jolly GA, Caterson B (1993) Immunohistochemical analysis of 3-B-3(-) and 7-D-4 epitope expression in canine osteoarthritis. Arthritis Rheum 36:1718–1725

37. Plaas AHK, WongPalms S, Roughley PJ, Midura RJ, Hascall VC (1997) Chemical and immunological assay of the nonreducing terminal residues of chondroitin sulfate from human aggrecan. J Biol Chem 272:20603–20610

38. Plaas AHK, West LA, Wong-Palms S, Nelson F (1998) Glycosaminoglycan sulfation in human osteoarthrtitis. Disease-related alterations at the non-reducing termini of chondroitin and dermatan sulfate. J Biol Chem 273:12642–12649

39. Hauser N, Geiss J, Neidhart M, Paulsson M, Häuselmann HJ (1995) Distribution of CMP and COMP in human cartilage. Acta Orthop Scand 66 [Suppl 266]:72–73

40. Wolfe GC, MacNaul KL, Buechel FF, McDonnell J, Hoerrner LA, Lark MW, Moore VL, Hutchinson NI (1993) Differential in vivo expression of collagenase messenger RNA in synovium and cartilage. Quantitative comparison with stromelysin messenger RNA levels in human rheumatoid arthritis and osteoarthritis patients and in two animal models of acute inflammatory arthritis. Arthritis Rheum 36:1540–1547

41. Roos H, Dahlberg L, Hoerrner LA, Lark MW, Thonar EJ-MA, Shinmei M, Lindquist U, Lohmander LS (1995) Markers of cartilage matrix metabolism in human joint fluid and serum – The effect of exercise. Osteoarthritis Cartilage 3:7–14

42. Laurent TC, Fraser RE (1992) Hyaluronan. FASEB Journal 6:2397–2404

43. Thonar EJ-MA, Lenz ME, Klintworth GK, Caterson B, Pachman LM, Glickman P, Katz R, Huff J, Kuettner KE (1985) Quantification of keratan sulfate in blood as a marker of cartilage catabolism. Arthritis Rheum 28:1367–1376

44. Spector TD, Woodward L, Hall GM, Hammond A, Williams A, Butler MG, James IT, Hart DJ, Thompson PW, Scott DL (1992) Keratan sulphate in rheumatoid arthritis, osteoarthritis, and inflammatory diseases. Ann Rheum Dis 51:1134–1137

45. Thonar EJ-MA, Shinmei M, Lohmander LS (1993) Body Fluid Markers of Cartilage Changes in Osteoarthritis. Rheum Dis Clin North America 19:635–657

46. Lohmander LS, Thonar EJ-MA (1994) Serum keratan sulfate concentrations are different in primary and posttraumatic osteoarthrosis of the knee (abstract). Trans Orthop Res Soc 19:459

47. Petersson IF, Sandquist L, Svensson B, Saxne T (1997) Cartilage markers in synovial fluid in symptomatic knee osteoarthritis. Ann Rheum Dis 56:64–67

48. Saxne T, Heinegård D, Wollheim FA (1987) Cartilage proteoglycans in synovial fluid and serum in patients with inflammatory joint disease. Arthritis Rheum 30:972–979

49. Belcher C, Yaqub R, Fawthrop F, Bayliss M, Doherty M (1997) Synovial fluid chondroitin and keratan sulphate epitopes, glycosaminoglycans, and hyaluronan in arthritic and normal knees. Ann Rheum Dis 56:299–307

50. Saxne T, Heinegård D (1992a) Synovial fluid analysis of two groups of proteoglycan epitopes distinguishes early and late cartilage lesions. Arthritis Rheum 35:385–390

51. Sharif M, George E, Shepstone L, Knudson W, Thonar EJ, Cushnagan J, Dieppe P (1995a) Serum hyaluronic acid level as a predictor of disease progression in osteoarthritis of the knee. Arthritis Rheum 38:760–767

52. Sharif M, Saxne T, Shepstone L, Kirwan JR, Elson CR, Heinegård D, Dieppe PA (1995b) Relationship between serum cartilage oligomeric matrix protein levels and disease progression in osteoarthritis of the knee joint. Br J Rheumatol 34:306–310

53. Månsson B, Carey D, Alini M, Ionescu M, Rosenberg LC, Poole AR, Heinegård D, Saxne T (1995) Cartilage and bone metabolism in rheumatoid arthritis. Differences between rapid and slow progression of disease identified by serum markers of cartilage metabolism. J Clin Invest 95:1071–1077

54. Spector TD, Hart DJ, Nandra D, Doyle DV, Mackillop N, Gallimore JR, Pepys MB (1997) Low-level increases in serum C-reactive protein are present in early osteoarthritis of the knee and predict progressive disease. Arthritis Rheum 40:723–727

55. Clark IM, Powell LK, Ramsey S, Hazleman BL, Cawston TE (1993) The measurement of collagenase, tissue inhibitor of metalloproteinases (TIMP), and collagenase-TIMP complex in synovial fluids from patients with osteoarthritis and rheumatoid arthritis. Arthritis Rheum 36:372–379

56. Manicourt DH, Fujimoto N, Obata K, Thonar EJ (1994) Serum levels of collagenase, stromelysin-1, and TIMP-1. Age- and sex-related differences in normal subjects and relationship to the extent of joint involvement and serum levels of antigenic keratan sulfate in patients with osteoarthritis. Arthritis Rheum 37:1774–1783

57. Zucker S, Lysik RM, Zarrabi MH, Greenwald RA, Gruber B, Tickle SP, Baker T, Docherty AJP (1994) Elevated plasma stromelysin levels in arthritis. J Rheumatol 21:2329–2333

58. Yoshihara Y, Obata KI, Fujimoto N, Yamashita K, Hayakawa T, Shimmei M (1995) Increased levels of stromelysin-1 and tissue inhibitor of metalloproteinases-1 in sera from patients with rheumatoid arthritis. Arthritis Rheum 38:969–975

59. Sandy JD, Flannery CR, Neame PJ, Lohmander LS (1992) The structure of aggrecan fragments in human synovial fluid: Evidence for the involvement in osteoarthritis of a novel proteinase which cleaves the glu 373-ala 374 bond of the interglobular domain. J Clin Invest 89:1512–1516

60. Lohmander LS, Neame P, Sandy JD (1993b) The structure of aggrecan fragments in human synovial fluid: Evidence that aggrecanase mediates cartilage degradation in inflammatory joint disease, joint injury and osteoarthritis. Arthritis Rheum 36:1214–1222

61. Lark MW, Bayne EK, Flanagan J, Harper CF, Hoerrner LA, Hutchinson NI, Singer II, Donatelli SA, Weidner JR, Williams HR, Mumford RA, Lohmander LS (1997) Aggrecan degradation in human cartilage. Evidence for both aggrecanase and matrix metalloproteinase activity in normal, osteoarthritic and rheumatoid joints. J Clin Invest 100:93–106

62. Saxne T, Heinegård D, Wollheim FA (1986) Therapeutic effects on cartilage metabolism in arthritis as measured by release of proteoglycan structures into the synovial fluid. Ann Rheum Dis 45:491–497

63. Sharif M, Salisbury C, Taylor DJ, Kirwan JR (1998) Changes in biochemical markers of joint tissue metabolism in a randomized controlled trial of glucocorticoid in early rheumatoid arthritis. Arthritis Rheum 41:1203–1209

64. Brennan FM, Browne KA, Green PA, Jaspar JM, Maini RN, Feldmann M (1997) Reduction of serum matrix metalloproteinase 1 and matrix metalloproteinase 3 in rheumatoid arthritis patients following anti-tumour necrosis factor-alpha (cA2) therapy. Br J Rheumatol 36:643–650

65. Lindqvist E, Saxne T (1997) Cartilage macromolecules in knee joint synovial fluid. Markers of the disease course in patients with acute oligoarthritis. Ann Rheum Dis 56:751–753

66. Lohmander LS, Dahlberg L, Eyre D, Lark M, Thonar EJ-MA, Ryd L (1998b) Longitudinal and cross-sectional variability in markers of joint metabolism in patients with knee pain and articular cartilage abnormalities. Osteoarthritis Cartilage 6:351–361

67. Lohmander LS, Dahlberg L, Ryd L, Heinegård D (1989) Increased levels of proteoglycan fragments in knee joint fluid after injury. Arthritis Rheum 32:1434–1442

68. Campion GV, Delmas PD, Dieppe PA (1989) Serum and synovial osteocalcin (bone Gla protein) levels in joint disease. Br J Rheumatol 28:393–398

69. Mehraban F, Finegan CK, Moskowitz RW (1991) Serum keratan sulfate – quantitative and qualitative comparisons in inflammatory versus noninflammatory arthritides. Arthritis Rheum 34:383–392

70. Hazell PK, Dent C, Fairclough JA, Bayliss MT, Hardingham TE (1995) Changes in glycosaminoglycan epitope levels in knee joint fluid following injury. Arthritis Rheum 38:953–959

71. Slater Jr RR, Bayliss MT, Lachiewicz PF, Visco DM, Caterson B (1995) Monoclonal antibodies that detect biochemical markers of arthritis in humans. Arthritis Rheum 38:655–659

72. Shinmei M, Miyauchi S, Machida A, Miyazaki K (1992) Quantitation of chondroitin 4-sulfate and chondroitin 6-sulfate in pathologic joint fluid. Arthritis Rheum 35:1304–1308

73. Witsch-Prehm P, Miehlke R, Kresse H (1992) Presence of small proteoglycan fragments in normal and arthritic human cartilage. Arthritis Rheum 35:1042–1052

74. Saxne T, Heinegård D (1992b) Cartilage oligomeric matrix protein: a novel marker of cartilage turnover detectable in synovial fluid and blood. Br J Rheumatol 31:583–591

75. Shinmei M, Ito K, Matsuyama S, Yoshihara Y, Matsuzawa K (1993) Joint fluid carboxyterminal type II procollagen peptide as a marker of cartilage collagen biosynthesis. Osteoarthritis Cartilage 1:121–128

76. Hollander AP, Heathfield TF, Webber C, Iwata Y, Bourne R, Rorabeck C, Poole AR (1994) Increased damage to type II collagen in osteoarthritic cartilage detected by a new immunoassay. J Clin Invest 93:1722–1732

77. Billinghurst RC, Dahlberg L, Ionescu M, Reiner A, Bourne R, Rorabeck C, Mitchell P, Hambor J, Diekmann O, Tschesche H, Chen J, Van Wart H, Poole AR (1997) Enhanced cleavage of type II collagen by collagenases in osteoarthritic articular cartilage. J Clin Invest 99:1534–1545

78. Atley LM, Shao P, Shaffer K, Ochs V, Clemens JD, Eyre DR (1998) Collagen type II crosslinked telopeptides, a promising marker of cartilage degradation in arthritis (abstract). Transactions of Combined Orthopedic Research Societies Meeting, in press

79. Goldberg RL, Lenz ME, Huff J, Glickman P, Katz R. Thonar EJ-MA (1991) Elevated plasma levels of hyaluronate in patients with osteoarthritis and rheumatoid arthritis. Arthritis Rheum 34:799–807

80. Hedin P-J, Weitoft T, Hedin H, Engström-Laurent A, Saxne T (1991) Serum concentrations of hyaluronan and proteoglycan in joint disease. Lack of association. J Rheumatol 18:1601–1605

81. Sharif M, George E, Dieppe PA (1996) Synovial fluid and serum concentrations of aminoterminal propeptide of type III procollagen in healthy volunteers and patients with joint disease. Ann Rheum Dis 55:47–51

82. Lohmander LS, Saxne T, Heinegård D (1996b) Increased concentrations of bone sialoprotein in joint fluid after knee injury. Ann Rheum Dis 55:622–626

83. Sharif M, George E, Dieppe PA (1995c) Correlation between synovial fluid markers of cartilage and bone turnover and scintigraphic scan abnormalities in osteoarthritis of the knee. Arthritis Rheum 38:78–81

84. Astbury C, Bird HA, McLaren AM, Robins SP (1994) Urinary excretion of pyridinium crosslinks of collagen correlated with joint damage in arthritis. Br J Rheumatol 33:11–15

85. Thompson PW, Spector TD, James IT, Henderson E, Hart DJ (1992) Urinary collagen crosslinks reflect the radiographic severity of knee osteoarthritis. Br J Rheumatol 31:759–761

CHAPTER 6

Evolution and Prognosis of Osteoarthritis

E. VEYS and G. VERBRUGGEN

6.1
Introduction

The prediction of the outcome of the osteoarthritic disease of involved joints in individual patients actually is nearly impossible since in general little is known about the natural course of the disease. The technical investigations, nowadays available, do not allow an individualised approach of prognostic factors. The most recent technics, as magnetic resonance imaging [1, 2], bone scintigraphy [2–5] and serum markers of cartilage loss [6] are still in investigation and before they can be accepted as prognostic markers their correlation with the conventional radiographs [7–9], the golden standard, has to be proven. Further on the actually available data on conventional radiographs are scarse and limited to hand [9–15], knee [5, 14, 16–23] and hip joints [24–29].

The heterogeneity of the osteoarthritic conditions is the major reason why it remains so hazardous to make prognostic speculations in individual patients. The recognition of prognostic factors will depend on the better knowledge of the natural course of the disease. The sequential analysis of large populations of patients, the comparison of populations which only differ by minimal number of variables (age or sex or occupation or symptom) and the better understanding of the etiologic moments of the disease are key investigations by which the physician will be capable to predict the outcome of the disease.

6.2
Heterogeneity of Osteoarthritis

Osteoarthritis is the common name given to a heterogeneous group of conditions resulting in similar pathological and radiographic changes. The clinical features are characterized by similar subjective complains and by decrease of the joint mobility and subsequent functional loss. Although some authors reported an increased prevalence of pain in more progressive cases of osteoarthritis [10, 30], there is no strict parallelism between the anatomical changes and the clinical findings: this is one of the key problems to predict the outcome of the disease in one particular patient when the physician only depends on the radiographs.

The heterogeneity of osteoarthritis is well recognised, but a largely accepted list of subsets is not yet available and frequently different concepts are associated to identical items.

Starting from the premise that all osteoarthritic conditions in fact are caused by biomechanical stress, we can subdivide them in **primary** osteoarthritis when the anatomical status of the joint tissues was intact at the moment of the initiation of the disease and in **secondary** osteoarthritis when the joint tissues were already altered at the moment of the initiation of the osteoarthritic disease.

Primary osteoarthritis will occur in all subjects in those joints which are compromised by their localization so that, with normal use and with increasing age, they will present anatomical changes compatible with the features which are considered as characteristic for osteoarthritis: e.g. the intervertebral disks between the 5th and the 6th cervical vertebral bodies, the 4th and the 5th lumbar vertebrae, the 5th lumbar and the 1st sacral vertebral bodies, the carpometacarpal joint of the thumbs and the first metatarsophalangeal joint. Primary osteoarthritis due to postural abnormalities is more relevant for the clinician: osteoarthritis of the knee or hip joints due to varus or valgus deformities of these joints, lipping of the "forside" of the dorsal vertebrae in patients with a hyperkyfosis, and osteoarthritis of the dorsolateral zygapophyseal joints of the lumbar spine in patients with a lumbar hyperlodosis.

Secondary osteoarthritis will occur in patients with preexisting abnormalities in the joint tissues. This type of osteoarthritis can occur in joints with previously affected articular cartilage after transient but recurrent inflammation of the synovial membrane as seen in haemochromatosis, in chondrocalcinosis, in burned-out rheumatoid arthritis, in spondyloarthropathies especially at the hip joints. Cartilage dysfunction may result from inherited disorders of collagen molecules [32, 32] and will occur in various metabolic diseases such as acromegaly, haemochromatosis, chondrocalcinosis, ochronosis. Secondary osteoarthritis also will occur in subjects with previously affected subchondral bone, e.g. in the congenital epiphyseal dysplasia's, in Paget disease or after intraarticular fractures.

These examples are given to document the heterogeneity in the osteoarthritis population due to the cause of the disease. One of the problems in classifying osteoarthritic patients according to that issue is due to the fact that a patient frequently consult the physician in a late stage of the disease at the moment the symptoms become obvious. At that stage the disease became already multifactorial, all joint tissues being involved in the disease process: articular cartilage, subchondral bone, synovial membrane and adjacent muscles. It becomes then hazardous to speculate on the origin of the disease.

The classification of osteoarthritic patients in different subsets is possible on the basis of the presumed initiating factors of the disease, subsets also can be proposed according to the number and the pattern of joints involved or the distribution within joints. Further on, weight bearing joints will undergo another evolution than non weight bearing joints.

The radiographic aspect of the affected joint is another cause of heterogeneity: when the repair phenomena are pronounced (hypertrophic osteo-

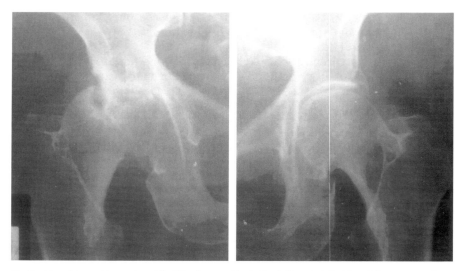

Fig. 1. Atrophic and hypertrophic OA of respectively the left and right hip of the same patient. The joint space of the right hip joint is narrowed, subchondral sclerosis is present at the upper part of the acetabulum and discrete osteophytosis has installed as a part of the remodeling process. At the left side, the joint space has disappeared and huge cysts have been formed in the acetabulum and in the femoral head. No signs of remodeling are apparent

arthritis) one can speculate that the outcome of the disease will be different from a joint which presents practically no signs of repair (atrophic osteo-arthritis) (Fig. 1).

In each case, we must consider that several factors will influence the out-come; as an example, the evolution of the osteoarthritis of the knee in a patient who underwent a medial meniscectomy, will depend from the inherited quality of its joint tissues [33], from his body weight [18, 34 – 35] and occupation, from the vascularization of the subchondral bone and from the previous bio-mechanical status of the joint. The influence of these factors is assumed but their association with the evolution is less clear, there are still a number of unknowns as well.

The influence of biomechanical abnormalities in adjacent joints is another factor which can influence the evolution of osteoarthritis in a considered joint, so the genu varum is deleterious for the knee joint but obviously presents some biomechanical beneficial effect on the hip joint. This point can be the reason why authors looking for subsets of patients with osteoarthritis according to the localisation of involved joints report a separate subset of patients presenting hip joint as unique manifestation of the disease in contrast to patients with osteoarthritis of the knee joints who simultaneously present osteoarthritis of the hands and spine.

6.3
Population Studies

Two different ways can be followed to collect data from population studies to improve the knowledge of the final outcome of osteoarthritis, the final issue being to give the possibility to the physician to predict the prognosis of osteoarthritis at single joint level or for several joints in cases of generalized osteoarthritis. Ideally, the prognosis should be predicted at the first contact with the patients, based on imaging techniques and on serum levels of specific markers. Unfortunately, we are far from this optimal situation since data on the natural course of the disease in population studies are scarse and limited to some joints as the hands, the knees and the hips. The first possibility to improve this knowledge, is to follow a cohort of patients over the time and to collect as much data as possible at each visit. Since osteoarthritis is a slow progressing disease the cohort should be followed for a rather long time, even the time interval between two analyses must be long enough: changes must be detectable with conventional techniques. The second possibility is to perform a cross sectional analyse of two populations which only differ by one variable in order to approach the influence of this variable on the evolution of the disease. The populations can be different either in age, in sex, in occupation, or in the presence or absence of symptoms, … but they should be as homogeneous as possible for variables other than the variable selected for the study.

6.3.1
Sequential Population Studies

The number of studies dealing with the natural course of the disease are scarse and they are all focussed on hands, knees and hips. The evolution and outcome of knee and hand osteoarthritis will be dicussed in this chapter.

6.3.1.1
Radiographic Progression of Knee Osteoarthritis

Most authors agree that separate scoring of different osteoarthritis-associated variables give more accurate data than when a general joint score as proposed in the Kellgren and Lawrence method [36] is allocated to the joint. The involvement of the different compartments is another variable considered in a few investigations [8, 37]. In most studies the following variables were evaluated: joint space narrowing, osteophytes, cyst formation, subchondral bone sclerosis. In some studies the loss of cortical integrity was also noticed as attrition and chondrocalcinosis and desaxation were also evaluated. Most often, semiquantitative assessment was used to grade the severity of the anatomical changes. Microfocal radiography was proposed to measure the changes in some of these osteoarthritis-associated features more accurately [14, 23].

6.3.1.1.1
Joint Space Narrowing

The narrowest point of the tibiofemoral joint space can be measured in millimeters with a ruler or a caliper [5, 21], but the narrowing can also be graded 0–3 in the separate compartments of the knee joint [5, 16, 17, 19]. In a general population study, Schouten et al. [18] used a nine point score for the evaluation of the joint space, from −4 over 0 to +4. For others [38] the joint space was one variable included in a summative quantitative score, presence of joint space narrowing being scored as +1.0 at inclusion in the study and further narrowing or widening during follow up being scored as a supplementary + or −1.0.

6.3.1.1.2
Osteophytes

Some authors did not evaluate the osteophytes in their scoring system [18]. Others scored them as present or absent [16] or on a 3- (absent, present, severe) [5, 21], or 4-point (absent, dubious, moderate, severe) scale [20]. Finally osteophytes at different sites of the joint were be quantitated separately, the presence of each ostephyte at the inclusion in the study being scored as +0.2. During follow up the appearance or disappearance of an osteophyte was then scored as + or −1.0, the enlargement or decrease in size of an existing osteophyte as + or −0.5. These numbers were then included in a general quantitative joint score [38].

6.3.1.1.3
Subchondral Bone Sclerosis

In the majority of the studies bone sclerosis was noticed as present or absent [5, 21] and during follow up as 'not changed', 'minor change' or 'major change'. In other studies a score between 0 and 3 was allocated for bone sclerosis [17, 19]. Other authors did not consider this variable [18]. As a matter of fact everybody agrees that subchondral bone sclerosis is difficult to quantitate. In a recently proposed quantitative score system [38] a value of +1.0 was attributed to the presence of subchondral bone sclerosis at the inclusion of the subjects in the study and during follow up on the roentgenograms a score of +1.0 or −1.0 was given in cases of appearance or disappearance of this feature.

6.3.1.1.4
Cysts, Attrition and Desaxation

In most studies the absence or presence was recorded for these three variables [5, 16, 17, 19 – 21]. In a recent survey, the presence of each of these features added +1.0 point to the patient's overall quantitative score at its inclusion. Appearance or disappearance during follow up was scored + or −1.0 [38].

6.3.1.1.5
Summative, Global or Overall Scores

In most prospective studies the presence and severity of the separately evaluated variables are recorded as such [5, 16 – 21]. A somewhat modified summative quantitative score for the knee joint was proposed more recently [38] in which the presence of each of these variables was recorded at multiple sites of the joint and quantified as reported above. Overall knee joint scores were obtained at inclusion and after each consecutive evaluation (Fig. 2).

6.3.1.1.6
Analysis of the Reported Populations

A number of populations have been recently reported with sufficient duration of follow up to allow some conclusions about the prognosis of OA of the knee joint. All of them were prospective studies and most of them focussed on radiographic data (Table 1).

Massardo et al. [16] reported a follow up study of 32 patients, in which roentgenograms were taken at start and after 8 years. The authors separately evaluated the different radiographic signs: osteophytosis, loss of cortical integrity, joint space narrowing, subchondral bone reaction and the presence of chondrocalcinosis. Their major conclusion was that the presence of OA of the hands was a predictive sign for deterioration of the status of the knee joint. Spector et al. [17] analysed 63 patients in a 11 years long follow up study. Radiographs were taken at start and after 11 years. They used the Kellgren and Lawrence score, but scored also separately joint space narrowing in a 0 – 5 scale. The osteophytes and the subchondral bone sclerosis was evaluated per compartment in an overall 0 – 3 score. They considered joints which showed an increase of 1 grade or more, or a additional reduction of joint space of 10 % or more, to be progressive. Their major conclusions were that in general the disease had a slow progression, that the body weight at entry was not a major sign of disease progression and that patients with rapid progression were found between those who had knee pain at the entry of their prospective study. The overall good prognosis in this population is in contradiction with the data reported by Hernborg and Nilsson [22]. In this study 60 % of the patients showed deterioration after 13 years, but a major bias might have been the exclusion of patients presenting osteophytes as unique radiological manifestation of OA. So, the authors possibly selected more progressive cases at the inclusion. Starting from a population study, Schouten et al. [18] did a follow up analysis of the evolution of OA of the knee in 142 patients with a duration of follow up of 12 years. Roentgenograms were taken at start and at the end of this study. The authors used the Kellgren and Lawrence score but also graded the joint space narrowing on a 9-point scale (from – 4 to + 4). They also looked to the presence of chondrocalcinosis. The variables which appeared to be significantly related to cartilage loss were: body mass index, repetitive impulse loading, valgus or varus deformity, chondrocalcinosis and the presence of Heberden's nodes. Surprising was the finding that injury of the knee and especially meniscectomy

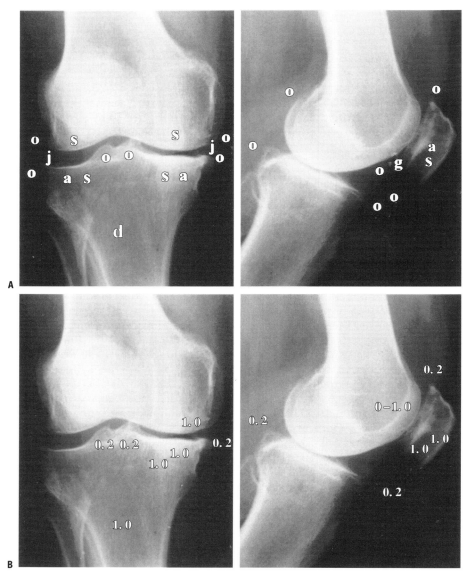

Fig. 2A, B. Osteoarthritis of the knee; scoring system developed at the Ghent University Hospital. **A** The system is based on the recognition of five OA-associated features sought for at different sites of the joint on the anteroposterior and laterolateral roentgenograms. **B** Scores attributed to 'presence' of the abnormalities (Table 3) are added to obtain an 'overall severity score'. In this case the 'overall severity score' amounts to 7.2 or 8.2 depending on the reader's personal bias about the femoropatellar joint space. After a given interval of time the changes in the appearance of the OA-associated features are added to obtain the 'overall progression score'. Overall severity score at the start of a study and overall progression score after completion of a study can be cumulated to a severity score at the end of the follow up period

Table 1. Cohort studies of the natural evolution of knee osteoarthritis

Authors	Ref.	Number of patients	Follow-up (years)
Dieppe et al.	[5]	75	5
Massardo et al.	[16]	32	8
Spector et al.	[17]	63	11
Schouten et al.	[18]	142	13
Ledingham et al.	[19]	188	2
Doherty et al.	[20]	135	2.5
Dieppe et al.	[21]	415	3
Hernborg and Nilsson	[22]	84	15
Buckland-Wright	[23]	33	1.5
Verbruggen et al.	[38]	36	3 and 5

were unrelated to cartilage loss. Dieppe et al. [5] followed 75 patients with OA of the knee during 5 years. Actually, the authors started with 94 patients but 19 of them were lost of follow up or died. They looked to the following outcomes: need of surgery, joint space narrowing of 2 mm, ostephytes (on a 3-point scale) and the presence of sclerosis. Age, sex, obesity and duration of symptoms were only weakly related to outcome. Presence of crepitus, joint swelling and instability at intrance achieved highly significant correlations with outcome. The strongest positive correlation was the association of severe pain at entry and a subsequent operation of the knee (15 patients).

The authors also performed bone scintigraphy on these cohort, all patients who progressed had a positive scan, but nearly half of the patients who did not progress also had a positive scan. Ledingham et al. [19] evaluated the prognostic significance of radiographic features for outcome of knee osteoarthritis; The data were obtained from 188 patients, from which 350 joints were analysed with a medium duration of follow up of 2 years. The Kellgren and Lawrence score was evaluated altough the separate features also were recorded. An increase of the osteophyte size did not correlate with clinical status. Narrowing of joint space and bone attrition, which are variables reflecting bone and cartilage loss were correlated with deterioration of the clinical condition of the patients. Also knee effusion and the presence of chondrocalcinosis reflected a deterioration of the radiologic pictures. In fact 72 % of the patients presented changes of at least one radiographic feature: increase in joint space narrowing occured in 52 % of the patients, osteophyte evolution in 32 %, cysts in 19 %, sclerosis in 14 % and attrition in 30 %. Nearly the same numbers were reported by Doherty et al. [20], in a follow up study of 2.4 years of 135 patients. The authors evaluated the radiographs in the same way as in the previous study and described also a close correlation between the evolution of both knees in individual cases. Dieppe et al. [21] following the same procedure as in their previous study [5], confirmed the strong association between the 'right-left knee' evolution in the same patient. They also described a strong association between joint space narrowing and increase in osteophyte size or in appearance of subchondral sclerosis. There was little evidence of correlation between any clinical outcomes and any changes on radiographs.

6.3.1.1.7
The Natural Evolution of Knee Osteoarthritis: Conclusions

There is significant progression of osteoarthritis of the knee during follow up. Although this evolution was reported to be slow in some studies [5, 17, 21], others reports showed a less optimistic picture [19, 20]. Evolution on both sides was found to be strongly associated [20, 21]. Age, sex, body weight, duration of symptoms and the presence of generalized osteoarthritis are associated to the outcome of the knee joint disease [5, 17, 21, 34].

The presence of symptoms at entry is correlated with increase of joint space narrowing on follow up [17, 19], with increasing bone attrition [19], but not with increase of the osteophytosis [19]. Another study showed a strong association between narrowing of the joint space and increase in osteophyte size and appearance of subchondral sclerosis [21]. The patients who presented finger joint osteoarthritis were more at risk to show a rapid progression of their osteoarthritis of the knees [16, 33].

6.3.1.2
Radiographic Progression of Finger Joint Osteoarthritis

6.3.1.2.1
Non Erosive Versus Erosive Osteaoarthritis of the Finger Joints

The incidence, pattern of joint involvement and severity of degenerative joint disease are comparable in men and women to their early fifties. After this age, the disease becomes more generalized and progressive in women [39, 40]. The interphalangeal (IP) joints, and the first carpometacarpal (CMC) joints become more frequently involved [39, 40]. Distal interphalangeal joints (DIP) were reported to be more frequently involved than the proximal interphalangeal joints (PIP) or the metacarpophalangeal joints (MCP) [41–43]. Several studies have shown 70–80% of the DIP joints, and about 50% of the PIP joints to be affected in individuals with a history of symptom producing osteoarthritis of their finger joints for several years. These patients who effectively sought medical advise for their osteoarthritis, had rapidly developed symmetric involvement of the finger joints and the above-mentioned incidence rates were seen in patients with a clinical history of over 5 years. Furthermore, the progression of the disease is completely different in IP and in MCP joints. The destructive evolution characteristic for what is classically coined as 'erosive' [42] or 'inflammatory' [43, 44] osteoarthritis of the finger joints is exclusively seen in the distal and proximal interphalangeal joints. These observations suggest that in women of menopausal age, factors other than exclusively mechanical ones are operational when the disease comes to expression. Changes in the hormonal balance might increase the risk of inflammatory processes in synovial joints, and osteoarthritic (OA) DIP and PIP joints can become severely inflamed in the perimenopausal period [41–47]. Hence, the functional outcome of the disease depends largely on the occurence eventually of the 'erosive' or 'inflammatory' form of the disease.

MCP joints were less frequently affected and the pattern of involvement allowed to suggest that mechanical factors probably were the main initiators of osteoarthritis of the MCP joints. The second MCP joint was significantly more affected than the third MCP. There was only minor involvement of MCP4 and 5 [15].

6.3.1.2.2
Progression of Non Erosive Osteoarthritis of the Finger Joints

Roentgenograms are still commonly accepted to judge the morbidity and the progression of osteoarthritis of the finger joints. Non erosive and erosive osteoarthritis differ in their clinical outcome and radiographic characteristics. The measurement of progression of both types of osteoarthritis has to be done by different scoring systems. As in most other joints, non erosive osteoarthritis of the finger joints is characterized by the classical features of osteoarthritis e. g. narrowing of the joint space together with the changes in the bony compartments of the joint such as osteophytes, subchondral sclerosis and cysts.

A 'Global Estimate' of Progression

A global estimate of osteoarthritis of the finger joints was developed by Kellgren and Lawrence in 1957 and for many years was accepted to be the golden standard for measuring the progression of finger joint osteoarthritis [36]. This grading system was based on the assumption that progression of osteoarthritis in these joints follows a sequence of events in which osteophyte formation was the pathognomonic event and all other signs of osteoarthritis were considered as less specific. However, joint space narrowing and the changes in the subchondral bone architecture can occur before osteophytes develop. Furthermore, changes in the anatomy of the affected joint tissues progress at different rates during different intervals of time. The system was thus unsensitive to change. Assessment of the progression of osteoarthritis of the DIP joints showed that it took 11 years on average to progress 1 Kellgren/Lawrence scale grade for these particular joints [48].

Semiquantitative Assessment of Progression of Osteoarthritis-Associated Features

More recently, attempts have been made to define the clinical criteria for the diagnosis of symptomatic primary osteoarthritis of the hands [49] and to score the progression of the different osteoarthritis associated items within certain time limits [9]. In a series of hand roentgenograms taken with an interval of 12 to 60 months progression was scored in 12 sites of both hands: the 4 DIP and 4 PIP joints, the first IP joint, the first trapeziometacarpal joint, the scaphotrapezoid joint and the widening of the distance between the bases of the first and second metacarpals. Radiographic variables assessed were joint space width, osteophytes, sclerosis, cysts or erosions and alignment (Table 2). The degree of abnormality was scored in a 4-point scale, and for each parameter the extent of difference between the 2 films was marked on a 10-cm analog scale, for which the center mark indicated no difference. Osteophytes were rated as the

Table 2. Osteoarthritis of the finger joints: measurement of progression

	Assay system	Severity scale	Progression	Time interval	Ref.
Non erosive osteoarthritis					
Kellgren	Reference picture	Semiquantitative ?	Comparative	Not sensitive	[11]
Altman et al.	OA-associated items	Semiquantitative	Comparative (2 films)	12–60 months	[14]
	Joint space width	4-point scale '0–3'	10 cm VAS		
	Osteophytes	4-point scale '0–3'	10 cm VAS		
	Sclerosis	4-point scale '0–3'	10 cm VAS		
	Cysts/erosions	4-point scale '0–3'	10 cm VAS		
	Alignment	4-point scale '0–3'	10 cm VAS		
	MC widening	4-point scale '0–3'	10 cm VAS		
Kallman et al.	OA-associated items	Semiquantitative	Comparative	7.6 years[a]	[15]
	Joint space width	4-point scale '0–3'	'P/A'[b]		
	Osteophytes	4-point scale '0–3'	'P/A'[b]		
	Sclerosis	2-point scale'P/A'[b]	'P/A'[b]		
	Cysts	2-point scale'P/A'[b]	'P/A'[b]		
	Lateral deformity	2-point scale'P/A'[b]	'P/A'[b]		
	Collapse cortical bone	2-point scale'P/A'[b]	'P/A'[b]		
Verbruggen and Veys	OA-associated items	Not done	Comparative	3–5 years[c]	[16]
	Joint space width	Not done	see Table 3		
	Osteophytes	Not done	see Table 3		
	Subchondral cysts	Not done	see Table 3		
Buckland-Wright et al.	OA-associated items	Quantitative[d]	Quantitative	18 months	[17, 18]
	Joint space width	Quantitative[d]	Quantitative		
	Osteophytes	Quantitative[d]	Quantitative		
	Juxtaarticular radiolucencies	Quantitative[d]	Quantitative		
	Subchondral sclerosis	Quantitative[d]	Quantitative		
Erosive osteoarthritis					
Verbruggen and Veys	Reference picture	Anatomical phases	Comparative	3–5 years[e]	[16]

[a] On average.
[b] P/A: present/absent.
[c] Radiographs taken with one-year intervals, sensitive to change within 2 years.
[d] Smallest object recorded: 25–50 μm; 4% changes in joint space width or in osteophyte length were considered to be significant.
[e] Radiographs taken with one-year intervals, sensitive to change within 1 year.

most important feature in identifying osteoarthritis progression in the hand. Erosions were the second most important variable for determining progression and joint space narrowing was rated third in importance. Although osteophyte scores most often identified the correct time sequence between two roentgenograms, no single variable highly sensitively identified osteoarthritis progression. Added combinations of radiographic findings (osteophytes plus narrowing plus erosions) increased the sensitivity scores and scores that combined both hands were superior to those of one hand alone. In summary, this score system enabled clinicians to grade the severity of osteoarthritis of the hands at one particular time, and to assess the progression of the disease during a variable time interval. However, the 4-point scale system (normal, mild, moderate and severe) to assess morbidity and the visual analogue scale used to measure progression leaves some room for interpretation and subjectivity.

A similar grading system [10] used almost identical variables to score the severity of osteoarthritis in a somewhat different scale alignment (Table 3). Kallman et al. graded subchondral sclerosis, cysts, lateral deformity and collapse of central joint cortical bone as 'absent or present'. Osteophytes and joint space narrowing on a 4-point scale are again leaving some room for interpretation. On average, the roentgenograms were taken 7.6 years apart. Progression was significant within this long period of follow-up. Close agreement between readers was obtained when changes in osteophytes, joint space width, alignment and collapse of central joint cortical bone were considered. There was no agreement on the changes in the subchondral bone, e.g., sclerosis and cysts.

More recently, 46 patients with osteoarthritis of their finger joints were followed up for 3 years; 36 of them were followed up for 5 years [15]. Posteroanterior radiographs of the hands were obtained at the start of this prospective study and at yearly intervals. Progression over time was assessed in the DIP, PIP and MCP joints and the scoring system used were based on the increase in incidence of osteoarthritis during consecutive years in previously normal joints and the radiological progression of the anatomical lesions in the pathological finger joints (Table 3). As mentioned earlier [10], readers of roentgenograms are confronted with their own inherent bias about what they consider a positive radiological finding. To avoid problems in interpretation when defining 'presence or absence' of an abnormality at the start and at the finish of the follow up period, only changes during fixed time intervals were recorded. To facilitate the readings, documents were compared during the same reading session. The assay system was based on the changes in osteophytes or small ossification centers (ossicles) occurring at the joint margins, joint space and subchondral bone (cyst formation). Subchondral sclerosis was not considered since it was difficult to quantify. When roentgenograms were compared at one-year intervals, it appeared that the minute changes in the size of osteophytes, in joint space width or in the structure of the subchondral plate were to often disputable. It was decided to increase the interval between two readings to obtain more definite changes. On completion of the study only the posteroanterior roentgenograms obtained at the start and after 3 and 5 years were used to evaluate the incidence and progression of the disease.

24 joints (8 MCP, 8 PIP and 8 DIP joints) per roentgenogram were studied. The condition at the time of patient inclusion was compared with the appearance 3 or 5 years later. Points were attributed to changes in the aforementioned items as illustrated in Table 3. The scores for the 8 DIP, 8 PIP and 8 MCP joints were combined for each patient. Significant increases both in the numbers of affected DIP, PIP and MCP joints per subject, and in the anatomical progression of the OA in the different finger joints of each individual patient were recorded during 3 and 5 years of follow-up.

Table 3. Scores attributed to changes in osteoarthritic joints

Osteophytes[a]		Joint space		Subchondral cysts	
Appearance	+ 1.0	Narrowing	+ 1.0	Appearance	+ 1.0
Disappearance	– 1.0	Widening	– 1.0	Disappearance	– 1.0
Increase in size	+ 0.5			Increase in size	+ 0.5
Decrease in size	– 0.5			Decrease in size	– 0.5

[a] Small ossification centers at the joint margins were regarded as OA-related changes and they were evaluated as osteophytes.

Quantitative Microfocal Radiography: Progression of Osteo-Arthritis

The best results with the above-mentioned assay procedures are obtained when the changes in the different features in a set of finger joints are grouped in a global summative score. Even then, it takes years to obtain interpretable changes in the anatomy of these finger joints. Measurement of the changes over 18 months of each different radiologic feature of so-called 'non erosive' osteo-arthritis in finger joints was made possible by quantitative microfocal radiography [11, 12] (Table 2). Significant progression in the anatomical changes were detected within this short period of time.

The fact that this technique enabled the detection of changes associated with the earliest phases of osteoarthritis is of particular interest. An increase of the joint space width in a significant proportion of these patients was logically interpreted as a possible consequence of the increase of cartilage water content associated with early disease [50, 51]. In the more progressed stages of the disease narrowing of the joint space became obvious [11]. In most of the osteoarthritic finger joints, changes in the bony compartments: e. g. osteophyte formation and subchondral sclerosis became appearant before narrowing or widening of the joint space had occurred.

This accurate method of measurement showed that narrowing of the joint space of patients with finger joint osteoarthrosis was generalized and symmetrical. The changes were first observed in the DIP joints and extended through the PIP joints to the MCP and wrist joints. This observation agrees with the earliest and more recent descriptions of the disease.

6.3.1.2.3
Non Erosive Osteoarthritis of the Finger Joints: Discussion

Different observers have agreed that progression of finger joint osteoarthritis could be measured within a reasonably short period of time when progression was assayed by studying different osteoarthritis-associated features (Table 3). Conventional roentgenograms showed osteophytes and erosions or collapse of the subchondral bone plate as the most reliable variables to be followed up. Joint space narrowing has not been considered as sensitive to change. Most readers have difficulties to grade subchondral sclerosis. However, the intro-duction of quantitative microfocal radiography has allowed to use joint space width as a very sensible variable to measure disease progression in much shorter intervals of time. The reliability of most of the grading systems proposed to grade the morbidity of osteoarthritis of the finger joints is increased when the changes in different OA-associated items are combined and when selected combinations of finger joints are taken into consideration.

According to our own experience, classification of the pathological changes in multiple categories; e.g. 'normal', 'doubtful', 'moderate', 'severe', ... leaves much room for personal biases. Therefore, it was proposed to consider the occurence of changes in the above-mentioned OA-associated features as a method of choice to compare the progressive nature of the disease in cohorts of patients under different therapeutic regimes.

6.3.1.2.4
Progression of 'Inflammatory' or 'Erosive' Osteoarthritis of the Finger Joints

Follow-up of the patients disclosed that the disease pattern followed in IP and MCP joints was completely different. The IP joints frequently showed clinically appearant signs of inflammation. This was never the case in MCP joints. Roentgenograms taken during or after these inflammatory episodes showed an 'erosive' type of osteoarthritis classically described in the literature [42–47]. A prospective study was done to assess and to score the progressive nature of osteoarthritis in the DIP and PIP and MCP joints of forty-six patients who were followed for three to five years. Posteroanterior radiographs of the hands were obtained at the start of this prospective study and at yearly intervals. In approx. 40% of these patients the classical picture of OA was complicated by manifest erosive changes, which preceded a period in which repair phenomena in the 'eroded' finger joints led to the generation of a new subchondral plate covered by cartilaginous tissue. Huge osteophytes were then responsible for the nodular aspect of the affected finger joints (Fig. 3).

Five distinct phases in disease progression in the IP joints were defined: the nonaffected joint (N), the stationary osteoarthritic joint (S), the disappearance of the joint space (J), the erosive joint (E) and finally the remodeled (R) or fused (F) joint. J and E phases were only observed in hands with radiological signs of OA; these inflammatory events mainly occurred in joints that already were in the S phase. J or E joints regressing to the S phase were never encountered. Most of the joints in the J or E phases at the start of this prospective study remodeled during the 5 years' observation period. Contrary to what is seen in most chronically progressive rheumatic disorders, the inflammatory episodes spontaneously subsided and were followed by distinct repair. R joints never returned to J or E phases, and no longer showed any evolution. The R joint is the final stage of the disease and clinically appears as a Heberden (DIP) or Bouchard (PIP) node. It can safely be stated that the sequence 'N → S → J → E → R' reflects the natural history of OA of the finger joints in perimenopausal women. Proportions of patients that went through a particular phase are given in Fig. 4.

Roentgenologically, the erosive lesions are identical to those described earlier in so-called 'erosive osteoarthritis' of the finger joints [46, 47]. This disease has been considered a variant form or an entity distinct from other

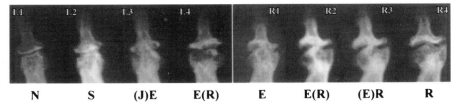

N   S   (J)E   E(R)   E   E(R)   (E)R   R

Fig. 3. Erosive osteoarthritis of the interphalangeal finger joints. The progression through the successive anatomical phases is illustrated. Four pictures on the *left*: roentgenograms of the same DIP2 of the left hand (L1-L4) taken with one-year intervals; L1: not affected (*N*) – L2: the joint became osteoarthritic (stationary phase) showing joint space narrowing, subchondral sclerosis and cysts (without obvious osteophytosis). The joint space has not disappeared (*S*). – L3: Subchondral erosions braking through the subchondral plate; the joint has entered the erosive phase and apparently did not go through the 'lost joint space' phase: (*J*) E – L4: a huge cyst has broken through the subchondral plate of the distal end of the mid phalanx; the base of the terminal phalanx is being remodeled and huge 'nodal' osteophytes appear; the joint is still considered to be in the erosive phase although signs of remodeling are obvious: E(*R*). Four pictures on the *right*: roentgenograms of the DIP2 joint of the right hand of the same patient (R1-R4) taken with one-year intervals; R1: joint in the erosive phase (E) – R2: the DIP joint is still in the E-phase although the base of the terminal phalanx is being remodeled and osteophytes which were already present the year before are increasing in size: E(R) – R3: one year later, the joint is being remodeled further on but remodeling is not completed: (E)R – R4: completely remodeled DIP joint

degenerative diseases affecting the finger joints in women, e. g. menopausal OA [45], inflammatory OA [42], primary generalized OA [52], nodal OA [53]. The earlier recognition of 'erosive' OA in some patients was based on the interpretation of one or at the most two roentgenograms obtained at varying intervals. Our 5 years' follow-up – with roentgenograms made every year – discloses that 'erosive OA' represents merely an episode in the evolution of OA, rather than a separate form of OA. In our population 'erosive osteoarthritis' affected about half of the patients. We would conclude that all clinically manifest Heberden's and Bouchard's nodes with clinical and roentgenological evidence of hard tissue enlargement went through that erosive phase.

6.3.1.2.5
Radiographic Progression and Functional Outcome

A considerable number of patients with osteoarthritis of their finger joints, fortunately do not enter into the 'erosive' phase of the disease. The IP finger joints of these patients remain in the 'stationary' phase and the progresion of this type of osteoarthritis is not different from that seen in the MCP or in any other joint. However, OA of the finger joints is progressive in nature and a proportion of these patients will develop 'inflammatory' or 'erosive' osteoarthritis. Their finger joints will pass through predictable anatomical phases. The recognition of and the attribution of a score to these respective phases, made it possible to assess the progression of 'inflammatory' OA of the IP finger joints.

% of patients

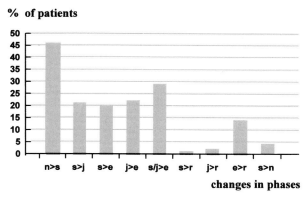

changes in phases

Fig. 4. A cohort of 85 patients with OA of the finger joints has been followed over 3 years. Proportions of patients showing a change in one of the different anatomical phases of OA in their interphalangeal joints are represented. Approx. 45% of the patients developed OA in one or more previously normal finger joints. In 20–30% of the patients, osteoarthritic interphalangeal joints went through the destructive 'J' or 'E' phases characteristic of 'erosive' or 'inflammatory OA. These patients will develop the Heberden's and Bouchard's nodes

The destructive evolution characteristic for what is classically coined as 'erosive' [44] or 'inflammatory' [42, 43] osteoarthritis of the finger joints is exclusively seen in the distal and proximal interphalangeal joints.

The development of franc 'erosive' osteoarthritis in previously 'stationary' osteoarthritic joints is of clinical interest. Osteoarthritis of the finger joints is asymptomatic when the disease is 'non erosive' and becomes symptomatic during the inflammatory episodes associated with the onset of 'erosive' osteoarthritis. Sequential roentgenograms showed that remodeling always occurred in interphalangeal joints after they went through destructive phases [15]. Remodeled distal and proximal interphalangeal finger joints present the typical nodal appearance of Heberden's and Bouchard's noduli and limit the daily activities of the hands.

References

1. Hutton CW, Vennart W (1994) Osteoarthritis and magnetic resonance imaging: potential and problems. Ann Rheum Dis 54:237–243
2. McAlindon TE, Watt I, McCrae FM, Goddard P, Dieppe PA (1991) Magnetic resonance imaging in osteoarthritis of the knee: correlation with radiographic and scintigraphic findings. Ann Rheum Dis 50:14–19
3. Hutton CW, Higgs ER, Jackson PC, Watt I, Dieppe PA (1986) 99TC-HMDP bone scanning in generalized nodal osteoarthritis. 2. The 4-hour bone scan image predicts radiographic change. Ann Rheum Dis 45:622–626
4. McCrae F, Shoels J Dieppe P, Watt I (1992) Scintigraphic assessment of osteoarthritis of the knee joint. Ann Rheum Dis 51:938–942
5. Dieppe PA, Cushnaghan J, Young P, Kirwan J (1993) Prediction of the progression of joint space narrowing and osteoarthritis of the knee by bone scintigraphy. Ann Rheum Dis 52:557–563

6. Lohmander LS (1991) Markers of cartilage metabolism in arthrosis: A Review. Acta Orthop Scand 62 : 623 – 632

7. Dieppe PA (1995) Recommended methodology for assessing the progression of osteo-arthritis of the hip and knee joints. Osteoarthritis Cart 3 : 73 – 77

8. Altmann RD, Hochberg M, Murphy WA, Wolfe F, Lequesne M (1995) Atlas of individual radiographic features in osteoarthritis. Osteoarthritis Cartilage 3 (suppl A): 3 – 70

9. Altman RD, Fries JF, Bloch DA, Carstens J, Cooke TD, Genant H, Gofton P, Groth H, McShane DJ, Murphy WA, Sharp JT, Spitz P, Williams CA, Wolfe F (1987) Radiographic assessment of progression in osteoarthritis. Arthritis Rheum 30 : 1214 – 1225

10. Kallman DA, Wigley FM, Scott WW, Hochberg MC, Tobin JD (1989) New radiographic grading scales for osteoarthritis of the hand. Arthritis Rheum 32 : 1584 – 1591

11. Buckland-Wright JC, MacFarlane DG, Lynch JA, Clark B (1990) Quantitative microfocal radiographic assessment of progression of osteoarthritis of the hand. Arthritis Rheum 33 : 57 – 65

12. Buckland-Wright JC, MacFarlane DG, Lynch JA (1991) Osteophytes in the osteoarthritic hand: their incidence, size, distribution and progression. Ann Rheum Dis 50 : 627 – 630

13. Buckland-Wright JC, MacFarlane DG, Lynch JA (1992) Relationship between joint space width and subchondral sclerosis in the osteoarthritic hand: a quantitative microfocal radiographic study. J Rheumatol 19 : 788 – 795

14. Buckland-Wright JC (1994) Quantitative radiography of osteoarthritis. Review. Ann Rheum Dis 53 : 268 – 275

15. Verbruggen G, Veys EM (1996) Numerical scoring systems for the anatomic evolution of osteoarthritis of the finger joints. Arthritis Rheum 39 : 308 – 320

16. Massardo L, Watt I, Cushnaghan J, Dieppe P (1989) Osteoarthritis of the knee joint: an eight year prospective study. Ann Rheum Dis 48 : 893 – 897

17. Spector TD, Dacre JE, Harris PA, Huskisson EC (1992) Radiological progression of osteo-arthritis: an 11 year follow up study of the knee. Ann Rheum Dis 51 : 1107 – 1110

18. Schouten JSAG, Van den Ouweland FA, Valkenburg HA (1992) A twelve-year follow-up study in the general population on prognostic factors of cartilage loss in osteoarthritis of the knee. Ann Rheum Dis 51 : 932 – 937

19. Ledingham J, Regan M, Jones A, Doherty M (1995) Factors affecting radiographic progression of the knee. Ann Rheum Dis 54 : 53 – 58

20. Doherty M, Belcher C, Regan M, Jones A, Ledingham J (1996) Association between synovial fluid levels of inorganic pyrophosphate and short term radiographic outcome of knee osteoarthritis. Ann Rheum Dis 55 : 432 – 436

21. Dieppe PA, Cushnaghan J, Shepstone L (1997) The Bristol 'OA500' Study: progression of osteoarthritis (OA) over 3 years and the relationship between clinical and radiographic changes at the knee joint. Osteoarthritis Cartilage 5 : 87 – 97

22. Hernborg JS, Nilsson BE (1977) The natural course of untreated osteoarthritis of the knee. Clin Orthop Rel Res 123 : 130 – 137

23. Buckland-Wright JC, MacFarlane DG, Lynch JA, Jasani MK (1995) Quantitative microfocal radiography detects changes in OA knee joint space width in patients in placebo con-trolled trial of NSAID therapy. J Rheumatol 22 : 937 – 943

24. Danielsson L (1964) Incidence and prognosis of coxarthrosis. Acta Orthop Scand 66 (suppl): 9. 87

25. Seifert MH, Whiteside CG, Savage O (1969) A 5-year follow-up of fifty cases of idiopathic osteoarthritis of the hip. Ann Rheum Dis 28 : 352 – 356

26. Macys JR, Bullough PG, Wilson PD Jr (1980) Coxarthrosis: a study of the natural history based on a correlation of clinical, radiographic, and pathological findings. Semin Arthritis Rheum 10 : 66 – 80

27. Ledingham J, Dawson S, Preston B, Milligan G, Doherty M (1993) Radiographic progres-sion of hospital referred osteoarthritis of the hip. Ann Rheum Dis 52 : 263 – 267

28. Dougados M, Gueguen A, Nguyen M, Berdah L, Lequesne M, Mazieres B, Vignon E (1996) Radiological progression of hip osteoarthritis: definition, risk factors and correlations with clinical status. Ann Rheum Dis 55 : 356 – 366

29. Dougados M, Gueguen A, Nguyen M, Berdah L, Lequesne M, Mazieres B, Vignon E (1997) Radiographic features predictive of radiographic progression of hip osteoarthritis. Rev Rheum 64:795–803

30. Croft P, Cooper C, Wickham C, Coggon D (1990) Defining osteoarthritis of the hip for epidemiologic studies. Am J Epidemiol 132: 514–522, 1990

31. Williams CJ, Jimenez SA (1993) Heredity, genes and osteoarthritis. Rheum Dis Clin North Am 19 : 523–543

32. Jimenez SA, Dharmavaram RM (1994) Genetic aspects of familial osteoarthritis. Ann Rheum Dis 53:789–797

33. Doherty M, Watt I, Dieppe P (1983) Influence of primary generalized osteoarthritis on development of secondary osteoarthritis. The Lancet ii: 8–11

34. Dougados M, Gueguen A, Nguyen M, Thiesce A, Listrat V, Jacob L, Nakache JP, Gabriel KR, Lequesne M, Amor B (1992) Longitudinal radiologic evaluation of osteoarthritis of the knee. J Rheumatol 19 : 378–383

35. Spector TD, Hart DL, Doyle DV (1994) Incidence and progression of osteoarthritis in women with unilateral knee disease in the general population: the effect of obesity. Ann Rheum Dis 53:565–568

36. Kellgren JH, Lawrence JS (1957) Radiological assessment of osteoarthritis. Ann Rheum Dis 16 : 494–501

37. McAlindon TE, Snow S, Cooper C, Dieppe P (1992) Radiographic patterns of knee osteo-arthritis in the community: the importance of the patellofemoral joint. Ann Rheum Dis 51:844–849

38. Verbruggen G, Goemaere S, Veys EM (1998) Effects of two chondroitinsulfates on the anatomical evolution of osteoarthritis of the human knee joint. Osteoarthritis Cartilage: submitted

39. Kellgren JH, Lawrence JS, Bier F (1963) Genetic factors in generalized osteoarthrosis. Ann Rheum Dis 22 : 237–245

40. Moskowitz RW (1972) Clinical and laboratory findings in osteoarthritis. Arthritis and allied conditions. Edited by JL Hollander, DJ McCarty Jr. Philadelphia, Lea & Febiger

41. Stecher RM (1955) Heberden's nodes: a clinical description of osteoarthritis of the finger joints. Ann Rheum Dis 14:1–10

42. Ehrlich GE (1972) Inflammatory osteoarthritis: I. The clinical syndrome. J Chron Dis 25:317–328

43. Ehrlich GE (1975) Osteoarthritis beginning with inflammation. Definitions and cor-relations. J Amer Med Ass 232:157–159

44. Peter JB, Pearson CM, Marmor L (1966) Erosive arthritis of the hands. Arthritis Rheum 9:365–88

45. Cecil RL, Archer BH (1926) Classification and treatment of chronic arthritis. JAMA 87:741–746

46. Stecher RM, Hauser H (1948) Heberden's nodes. VII. The roentgenological and clinical appearance of degenerative joint disease of the fingers. Am J Roentgenol 59:326–337

47. Crain DC (1961) Interphalangeal osteoarthritis. Characterized by painful, inflammatory episodes resulting in deformity of the proximal and distal articulations. JAMA 175:1049–1053

48. Busby J, Tobin JT, Ettinger W, Plato CC (1986) Progression of osteoarthritis: significance of starting level, age, and length of follow-up. Gerontologist 26 (suppl): 141 A

49. Altman R, Alarcon G, Appelrouth D, Bloch D, Borenstein D, Brandt K, Brown C, Cooke TD, Daniel W, Gray R, Greenwald R, Hochberg M, Howell D, Ike R, Kapila R, Kaplan D, Koop-man W, Longley S, McShane DJ, Medsger T, Michel B, Murphy W, Osial T, Ramsey-Gold-man R, Rotschild B, Stark K, Wolfe F (1990) The American College of Rheumatology criteria for the classification and reporting of osteoarthritis of the hand. Arthritis Rheum 33:1601–1610

50. Maroudas A, Evans H, Almeida L (1973) Cartilage of the hip joint: Topographical variations of glycosaminoglycan content in normal and fibrillated tissue. Ann Rheum Dis 32:1–9

51. McDevitt CA, Muir H (1976) Biochemical changes in the cartilage of the knee in experimental and natural osteoarthritis in the dog. J Bone Jt Surg 58B: 94–101
52. Kellgren JH, Moore R (1952) Generalized osteoarthritis and Heberden's nodes. Br Med J i: 181–187
53. Jones AC, Pattrick M, Hopkinson ND, Doherty M (1993) Towards a radiographic definition of nodal osteoarthritis (OA). Osteoarthritis Cartilage 1:19

CHAPTER 7

Impact of Osteoarthritis on Quality of Life

J. POUCHOT, J. COSTE and F. GUILLEMIN

7.1
Introduction

Osteoarthritis (OA) is characterized by alteration in the structure and function of a joint, and results from changes in articular cartilage, underlying bone and soft tissues [1]. Osteoarthritis is the most common rheumatic disorder, and the aging of the population will result in a significant increase in its prevalence [2]. In Western population, as much as one third of the adults aged 25–75 years have evidence of radiographic OA [2]. Although it does not reduce life expectancy significantly, OA results in pain, disability and quality of life (QoL) impairment. To a certain extent only these outcomes are accounted for by radiographic evidence of articular degeneration. Indeed, pain and disability are not always correlated with radiographic disease severity [3, 4]. Yet, only about 60% of patients with radiographic evidence of OA are symptomatic. The sensitivity of radiographic assessment to detect pathological changes of OA is low [5], and this may partly explain the discrepancy between radiographic changes and symptoms found in epidemiological studies. However, our understanding of the determinants of the disability in OA remains poor. The pathways that depict OA from biomechanical factors and pathology to pain and disability, and include the various factors and interventions that may intervene at every step of the illness have been recently reviewed [2, 6].

Candidate variables for assessing outcome of OA have been recently reviewed [7]. Up to recently, traditional evaluation of OA was based upon assessments of joint range of motion, pain intensity and radiographic disease severity. However, accumulating evidence that functional disability and QoL measures are valid, reliable, and sensitive to significant clinical changes has generated a growing interest in these new methods of assessment. The purpose of these measures is to assess the patient's experiences of illness. They have a wide range of applications in OA, and supplement traditional clinical and biological measures of health status. Quality of life and functional impairment assessments are increasingly used as outcomes in clinical trials and evaluation studies, and have been included in recent recommendations at OMERACT III [8]. They provide epidemiologic data concerning the natural history of OA, and may aid to the individual patient care and clinical decision making. Although OA may involve any joint, this chapter will be dedicated to the weight-bearing joints of the lower extremities.

7.2
Definition and Conceptual Issues

The need to consider outcomes other than morbidity and mortality was heralded by the 1947 World Health Organisation who defined health as being the presence of physical, mental and social well-being and not only the absence of disease or infirmity. Patients do not really care about their erythrocyte sedimentation rate, or the accurate measurement of radiographic joint space narrowing, or limitation of range of motion of their diseased joint. As health status assessment naturally evolves to allow insight into patient's experience, QoL has emerged as an attractive but somewhat misleading term to describe this new domain of measure [9]. Indeed, although related to health, the concept of QoL is quite distinct from it. Most approaches used in medical field do no attempt to include widely valued aspects of life that are not generally considered to fall under the purview of the health care systems such as income, freedom, personal relationships, self-image, work status, environment or other living standards. As a consequence, the concept of QoL has generated much controversy in the field of health care. Some of the terms used for QoL, including health status, functional status, subjective health status or health related quality of life (HRQL) convey more accurately the content and purpose of these types of measure, and are commonly used interchangeably.

Although this can be challenged [9], QoL is usually considered to be a multi-dimensional concept, and several models and operational definitions have been proposed [10–13]. Quality of life conceptually refers to the physical, psychological, and social components of health that are influenced by own experience, beliefs, expectations and perceptions, or duration of illness. Since own expectations, perceptions, preferences and values regarding health and satisfaction with life may vary greatly, two individuals with the same health status may express very different quality of life. Indeed, for some individuals, suffering a chronic illness may paradoxically have enriching effect on their lives. It is commonly assumed that the process of measurement will result in a continuum between death (albeit some health states could be rated worse than death) and a fully healthy life. Variation among the numerous available QoL questionnaires is related to the extent to which various health domains are covered and the format of items. There is usually an overwhelming emphasis on the physical function component. Discrepancies between the patient and his/her physician in the assessment of QoL may be substantial. Although it could be argued that in certain health policy decision making, the point of view taken into account should be that of the society, in most cases the primacy of the patient's perspective is warranted [9, 11].

7.3
Available Instruments

Despite the ambiguity of the QoL term, it will be used all along this review to refer to the instruments assessing at least one health dimension. Many QoL instruments have been used in patients with OA. With respect to the taxonomy, two basic types of instruments, generic and disease-specific, could be characterized. More recently, patient-specific questionnaires have been elaborated and used in OA. Although some instruments are administered by clinicians or interviewers, most often they are self-completed. Most of the instruments provide a separate score for each of the different components of QoL that they explore. Such health profiles usually do not allow to aggregate these scores, because contradictory trends for differents aspects of health would be missed, and could result in the same global score. However, a few instruments combine various health-related QoL domains to yield a single number. These index or utility/preference measures are used in medico-economic studies. Only those QoL instruments that have been used widely in the field of OA will be detailed below.

7.3.1
Generic Instruments

Generic QoL instruments are intended to be applicable across a wide spectrum of diseases, and to assess different interventions. This imply a more comprehensive assessment of QoL domains. However, one limitation of these generic instruments is that inevitably they cover each health area superficially. This may limit their responsiveness, and it has been demonstrated that generic instruments were less powerful in detecting treatment effects than specific ones. On the other hand, the advantage of generic measures is to allow comparison of the impact of treatment on QoL across diseases or conditions. The widespread use of generic instruments provides considerable information about norms and benchmarks useful to compare different diseases and estimate their respective burden. There are a number of well-established generic health measures, including the Sickness Impact Profile (SIP), the Nottingham Health Profile (NHP) and the short forms of the instruments used in the Medical Outcomes Study that have advantages of simplicity and self-administration. They have all been used in OA.

7.3.1.1
The Sickness Impact Profile

The sickness impact profile (SIP) consists of 136 items describing health-related behavior to which the respondent gives a yes/no response [14]. These items correspond to 12 dimensions (walking, body care and movement, mobility, work, sleeping and rest, eating, housework, recreation, emotions, social interaction, alertness and communication). Scores may be expressed by dimension or may be summed up to give a unique total global score. Scores for items use predetermined weights based on rater panel estimates of relative severity of dysfunction. The global score is computed by summing dimensions and then standardized to a percentage of the maximum possible score. This instrument therefore provides both an index and a profile. Three dimensions (walking, body care, and mobility) may be aggregated into a physical component; and four dimensions (emotions, social interaction, alertness and communication) may be aggregated into a psychosocial component. It requires approximately 30 minutes to complete. The SIP is available in a self-administered form or can be administered with an interviewer.

7.3.1.2
The Short Form-36 items

The short form-36 items (SF-36) is one of the most popular generic health status instruments to date [15–17]. This instrument is derived form a larger battery of questions administered in the Medical Outcomes Study. It has been widely adopted because of its brevity and its comprehensiveness. Across 36 multiple choice questions, this questionnaire provides a profile of 8 dimensions (physical functioning, role physical, bodily pain, general health, vitality/energy, social functioning, role emotional, mental health) and summary physical and mental health measures. The SF-36 also yield a self-assessment of health transition over the past year. The questionnaire is suitable for self-administration or administration by a trained interviewer in person or by telephone. The SF-36 can be administered in 5–10 minutes and the scores for each dimension range from 0 (the worse) to 100 (the best).

7.3.1.3
The Nottingham Health Profile

The Nottingham health profile (NHP) is another widely used generic QoL instrument that measures perceived health [18]. It has 38 items that are answered by a simple yes or no. Positive responses are rated with weights obtained from panel's judgments of the severity of the items. There are 6 dimensions: physical, mobility, pain, emotional reactions, energy level, sleep and social isolation. The authors who developed the NHP considered that it would be meaningless to combine the score in an index, and each of the 6 sections of the instrument had to be scored separately. The questionnaire is self-administered and takes approximately 5 minutes to complete. As for SF-36 reference values are available. The possible range for the 6 dimensions is 0 (the best score) to 100 (the worst score).

7.3.1.4
The Quality of Well Being

The quality of well being (QWB) defines function by 3 scales with ordinal categories, physical activity, mobility, and social activity [19]. A trained interviewer determines what the patient did and did not do because of his/her illness during the past week. There is an associated list of symptoms or problems used to generate a unique weighted score. The administration of the questionnaire takes approximately 20 minutes. Major limitations of the QWB include the complexity of the instrument and the requirement of a trained interviewer. This instrument is used in medico-economic studies.

7.3.1.5
The European Quality of Life Scale

The European quality of life scale (EuroQoL) is a self-administered multi-dimensional measure of health-related QoL [20]. Dimensions of this instrument have been mainly selected from existing instruments including the QWB, the SIP and the NHP. The instrument has 5 dimensions: mobility, self-care, usual activities, pain/discomfort, anxiety/depression, and assesses health transition over the past 12 months. The EuroQoL gives both a profile and a single index value. In addition, this instrument asks respondents to indicate on a 20-cm thermometer their rating of their current health status. The EuroQoL has been developped in many European and Nordic countries.

7.3.2
Disease-specific Instruments

Disease-specific instruments have been developed for one disease or a narrow range of diseases. They focus on aspects of health status that are specific to the area or primary interest. These instruments may be specific to a disease (i. e. OA, rheumatoid arthritis), a patient population (i. e. children, frail elderly), a function (i. e. sleep) or a problem (i. e. pain). Clinicians usually prefer the use of the disease-specific instruments as they are closely related to the domains they routinely explore in patient care. Moreover, these specific measures may be more responsive in the explored dimensions to significant clinical changes than the generic instruments, although they may miss unexpected health outcomes. Some scales were specifically designed to assess functional activities of patients rather than the broader aspects of the health status which are encompassed within the much broader QoL concept.

7.3.2.1
The Health Assessment Questionnaire

The health assessment questionnaire (HAQ) [21] is an arthritis-specific scale that has been mainly developed and centered on rheumatoid arthritis, but this disability index has also been used successfully in OA. This instruments consists of 20 items which measures performance in 8 activities of daily living over the past week (dressing and grooming, rising from a chair or bed, eating, walking, hygiene, reach, grip and outside activities), emphasizing difficulty and the need for aids and devices to complete the tasks. Scores from these 8 subscales are averaged to provide a disability index with a range from 0 (the best score) to 3 (the worst score). It also includes a visual analogue scale to measure pain intensity. It takes approximately 5 to 10 minutes to complete and it has been shown that responses are closely similar when the instrument is selfcompleted or administered by an interviewer. The HAQ is primarily centered on physical function and pain, while other QoL dimensions are not adressed.

7.3.2.2
The Western Ontario and McMaster Universities Osteoarthritis index

The Western Ontario and McMaster Universities osteoarthritis index (WOMAC) is a disease-specific questionnaire developed to evaluate patients with OA of the hip or knee [22, 23] that has been shown to be valid and reliable. The WOMAC may be self-administered, but may also be administered by interview or telephone. Recently a computerized version has been validated [24]. It has 24 items across 3 dimensions: pain, stiffness, and physical function. The items of social and emotional dimensions that were included in the initial version of the WOMAC were excluded in the final version because they were not enough responsive. Using 5-point category rating scales, patients rate 5 pain items, 2 stiffness items, and 17 physical function items. Aggregate scores for each dimension are determined by summing the component item scores for each dimension. A signal measurement strategy has also been applied to the WOMAC in an approach comparable to that used in the patient-specific instruments (vide infra) [25].

7.3.2.3
The Lequesne's Knee and Hip Index

The indices of severity for OA of the hip or the knee have been validated [26–28]. They are administered by interview and contain 11 items assessing pain, stiffness, maximum distance walked and activities of daily living. The possible scores ranges from 0 to 24 for each index. The index of severity for hip OA contains an additional item concerning sexual activity in sexually active women when hip prosthesis is considered. It takes approximately 3–4 minutes to complete with an interviewer.

7.3.2.4
The Arthritis Impact Measurement Scales

The arthritis impact measurement scales (AIMS) consists of 45 items grouped into 9 component scales: mobility, physical activity, activities of daily living, dexterity, household activities, pain, depression, anxiety, and social activity [29, 30]. These 9 scales measure physical, social, and mental health status. The scales contain 4 to 9 items, and each item contains 2 to 6 possible responses. The possible range of scores on each subscale is 0 (the best score) to 10 (the worst score). This is a self-completed questionnaire that takes 15–20 minutes to complete. The AIMS has been extensively validated and used in patients with rheumatoid arthritis, and it has been demonstrated that this health status model is applicable to patients suffering from OA [31].

The AIMS2, a revised and expanded version of the AIMS has been published in 1992 and added 3 new dimensions, arm function, work, and social support [32]. Although this instrument has been claimed to be valid for patient with OA, it is possible that dimensions such as arm function, or hand and finger function may not be relevant for patients suffering from OA of the weight bearing joints of the lower extremities. This may require further investigations. Of conceptual importance are the added new assessments which allow the patient to rate for each of the 12 dimensions, how satisfied they have been and the impact of arthritis, and to prioritize up to 3 dimensions in which they particularly seek improvement. In this respect AIMS2 resembles new patient-specific QoL instruments. As the initial version, AIMS2 is a self-completed questionnaire that takes approximately 20 – 30 minutes to complete, and the possible range of score on each subscale is 0 – 10.

7.3.3
Patient-specific Instruments

Few existing instruments provide a mean of assessing the patient's priorities of a good and healthy life. This is a new approach to the investigations of health status by asking the patient to prioritize those domains that are directly affected by the illness and in which the patient particularly seeks improvement.

7.3.3.1
The McMaster Toronto Arthritis Patient Preference Disability Questionnaire

The McMaster Toronto arthritis patient preference disability questionnaire (MACTAR) was initially developed for use with patients who have rheumatoid arthritis [33] but has also been employed in hip OA [34]. Using a semi-structured interview, patients are asked to designate key functional activities based on their own preferences, and the five activities that rank highest are evaluated. At the end of the study period, patients are asked on a visual analogue scale if their ability to perform the selected activities has improved, deteriorated, or remained stable. This technique may be more sensitive to small changes when compared with conventional standardized questionnaire. This questionnaire is very appealing but major methodologic problems remained to be solved. Indeed, the possibility to assess each patient in different selected health status domains is challenging, and the main concern relates to between patients comparison. Also, this questionnaire should be administered by a trained interviewer.

7.3.3.2
The Schedule for the Evaluation of Individual Quality of Life

The schedule for the evaluation of individual quality of life (SEIQoL) [35] also avoids the imposition of an external value system on the patients by the use of standardized questionnaires. During a structured interview, patients are asked to select the five areas of life that they judge to be most important to their overall QoL. Then patients rate their current status on each of this five areas on a visual analogue scale. Patients are then asked to rate their overall QoL on a visual analogue scale. This questionnaire allows to quantify the relative weight of each elicited cue in the patient's overall judgment of QoL according to judgment theory. Scores in each elicited dimension can range from 0 to 100.

This technique brings up the same methodological problems than the MACTAR questionnaire, regarding the inter- and intra-patient comparisons. Both methods require trained interviewers and are therefore resource intensive.

7.4
Applications of Instruments

Different applications of QoL instruments need to be individualized as instruments that works well for one purpose may not in other situations.

7.4.1
Cross Sectional and Short Term Longitudinal Studies in Osteoarthritis

Although OA of the knee or the hip is associated with progressive and significant disability and QoL impairment, studies that have specifically addressed QoL measure in OA are scanty. Most available data are extracted from non-randomized longitudinal or cross-sectional studies that were clinical trials or validation studies of QoL instruments. Quality of life questionnaires that have been used in patients with OA, severe enough to justify a treatment with nonsteroidal antiinflammatory drugs (NSAID), demonstrate the severity of functional disability. In the validation study of the WOMAC [22] patients with symptomatic OA of the hip or knee "requiring" NSAID therapy were studied. Patients were of both gender and had a mean age of 66.5 years. They all had definite radiographic evidence of primary OA, and the mean disease duration was 9 years. Scores for the pain, stiffness and physical function were roughly median, but unfortunately hip and knee OA results were not contrasted (Table 1). The results obtained with the Lequesne's questionnaire in the same study were similar. Most of the items of the WOMAC significantly improved by 6 weeks of treatment with NSAID. These results were confirmed in a subsequent study by the same authors [23]. In a cross-sectional study using the SIP, subjects with more chronic and severe pain from OA of the hip or knee had relatively high levels of physical and psychosocial impairment compared to a control group [36]. These results have been confirmed in patients with OA in a family practice setting with the same QoL instrument [37].

However, data regarding long-term modification of QoL in patients with OA of the weight bearing joint are not available. Patients with internal femorotibial OA followed-up over one year by rheumatologists improved of approximately

Table 1. Scores obtained in patients with OA of the knee or hip "requiring" NSAID therapy

Health status instrument	Pain[a]	Stiffness[b]	Physical function[c]
WOMAC	10.3 (4.4)	4.4 (1.8)	32.2 (13.8)
Lequesne's questionnaire	4.4 (1.1)	1.5 (0.5)	5.7 (2.3)

Presented scores are means and (standard deviation). Scores could range from [a]0–20 and 0–6, [b]0–8 and 0–2, [c]0–68 and 0–16 for the WOMAC and Lequesne's questionnaires, respectively [22].

one point (9.7 to 8.8 for a range of 0–24) on the Lequesne's questionnaire [27]. However, this improvement could be partly explained by the inclusion of patients during a disease flare. In another longitudinal study conducted in OA patients (location of OA was not specified) with a mean age of 69 years, the HAQ scores, relatively low compared to those obtained in patients with rheumatoid arthritis (0.6 for a range of 0–3) remained stable over 20 months. The disability index was positively correlated to the age of patients [21].

There are no available data allowing to contrast QoL between OA of the hip and knee. However, in OA of the knee, involvement of the femorotibial compartment seems to be associated with a poorer QoL outcome assessed by the Lequesne's questionnaire than that observed in OA located to the femoropatellar compartment (9.6 versus 7.8) [38]. The SIP has been used in patients with moderate OA of the femorotibial compartment of the knee [39]. Sixty patients of both gender with a mean age of 63 years were included in this study. In this patient population, the SIP revealed both physical and psychosocial changes with scores that were reduced of 10.8% and 3.6% respectively. Patients considered that their knee OA had great influence physically on ambulation, during recreation and pastimes, during sleep and rest, and psychosocially on emotional behaviour. No correlation was found between SIP and age, weight or disease duration. The AIMS and its revised and expanded version AIMS2 have also been used in OA. Although the data are few, they illustrate the severity of OA in physical and pain domains of these QoL instruments (Table 2) [30, 32, 40]. As it could be expected, the dimensions of AIMS and AIMS2 exploring the upper limb may not be relevant for studying the outcome of OA.

Table 2. Mean scores of AIMS and AIMS2 in patients with osteoarthritis [30, 32, 40]

AIMS component or dimension	Mean score (355 patients)	AIMS2 dimension	Mean score (109 patients)
Physical domain	1.78	Mobility level	1.35
Mobility	0.82	Walking and bending	4.24
Physical activity	5.42	Hand and finger function	1.75
Dexterity	1.86	Arm function	0.68
Activities of daily living	0.20	Self care	0.39
Household activities	0.55	Household tasks	0.91
Psychological domain	2.96		
Anxiety	3.67	Level of tension	4.19
Depression	2.26	Mood	2.48
Pain	6.04	Arthritis pain	4.69
Social activity	3.37	Social activities	4.88
		Support from family	1.83
		Work	3.48
Arthritis Impact	4.81		

The scores for AIMS and AIMS2 could range from 0 (the best score) to 10 (the worst score). Arthritis impact is assessed by a 10-cm visual analogue scale.

Osteoarthritis may be severe enough to warrant joint replacement. The NHP has been used in patients who were waiting total hip replacement [18, 41]. As expected impairment was marked in the dimensions referring to physical mobility and pain, but this study also highlights the impairment in sleep and energy dimensions. The remaining two dimensions of the NHP, emotional reactions and social isolation were less affected by the disease (Table 3). Better scores were obtained by younger patients for energy and physical mobility dimensions. Other studies using the NHP before and after total hip replacement confirm these data [42].

7.4.2
Osteoarthritis Contrasted to Other Diseases

Quality of life as an outcome has been rarely compared between patients with OA or other conditions. In one study [43] contrasted patients with rheumatoid arthritis, low back pain, fibromyalgia, degenerative cervical spine disease, and OA of the knee or the small joints of the hands (Table 4). The authors used the HAQ, and the anxiety and depression scales of the AIMS questionnaire. In addition, pain was evaluated by a visual analogue scale. Patients with

Table 3. Mean scores of NHP in patients awaiting total hip replacement

Nottingham Health Profile	Mean score (58 patients) (Hunt et al. [18])	Mean score (71 patients) (Thorsen et al. [41])
Energy	63.2	69.0
Pain	70.8	80.5
Emotional reactions	21.3	32.6
Sleep	48.7	44.5
Social isolation	12.5	16.9
Physical mobility	54.8	59.5

The scores of the 6 dimensions of the Nottingham Health Profile could range from 0 (the best score) to 100 (the worst score).

Table 4. Mean scores of HAQ, and anxiety and depression dimensions of AIMS in various rheumatologic disorders (Hawley and Wolfe [43])

Disorder	HAQ	AIMS Anxiety	AIMS depression
Rheumatoid arthritis	1.2	3.5	2.6
Low back pain	0.8	4.2	2.9
Hand osteoarthritis	0.8	3.5	2.5
Knee osteoarthritis	0.9	3.6	2.5
Fibromyalgia	1.1	4.7	3.2
Degenerative cervical spine disease	0.7	4.5	2.9

The scores could range from 0 to 3 (worst score) for the HAQ and from 0 to 10 (worst score) for AIMS scales.

rheumatoid arthritis rated the worst scores on the HAQ disability index. However, they scored better than the other conditions in the anxiety and depression dimensions of AIMS, and they had lower pain scores. Conversely, pain and psychological outcomes were less favourable in patients suffering low back pain, degenerative cervical spine disease, and fibromyalgia.

In the validation study of the HAQ, disability index was better in OA than in rheumatoid arthritis (0.6 versus 0.8 for a range of 0 to 3) and the follow-up study showed a deterioration of health status in rheumatoid arthritis patient (disability index of 1.2) while it remained stable in OA at 20 months [21]. Severity of disability index score correlated with age in OA, and with disease duration in rheumatoid arthritis. Another study assessed the impact on health status of rheumatoid arthritis and OA [44]. Compared to controls matched for age and sex, patients with rheumatoid arthritis had the severest scores in the 8 domains of activities of the HAQ. Conversely, only 3 of the explored activities (household chores, shopping and errands, and leisure activities) were affected in OA compared to control patients. A study using the modified HAQ showed that the health status outcome of OA was intermediate between that of rheumatoid arthritis and systemic lupus erythematosus [45]. Disability index in OA patients was more or less similar to that of those suffering scleroderma.

In the study of validation of the AIMS2 [32] it may be possible to contrast the results of patients with OA and rheumatoid arthritis (Table 5). In all but one dimension, health status was better in OA, and as expected this was significant in the hand and finger function, arm function, activity of daily living, and household tasks dimensions. The score differences were even worse when compared with patients suffering rheumatoid arthritis severe enough to justify the initiation of methotrexate therapy [46]. These studies as others confirmed that rheumatoid arthritis is associated with a more severe health status outcome than OA [21, 40].

Table 5. AIMS2 dimension scores in patients with rheumatoid arthritis and osteoarthritis

AIMS2 dimension	Rheumatoid arthritis (Meenan et al. [32])	Rheumatoid arthritis (Pouchot et al. [46])	Osteoarthritis
Mobility level	1.69	2.9	1.35
Walking and bending	4.58	5.6	4.24
Hand and finger function	3.16	3.5	1.75
Arm function	2.01	3.5	0.68
Self-care	0.73	2.2	0.39
Household tasks	1.67	4.0	0.91
Level of tension	4.05	4.9	4.19
Mood	2.63	3.5	2.48
Arthritis pain	4.69	7.3	4.69
Social activities	4.91	5.7	4.88
Support from family and friends	1.84	3.2	1.83
Work	3.80	4.4	3.48

The scores could range from 0 to 10 (worst score) for AIMS2 scales.

Table 6. Mean scores of the NHP in patient with hip osteoarthritis compared to chronic conditions (Wiklund et al. [47])

NHP dimension	Hip osteo-arthritis (71 patients)	Stroke (23 patients)	Chronically ill patients > 65 years (24 patients)	Peripheral vascular disease (25 patients)
Energy	65	35	38	30
Pain	73	11	29	23
Emotional reaction	31	21	15	14
Sleep	52	22	32	25
Social isolation	15	20	13	9
Physical mobility	49	21	29	22

The scores could range from 0 to 100 (worst score) for NHP scales.

Generic QoL instruments allow to compare the health outcome of OA with various disorders having a chronic course. Indeed, the NHP was used to contrast QoL of patients with hip OA on a waiting list for a total hip replacement with that of patients suffering other chronic conditions (Table 6) [47]. The EuroQoL which is a validated QoL scale was recently used to survey patients with rheumatic diseases [48]. Quality of life was similar in patients with rheumatoid arthritis and OA, but was lower in patients with fibromyalgia.

7.4.3
Medical Treatment of OA

7.4.3.1
Nonsteroidal Antiinflammatory Drugs and Analgesics

Management of OA should alleviate symptoms and maintain or improve functional status and ultimately QoL. In OA of the weight-bearing joints, weight loss can reduce symptoms, but NSAIDs, analgesics, and intraarticular injections of corticosteroids are often required during the course of the disease and appear to be beneficial. Evaluation of these treatments is usually based upon traditional endpoints including pain assessment, global patient and physician judgment. Nevertheless, several studies have used QoL questionnaires to compare NSAIDs or NSAIDs and analgesics. In patients with primary OA of the femorotibial compartment, a 6 week therapy with NSAIDs results in a significant improvement of disability with a decrease of approximately 50% in the three dimensions of the WOMAC, and of about 4.5 points of the score of the Lequesne's questionnaire [23]. In this study, the WOMAC was also used to compare two NSAIDs, and between drug differences favored meclofenamate over diclofenate sodium. Another study showed evidence of QoL improvement in patients suffering from OA (location was not defined) and treated with NSAIDs [40]. The AIMS results showed substantial improvements in physical function, psychological status and pain components of the instrument, as well as in overall arthritis impact. These improvements closely paralleled the changes demonstrated by standard clinical measures, were noted by the time of the first outcome assessment at 8 weeks, and were maintained over the course of this 24-week trial. The health status changes were similar for patients with OA and rheumatoid arthritis. Another study with a similar design resulted in the same conclusions [49]. Health Assessment Questionnaire has been used to compare the efficacy of a NSAID given at either an antiinflammatory dose or an analgesic dose, with that of a pure analgesic in patient with OA of the knee [50]. All three groups had improvement in the HAQ score of a magnitude of 0.3 – 0.5 points from a baseline value of 1.46 – 1.61 at entry into the study.

7.4.3.2
Rehabilitation and Education

With progression of OA, chronic pain and disability may lead to an increasing need for medical services. One study addressed the efficacy and safety of supervised fitness walking in the clinical management of patients with OA of the knee [51]. Patients randomly assigned to the fitness program had a significant increase in their walking distance, and also obtained improvement in QoL as measured by the physical activity and the arthritis pain subscales of the AIMS. Aside exercice programs, it has been suggested that social support interventions could also be beneficial for patients with OA. Indeed, informations provided by telephone contact improved by 6 months, physical, pain, and psychological components of the AIMS [52]. The telephone intervention consisted of brief interviews with patient, mainly to discuss medications and their side-effects, joint pain, and problem to attend the scheduled outpatients visits. A self-care education for inner-city patients with OA of the knee, as complement of primary care was found to result in relative preservation of function as assessed by the HAQ, while the overall effect on general health status evaluated by QWB was not significant [53]. Lequesne's questionnaire and AIMS2 have been used to assess the prolonged effects of spa therapy of 3 weeks duration in patients with OA of the hip or knee and supported the existence of a beneficial symptomatic effect [54].

7.4.3.3
Symptomatic Slow Acting Drugs (SSADs) and Disease-modifying Drugs (DMDs)

Current treatment of OA is based chiefly on the use of analgesics, NSAIDs and intraarticular injections of corticosteroids. Because of the limitations of the medical treatment of OA, SSADs with disease-modifying properties that are not yet demonstrated, are currently under development [55, 56]. DMDs should prevent, delay or reverse pathologic changes that are observed in the cartilage. No one exists currently. The pathologic changes of OA usually progress rather slowly. Nevertheless, the mean cartilage loss may be in fact quite easily demonstrated by the reduction of the joint space width in radiographs, and this is the cornestone of the evaluation of new slow acting drugs in OA [55, 57]. However, this endpoint may be limited since symptoms and radiographs often did not correlate. Indeed, from the patient's point of view, functional ability and QoL outcomes are certainly the main variables of interest. A few studies have included a QoL assessment in the evaluation of a SSAD. The Lequesne's questionnaire and the AIMS2 have been used in evaluation studies of intra-articular sodium hyaluronate in OA of the knee and demonstrated improvement [58, 59].

7.4.4
Surgical Treatment of OA

Unfortunately, medical treatment of OA is only moderately effective, and many patients report chronic pain and severe disability. Total joint replacement has been a major advance in the treatment of patients with OA. Hip and knee arthroplasties are common surgical procedures in Western countries, and are associated with low rates of morbidity and mortality. However, it still remains a difficult task to determine the right moment to recommend a surgical procedure to a patient suffering from severe OA.

7.4.4.1
QoL Measures as an Aid to Surgical Decision

In severe OA of the knee or hip, decision of a joint replacement is usually based upon the importance of the limitation of the joint range of motion appreciated by clinical examination, and the severity of the joint space narrowing on radiographs. However, physician and patient global judgments are of utmost importance in the decision process. Therefore, assessment of joint pain severity, disability, and QoL are cornerstones to the surgical decision. In order to diminish the subjectivity of this process it has been proposed to incorporate QoL results in the discussion. Lequesne' questionnaire may be used for this purpose, and total joint replacement could be reasonably considered for scores between 8 and 12 in patients who received an adequate conservative therapy [38]. This proposed range allows to take into account individual characteristics of patients, including age, psychological status, comorbidity and physical needs.

Knowledge of the scores obtained with other QoL instruments in patients suffering severe OA, immediately before joint replacement may be helpful to clinicians to decide a surgical procedure. Scores of the WOMAC in patients waiting total hip replacement have been published [34]. Other specific or generic QoL instruments, including the NHP [42], the SIP [14, 34], the AIMS and the AIMS2 [60] have been used in patients waiting surgery for total joint replacement.

7.4.4.2
Evaluation of the Results of Joint Replacement

Several specific or generic QoL instruments have been used to evaluate the results of total joint replacement. The preoperative assessments indicate that advanced OA not only causes severe pain, but also markedly affects the other health components, including psychologic and social components. The improvement in QoL is rapid and very substantial after surgery, and affects all components of health, most patients returning to nearly normal health. Generic instruments, such as the NHP have been used to compare QoL before and after total joint replacement (Table 7) [42]. The NHP scores clearly demonstrated that the QoL of the patient waiting a total hip replacement was severely impaired compared with that of a healthy population of similar age and sex distribution. Neither age nor duration of symptoms were related to the one year postoperative outcome. One year after total hip replacement, the patients rated their QoL very close to that of the control group. In another study with similar design [34], significant improvement in QoL measures was also noted. Most of the improvement had occurred by three months postoperatively and was maintained at

Table 7. Mean scores of various QoL instruments before and after total hip replacement (Wiklund et al. [42])

NHP dimension	Preoperative scores	Postoperative scores	Healthy control patients
Nottingham Health Profile			
Energy	63	20	15
Pain	75	15	8
Emotional reaction	30	10	9
Sleep	55	19	16
Social isolation	14	7	5
Physical mobility	48	18	6
Harris Hip score	44	98	NA
Merle d'Aubigné Hip score	10	18	NA
Sickness Impact Profile			
Sleep and rest	31.0	3.3	NA
Emotional behavior	22.2	2.1	NA
Body care and movement	22.3	3.2	NA
Home management	28.4	3.2	NA
Mobility	9.4	0.7	NA
Social interaction	14.6	0.8	NA
Ambulation	36.4	5.4	NA
Recreation and pastimes	41.5	3.8	NA
Work	21.8	9.3	NA
Global physical score	23.1	3.2	NA
WOMAC			
Pain	4.9	0.7	NA
Stiffness	5.9	1.0	NA
Physical function	5.7	0.7	NA
MACTAR	7.7	0.8	NA

The scores range from 0 to 100 (worst score) for the NHP scales. Harris Hip score: the best possible score is 100. Merle d'Aubigné score: the best possible score is 18. SIP: for each domain the score could range from 0 to 100 (worst score). WOMAC: for each domain the score ranges from 0 to 10 (worst score). MACTAR: the score ranges from 0 to 10 (worst score). Patients were evaluated one year after total hip replacement for the NHP and after two years for the other instruments.

Table 8. Mean preoperative and postoperative scores of 5 QoL instruments in patients undergoing total joint arthroplasty (Liang et al. [61])

Health component		AIMS	FSI	HAQ	QWB	SIP
Mobility	preop	55.1	19.1	45.7	33.3	22.3
	postop	19.4	13.6	19.3	13.4	11.9
Pain	preop	57.6	24.4	46.4	NA	NA
	postop	25.0	14.6	21.3	NA	NA
Social	preop	24.1	22.5	47.0	45.4	21.4
	postop	2.6	10.7	12.3	15.3	6.4

For the 5 instruments the scores have been normalized to a common range of possible values from 0 to 100 (worst score).

2 years. These authors used the SIP as a generic instrument, several disease-specific instruments (the Harris Hip score, the Merle d'Aubigné Hip score, and the WOMAC), and a patient-specific instrument, the MACTAR. In a comparative study of the measurement properties of five QoL instruments (Functional Status Instrument [FSI], HAQ, AIMS, QWB, and SIP), no single instrument consistently outperformed the others [61]. These five instruments were administered to patients before and after total joint arthroplasty of the hip or knee and the results also highlight the major QoL improvement that was obtained after surgery (Table 8). Because the proliferation of instruments to evaluate the results of total hip joint replacement makes it difficult to compare the results of different investigators, the American Academy of the Orthopaedic Surgeons decided to develop the Total Hip Arthroplasty Outcome Evaluation Questionnaire. This instrument assesses the results of hip replacement from the perspective of the patient and provides data on pain, function and satisfaction. Its psychometric properties have been studied carefully [62]. A review that assesses the health related QoL after total hip replacement concluded that all 20 analyzed studies provided consistent results showing beneficial and often rapid and dramatic improvement after elective total hip replacement [63]. The SF-36 appears to be preferable to the SIP as a generic QoL instrument in patients undergoing total hip replacement [64]. The SF-36 is shorter, more relevant, and more responsive. Recently, a specific instrument to assess disability in patients with total knee replacement has been developed [65]. This 12-item self-administered questionnaire has been shown to be reliable, valid and sensitive to clinically important changes over a 6-month period of follow-up after surgery.

7.4.4.3
Medicoeconomic Studies

The most controversial use of QoL measures is in health economics. In this field, QoL measures are used to assess the results of health care interventions, and could be also a very controversial mean of prioritising funding. A common design is the study of cost-effectiveness, which estimates the increase of cost of a treatment compared with the beneficial effect on health, which is commonly assessed by adjusting the survival by the QoL (QALYs: Quality Adjusted Life Years). Total joint replacement has certainly been a major advance in the treatment of patients with end-stage OA. It improves pain, function and overall QoL. However, its cost-effectiveness may be questioned by health policy makers. A prospective cost-effectiveness analysis of total joint replacement using the QWB as a QoL measure has been reported [60]. Six months after total joint replacement of the hip or knee in patients with OA, there was significant improvement in global health and in functional status. The overall health improvement was similar for hip and knee total joint replacement. As the mean age of the patients was 66 years, the surgery did not change work status. The authors concluded that total joint replacement was more cost-effective for those patients with the poorest initial health. A utility measure derived from a time trade-off technique has been applied to patients with OA of the hip [34]. This technique is based upon the number of years of life that the patients would be willing to give up in order to achieve a full health, according to various clinical scenarios. In this study, utility scores [range from 0 (no difference between life and death) to 1.0 (full health)], markedly improved from a mean time trade-off score of 0.32 preoperatively to 0.87 two years postoperatively. This could be translated in a significant increase in QALYs. Other cost-utility studies in patients after hip arthroplasty, came to the same conclusions [66, 67]. Conversely, it has been suggested that the gain of QALYs in knee arthroplasty was very low, about the tenth of that obtained after total hip joint replacement [68]. Using the McKnee system, a new developed utility measure, there was no significant changes in health-utility index before and three months after knee joint replacement [69]. However these pessimistic studies have been recently disputed in another one using the QWB [70]. Cost of health care is increasing steadily and the methods to assess the economic benefits of health interventions using QoL measures will certainly be used more widely in a near future. A recent study outline a method to evaluate cost-effectiveness assessment in the field of rheumatology, including OA [71].

7.4.4.4
Health Care Access

Recent studies have shown disparities in utilization of health care between men and women. The age-adjusted frequency of total joint replacement of hip or knee is higher in women than in men. The observed differences in functional status demonstrated that women are operated on at a more advanced stage in the course of their OA [62].

7.5
Methodological Problems

7.5.1
Selection of QoL Instruments in OA

A particular issue in studies measuring QoL is the selection of a suitable instrument. This may vary according to the study design. However, it remains a difficult task, influenced by the severity and nature of the disease, and the expected benefits and deleterious effects of the health intervention. Quality of life questionnaires administration vary from a self-completion, interview, telephone query or mail-back survey. The strengths and weaknesses of these various modes of administration have been detailed [72]. One of the most important problem with questionnaires administered by interview is their cost, and a common approach is to use self-completed questionnaires with supervision.

The few disease-specific instruments to be used in OA, have not been compared face to face, and the available studies which have addressed the selection of QoL instruments in OA have contrasted disease-specific and generic instruments. The results summarized below do not provide a clear-cut answer to this issue. In longitudinal study, a generic measure, the SIP and a specific one, the AIMS were compared in patients with symptomatic OA of the hip or knee [73]. The SIP and the AIMS were significantly correlated for physical domain (2 out of the 12 dimensions of the SIP, and 5 out of the 9 dimensions of the AIMS) and global health (12 dimensions of the SIP, and 7 dimensions of the AIMS). Correlations for psychological health were weaker. The authors concluded that the health related data obtained with both instruments were similar. Nevertheless it should be noted that pain assessment is missing in the SIP which is a major caveat to use it alone in OA. Another study has compared the generic SF-36 instrument with a specific version of this questionnaire adapted for patients having OA of the knee [74]. As it was expected, adapted SF-36 was more specific than SF-36 among patients with other morbid conditions, and less so in patients having only OA of the knee. Other generic and disease specific QoL instruments have been contrasted in OA (FSI, HAQ, AIMS, QWB, SIP), and none outperformed the other in terms of responsiveness and relative efficiency (Table 8) [61]. The SF-36 and WOMAC have been compared in patients after knee replacement surgery [75, 76], and results supported the inclusion of both a generic and a disease specific QoL instrument in cross sectional studies, as it has been previously recommended [77].

7.5.2
Psychometric Properties of the QOL Instruments

Parallel to the QoL instrument selection, the most important issue is to verify how well the instrument will perform in the considered situation. This can be appreciated from the psychometric properties of the instruments [72, 78–80].

7.5.2.1
Validity

A QoL instrument is valid if it actually measures what it is intended to measure. This is very difficult to assess because QoL instruments are measuring an inherently subjective phenomenon for which there is no reference. In a first empirical approach, the content validity examines to what extent the domains of interest are covered by the questionnaire, and reflect the patients' perspectives. The construct validity involves comparisons between QoL scores and the results of other more established clinical or laboratory measures, according to logical relationships that should exist between these measures. Exact agreement is not compulsory since it would signify that QoL measures are redundant. Also, a discriminative QoL instrument should distinguish between patient groups considered to have different health status (principle of known extreme patient groups).

7.5.2.2
Reliability

An instrument is reliable if it produces the same results on repeated use under similar conditions. This is essentially examined by a test-retest procedure and computation of the intraclass correlation (for quantitative data) or Kappa (for qualitative data) coefficients. Reliability is also often assessed by the evaluation of the internal consistency of multi-items scales by computation of Cronbach's alpha coefficients, which assess the degree of agreement of item addressing the same concepts.

7.5.2.3
Responsiveness and Interpretability

Responsiveness or sensitivity refers to the ability of the QoL measure to detect a meaningful change in QoL. If an instrument lacks sensitivity, an intervention that actually improves or deteriorates health status may show no apparent difference between treated and untreated patients. Inadequate range of scaling or the presence of a ceiling or a floor phenomenon may mask meaningful changes in QoL. Indeed, for patients who have minimum QoL scores before an health intervention, it would be impossible to detect any further deterioration with the considered instrument, and vice versa [72]. Disease-specific scales have generally been reported to be more responsive than generic health status measures. Indeed, generic QoL measures include items that are not expected to change with the planned intervention. It is possible that patient-specific scales would be the most responsive type of scale. A recent study compared the responsiveness of a patient-specific scale (MACTAR), a disease-specific scale (WOMAC), and a generic QoL measure (SF-36) in patients with OA of the hip [81]. All the scales were administered before and 6 months after total hip replacement. This study showed that disease- and patient-specific instruments were the most responsive. However, different indices of responsiveness provided different rank ordering among the tested instruments.

In studies with traditional outcomes there is usually a consensus on what constitutes a meaningful clinical effect. However, because of limited experience, this is not the case when QoL outcomes are used, and one must make the distinction between clinically and statistically significant variation in health status. Indeed, of the utmost importance is to determine whether the observed variation in health status makes sense from a clinical standpoint of view, and constitutes a trivial, a small, a medium or a large difference. This property that is called interpretability remains elusive for most QoL instruments [72]. Because they have a wide range of application, generic QoL instruments have often a better interpretability than disease-specific instruments.

7.5.2.4
Acceptability

Acceptability of the QoL questionnaires directly depends on the number of items. All the QoL questionnaires that have been cited in this chapter are acceptable to patients. However, to maximise the response rate and reduce the missing answers, one should give preference to short questionnaires [82]. This explain the tendency to develop shorter QoL questionnaires, and for example several shortened versions of the AIMS and AIMS2 have been reported [83–85]. However, an excess of shortness could be detrimental to the psychometric properties of the instrument. Currently, QoL instruments are used preferentially in clinical trials and evaluation studies, usually in association with other more traditional outcome measures. These instruments are not yet used in routine clinical care as they have many caveats including difficulty to administer and process. Moreover, individual patient' score would be difficult to interpret. Future instruments that will be used routinely will need to be simple and short.

7.5.3
Cross-cultural Issues

As it has been shown for painful sensations, cross-cultural differences in subjective reports of well-being and other dimensions of health are likely to be significant. Most of the QoL instruments have been developed in English language. Development of a new QoL instrument is an enormous task, and usually requires several years of investment. A more simple approach has been to translate existing QoL questionnaire in foreign language. This technique which has many advantages including simplicity, allows international comparisons and is less resources consuming. However, a simple translation is unlikely to be adequate, and in order to take into account the cross-cultural differences, standardized guidelines have been proposed [86]. These guidelines include recommendations for obtaining semantic, idiomatic, experiential and conceptual equivalence during the translation process by using back-translation techniques and committee review, and pre-testing techniques. Moreover a complete repetition of the validation process is required for the instruments that have been cross-culturally adapted [46, 87].

7.6
Conclusions

During the past decades, advances in health care resulted, at least in Western countries, in a shift in the focus of modern medicine to the management of chronic conditions, and QoL became an increasingly important outcome measure. Certainly OA of weight bearing joint not only causes pain and disability, but is also associated with QoL impairment that may be severe. From this review, it is clear enough that QoL instruments have a wide range of applications in this disease, including epidemiologic studies, evaluation of medical therapy and surgery, and aids to the choice of optimal treatment for individual patients. However, despite the widespead interest in QoL, conceptual and methodological barriers limit their use in routine clinical care. Many researchers place too much confidence in the so called objective "hard" radiographic and laboratory data, claiming that there are more reliable than the "soft" clinical and social sciences data. Such confidence is certainly unwarranted. Conversely, because of the tremendous number of so called QoL instruments, and infatuation for this research field, caution should be given against uncontrolled use of instruments with unverified psychometric properties in inappropriate study designs.

Beyond the traditional outcome evaluation, the development of QoL assessment constitutes a major advance and corresponds to a real progress towards a more humanist practice of medical care. However, QoL questionnaires should not replace the traditional patient-physician relationships, and the usual inquiry needed to ascertain the patient's expectations and values remains essential in routine clinical care.

References

1. Altman RD (1997) The syndrome of osteoarthritis. J Rheumatol 24:766–767
2. Creamer P, Hochberg MC (1997) Osteoarthritis. Lancet 350:503–509
3. Summers MN, Haley WE, Reveille JD, Alarcon GS (1988) Radiographic assessment and psychological variables as predictors of pain and functional impairment in osteoarthritis of the knee or hip. Arthritis Rheum 31:204–209
4. McAlindon TE, Cooper C, Kirwan JR, Dieppe PA (1993) Determinants of disability in osteoarthritis of the knee. Ann Rheum Dis 52:258–262
5. Rogers J, Watt I, Dieppe (1990) Comparison of visual and radiographic detection of bony changes at the knee joint. BMJ 300:367–368
6. Sharma L, Felson DT (1998) Studying how osteoarthritis causes disability: nothing is simple. J Rheumatol 25:1–4
7. Bellamy N (1997) Osteoarthritis clinical trials: candidate variables and clinimetric properties. J Rheumatol 24:768–778
8. Bellamy N, Kirwan J, Boers M, Brooks P, Strand V, Tugwell P, Altman R, Brandt K, Dougados M, Lequesne M (1997) Recommendations for a core set of outcome measures for future phase III clinical trials in knee, hip and hand osteoarthritis. Consensus development at OMERACT III. J Rheumatol 24:799–802
9. Leplège A, Hunt S (1997) The problem of quality of life in medicine. JAMA 278:47–50
10. Patrick DL, Bush JW, Chen MM (1973) Toward an operational definition of health. J Health Soc Behav 14:6–23
11. Ware JE Jr (1984) Conceptualizing disease impact and treatment outcomes. Cancer 53:2316–2326

12. Bergner M (1985) Measurement of health status. Med Care 23:696–704
13. Ware JE Jr (1987) Standards for validating health measures: definition and content. J Chron Dis 40:473–480
14. Bergner M, Bobbitt RA, Carter WB, Gilson BS (1981) The sickness impact profile: development and final revision of a health status measure. Med Care 19:787–805
15. Ware JE Jr, Sherbourne CD (1992) The MOS 36-item short-form health survey (SF-36), I: conceptual framework and item selection. Med Care 30:473–483
16. McHorney CA, Ware JE, Lu JFR, Sherbourne CD (1994) The MOS 36-item short-form health survey (SF-36), III: tests of data quality, scaling assumptions, and reliability across diverse patient groups. Med Care 32:40–66
17. McHorney CA, Ware JE Jr, Raczek AE (1993) The MOS 36-item short-form health survey (SF-36), II: psychometric and clinical tests of validity in measuring physical and mental health conditions. Med Care 31:247–263
18. Hunt SM, McKenna SP, McEwen J, Williams P, Papp E (1981) The Nottingham health profile: subjective health status and medical consultations. Soc Sci Med 15 A:221–229
19. Kaplan RM, Bush JW, Berry CC (1976) Health status: types of validity for an index of well-being. Health Serv Res 11:478–507
20. Kind P (1996) The EuroQoL instrument: an index of health-related quality of life. In: Spilker B. Quality of Life and Pharmacoeconomics in Clinical Trials. Second edition. Lippincott-Raven Publishers pp 191–201
21. Fries JF, Spitz PW, Young DY (1982) The dimensions of health outcomes: the health assessment questionnaire, disability and pain scales. J Rheumatol 9:789–793
22. Bellamy N, Buchanan WW, Goldsmith CH, Campbell J, Stitt LW (1988) Validation study of WOMAC: a health status instrument for measuring clinically important patient relevant outcomes to antirheumatic drug therapy in patients with osteoarthritis of the hip or knee. J Rheumatol 15:1833–1840
23. Bellamy N, Kean WF, Buchanan WW, Gerecz-Simon E, Campbell J (1992) Double blind randomized controlled trial of sodium meclofenamate (meclomen) and diclofenac sodium (voltaren): post validation reapplication of the WOMAC osteoarthritis index. J Rheumatol 19:153–159
24. Bellamy N, Campbell J, Stevens J, Pilch L, Stewart C, Mahmood Z (1997) Validation study of a computerized version of the Western Ontario and McMaster Universities VA3.0 Osteoarthritis Index. J Rheumatol 24:2413–2415
25. Bellamy N, Buchanan WW, Goldsmith CH, Campbell J, Duku E (1990) Signal measurement strategies: are they feasible and do they offer any advantage in outcome measurement in osteoarthritis? Arthritis Rheum 33:739–745
26. Lequesne MG, Méry C, Samson M, Gérard P (1987) Indexes of severity for osteoarthritis of the hip and knee. Scand J Rheumatol [Suppl] 65:85–89
27. Lequesne M, Samson M (1991) Indices fonctionnels pour la coxarthrose et la gonarthrose. In: De Sèze S, Ryckewaert A, Kahn MF, Kuntz D, Dryll A, Guérin C (eds) L'actualité rhumatologique présentée au praticien. Expansion Scientifique Française, pp 195–206
28. Lequesne M (1997) The algofunctional indices for the hip and knee osteoarthritis. J Rheumatol 24:779–781
29. Meenan RF, Gertman PM, Mason JH (1980) Measuring health status in arthritis: the arthritis impact measurement scales. Arthritis Rheum 23:146–152
30. Meenan RF, Gertman PM, Mason JH, Dunaif R (1982) The arthritis impact measurement scales: further investigations of a health status measure. Arthritis Rheum 25:1048–1053
31. Mason JH, Anderson JJ, Meenan RF (1989) Applicability of a health status model to osteoarthritis. Arthritis Care Res 2:89–93
32. Meenan RF, Mason JH, Anderson JJ, Guccione AA, Kazis LE (1992) The content and properties of a revised and expanded arthritis impact measurement scales health status questionnaire. Arthritis Rheum 35:1–10
33. Tugwell P, Bombardier C, Buchanan WW, Goldsmith CH, Grace E, Hanna B (1987) The MACTAR patient preference disability questionnaire. An individualized functional priority approach for assessing improvement in physical disability in clinical trials in rheumatoid arthritis. J Rheumatol 14:446–451

34. Laupacis A, Bourne R, Rorabeck C, Feeny D, Wong C, Tugwell P, Leslie K, Bullas R (1993) The effect of elective total hip replacement of health-related quality of life. J Bone Joint Surg 75-A:1619–1626
35. O'Boyle CA, McGee H, Hickey A, O'Malley K, Joyce CRB (1992) Individual quality of life in patients undergoing hip replacement. Lancet 339:1088–1091
36. Hopman-Rock M, Bijlsma JW, Kraaimaat FW, Hofman A, Odding E (1996) Physical and psychosocial disability in elderly subjects in relation to pain in the hip and/or knee. J Rheumatol 23:1037–1044
37. De Bock GH, Mulder JD, Touw-Otten F, Kaptein AA (1995) Health-related quality of life in patients with osteoarthritis in a family practice setting. Arthritis Care Res 8:88–93
38. Lequesne M, Samson M, Gérard P, Méry (1990) Indices algo-fonctionnels pour le suivi des arthroses de la hanche et du genou. Rev Rhum Mal Osteoartic 57:32S–36S
39. Mattsson E, Brostrom LA (1991) The physical and psychosocial effect of moderate osteoarthrosis of the knee. Scand J Rehabil Med 23:215–218
40. Anderson JJ, Firschein HE, Meenan RF (1989) Sensitivity of a health status measure to short-term clinical changes in arthritis. Arthritis Rheum 32:844–850
41. Thorsen H, McKenna SP, Gottschalk L (1993) The Danish version of the Nottingham health profile: ist adaptation and reliability. Scand J Prim Health Care 11:124–129
42. Wiklund I, Romanus B (1991) A comparison of quality of life before and after arthroplasty in patients who had arthrosis of the hip joint. J Bone Joint Surg 73-A:765–769
43. Hawley DJ, Wolfe (1991) Pain, disability and pain/disability relationships in seven rheumatic disorders: a study of 1522 patients. J Rheumatol 18:1552–1557
44. Yelin E, Lubeck D, Holman H, Epstein W (1987) The impact of rheumatoid arthritis and osteoarthritis: the activities of patients with rheumatoid arthritis and osteoarthritis compared to controls. J Rheumatol 14:710–717
45. Callahan LF, Smith WJ, Pincus T (1989) Self-report questionnaires in five rheumatic diseases. Comparisons of health status constructs and associations with formal education level. Arthritis Care Res 2:122–131
46. Pouchot J, Guillemin F, Coste J, Brégeon C, Sany J, and the French "Quality of Life in Rheumatology" Group (1996) Validity, reliability, and sensitivity to change of a French version of the Arthritis Impact Measurement scales 2 (AIMS2) in patients with rheumatoid arthritis treated with methotrexate. J Rheumatol 23:52–60
47. Wiklund I, Romanus B, Hunt SM (1988) Self-assessed disability in patients with arthrosis of the hip joint. Reliability of the Swedish version of the Nottingham health profile. Int Disab Studies 10:159–163
48. Wolfe F, Hawley DJ (1997) Measurement of the quality of life in rheumatic disorders using the EuroQoL. Br J Rheumatol 36:786–793
49. Gordon G (1988) Effects of piroxicam on quality of life of patients with osteoarthritis. Consultant (suppl) 28:4–10
50. Bradley JD, Brandt KD, Katz BP, Kalasinski LA, Ryan SI (1991) Comparison of an antiinflammatory dose of ibuprofen, an analgesic dose of ibuprofen, and acetaminophen in the treatment of patients with osteoarthritis of the knee. N Engl J Med 325:87–91
51. Kovar PA, Allegrante JP, MacKenzie CR, Peterson MGE, Gutin B, Charlson ME (1992) Supervised fitness walking in patients with osteoarthritis of the knee. Ann Intern Med 116:529–534
52. Weinberger M, Tierney WM, Booher P, Katz BP (1989) Can the provision of information to patients with osteoarthritis improve functional status? A randomized, controlled trial. Arthritis Rheum 32:1577–1583
53. Mazzuca SA, Hanna M, Byrd D, Chambers M, Katz BP, Brandt KD (1997) Effects of self-care education on the health status of inner-city patients with osteoarthritis of the knee. Arthritis Rheum 40:1466–1474
54. Nguyen M, Dougados M, Revel M (1997) Prolonged effects of 3 week therapy in a spa resort on lumbar spine, knee and hip osteoarthritis: follow-up after 6 months. A randomized controlled trial. Br J Rheumatol 36:77–81

55. Lequesne M, Brandt K, Bellamy N, Moskowitz R, Menkès CJ, Pelletier JP, Altman R (1994) Guidelines for testing slow-acting and disease-modifying drugs in osteoarthritis. J Rheumatol [Suppl] 41:65–71
56. Burkhardt D, Ghosh P (1987) Laboratory evaluation of antirheumatic drugs as potential chondroprotective agents. Semin Arthritis Rheum 17:3–34
57. Ravaud P, Dougados M (1997) Radiographic assessment in osteoarthritis. J Rheumatol 24:786–791
58. Puhl W, Bernau A, Greiling H, Köpcke W, Pförringer W, Steck KJ, Zacher J, Scharf HP (1993) Intra-articular sodium hyaluronate in osteoarthritis of the knee: a multicenter, double-blind study. Osteoarthritis Cartilage 1:233–241
59. Listrat V, Dougados M, Amor B, Simonnet J, Bonvarlet JP, Patarnello F, Ayral X (1997) Arthroscopic evaluation of potential structure modifying activity of hyaluronan (Hyalgan) in osteoarthritis of the knee. Osteoarthritis Cartilage 5:153–160
60. Liang MH, Cullen KE, Larson MG, Thompson MS, Schwartz JA, Fossel AH, Roberts WN, Sledge CB (1986) Cost-effectiveness of total joint arthroplasty in osteoarthritis. Arthritis Rheum 29:937–943
61. Liang MH, Larson MG, Cullen KE, Schwartz JA (1985) Comparative measurement efficiency and sensitivity of five health status instruments for arthritis research. Arthritis Rheum 28:542–547
62. Katz JN, Phillips CB, Poss R, Harrast JJ, Fossel AH, Liang MH, Sledge CB (1995) The validity and reliability of a total hip arthroplasty outcome evaluation questionnaire. J Bone Joint Surg 77-A:1528–1534
63. Towheed TE, Hochberg MC (1996) Health-related quality of life after total hip replacement. Semin Arthritis Rheum 26:483–491
64. Stucki G, Katz JN, Philipps C, Liang MH (1995) The Short Form-36 is preferable to the SIP as a generic health status measure in patients undergoing elective total hip arthroplasty. Arthritis Care Res 8:174–181
65. Dawson J, Fitzpatrick R, Murray D, Carr A (1998) Questionnaire on the perceptions of patients about total knee replacement. J Bone Joint Surg 80-B:63–69
66. Garellick G, Malchau H, Herberts P, Hansson E, Axelsson H, Hansson T (1998) Life expectancy and cost utility after total hip replacement. Clin Orthop 346:141–151
67. Chang RW, Hazen GB, Pellisier JM (1996) A cost-effectiveness analysis of total hip arthroplasty for osteoarthritis of the hip. JAMA 275:858–865
68. Drewett RF, Minns RJ, Sibly TF (1992) Measuring outcome of total knee replacement using quality of life indices. Ann R Coll Surg Engl 74:286–290
69. Bennett KJ, Goldsmith CH, Smith F, Moran LA, Torrance GW (1997) Health state utilities in knee replacement surgery: the development and evaluation of McKnee. J Rheumatol 24:1796–1805
70. Lavernia CJ, Gachupin-Garcia A, Guzman JF (1997) Cost effectiveness and quality of life in knee arthroplasty. Clin Orthop 345:134–139
71. Ruchlin HS, Paget SA, Elkin EB (1997) Assessing cost-effectiveness analyses in rheumatoid arthritis and osteoarthritis. Arthritis Care Res 10:413–421
72. Guyatt GH, Feeny DH, Patrick DL (1993) Measuring health-related quality of life. Ann Intern Med 118:622–629
73. Weinberger M, Samsa GP, Tierney WM, Belyea MJ, Hiner SL (1992) Generic versus disease specific health status measures: comparing the Sickness Impact Profile and the Arthritis Impact Measurement Scales. J Rheumatol 19:543–546
74. Kantz ME, Harris WJ, Levitsky K, Ware J, Ross Davies A (1992) Methods for assessing condition-specific and generic functional status outcomes after total knee replacement. Med Care 30:MS240–MS252
75. Hawker G, Melfi C, Paul J, Green R, Bombardier C (1995) Comparison of a generic (SF-36) and a disease specific (WOMAC) instrument in the measurement of outcomes after knee replacement surgery. J Rheumatol 22:1193–1196
76. Bombardier C, Coyte P, Wright J, Hawker G, Green R, Paul J, Melfi CA (1995) Comparison of a generic and a disease-specific measure of pain and physical function after knee replacement surgery. Med Care (suppl) 33:AS131–AS144

77. Patrick DL, Deyo RA (1989) Generic and disease-specific measures in assessing health status and quality of life. Med Care 27:S217–S232
78. Kirshner B, Guyatt G (1985) A methodological framework for assessing health indices. J Chron Dis 38:27–36
79. Fitzpatrick R, Fletcher A, Gore S, Jones D, Spiegelhalter D, Cox D (1992) Quality of life measures in health care. I: applications and issues in assessment. BMJ 305:1074–1077
80. Coste J, Fermanian J, Venot A (1995) Methodological and statistical problems in the construction of composite measurement scales. A survey of six medical and epidemiological journals. Stat Med 14:331–345
81. Wright JG, Young NL (1997) A comparison of different indices of responsiveness. J Clin Epidemiol 50:239–246
82. Coste J, Guillemin F, Pouchot J, Fermanian J (1997) The methodological approaches to shortening composite measurement scales. J Clin Epidemiol 50:247–252
83. Wallston KA, Brown GK, Stein MJ, Dobbins CJ (1989) Comparing the short and long versions of the Arthritis Impact Measurement Scales. J Rheumatol 16:1105–1109
84. Lorish C, Abraham N, Austin JS, Bradley LA, Alarcon GS (1991) A comparison of the full and short versions of the Arthritis Impact Measurement Scales. Arthritis Care Res 4:168–173
85. Guillemin F, Coste J, Pouchot J, Ghézail M, Brégeon C, Sany J, and the French Quality of Life in Rheumatology Group (1997) The AIMS2-SF. A short form of the Arthritis Impact Measurement Scales 2. Arthritis Rheum 40:1267–1274
86. Guillemin F, Bombardier C, Beaton D (1993) Cross-cultural adaptation of health-related quality of life measures: literature review and proposed guidelines. J Clin Epidemiol 46:1417–1432
87. Guillemin F (1995) Cross-cultural adaptation and validation of health status measures. Scand J Rheumatol 24:61–63

CHAPTER 8

Medical Management of Osteoarthritis

8.1
Medical Aspects

8.1.1
Basic Principles in Osteoarthritis Treatment

D. CHOQUETTE, J. P. RAYNAULD and E. RICH

8.1.1.1
Introduction

As the most common form of joint disease, osteoarthritis (OA) represents a major cause of morbidity and disability, as well as a significant burden on health-care resources. Medical interventions can be directed to different stages of the disease process: primary prevention, screening at an asymptomatic stage to avoid progression to overt disease, and treatment of an established condition. Although important advances in understanding the pathophysiological process of osteoarthritis have been made through epidemiology, biomechanics and molecular level studies, we are still mainly involved in treating the established disease [1] and this will be the principal focus of this chapter.

Management of OA requires careful diagnostic evaluation, appreciation of the severity of the articular process, establishment of the level of necessary or desired therapy and a judgment on general health status before initiating any type of intervention. Many therapeutic modalities can be offered to patients suffering from OA, although none has yet been proven to be disease-modifying. A comprehensive treatment program tailored to the disease severity should be developed for each individual.

8.1.1.2
Goals and Categories of Treatment

The main objectives in the management of OA are to reduce symptoms, minimize functional disability and limit progression. These goals can be reached through a pyramidal treatment approach (Fig. 1) [2] which, in the years to come,

Fig. 1. Pyramid approach to the management of osteo-arthritis. (Modified from [2])

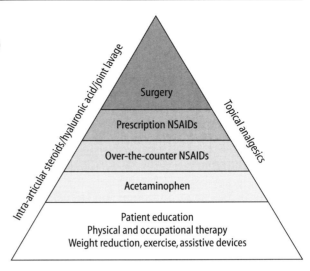

Surgery

Prescription NSAIDs

Over-the-counter NSAIDs

Acetaminophen

Patient education
Physical and occupational therapy
Weight reduction, exercise, assistive devices

Intra-articular steroids/hyaluronic acid/joint lavage

Topical analgesics

may evolve with the advent of potentially disease-modifying drugs. Three main categories of treatment which can overlap are nonpharmacological, pharmacological and surgical management. The latter topic is thoroughly reviewed in Chap. 9.

8.1.1.2.1
Nonpharmacological Management

Patient Education and Social Support

This is an essential part of any treatment plan for patients with OA. There is mounting evidence for the effectiveness of patient education programs such as the "Arthritis Self-Management Course" in reducing pain, decreasing the frequency of visits to a physician, improving the quality of life and maintaining function [3–5]. A recent meta-analysis comparing controlled patient education trials with placebo-controlled trials of nonsteroidal anti-inflammatory drugs (NSAID) showed that the former had beneficial effects on pain, although of slightly inferior magnitude than NSAID [6].

The efficacy of educational programs in OA may be enhanced by involving the spouse [7]. Even a mail-delivered self-management program has made significantly positive changes in self-care behavior, reducing helplessness, pain and depression [8]. Health professional social support via telephone is another approach found to relieve pain and improve functional status in patients with OA [9, 10]. There are data indicating that all of the above measures are cost-effective [4, 11].

Weight

Overweight persons are more prone to knee OA, regardless of whether OA is defined by symptoms or by radiograph [12]. Furthermore, obese patients with knee

OA are at a higher risk of developing a progressive disease than are non-overweight patients [13, 14]. Inversely, a weight loss of 5 kilograms in women is associated with a 50 % reduction in the risk of developing symptomatic knee OA [15].

There is a surprising scarcity of data on weight loss as a treatment for OA. In a small clinical trial of an appetite suppressant in patients with knee or hip OA, weight loss (3–6 kg on average) correlated strongly with a reduction in symptoms, more so for knee than hip OA [16]. Preliminary data indicate that obese women suffering from knee OA [17] experience a reduction in pain and functional impairment in association with weight loss.

Physical Therapy

Physical therapy plays an important role in the treatment of OA. This involves aerobic exercise, range of motion and strengthening exercises of the concerned muscle groups, thermal modalities, transcutaneous electrical nerve stimulation (TENS), ultrasound, diathermy, devices to assist ambulation, and other analgesic modalities (i. e. acupuncture). It is essential to inform the patient with knee and/or hip OA of the definite data on pain reduction and function improvement achieved with quadriceps-strengthening and aerobic exercises [18, 19] (further detailed in Chapter 10). This effect is likely the result of an increase in the joint-stabilizing and shock-absorbing properties of the periarticular muscles, and improved muscle sensorimotor function, thereby improving joint proprioception [20]. Controlled clinical trials suggest that TENS may be beneficial to patients with knee OA, but sample sizes are small and study designs do have limitations [18].

In patients with knee OA who have patellofemoral involvement, a small study found that medial taping of the patella provided significant short term pain relief [21]. To diminish joint loading, shock-absorbing shoes and the proper use of a cane can be of benefit; the latter may reduce loading forces on the OA hip by as much as 50 % [22]. Heel wedges with a 5° to 10° angle inducing a calcaneo-valgus have been shown to be helpful in medial compartment knee OA, particularly in patients with mild disease severity [23]. Knee braces may also be helpful in knee OA when there is joint instability or unicompartmental disease. A knee sleeve or bandage improves proprioception in knee OA, giving a sense of less instability in some patients [24].

Occupational Therapy

The occupational therapist evaluates the patient's limitations in the activities of daily life and proposes adaptive devices. For patients with OA of the lower limbs, information on how to overcome difficulties with sexual activities can also be provided.

Epidemiological studies have identified particular repetitive joint activities as a risk factor for developing OA at specific sites: OA of the hand is more prevalent in employees of a textile mill that use a repeated pincer grip; jobs that require kneeling and squatting favor the appearance of knee OA; and farmers have a definite increase in the incidence of hip OA [1]. It therefore seems reasonable to avoid as much as possible those particular activities that may aggravate OA in the related joint, or at least alter the way these tasks are performed.

8.1.1.2.2
Pharmacological Management of Osteoarthritis (Excluding NSAID)

Systemic Treatment

The first pharmacological line of treatment is analgesics. In OA, purely analgesic agents (acetaminophen being the prototype) should be considered first, and before the use of NSAID, in view of the higher incidence of toxicity associated with the latter. The mechanism of action of acetaminophen is not yet fully known, and evidence implicates direct effects on the central nervous system [25].

In recent publications, up to 30% of patients suffering from knee OA have demonstrated a substantial benefit from acetaminophen, even those previously treated with NSAID [26, 27]. Bradley et al., in a study on OA patients with chronic knee pain and moderate radiographic changes treated for four weeks with either ibuprofen 2400 mg/d, ibuprofen 1200 mg/d or acetaminophen 4000 mg/d, demonstrated no superiority of ibuprofen at either dosage over acetaminophen [28]. Stamp et al. compared flurbiprofen to nefopam with similar results [29].

NSAID are generally overprescribed in elderly patients. Withdrawal studies have demonstrated that a substantial percentage of elderly patients were able to stop NSAID therapy, and were still off these drugs up to 6 months later [30].

As previously mentioned, the major advantage of acetaminophen use is its lack of upper and lower gastrointestinal toxicity. However, drug overdose (over 10 g/d) is associated with hepatotoxicity. Such dosages represent twice the maximum recommended therapeutic dose for adults [31]. With the usual acetaminophen dosage, there is also an increased incidence of hepatotoxicity in patients with preexistent liver disease and alcoholism; fatal hepatic damage in association with a moderate intake of alcohol has been reported [32]. Current literature suggests careful monitoring of daily dosage aiming at the lowest effective dosage. It is advisable to discourage regular analgesic use in patients with chronic alcohol consumption.

The risk of nephrotoxicity with chronic acetaminophen usage is not clearly established and likely remains very low. The absence of peripheral inhibition of prostaglandin synthesis is the presumable reason for this low incidence of renal toxicity. Acute acetaminophen nephrotoxicity has been documented in overdose cases, the majority in association with hepatic failure [33, 34]. Murray et al. looked at the incidence of end-stage renal disease and analgesic use [35], and found no evidence of association. Perneger et al. reported the results of a case-control study on the risk of developing end-stage renal disease with over-the-counter analgesic usage [36]. An intake of more than one daily tablet, and a cumulative acetaminophen consumption of more than a thousand pills, double the odds of end-stage renal disease. Surprisingly, acetylsalicylic acid tablet usage revealed no association with chronic renal disease. Caution should be used when analyzing this type of publication as case-control studies are subject to recall bias. There are also concerns about the sequence in which drug exposure and renal insufficiency supervened. Clinical events associated with the renal problem, rather than the cause of the nephropathy, may have been the determining factor in taking analgesia. Recently, in a case-control study, Hylek et al. reported an increase of INR in patients on anticoagulotherapy in association with acetaminophen usage [37]. It was suggested that acetaminophen could be an unrecognized cause of overanticoagulation.

Narcotic use in the chronic management of OA is not recommended. The target age-group being the elderly, the incidence of side effects including nausea, vomiting, constipation, urinary retention, mental confusion and drowsiness is far from negligible. The possible psychological and physical dependencies associated with these agents are also a concern for health professionals. Conversely, rigid opposition to the use of opioids in specific and limited clinical situations is also not advised. These agents may have their place in the armamentarium against OA for short periods of administration.

Tramadol hydrochloride, a new analgesic agent, has two modes of action. This synthetic amino-cyclohexanol binds to μ-opioid receptors and inhibits the reuptake of norepinephrine and serotonin. One hundred mg of tramadol is more effective than 60 mg of codeine, and as effective as combinations of codeine with aspirin or acetaminophen [38, 39]. A two-week trial comparing tramadol (300 mg/d) and dextropropoxyphene (300 mg/d) showed them to be equipotent [40]. Respiratory depression has not been noted with recommended doses, and titration from 50 mg/d up to a full dose over four to five days may minimize the incidence of nausea and vomiting. The potential for abuse and addiction associated with this compound appears notably low. However, due to its mode of action, it should not be administered in combination with a tricyclic antidepressant or monoamine oxidase inhibitor. In OA patients with insufficient clinical response to the maximal dose of acetaminophen and definitive contraindications to NSAID usage, such as prior upper gastrointestinal bleeding episodes, a trial with tramadol may certainly be a therapeutic option.

Newer highly selective cyclooxygenase-2 inhibitors may eventually offer a safer alternative to the classic NSAID, which are well-known offenders of the gastrointestinal mucosa, and would make the opioid alternative to NSAID (or non-narcotic analgesic) usage less attractive.

The use of NSAID, which will be discussed in Chapter 8.1.2, is certainly associated with a non-negligible burden of toxic side effects that are more frequently found in the predominant OA patient group, the aging population. In our society, the percentage of these patients is steadily increasing. Moreover, this group of patients requires additional medication for associated diseases such as hypertension, diabetes mellitus and heart disease. Therefore, there is an important risk of drug interaction to consider, and an associated compliance problem.

For these reasons, topical agents in the management of OA pain is an attractive therapeutical option. Numerous topical NSAID preparations are available in Europe, but none of these have yet been released on the North American market. Some over the counter salicylate-containing preparations are available; however, clear evidence of their efficacy is still lacking. The resulting benefit may be mediated through a pharmacological action, a placebo effect or their action as a rubbing compound. A 1998 report reviewed 86 studies to evaluate the efficacy and toxicity of topical agents for acute and chronic painful conditions

[41] (including OA), and concluded that they are effective and safe in the management of these conditions. Some studies on hand and knee OA are currently in progress with results forthcoming shortly. Hewitt et al. recently reported an enhancing effect of DMSO for transcutaneous absorption of NSAID [42]. Additional data are needed to establish a clinical efficacy and safety profile of DMSO.

Capsaicin (Trans-8-Methyl-N-vanillyl-6-nonenamide) is an alkaloid derived from the seeds and membranes of the nightshade family of plants, including the common pepper plant. Substance P is responsible for the transmission of nociceptive stimuli from the periphery to the central nervous system. On topical application, capsaicin provokes the release of substance P by peripheral nerves. It also prevents the substance P reaccumulation in the neurons and terminal endings. Indications for its use include postmastectomy pain, phantom limb syndrome, diabetic neuropathy, cluster headaches and post-herpetic neuralgia.

Articular cartilage does not have nerve endings. Joint capsule, tendons, ligaments, and periosteum are, on the other hand, extensively innervated [43, 44]. Nerve endings of the synovium contain substance P [45], and the content of substance P may even be increased in certain clinical situations such as OA. Finally, trials using capsaicin have demonstrated beneficial effects on pain caused by OA [46].

A thin layer of capsaicin should be applied on all aspects of the target joint. This should be repeated three to four times daily. Patients should be instructed to wash their hands after each application, and to avoid contact with inflamed skin, eyes and mucous membranes.

Intra-articular Injections as Treatment in Osteoarthritis

Corticosteroids

Intra-articular corticosteroid injections have been used by rheumatologists, orthopedic surgeons and other practitioners for more than four decades. Despite extensive clinical experience, certain aspects of local corticosteroid treatment remain controversial (e.g. relative efficacy, possible deleterious effects, potential chondroprotective properties).

Different steroid formulations have been used since 1966: triamcinolone hexacetonide [47–51], methylprednisolone [47, 52], prednisolone acetate [47, 53, 54]. Single corticosteroid injection [50, 51, 53] or repetitive injections [47–49, 52] were administered intra-articularly, and when present, synovial fluid was aspirated. Sambrook et al. [52] investigated an injection technique of the corticosteroid around the patella.

Local corticosteroid injections are a relatively safe and effective adjunct in managing knee OA; however, there is no definitive answer regarding long-term beneficial or deleterious effects. Triamcinolone hexacetonide (THA) provided short–term pain relief in knee OA, and an increased benefit was associated with both clinical evidence of joint effusion and successful aspiration of synovial fluid at the time of injection [50]. Dieppe et al. reported that steroid injections caused a significantly greater reduction in pain and tenderness than placebo, and were preferred by patients [48]. A randomized clinical trial conducted in Finland showed that THA had a pronounced effect of long duration. The results confirmed that intra-articular treatment of OA with THA was highly effective and provided a significantly prolonged duration of benefit compared to beta-methasone [51]. However, Friedman noted differences between groups at one week and no significant differences thereafter [49]. Intra-articular predniso-lone injection was assessed by conducting a placebo-controlled trial [53]. Steroid injection provided greater pain relief at one week, but results at four, six, and eight weeks were similar. A retrospective observational study evaluated in-tra-articular steroid injections repeated over a period extending from four to 15 years [47]. This study was based on radiological assessment, and the authors are of the opinion that intra-articular corticosteroid therapy, if used judiciously, has an important part to play in the management of chronic arthritis. They found no real evidence supporting the suggestion that repeated intra-articular injec-tions inevitably lead to rapid joint destruction.

Hyaluronic Acid

Hyaluronic acid (hyaluronan), a polysaccharide consisting of a long chain of di-saccharides (β-D-glucuronyl-β-D-N-acetylglucosamine), is a natural compo-nent of cartilage and plays an essential role in the articular milieu. It is consi-dered not only a joint lubricant, but also a physiological factor in the trophic status of cartilage. Balazs proposed hyaluronic acid (HA) as an effective agent in the treatment of patients with arthritic diseases. Its clinical use was consid-ered after determining that HA was reduced in concentration and in chain length in the synovial fluid of arthritis patients. Preliminary human clinical studies of sodium hyaluronate in human arthritic joints were performed by Peyron and Balazs in the early 1970's. Several studies with various preparations of hyaluronan from different sources and molecular weights have since been conducted.

The efficacy of viscosupplementation – the replacement of pathological sy-novial fluid with a hyaluronan-based elastoviscous solution – depends on the physical properties of the solution used and its residence time in the joint. Pre-parations of hyaluronic acid or sodium hyaluronate with a molecular weight be-tween 500–700 KD, 600–1200 KD and 4000–5000 KD have been used in clini-cal studies.

Intra-articular injections of hyaluronan or sodium hyaluronate with a mole-cular weight between 500,000 and 750,000 Daltons have been studied using corticosteroid injections [55–58] or NSAIDs [59] as control treatment, and by conducting placebo-controlled clinical trials [60–65]. A prospective study in-cluding 43 patients with knee OA showed good tolerance to treatment, without adverse side effects. This therapy was effective if OA was less than moderate in grade; it was not effective in cases with considerable effusion or in those with gross architectural changes [65]. A single-blind parallel trial used two dosage regimens of HA (40 mg and 20 mg) to assess its efficacy [50]. The active treat-ments were shown to be equally highly effective in reducing pain; both were sig-nificantly superior to placebo, and beneficial effects lasted for more than a month demonstrating the long-term action of the drug. Several double-blind placebo-controlled trials suggest that intra-articular injection of sodium hyal-uronate (Hyalectin) may improve the clinical condition and have a long-term beneficial effect in patients with knee OA [61–63]. However, a double-blind placebo-controlled study involving 91 patients with radiologically confirmed knee OA concluded that intra-articular administration of 750 KD hyaluronan offered no significant benefit over placebo during a five-week treatment period, but incurred a significantly higher morbidity [64]. The principal side effects were a transient increase in pain and swelling in the affected knee that was observed in 47% of the treatment group compared with 22% of the placebo group. Graf et al. conducted a single-blind, randomized clinical trial to compare both the efficacy and safety of HA with that of mucopolysaccharide polysulfuric acid ester (MPA) in patients with OA [66]. Both HA and MPA demonstrated efficacy, with hyaluronic acid superior in the parameters investigated.

Furthermore, in a study that evaluated the effect of joint lavage with lactated Ringer's solution in 23 patients, the secondary goal was to determine if any additional benefit could be obtained by injecting the knee with HA following washout treatment [67]. Improvement was noted at one- and two-year follow-ups, however there were no statistically significant differences in outcome for the hyaluronan and placebo groups.

Others have used methylprednisolone acetate as the drug of comparison. The results showed that on a short-term basis, both HA and 6-methylprednisolone acetate were efficacious in controlling OA symptoms. In the long-term assessment, the results obtained at the end of treatment in the HA group persisted, and in some cases even improved [56, 58]. It was concluded that sodium hyaluronate would appear to offer an alternative to steroids in intra-articular treatment of OA [57]. Grecomoro et al. evaluated the therapeutic synergism between HA and dexamethasone in intra-articular treatment by conducting a open randomized study [55]. Dexamethasone notably potentiated the clinical effectiveness of hyaluronic acid, even if used only during the first weekly infiltration of a five-week treatment regimen.

A one-year double-blind control study involving 52 patients compared the effect of intra-articular injections of hyaluronan (600–1200 KD) and placebo, both administrated weekly for five weeks [68]. Though both groups improved from baseline, there was no statistically significant difference in any of the relevant variables at any time point. Recently, a large randomized double-blind placebo-control trial also found no significant difference at 20 weeks between the two groups when compared to their baseline evaluation; however, once stratified according to age and disease severity, HA proved more efficacious than placebo in patients over 60 years of age who had the most severe knee OA [69].

The long-term structure-modifying properties of HA (Hyalgan) were investigated through a double-blind randomized placebo-controlled trial using a standardized arthroscopic score after one year of follow up. HA proved superior to placebo in two out of three parameters used to quantify the severity of lesions [70].

The efficacy of a weekly therapeutic regimen of either two or three injections of hylan GF-20 (a higher molecular weight compound) was further demonstrated by Scale et al. in a randomized double-blind placebo-controlled clinical trial that included a six-month follow-up [71]. Compared to the control group, the two-injection and three-injection hylan treatment groups both showed statistically significantly greater improvement in pain outcome measures, as well as overall evaluation of treatment at the 12-week point. At six-month follow-up, results in both hylan treatment groups were superior to those in the control group. Adams et al. evaluated the safety and effectiveness of three weekly intra-articular injections of hylan G-F20 (Synvisc) in patients with knee OA, and compared this treatment to continuous oral NSAID therapy in both the presence and absence of hylan G-F 20 viscosupplementation [59]. The results support the hypothesis that treatment of knee OA pain with hylan is at least as effective as treatment with NSAID. Hylan G-F 20 is a safe and effective treatment for knee OA, and can be used either as a replacement for or an adjunct to NSAID therapy.

Intra-articular injection with hyaluronan is a relatively safe approach; however, some adverse events have been reported. One patient developed an haemarthrosis after sodium hyaluronate injection [61]. Other observed events were local reactions such as effusion, feeling of warmth, sensation of heat, tingling and pain following HA injections [66]. A transient adverse event of muscle pain was also mentioned [71].

In conclusion, in the majority of studies, a clinical benefit of treatment was reported compared to the control injected group. Compared to treatment with local corticosteroids, the benefit of hyaluronan was somewhat less dramatic but longer lasting.

Other Intra-articular Therapies in Knee Osteoarthritis

Corticosteroid and hyaluronan intra-articular injections have been widely used in the last few decades for treatment of knee OA. However, other substances such as orgotein, yttrium–90, silicone, somatostatin and tenoxicam have been investigated as potentially therapeutic in the treatment of arthritic joints.

Orgotein is the pharmaceutical form of the bovine enzyme Cu-Zn superoxide dismutase. The anti-inflammatory properties of orgotein were discovered in 1965. Intra-articular injection of orgotein presents a potentially therapeutic advance, especially in the treatment of OA [72]. This study showed that four weekly injections of 4 mg orgotein were superior to four weekly injections of saline, and orgotein was safe and well tolerated. Furthermore, three orgotein dose/regimens were compared with a placebo in terms of efficacy, safety and duration of effect in 139 patients with knee OA. Orgotein was effective in reducing symptoms for up to three months after treatment; 16 mg given twice was the most effective and best-tolerated regimen [73].

A randomized double-blind study was conducted to compare orgotein injections with intra-articular methylprednisolone acetate injections. It was found that orgotein could be used safely and effectively without serious adverse reactions [74]. The efficacy of orgotein was compared to that of betamethasone over a one-year period in 419 patients with knee OA [75]. Though betamethasone acted more quickly, orgotein at low doses (4 or 8 mg) was comparable with the corticosteroid from week four, and up to a year after the beginning of the study.

The main adverse reactions to orgotein were pain, swelling and stiffness [74]. Pain, prickling or burning sensations, or a feeling of heaviness at the injection site, were the adverse effects most frequently reported [75]. Skin eruption and/or pruritus were also mentioned [73].

An observational prospective study evaluating the effects of both radiation synovectomy and triamcinolone acetonide was conducted in 40 patients with knee OA over a one-year period [76]. A marked improvement in pain and evaluation scores occurred at three months, but had disappeared by six months post treatment. The safety and efficacy of Disprosium-165 Hydroxide Macroaggregate (165 Dy) was compared with Yttrium–90 Silicate for radiation synovectomy of the knee in a multicentre double-blind clinical trial conducted in Australia [77]. There was no significant difference in clinical response in the two treatment groups, and there were no clinically significant side effects.

Wright et al. conducted a pilot study in five patients, with a control of 25 outpatients, to evaluate silicone as an artificial lubricant for OA joints [78]. Sequential analyses showed a significant benefit from saline compared to silicone at one week follow-up, and no significant difference at one month.

A randomized placebo-controlled study to assess saline lavage of knee OA in 20 patients was carried out [79]. Though both groups showed improvement, knee washout conferred no further benefit than intra-articular saline injection. However, in a recent randomized single-blind study, tidal knee irrigation with saline on 77 patients with knee OA showed a greater improvement in pain reduction than did conservative medical management [80].

Glucosamine was evaluated in 54 patients with gonarthrosis in a double-blind controlled study [81]. The results showed that glucosamine was safe and provided a greater improvement than placebo injections.

An open six-month pilot study of intra-articular tenoxicam was conducted by Papathanassiou [82] in 28 patients with knee OA. Results of this preliminary study indicated that a single administration of tenoxicam injected intra-articularly could provide long-lasting beneficial effects without the problems of local tolerance.

Intra-articular injection of somatostatin in knee OA was evaluated by Silveri et al. in an observational prospective study involving 20 patients [83]. The results revealed an improvement in pain and joint function after intra-articular injection. This was confirmed with statistical analysis, and no side effects were reported.

Summary and Guidelines Regarding Intra-Articular Therapies for Osteoarthritis

In summary, the literature regarding intra-articular injections as treatment for knee OA is scant. There are no long-term studies on efficacy (six months of follow-up or more), and no functional evaluation using validated instruments (i. e. WOMAC or the like) has been carried out. No anatomical evaluation data on the progression of disease, nor the disease cost assessment are available. Therefore, one cannot really derive evidence-based medicine from the information currently available on intra-articular injection as treatment for knee OA. The following recommendations for the use of intra-articular modalities reflect the authors' experience more than solid evidence based on medical literature.

A clinician should consider intra-articular therapies for knee OA when simple therapeutic (pharmacological and non-pharmacological) modalities are not successful or may be potentially harmful. The authors feel that, if moderate or severe OA of the knee does not respond to a trial of acetaminophen (Tylenol) and/or NSAID, intra-articular injections should be considered.

If the knee presents signs of inflammation (warmth or effusion), a joint tap to remove as much fluid as possible should be performed. If the fluid does not indicate infection, corticosteroids should be injected into the articulation. A good decrease in pain and effusion is usually achieved, and will last for some period of time.

If a relapse occurs 3 months after the injection, a second injection of corticosteroids may be given. However, there is no clear consensus on any harmful effect of repeated injections of steroids on the structure of the knee. Therefore, we feel that until proven otherwise, if more than three or four injections per year are needed regularly, other therapies should be considered.

Should a relapse occur before 3 months, or the knee does not present signs of inflammation (warmth or effusion),viscosupplementation could offer a longer period of relief if effective. Three injections on a weekly basis are needed, and the cost of this product should also be considered.

8.1.1.3
Conclusion

In conclusion, before using non-steroidal antiinflammatory drugs (NSAID) in osteoarthritis (OA), several modalities should seriously be considered as discussed previously. These approaches offer the clinician valuable alternatives for OA management.

References

1. Felson DT, Zhang Y (1998) An update on the epidemiology of knee and hip osteoarthritis with a view to prevention. Arthritis Rheum 41:1343–1355
2. Creamer P, Hochberg MC (1997) Osteoarthritis. Lancet 350:503–508
3. Lorig K, Lubeck D, Kraines RG, Seleznick M, Holman HR (1985) Outcomes of self-help education for patients with arthritis. Arthritis Rheum 28:680–685
4. Lorig KR, Mazonson PD, Holman HR (1993) Evidence suggesting that health education for self-management in patients with chronic arthritis has sustained health benefits while reducing health care costs. Arthritis Rheum 36:439–446
5. Hawley DJ (1995) Psycho-educational interventions in the treatment of arthritis. Bailleres Clin Rheumatol 9:803–823
6. Superio-Cabuslay E, Ward MM, Lorig KR (1996) Patient education interventions in osteoarthritis and rheumatoid arthritis: a meta-analytic comparison with nonsteroidal antiinflammatory drug treatment. Arthritis Care Res 9:292–301
7. Keefe FJ, Caldwell DS, Baucom D, Salley A, Robinson E, Timmons K, Beaupre P, Weisberg J, Helms M (1996) Spouse-assisted coping skills training in the management of osteoarthritic knee pain. Arthritis Care Res 9:279–291
8. Goeppinger J, Macnee C, Anderson MK, Boutaugh M, Stewart K (1995) From research to practice: the effects of the jointly sponsored dissemination of an arthritis self-care nursing intervention. Appl Nurs Res 8:106–113
9. Weinberger M, Tierney WM, Booher P, Katz BP (1989) Can the provision of information to patients with osteoarthritis improve functional status? A randomized, controlled trial. Arthritis Rheum 32:1577–1583

10. Maisiak R, Austin J, Heck L (1996) Health outcomes of two telephone interventions for patients with rheumatoid arthritis or osteoarthritis. Arthritis Rheum 39:1391–1399

11. Weinberger M, Tierney WM, Cowper PA, Katz BP, Booher PA (1993) Cost-effectiveness of increased telephone contact for patients with osteoarthritis. A randomized, controlled trial. Arthritis Rheum 36:243–246

12. Felson DT, Anderson JJ, Naimark A, Walker AM, Meenan RF (1988) Obesity and knee osteoarthritis. Ann Intern Med 109:18–24

13. Dougados M, Gueguen A, Nguyen M, Thiesce A, Listrat V, Jacob L, Nakache JP, Gabriel KR, Lequesne M, Amor B (1992) Longitudinal radiologic evaluation of osteoarthritis of the knee. J Rheumatol 19:378–384

14. Schouten JS, Van den Ouweland FA, Valkenburg HA (1992) A 12 year follow up study in the general population on prognostic factors of cartilage loss in osteoarthritis of the knee. Ann Rheum Dis 51:932–937

15. Felson DT, Zhang Y, Anthony JM, Naimark A, Anderson JJ (1992) Weight loss reduces the risk for symptomatic knee osteoarthritis in women. The Framingham Study. Ann Intern Med 116:535–539

16. Willims RA, Foulsham BM (1981) Weight reduction in osteoarthritis using phentermine. Practitioner 225:231–232

17. Martin K, Nicklas BJ, Bunyard LB et al. (1996) Weight loss and walking improve symptoms of knee osteoarthritis. Arthritis Rheum 39:S225 (Abstract)

18. Puett DW, Griffin MR (1994) Published trials of nonmedicinal and noninvasive therapies for hip and knee osteoarthritis. Ann Intern Med 121:133–140

19. Ettinger WH Jr, Burns R, Messier SP, Applegate W, Rejeski WJ, Morgan T, Shumaker S, Berry MJ, O'Toole M, Monu J et al. (1997) A randomized trial comparing aerobic exercise and resistance exercise with a health education program in older adults with knee osteoarthritis. The Fitness Arthritis and Seniors Trial (FAST). JAMA 277:25–31

20. Hurley MV, Scott DL, Newman DJ (1997) A clinically practicable rehabilitation regime that improves quadriceps sensorimotor function and reduces disability of patients with knee osteoarthritis. Arthritis Rheum 40:S281 (Abstract)

21. Cushnaghan J, McCarthy C, Dieppe P (1994) Taping the patella medially: a new treatment for osteoarthritis of the knee joint? BMJ 308:753–755

22. Neumann DA (1989) Biomechanical analysis of selected principles of hip joint protection. Arthritis Care Res 2:146–155

23. Sasaki T, Yasuda K (1987) Clinical evaluation of the treatment of osteoarthritic knees using a newly designed wedged insole. Clin Orthop 181–187

24. Barrett DS, Cobb AG, Bentley G (1991) Joint proprioception in normal, osteoarthritic and replaced knees. J Bone Joint Surg (Br) 73:53–56

25. Piletta P, Porchet HC, Dayer P (1991) Distinct central nervous system involvement of paracetamol and salicylate. In: Bond MR, Charlton JE, Woolf CJ (eds) Proceedings of the 5th World Congress on Pain. Elsevier, Amsterdam, pp 181–184

26. Dieppe P, Cushnaghan J, Jasani MK, McCrae F, Watt I (1993) A two-year, placebo-controlled trial of non-steroidal anti-inflammatory therapy in osteoarthritis of the knee joint. Br J Rheumatol 32:595–600

27. March L, Irwig L, Schwarz J, Simpson J, Chock C, Brooks P (1994) N of 1 trials comparing a non-steroidal anti-inflammatory drug with paracetamol in osteoarthritis. BMJ 309:1041–1045

28. Bradley JD, Brandt KD, Katz BP, Kalasinski LA, Ryan SI (1991) Comparison of an antiinflammatory dose of ibuprofen, an analgesic dose of ibuprofen, and acetaminophen in the treatment of patients with osteoarthritis of the knee. N Engl J Med 325:87–91

29. Stamp J, Rhind V, Haslock I (1989) A comparison of nefopam and flurbiprofen in the treatment of osteoarthrosis. Br J Clin Pract 43:24–26

30. Griffin MR (1993) NSAID use in the elderly. Prevalence and problems. In: Baker JR, Brandt KD (eds) Reappraisal of the management of patients with osteoarthritis. Scientific Therapeutic Information, Springfield, NJ, pp 35–37

31. Farrell GC (1986) The hepatic side-effects of drugs. Med J Aust 145:600–604

32. (1996) Acetaminophen, NSAIDs and alcohol. The Medical Letter 38:55–58
33. Kincaid-Smith P (1986) Effects of non-narcotic analgesics on the kidney. Drugs 32 (Suppl) 4:109–128
34. Sandler DP, Smith JC, Weinberg CR, Buckalew VM,Jr., Dennis VW, Blythe WB, Burgess WP (1989) Analgesic use and chronic renal disease. N Engl J Med 320:1238–1243
35. Murray TG, Stolley PD, Anthony JC, Schinnar R, Hepler-Smith E, Jeffreys JL (1983) Epidemiologic study of regular analgesic use and end-stage renal disease. Arch Intern Med 143:1687–1693
36. Perneger TV, Whelton PK, Klag MJ (1994) Risk of kidney failure associated with the use of acetaminophen, aspirin, and nonsteroidal antiinflammatory drugs. N Engl J Med 331: 1675–1679
37. Hylek EM, Heiman H, Skates SJ, Sheehan MA, Singer DE (1998) Acetaminophen and other risk factors for excessive warfarin anticoagulation. JAMA 279:657–662
38. Sunshine A (1994) New clinical experience with tramadol. Drugs 47 (Suppl) 1:8–18
39. Barkin RL (1995) Focus on tramadol: centrally acting analgesic for mild to moderately severe pain. Hospital Formulary 30:321–325
40. Jensen JM, Ginsberg F (1994) Tramadol vs dextropropoxyphene in the treatment of osteoarthritis: short term, double-blind study. Drug Invest 8:211–218
41. Moore RA, Tramer MR, Carroll D, Wiffen PJ, McQuay HJ (1998) Quantitative systematic review of topically applied non-steroidal anti-inflammatory drugs. BMJ 316:333–338
42. Hewitt PG, Poblete N, Wester RC, Maibach HI, Shainhouse JZ (1998) In vitro cutaneous disposition of a topical diclofenac lotion in human skin: effect of a multi-dose regimen. Pharma Res 15:988–992
43. Samuel EP (1952) The autonomic and somatic innervation of the articular capsule. Anat Rec 113:84–93
44. Ralston HJ, Miller MR, Kasahara M (1990) Nerve endings in human fasciae, tendons, ligaments, periosteum and joint synovial membrane. Ann Rheum Dis 49:649–652
45. Kidd BL, Mapp PI, Blake DR, Gibson SJ, Polak JM (1990) Neurogenic influences in arthritis. Ann Rheum Dis 49:649–652
46. Deal CL, Schnitzer TJ, Lipstein E, Seibold JR, Stevens RM, Levy MD, Albert D, Renold F (1991) Treatment of arthritis with topical capsaicin: a double-blind trial. Clin Ther 13:383–395
47. Balch HW, Gibson JM, El-Ghobarey AF, Bain LS, Lynch MP (1977) Repeated corticosteroid injections into knee joints. Rheum Rehabil 16:137–140
48. Dieppe PA, Sathapatayavongs B, Jones HE, Bacon PA, Ring EF (1980) Intra-articular steroids in osteoarthritis. Rheum Rehabil 19:212–217
49. Friedman DM, Moore ME (1980) The efficacy of intraarticular steroids in osteoarthritis: a double-blind study. J Rheumatol 7:850–856
50. Gaffney K, Ledingham J, Perry JD (1995) Intra-articular triamcinolone hexacetonide in knee osteoarthritis: factors influencing the clinical response. Ann Rheum Dis 54:379–381
51. Valtonen EJ (1981) Clinical comparison of triamcinolonehexacetonide and betamethasone in the treatment of osteoarthrosis of the knee-joint. Scand J Rheumatol Suppl 41:1–7
52. Sambrook PN, Champion GD, Browne CD, Cairns D, Cohen ML, Day RO, Graham S, Handel M, Jaworski R, Kempler S (1989) Corticosteroid injection for osteoarthritis of the knee: peripatellar compared to intra-articular route. Clin Exp Rheumatol 7:609–613
53. Cederlof S, Jonson G (1966) Intraarticular prednisolone injection for osteoarthritis of the knee. A double blind test with placebo. Acta Chir Scand 132:532–537
54. Wada J, Koshino T, Morii T, Sugimoto K (1993) Natural course of osteoarthritis of the knee treated with or without intra-articular corticosteroid injections. Bull Hosp Jt Dis 53: 45–48
55. Grecomoro G, Piccione F, Letizia G (1992) Therapeutic synergism between hyaluronic acid and dexamethasone in the intra-articular treatment of osteoarthritis of the knee: a preliminary open study. Curr Med Res Opin 13:49–55
56. Leardini G, Mattara L, Franceschini M, Perbellini A (1991) Intra-articular treatment of knee osteoarthritis. A comparative study between hyaluronic acid and 6-methyl prednisolone acetate. Clin Exp Rheumatol 9:375–381

57. Leardini G, Franceschini M, Mattara L, Bruno R, Perbellini A (1987) Intra-articular so-dium hyaluronate in gonarthrosis. A controlled study comparing methylprednisolone acetate. Clin Trials Journal 24:341–350
58. Pietrogrande V, Melanotte PL, D'Agnolo B, Ulivi M, Benigni GA, Turchetto L, Pierfederici P, Perbellini A (1991) Hyaluronic acid versus methylprednisolone intra-articularly inject-ed for the treatment of osteoarthritis of the knee. Curr Therap Res 50:691–701
59. Adams ME, Atkinson MH, Lussier AJ, Schulz JI, Siminovitch KA, Wade JP, Zummer M (1995) The role of viscosupplementation with hylan G-F 20 (Synvisc) in the treatment of osteoarthritis of the knee: a Canadian multicenter trial comparing hylan G-F 20 alone, hylan G-F 20 with non-steroidal anti-inflammatory drugs (NSAIDs) and NSAIDs alone. Osteoarthritis Cartilage 3:213–225
60. Bragantini A, Cassini M (1987) Controlled single-blind trial of intra-articularly injected hyaluronic acid in osteo-arthritis of the knee. Clin Trials J 24:333–340
61. Dixon AS, Jacoby RK, Berry H, Hamilton EB (1988) Clinical trial of intra-articular injec-tion of sodium hyaluronate in patients with osteoarthritis of the knee. Curr Med Res Opin 11:205–213
62. Dougados M, Nguyen M, Listrat V, Amor B (1993) High molecular weight sodium hyal-uronate (hyalectin) in osteoarthritis of the knee: a 1 year placebo-controlled trial. Osteo-arthritis Cartilage 1:97–103
63. Grecomoro G, Martorana U, Di Marco C (1987) Intra-articular treatment with sodium hyaluronate in gonarthrosis: a controlled clinical trial versus placebo. Pharmatherapeu-tica 5:137–141
64. Henderson EB, Smith EC, Pegley F, Blake DR (1994) Intra-articular injections of 750 kD hy-aluronan in the treatment of osteoarthritis: a randomised single centre double-blind place-bo-controlled trial of 91 patients demonstrating lack of efficacy. Ann Rheum Dis 53:529–534
65. Namiki O, Toyoshima H, Morisaki N (1982) Therapeutic effect of intra-articular injection of high molecular weight hyaluronic acid on osteoarthritis of the knee. Int J Clin Pharm Ther Toxicol 20:501–507
66. Graf J, Neusel E, Schneider E, Niethard FU (1993) Intra-articular treatment with hyal-uronic acid in osteoarthritis of the knee joint: a controlled clinical trial versus mucopoly-saccharide polysulfuric acid ester. Clin Exp Rheumatol 11:367–372
67. Edelson R, Burks RT, Bloebaum RD (1995) Short-term effects of knee washout for osteo-arthritis. Am J Sports Med 23:345–349
68. Dahlberg L, Lohmander LS, Ryd L (1994) Intraarticular injections of hyaluronan in pa-tients with cartilage abnormalities and knee pain: A one-year double-blind, placebo-con-trolled study. Arthritis Rheum 37:521–528
69. Lohmander LS, Dalen N, Englund G, Hamalainen M, Jensen EM, Karlsson K, Odensten M, Ryd L, Sernbo I, Suomalainen O et al. (1996) Intra-articular hyaluronan injections in the treatment of osteoarthritis of the knee: a randomised, double blind, placebo controlled multicentre trial. Hyaluronan Multicentre Trial Group. Ann Rheum Dis 55:424–431
70. Listrat V, Ayral X, Patarnello F, Bonvarlet JP, Simonnet J, Amor B, Dougados M (1997) Arthroscopic evaluation of potential structure modifying activity of hyaluronan (Hyal-gan) in osteoarthritis of the knee. Osteoarthritis Cartilage 5:153–160
71. Scale D, Wobig M, Wolpert W (1994) Viscosupplementation of osteoarthritic knees with hylan: a treatment schedule study. Curr Therap Res 55:220–232
72. Huskisson EC, Scott J (1981) Orgotein in osteoarthritis of the knee joint. Eur J Rheumatol Inflamm 4:212–218
73. McIlwain H, Silverfield JC, Cheatum DE, Poiley J, Taborn J, Ignaczak T, Multz CV (1989) Intra-articular orgotein in osteoarthritis of the knee: a placebo-controlled efficacy, safety, and dosage comparison. Am J Med 87:295–300
74. Gammer W, Broback LG (1984) Clinical comparison of orgotein and methylprednisolone acetate in the treatment of osteoarthrosis of the knee joint. Scand J Rheumatol 13:108–112
75. Mazieres B, Masquelier AM, Capron MH (1991) A French controlled multicenter study of intraarticular orgotein versus intraarticular corticosteroids in the treatment of knee osteoarthritis: a one-year followup. J Rheum Suppl 27:134–137

76. Will R, Laing B, Edelman J, Lovegrove F, Surveyor I (1992) Comparison of two yttrium-90 regimens in inflammatory and osteoarthropathies. Ann Rheum Dis 51:262–265

77. Edmonds J, Smart R, Laurent R, Butler P, Brooks P, Hoschl R, Wiseman J, George S, Lovegrove F, Warwick A (1994) A comparative study of the safety and efficacy of dysprosium-165 hydroxide macro-aggregate and yttrium-90 silicate colloid in radiation synovectomy–a multicentre double blind clinical trial. Australian Dysprosium Trial Group. Br J Rheumatol 33:947–953

78. Wright V, Haslock DI, Dowson D, Seller PC, Reeves B (1971) Evaluation of silicone as an artificial lubricant in osteoarthrotic joints. BMJ 2:370–373

79. Dawes PT, Kirlew C, Haslock I (1987) Saline washout for knee osteoarthritis: results of a controlled study. Clin Rheumatol 6:61–63

80. Ike RW, Arnold WJ, Rothschild EW, Shaw HL (1992) Tidal irrigation versus conservative medical management in patients with osteoarthritis of the knee: a prospective randomized study. Tidal Irrigation Cooperating Group. J Rheumatol 19:772–779

81. Vajaradul Y (1981) Double-blind clinical evaluation of intra-articular glucosamine in outpatients with gonarthrosis. Clin Ther 3:336–343

82. Papathanassiou NP (1994) Intra-articular use of tenoxicam in degenerative osteoarthritis of the knee joint. J Int Med Res 22:332–337

83. Silveri F, Morosini P, Brecciaroli D, Cervini C (1994) Intra-articular injection of somatostatin in knee osteoarthritis: clinical results and IGF-1 serum levels. Int J Pharmac Res 14:79–85

8.1.2
Non-steroidal, Anti-inflammatory Drug Administration in the Treatment of Osteoarthritis

J.T. Dingle

8.1.2.1
Introduction

8.1.2.1.1
Cartilage Structure and Function

It sometimes takes a very long time for radical changes in medical/scientific ideas to be generally recognised and applied to clinical problems. Thus the recognition over 30 years ago [1] that chondrocytes were capable both of degradation and synthesis of the extracellular matrix of articular cartilage was not thought to have significant clinical relevance. It took 20 years before a clinical study showed that osteoarthritic cartilage was capable of repair [2]. For generations, the anatomical textbooks had maintained that cartilage was essentially a non-viable tissue incapable of renewal and repair. Clinicians, however, had for a number of years noted that some cartilages apparently heal spontaneously [3]. Perry et al. [4] reported on 14 patients whom joint recovery was shown radiographically, and Daniellson [5] found that, in 91 patients followed for 10 years, there was an apparent regression of arthritic changes in some of these patients. While there was anecdotal evidence at least that human cartilage was capable of repair even during disease activity, it was not until extensive work on the mechanisms of animal cartilage metabolism had been carried out that attention was paid to human articular tissues. The discovery of intrinsic and exogenous proteolytic enzymes capable of cartilage destruction [6, 7] and the demonstration that the indigenous cells of cartilage were capable of synthesising the principal components of the extracellular matrix led to the concept of a dynamic equilibrium that could be modulated by endogenous and exogenous factors [8].

Articular cartilage is a highly specialised tissue [9, 10] consisting of a two-phase matrix in which the chondrocytes are embedded and which has developed to withstand the compressive and tensile stresses characteristic of weight-bearing joints [11]. The fibrillar collagen provides the tensile strength principally in type II, while minor types VI, IX, X and XI are responsible for various matrix–matrix and cell–matrix interactions. The glycosaminoglycan chains (GAG) form a very high molecular weight complex with hyaluronic acid, which in turn is held within the basket weave of collagen fibres. The ability of the cartilage to withstand the stress imposed upon it is a property of the basket weave architecture of the collagen matrix, which imposes physical limitation on the water uptake by the highly charged GAG. This in turn allows a high swelling pressure to develop, which is very resistant to compressive forces. If the GAG is even partially lost, then the resistance of the cartilage matrix to physical forces is diminished and the articular surface becomes susceptive to mechanical damage. However, this partial loss of GAG can be replaced by the synthetic activity of the indigenous chondrocytes. On the other hand, if significant collagen breakdown occurs, it is unlikely that repair can then be achieved. This is usually the terminal stage of disease activity.

8.1.2.1.2
Cartilage Degeneration and Repair

Cartilage, like all other tissues, is remodelled during growth and development, and this involves both synthesis and degradation. The matrix components themselves have measurable half-lives, the GAG turning over several times more rapidly that the collagens. For the integrity of the cartilage to be maintained throughout life, it is necessary that the continued synthesis of GAG, collagen and hyaluronic acid must equal the amount lost through natural turnover [12]. Thus the synthetic activity of aged cartilage is maintained, and it has been demonstrated that cartilages in patients over 90 years of age still maintain the ability to synthesis GAG at up to half the rate of juvenile cartilage. In pathological situations, increased catabolic activity may not be compensated for by sufficient increased synthetic activity if the chondrocyte metabolism is modulated by the presence of indigenous co-factors or exogenous drugs. In the initial phases of human osteoarthritis (OA), damage to cartilage involves loss of matrix GAG in the areas where the lesions develop; this is followed – often over a long period – by more extensive changes, and extensive fissuring and ulceration develop [13]. Individual chondrocytes in the area of the lesion may also be seen to be synthesising GAG in their pericellular environment. Proliferation of chondrocytes is often seen and may be another attempt at repair. Later, more severe changes occur, including capillary invasion from subchondral bone, calcification and abnormal new bone formation. Once these changes start to take place, it is unlikely that any attempt at increased repair by the individual chondrocytes will lead to restoration of functional activity. For a number of years, it was considered that the increased catabolic activity was the major event leading to articular damage in OA [14]. Extensive work on the mechanisms of animal cartilage degradation both *in vitro* and *in vivo* supported this view and implicated a variety of proteolytic enzymes, including cathepsins and metalloproteinases. It is now thought that catabolic reactions are only a part of the osteoarthritic process and that failure of the synthetic repair activity of the indigenous chondrocytes are of at least equal or perhaps greater importance in the slow development of the osteoarthritic lesion [8].

8.1.2.1.3
Cytokines and Growth Factors

Whilst the cytokine interleukin IL-1 is very catabolic in terms of the breakdown of animal cartilages, on most human cartilage it has been shown that this cytokine has little catabolic activity [15]. However, all human cartilages are extremely sensitive (at sub-nanogram concentrations) to inhibition of matrix synthesis by IL-1 [16], and it seems likely that any agent that controls IL-1 activity might in turn have a significant effect on the development of the disease process. This has led to much research on the factors that may inhibit cytokine synthesis, release or action [17–19]. It has been suggested that in OA the local release of cytokines, and particularly IL-1, may be an episodic [20] process perhaps due to microinflammation or local mechanical trauma (see Fig. 1). The inhibitory action of IL-1 on chondrocyte synthesis may then be important for reducing the natural repair mechanism that can take place. The other important factor in the maintenance of cartilage integrity is the presence of growth hormones, in particular insulin-like growth factor IGF-1 [21]. The activity of this and similar agents is probably of fundamental importance in the maintenance of cartilage matrix equilibrium. The continuous synthesis of both GAG and collagen is dependent on the presence of such agents, but in the presence of very low concentrations of IL-1, this growth factor activity is seen to be suppressed. It is thought that *in vivo* this balance between cytokine and growth factor activity is fundamental in controlling the extracellular matrix equilibrium of human cartilage. If this is the case, it is important to consider the mechanism by which cytokine–growth factor interactions could be controlled by drug intervention. It has been pointed out that it is even more important to ensure that the therapy itself does not add to the problem.

8.1.2.1.4
Non-steroidal Anti-inflammatory Drugs and Chondroprotection

The effect of non-steroidal anti-inflammatory drugs (NSAIDs) on animal cartilage matrix metabolism has been studied by Brandt [22, 23] and others over a number of years, and evidence has accumulated that these agents may interfere with cartilage metabolism [24]. It is only recently that similar studies have been

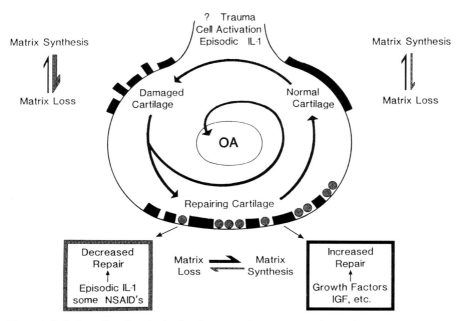

Fig. 1. Spiral of cartilage loss in the development of OA. Suggested episodic changes that may result in the cartilage damage characteristic of the disease. The diagram emphasises the matrix equilibrium between chondrocyte synthesis and chondrocyte degradation of the macromolecules of the extracellular matrix and the role of episodes of cytokine activity and the compensatory effect of growth factors

carried out on human cartilage. This is largely because there is at present no quantitative non-invasive method to determine the anabolic and catabolic reactions of human cartilage *in vivo*. Thus most information on the role of the cytokines, growth factors and NSAIDs has come from short-term organ culture experiments. The present chapter will deal with the use of this technique to study the *in vivo* and *in vitro* treatment of patients' cartilages with drugs, cytokines and growth factors in human non-arthritic and osteoarthritic cartilages. The improved understanding of the factors that control cartilage matrix synthesis and degradation in health and in disease have led us to reconsider the concept of chondroprotection. The earlier work on the enzymes that could degrade cartilage encouraged people to believe that enzyme inhibitors could prevent the disease process. However, claims for compounds that were inhibitors of cartilage damage were never substantiated by clinical trials, and the concept of chondroprotection fell into disrepute [25]. I would suggest now that any compound that promotes the long-term structural integrity of human articular cartilage could be considered to be chondroprotective. Such agents could achieve this not only by inhibiting degradation, but also by modulating synthetic processes that maintain cartilage structure. Thus certain drugs may modify the balance between the activity of cytokines and growth factors to give a chondroprotective function. Investigations of the effect on cartilage metabolism of a variety of NSAIDs have led some weight to this suggestion and will be discussed below.

8.1.2.2
Measurement of Human Cartilage Metabolism

As stated above, at present there is no clinically useful quantitative method for measuring the ability of human cartilage to repair and regenerate itself *in vivo*. Most of the information on the synthesis and turnover of human articular cartilage has come from the development of short-term *in vitro* organ culture methods. Much of the information on the action of growth factors, cytokines and other agents which control chondrocyte metabolism has come from the use of these techniques. They were developed from the original Strangeways Laboratory organ culture methods for embryonic chick cartilages [26]. These were subsequently modified for adult cartilages [7] and standardised some 12 years ago for use on human cartilage [27]. Most experiments have been done on arthritic and non-arthritic cartilages obtained from human femoral heads at operation. More recently, human femoral condyles have been the subject of investigation because an *in vivo* clinical trial using this material is under way to investigate the *in vivo* action of aceclofenac on patients' cartilage metabolism. The difference in metabolism between these two types of tissues will be commented on below.

The use of human cartilages is not simple because of both the variation in anatomical sites and the local nature of many of the pathological lesions. This necessitates the use of extensive numbers of replicates for each patient's cartilage (some 60 – 70 being used from each femoral head, for example) and also for the investigation of relatively large numbers of human patients' cartilages in order to obtain population means. In some studies of individual NSAIDs, for example, a total of 60 patients' cartilages have been investigated. Examples of individual variation have been published for 60 OA patients [28]. Non-arthritic cartilages were usually obtained from patients with fractures of the femoral head and were confirmed as being free from OA by histological examination; the variation in the non-arthritic cartilage population was unusually less than in the OA population. The measurement of GAG synthesis has been described elsewhere [27]; briefly, it involved the uptake of $^{35}SO_4$ under standard conditions (20 h pulse after a 5-day washout period) followed by CPC precipitation of the incorporated material. Collagen was measured in a similar fashion using ^3H-proline. Since the turnover (synthesis) of this collagen is much slower, incorporation times were as long as 16 days, as opposed to 20 h for GAG. The standardised methods for measuring GAG and collagen synthesis have been used on 200 non-arthritic cartilages and over 500 arthritic cartilages over a 12-year period [12]. It must be stressed that these measurements are relative measurements; synthesis of cartilage matrix in these patients can be compared to one another, but changes in the assay conditions would result in quantitative differences. Therefore, standardised incubation conditions using 5% serum in 200 µl DMEM medium with 5% CO_2 in the air at 37 °C were used throughout these studies. Cartilage replicates were full thickness and measured approximately 4×4 mm with a average dry weight of $3-5$ mg.

8.1.2.3
Relative Metabolism of Non-arthritic and Osteoarthritic Cartilages

Table 1 demonstrates the relative GAG synthetic activity of femoral head and condylar cartilage from 200 non-arthritic cartilages and 546 osteoarthritic cartilages. It is immediately apparent that the femoral head cartilage had a lower GAG synthetic activity than that from the femoral condyles, although only a relatively small number of femoral condyle metabolism studies have been carried out to date. Nevertheless, this finding is substantiated by the osteoarthritic cartilages, in which GAG synthesis was higher in the femoral condyle than in the femoral head material. The other significant observation shown in Table 1 is the variation in chondrocyte activity with diseased state. While there is a significant drop between the non-arthritic and the overall osteoarthritic cartilages, those that were most severely affected by the disease process showed the lowest GAG synthetic activity both in the femoral heads and the femoral condyles. This was not due to changes in cellularity. The tissues were graded histologically for this study. Slight OA was characterised as having local areas of erosion and some loss of metachromasia; moderate OA was characterised as having significant fibrillation, loss of metachromasia and evidence of structural damage; and severe OA showed substantial fibrillation and production of clefts and substantial

Table 1. Relative human cartilage matrix synthesis – a comparison of femoral head and condylar metabolism

Tissue	Femoral heads		Femoral condyles	
	Patients (n)[a]	Relative GAG synthesis (cpm/mg $\times 10^{-3}$) (mean ± SEM)	Patients (n)[a]	Relative GAG synthesis (cpm/mg $\times 10^{-3}$) (mean ± SEM)
Non-arthritic	185	3.63 ± 0.30	15	6.02 ± 0.41
Osteoarthritic				
Slight OA	101	2.45 ± 0.15	12	3.76 ± 0.16
Moderate OA	74	2.01 ± 0.14	15	2.39 ± 0.14
Severe OA	66	1.31 ± 0.14	5	1.95 ± 0.1
Total OA	486	1.88 ± 0.38	60	3.73 ± 0.36

GAG synthesis was measured as described in the text. The femoral condyles were shown to be histologically normal, but were obtained at knee replacement operations from patients clinically diagnosed as osteoarthritic. Disease severity in the cartilages from the arthritic patients was graded after histological observations as described in the text. Non-arthritic cartilages were obtained from patients after fracture of the femoral head and confirmed as being free from OA by histological examination. GAG synthesis was measured during a 20-h incubation period on day 6 in culture. Nine to ten replicate organs were set up for each estimation of a patient's cartilage. Results were expressed per milligram dry weight of cartilage.
[a] Number of patients from whom cartilage was obtained.

to complete loss of metachromasia with evidence of cellular cloning. Table 1 demonstrates the problems of both the individual variation and variation with disease state and emphasises the importance of assaying sufficient replicates and sufficient numbers of patients' cartilages when experiments are carried out with *in vitro* drug treatment.

The problem with inter-patient variation is also shown in Table 2, where patients who were not treated with NSAIDs before the operation were assayed for

Table 2. *Ex vivo* femoral head GAG synthesis of individual untreated OA patients

CRL no.	Age (years)	Sex	Diagnosis	Disease severity	GAG synthesis (cpm/mg × 10⁻³/20 h) (mean ± SEM)	
					Ex vivo	Post-incubation (3 days)
Np2/1	71	F	OA	3	0.92 ± 0.14	0.77 ± 0.13 [a]
2x/2	72	F	OA	2	2.06 ± 0.32	2.03 ± 0.23 [a]
9/4	64	F	OA	3	1.74 ± 0.2	1.82 ± 0.3 [a]
8/3	87	F	N? OA	3	0.65 ± 0.07	0.30 ± 0.04 [a]
2x/7	78?	M	RA	3	1.48 ± 0.29	1.63 ± 0.71 [a]
2x/8	81	F	OA	2	2.32 ± 0.45	2.18 ± 0.46 [a]
2x/9	72	F	OA	2	3.02 ± 0.56	3.46 ± 0.40 [a]
6x/7	67	F	OA	3	0.43 ± 0.08	1.50 ± 0.03 [b]
6x/10	72	M	OA	3	0.87 ± 0.15	1.28 ± 0.24 [a]
6x/12	75	F	OA	2	1.67 ± 0.12	2.84 ± 0.21 [d]
90/5	74	M	OA	3	0.84 ± 0.22	0.54 ± 0.2 [a]
7B/2	68	F	OA	3	1.94 ± 0.12	2.27 ± 0.22 [a]
5/16	82	F	N? OA	3	0.67 ± 0.13	0.34 ± 0.10 [a]
GP1	71	M	N? OA	3	1.35 ± 0.15	1.24 ± 0.11 [a]
GP3	75	F	OA	3	1.53 ± 0.14	1.10 ± 0.17 [a]
GP4	77	F	OA	1	2.17 ± 0.14	2.84 ± 0.23 [b]
HH1	70	F	OA	2	2.21 ± 0.11	2.01 ± 0.17 [a]
HH6	71	F	OA	2	2.48 ± 0.17	2.59 ± 0.22 [a]
HH9	64	M	OA	3	1.62 ± 0.08	2.00 ± 0.14 [a]
AD4	68	M	OA	2	1.97 ± 0.09	2.21 ± 0.09 [a]
C11	72	F	OA	2	2.11 ± 0.17	2.00 ± 0.11 [a]
C15	69	F	OA	3	2.08 ± 0.11	1.78 ± 0.13 [a]
L4	62	F	OA	3	1.69 ± 0.09	1.99 ± 0.14 [a]
L15	68	F	OA	2	2.48 ± 0.18	2.92 ± 0.22 [a]
L19	71	F	OA	1	2.56 ± 0.22	2.81 ± 0.24 [a]

The femoral heads were obtained at operation from 25 patients who were known not to have been treated with NSAIDs prior to operation. GAG synthesis was modified in these *ex vivo* experiments. The cartilage was assayed at two periods. Ten replicates from each cartilage were assayed immediately on transfer of the femoral head to the laboratory; they were incubated for 20 h with 5 µCi³⁵SO₄, and GAG synthesis incorporation was measured in the usual way. A further ten replicates from the same femoral head were incubated in DMEM+5% serum for 3 days as a washout procedure to remove any contaminating NSAID or other drugs. The cartilages were then pulsed in the same manner for 20 h and the data shown as post-incubation data. Disease severity was characterised as described in the text. The significance of difference between the *ex vivo* and the post-incubation assay was tested by Student's *t* test.
[a] not significant; [b] $p < 0.02$; [c] $p < 0.01$; [d] $p < 0.001$.

GAG synthetic activity. The *ex vivo* activity measured immediately on the tissue being taken to the laboratory varied between 0.43 and 3.02 cpm/mg per day $\times 10^{-3}$. Table 2 also shows the effect of incubating the paired tissue samples from each individual patient for 3 days as a washout procedure to remove any drug that was present. In these untreated OA patients, it will be seen that there was little difference between the post-incubated and the *ex vivo* assayed material, with only two out of 25 showing a significant difference. The population mean showed no significant difference. This technique was also used as an internal control on OA patients that had been treated *in vivo* with a variety of NSAIDs (see below).

8.1.2.4
Effect of In Vitro NSAID Treatment on GAG Synthetic Activity

The *in vitro* assessment of NSAID action on some 300 patients' femoral head cartilage GAG synthesis is shown in Fig. 2, where a variety of NSAIDs have been used at concentrations expected to occur in the plasma during treatment. In these experiments, the cartilage from each patient was incubated for 5 days in control or NSAID-containing medium and then pulsed with $^{35}SO_4$ for 20 h. The effect of NSAIDs on GAG synthesis is expressed as a percentage of the untreated control cartilage from each patients. It will be seen that the NSAIDs can be divided into three groups:

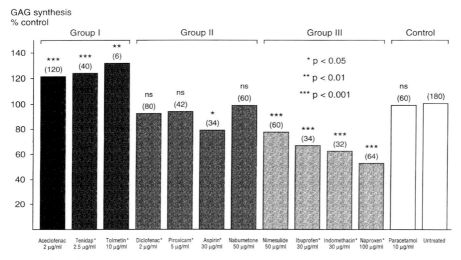

Fig. 2. Effect of NSAID on OA cartilage GAG synthesis. The data shown were collected over a 12-year period and represent relative GAG synthetic activity of human cartilage from some 250 individual patients. The data is expressed as the percentage of the untreated control in each individual patient. GAG synthesis was measured by incorporation of $^{35}SO_4$ into CPC precipital material as expressed on a dry-weight basis under standardised conditions. The number of patients' cartilages are shown in brackets. The statistical significance was derived from Students' *t* test. The results are the mean of the population for each NSAID treatment. These treatments were carried out *in vitro* over a 6-day period as described in the text

1. Those which are highly inhibitory, which include nimezulide, ibuprofen, indomethacin and naproxen, all of which depress GAG synthesis in a statistically highly significant manner.
2. Those such as diclofenac, piroxicam, aspirin and nabumetone, which at the concentrations shown were without major effect on the population mean. Diclofenac at the peak plasma level of 10 µg/ml, although not shown in Fig. 2, is significantly inhibitory.
3. A third group which were stimulatory include aceclofenac, tenidap and tolmetin.

Paracetamol was without effect on the population tested. An indication of the response of individual patients' cartilages to the NSAIDs is shown in Fig. 3, where, over the concentration range tested, the percentage of the patients' cartilages showing a significant increase and decrease from the control is indicated. It will be seen that, with aceclofenac, a large majority of the patients tested showed a significant increase and only a very small number showed any inhibitory effect. Tenidap, on the other hand, which was stimulatory at low levels and has been demonstrated to be inhibitory at high levels, showed at this range of concentrations approximately as many being inhibited as being stimulated. The same effect was seen with nabumetone. Aspirin and diclofenac, in this population, showed more cartilages to be inhibited than stimulated. Indomethacin, ibuprofen and naproxen were not stimulatory to any patients' cartilages. With naproxen, as much as 70% of the total population showed statistically significant inhibition of GAG synthetic activity.

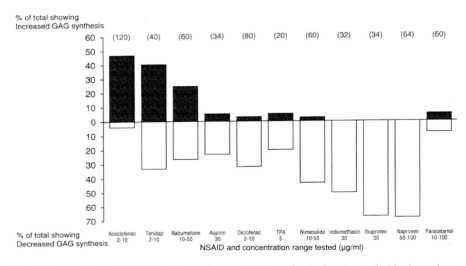

Fig. 3. Comparison of NSAID action on human GAG synthesis showing individual numbers of patients responding. GAG synthesis was measured under the same conditions as Fig. 1. The data is expressed as a percentage of those patients showing a significant ($p < 0.01$) increase or decrease in GAG synthesis in the population undergoing the specific NSAID treatment. The concentration range of NSAIDs tested are shown. Figures in *brackets* indicate the number of patients' cartilages tested. *TPA*, tiaprofenic acid

It was shown in Table 1 that synthetic activity of the cartilage from the femoral head and from the femoral condyles depended on the disease state. Figure 4 again shows this change of synthetic activity in 60 patients' femoral head cartilages. It also shows the effect of treatment with various doses of aceclofenac. The moderate to slightly osteoarthritic cartilages showed significant stimulation between 0.5 and 2 µg/ml. There was less stimulation with the severely arthritic cartilages, though this was significant. However, the non-arthritic cartilages showed no evidence of stimulation with aceclofenac. The effect of aceclofenac dosage on 14 individual OA patients' femoral condyle GAG synthetic activity is shown is Fig. 5. It will be seen that ten out of the 14 individuals showed a significant increase in GAG synthetic activity with increasing dosage of aceclofenac, one showed a slight decrease and three others did not show any significant change; however, these latter all had a low GAG synthetic activity, suggesting a severely arthritic disease state. Femoral condyle cartilage was also used in the studies shown in Fig. 6 from the same 14 individual patients. It may be noted that naproxen at 50 µg/ml was highly significantly inhibitory on all the patients' cartilages tested. This demonstration of three apparent groups of NSAIDs having different effects on matrix synthesis has been confirmed by studies of collagen synthesis using aceclofenac, diclofenac and naproxen as ex-

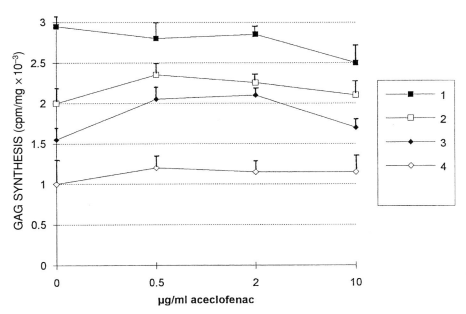

Fig. 4. Effect of aceclofenac on femoral head cartilages of varying disease states from 60 patients. GAG synthesis was measured in the conventional way, but the patients' cartilages were assessed histologically for the disease state. The grading is described in the text: 1, non-arthritic cartilages showing no obvious signs of osteoarthritic changes; 2, slight OA; 3, cartilages showing moderate osteoarthritic changes; 4, severely arthritic cartilages. Aceclofenac was added in concentrations between 0.5 and 10 µg/ml, 7.0 µg/ml being the peak value seen in plasma during treatment

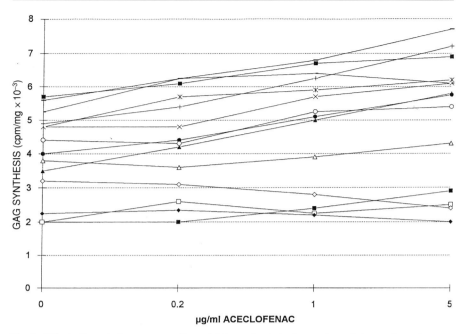

Fig. 5. Effect of aceclofenac on cartilage GAG synthesis in femoral condyle cartilage from 14 OA patients. The effect of between 0.2 and 5 µg aceclofenac/ml on the individual GAG synthesis in 14 patients is demonstrated. GAG synthesis is measured in the way set out in Fig. 1. The cartilage was moderately to severely arthritic

amples of these three groups. Aceclofenac again was stimulatory and naproxen highly inhibitory on collagen synthesis.

8.1.2.5
Effect of In Vivo Treatment with NSAIDs on Human Cartilage

Individual values of cartilage synthesis after *in vivo* treatment are shown in Table 3, and population means are shown in Table 4. It can be seen that the *ex vivo* assay for all NSAIDs of 1.12 cpm/mg × 10^{-3} was significantly lower than the *ex vivo* assay for the untreated OA patients (1.71 cpm/mg × 10^{-3}). Ibuprofen, indomethacin, diclofenac and naproxen were the agents used to treat the patients *in vivo* before the operation. Treatment for 7–10 days prior to operation was usual, and conventional levels of drug were employed. This was not a clinical study as such; the patients were selected from those who came to operation who had a known treatment regime. It can be seen that all those treated with NSAIDs showed a relatively low *ex vivo* synthesis, which doubled after washout incubation. The untreated patients' cartilages showed no significant increase. Also included in Table 4 are a small number of femoral condyle cartilages from 11 patients who had no NSAID treatment, and again it will be seen there was no

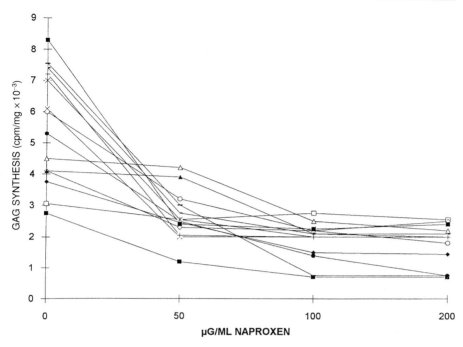

Fig. 6. Effect of naproxen on GAG synthesis on condyle cartilage from 14 patients. GAG synthesis was measured in the conventional manner, and the tissues were treated with between 50 and 200 µg naproxen/ml. The synthetic activity of the individual patients was seen

change in the level of GAG synthesis after the post-incubation washout period, suggesting that these cartilages were not inhibited by NSAID action. This work provides preliminary evidence that there is an effect of some NSAIDs on GAG synthetic activity when the patients have been treated *in vivo* prior to operation.

A comparison of *in vivo* and *in vitro* studies is shown in Table 5, in which aceclofenac is compared with indomethacin. *In vivo*, a total of nine patients were treated with aceclofenac prior to operation, and the GAG synthesis activity was 115% of the control value. In contrast, those treated with indomethacin showed 55% of the control value. *In vitro*, extensive studies have been carried out on both these agents. A total of 120 patients' cartilages were treated with aceclofenac at 2 µg/ml. A significant stimulation of GAG synthesis activity of 22% over the control was seen. Indomethacin again showed significant inhibition in 32 patients' cartilages tested. It is interesting to compare this with radiological studies that have been carried out in the LINK study with indomethacin, where 47% of patients showed deterioration of joint space on indomethacin treatment as compared with 22% on placebo, suggesting that our *in vitro* and *in vivo* results with indomethacin are comparable.

Table 3. *Ex vivo* femoral head cartilage GAG synthesis

CRL no.	Age (years)	Sex	Diagnosis	Disease severity	NSAIDs *in vivo*	GAG synthesis (cpm/mg × 10^{-3}/20 h) (mean ± SEM)	
						Ex vivo	Post-incubation (3 days)
21	80	M	OA	3	Indomethacin	1.12 ± 0.04	3.53 ± 0.25[c]
25	66	M	OA	1	Ketoprofen	2.70 ± 0.26	4.89 ± 0.37[c]
9/1	76	M	OA	2	Ibuprofen	1.89 ± 0.56	2.08 ± 0.25[a]
7/5	58	F	OA	3	Ibuprofen	0.81 ± 0.16	1.79 ± 0.16[c]
7/6	68	F	OA	3	Ibuprofen	0.86 ± 0.2	2.19 ± 0.3[c]
6x/1	60	M	OA	3	Aspirin	0.48 ± 0.1	1.95 ± 0.31[d]
6x/2	77	F	OA	2	Diclofenac	0.28 ± 1.06	2.60 ± 0.28[d]
6x/4	75	M	OA	3	Aspirin	0.71 ± 0.11	1.63 ± 0.13[d]
6x/5	67	F	OA	3	Ibuprofen	1.260 ± 0.16	1.20 ± 0.14[a]
6x/9	81	F	OA	2	Ibuprofen	1.03 ± 0.21	3.18 ± 0.29[d]
7B/3	75	F	OA	3	Diclofenac	0.53 ± 0.18	1.30 ± 0.15[d]
5/19	70	F	OA	3	Naproxen	0.51 ± 0.16	1.06 ± 0.13[b]
GP2	77	F	OA	3	Diclofenac	0.28 ± 0.06	0.90 ± 0.13[d]
7B/10	57	F	OA	3	Ibuprofen	0.66 ± 0.08	1.48 ± 0.04[b]
3R	66	F	OA	1	Indomethacin	1.70 ± 0.2	3.93 ± 0.09[c]
90/5	70	F	OA	2	Indomethacin	1.17 ± 0.4	1.79 ± 0.08[b]
91/1	70	M	OA	2	Indomethacin	1.60 ± 0.03	2.28 ± 0.31[c]
VV7	67	M	OA	3	Naproxen	0.87 ± 0.09	1.63 ± 0.12[c]
VV19	71	F	OA	3	Naproxen	1.46 ± 0.09	1.91 ± 0.11[a]
VV25	59	F	OA	3	Naproxen	0.46 ± 0.02	0.99 ± 0.05[b]
B21	70	F	OA	2	Naproxen	0.84 ± 0.04	1.82 ± 0.08[c]
P1	62	M	OA	3	Ibuprofen	1.22 ± 0.21	1.84 ± 0.20[b]
P3	68	M	OA	3	Ibuprofen	1.18 ± 0.31	2.46 ± 0.23[d]
P6	72	F	OA	3	Indomethacin	1.56 ± 0.20	2.51 ± 0.28[c]
A12	69	F	OA	2	Naproxen	1.63 ± 0.21	3.01 ± 0.27[d]
A13	71	F	OA	3	Naproxen	0.84 ± 0.09	1.41 ± 0.33[a]
A16	75	M	OA	2	Indomethacin	1.27 ± 0.21	2.87 ± 0.29[d]
A21	82	F	OA	2	Indomethacin	1.66 ± 0.19	3.16 ± 0.22[d]
A24	68	F	OA	2	Indomethacin	1.20 ± 0.14	1.83 ± 0.10[c]
P19	71	M	OA	2	Indomethacin	1.74 ± 0.21	1.96 ± 0.22[a]
H41	61	M	OA	3	Naproxen	0.76 ± 0.09	1.84 ± 0.20[c]
H44	67	F	OA	2	Naproxen	1.64 ± 0.15	2.09 ± 0.22[a]

Patients who had been treated with NSAIDs for 1–2 weeks prior to operation were selected. A total of 32 such patients were assayed, of whom eight had been treated with ibuprofen, nine with indomethacin, two with aspirin, four with diclofenac and nine with naproxen. The indomethacin dose was between 50 and 100 mg/day, the ibuprofen dose was between 1000 and 1500 mg/day, the diclofenac dose was between 100 and 150 mg/day and the naproxen dosage was between 500 and 750 mg/d. The *ex vivo* and the post-incubation GAG synthesis was measured as described in Table 2. The disease severity is indicated and was measured as described in the text.
[a] not significant; [b] $p < 0.02$; [c] $p < 0.01$; [d] $p < 0.001$.

Table 4. *Ex vivo* femoral cartilage GAG synthesis

Drug treatment	Patients (n)	GAG synthesis (cpm/mg $\times 10^{-3}$)	
		Ex vivo (mean ± SEM)	Post-incubation (3 days) (mean ± SEM)
Ibuprofen	8	1.11 ± 0.13	2.62 ± 0.22[a]
Indomethacin	9	1.45 ± 0.08	2.65 ± 0.26[a]
Aspirin	2	1.14 ± 0.16	2.17 ± 0.31
Diclofenac	4	0.55 ± 0.19	1.51 ± 0.37
Naproxen	9	1.00 ± 0.15	1.75 ± 0.20[b]
All NSAIDs	32	1.12 ± 0.10	2.15 ± 0.10[b]
No NSAID	25	1.71 ± 0.14	1.86 ± 0.17[c]
No NSAID (FC)	11	2.20 ± 0.28	2.31 ± 0.30[c]
Population mean	245	–	1.76 ± 0.4

Population summary of *in vivo* NSAID treatment of OA patients, summarising the individual data shown in Tables 2 and 3. The significant difference between the *ex vivo* and the post-incubation GAG synthetic activity was tested by Student's *t* test. Also included are 11 femoral condyle cartilages for comparison (FC).

[a] $p < 0.01$; [b] $p < 0.001$; [c] not significant.

Table 5. Comparison of *in vitro* and *in vivo* studies on aceclofenac and indomethacin in OA patients

Study type	Aceclofenac		Indomethacin	
	GAG synthesis (% of untreated control)	Patients (n)	GAG synthesis (% of untreated control)	Patients (n)
In vivo treatment (*ex vivo* assay)	115[b]	9	55[b]	9
In vitro assay	122[b]	120	63[c]	32
Clinical assessment	22% deterioration on placebo[a]		47% deterioration on on indomethacin[a,c]	

In the first study type, (*in vivo* treatment, *ex vivo* assay), aceclofenac was administered to patients at 100 mg/day before the operation and indomethacin at 50–100 mg/day. The *ex vivo* assays and the post-incubation assays were carried out as described in Table 2. The *in vitro* figures summarise the data shown previously; aceclofenac was administered at 2 µg/ml and indomethacin at 30 µg/ml.

[a] Radiological progression data obtained from the LINK study.

[b] $p < 0.01$; [c] $p < 0.001$ (difference from control).

8.1.2.6
Interaction of Cytokines and Growth Factors on Human Cartilage Metabolism

It was shown several years ago that human cartilage GAG and collagen synthesis is very sensitive to very low levels of the cytokine IL-1 [16, 29]. Cytokine inhibition of GAG synthesis occurred at levels below 0.1 ng/ml (concentrations exceeded in arthritic synovial fluid). Such low concentrations have no effect on the GAG turnover rate in human cartilage. It has also been known for some time that human cartilage is sensitive to growth factor stimulation of GAG synthetic activity, and it is thought that the balance of these two agents is fundamental in the maintenance of the equilibrium between synthesis and degeneration and thus of matrix structure and function. The continued synthesis of both GAG and collagen is probably dependent on the presence of several growth factors, of which IGF-1 is the best studied. Though no experiments have been carried out on human material, it seems likely that hyaluronic acid might also respond to such factors. In considering the action of NSAIDs in this system, the inhibitory effects of agents such as naproxen are readily explicable in terms of cytotoxic effects on chondrocyte metabolism. What is much more difficult to explain, however, is the apparent stimulatory action of agents such as aceclofenac, tenidap and tolmetin. The key to understanding these events was the observation that there was no stimulatory action of aceclofenac on arthritic cartilages in the absence of serum and that the serum could be replaced by the growth factor IGF-1 [29]. A further important fact was that aceclofenac did not stimulate non-arthritic human cartilage, GAG or collagen synthesis. Consideration of these facts has led to a hypothesis for the mode of action of aceclofenac:

1. Human cartilage matrix is continually synthesised and degraded throughout life by indigenous chondrocytes. This equilibrium is controlled by the presence of cytokines and growth factors and may be disturbed in disease, resulting in loss of articular cartilage.
2. Aceclofenac has been shown by Gonzales et al. [30] to reduce IL-1 and tumour necrosis factor (TNF) levels in arthritic patients where cytokine levels were high.
3. In human arthritic cartilage, the cytokine IL-1 prevents the expression of growth factor activity. The resulting inhibition of matrix synthesis is a major component of the slow development of articular damage in OA. In the presence of growth factors, aceclofenac increases GAG and collagen synthesis by partially reversing the action of IL-1.
4. In non-arthritic human cartilage, cytokine activity was thought to be minimal, and the presence of growth factors results in high matrix synthesis activity and hence the continual renewal and repair of articular cartilage. In these cartilages, aceclofenac has been shown not to stimulate matrix synthesis.
5. Unlike a number of NSAIDs, aceclofenac at peak plasma concentrations did not inhibit matrix synthesis in non-arthritic or arthritic cartilages and thus allowed the expression of growth factor activity. The low chondrocyte toxi-

city of aceclofenac would appear to distinguish it from some other NSAIDs, many of which inhibit cartilage matrix synthesis and hence diminish repair.

6. In summary, aceclofenac is not itself a growth factor but allows the natural repair process to continue in the presence of arthritic disease. It does not affect non-arthritic cartilage and would appear to be advantageous for the long-term treatment of damage to articular tissues.

8.1.2.7
Conclusion

It has been suggested that OA development is due, at least in part, to episodes of IL-1 activity. While the experiments reported above are very short-term, it is possible that similar events occur *in vivo*; thus the extent of the recovery after an episode of cytokine activity may be diminished by some NSAIDs. Naproxen and diclofenac, for example, inhibit recovery after an episode of exogenous IL-1. The toxicity of diclofenac may be due to the presence of a 5-OH metabolite which is not produced from aceclofenac [29]. One must of course exercise considerable caution in extrapolating from *in vitro* experiments to the *in vivo* situations, although the limited number of *in vivo* treatments of patients' cartilages followed by *ex vivo* assays tend to confirm *in vitro* work.

There is also evidence from studies on patients treated with indomethacin by Raschad et al. [31] and Huskinson et al. [32] that suggest that this NSAID has a deleterious effect on cartilage. The finding is compatible with the present *in vitro* and *in vivo* studies. It is possible to suggest that modification of the cytokine–growth factor interactions in arthritic cartilage (but not in non-arthritic cartilage), which has been demonstrated in the short-term organ culture experiments, may also occur *in vivo* during treatment with agents such as aceclofenac and *in vivo* could lead to stimulation of matrix synthesis and possible repair. This hypothesis needs to be tested *in vivo*, and further studies are under way to investigate the action of aceclofenac and a comparable NSAID on human cartilage treated *in vivo* followed by *ex vivo* assay of the cartilage metabolism similar to those preliminary experiments shown in work above. Thus, if *in vitro* work is confirmed by *in vivo* studies, this suggests that, when specific therapy for reducing pain and inflammation in osteoarthritic cartilage is considered, the effect of these same treatment schedules on the underlying integrity of the joint cartilage should also be considered. The concept of chondroprotection in these terms would be the use of agents which at the very least did not increase the joint damage in the arthritic patient and at best reinstated the natural repair mechanisms that these tissues appear to have and which appear to be suppressed during the more acute phases of the arthritic condition.

Acknowledgements. I should like to thank most sincerely Mrs. Dawn Ward and Mrs. Eileen Lean for many years of high-quality technical assistance. Support for these studies over a 12-year period was provided by the MRC, ARC, Nuffield, Strangeways Laboratory, CARE, Sybil Eastwood Trust, Pfeizer, Ciba-Geigy, Almirall-Prodesfarma and Searle.

References

1. Dingle JT (1966) The role of lysosomes in connective tissue disease. In: Hill AG (ed): Modern trends in rheumatology, London, Butterworth, p 110–120
2. Nakata K, Bullough PG (1986) The injury and repair of human articular cartilage: a morphological study of 192 cases of osteoarthritis, J Jpn Orthop Assoc 60:763–775
3. Dieppe P (1988) Osteoarthritis; the scale and scope of the clinical problem. In: Dieppe P(ed): Osteoarthritis: current research and prospectus for pharmacological intervention, London, IPC Technical Services, p 1–6
4. Perry GH, Smith MJG, Whiteside CG (1972) Spontaneous recovery of the joint space in degenerative hip disease. Ann Rheum Dis 31:440–448
5. Danielsson LG (1964) Instance and prognosis of coxarthrosis. Acta Orthop Scand; Suppl 66:1–114
6. Barrett AJ, Saklatvala J (1985) Proteinases in joint disease. In: Kelly WN, Harris ED, Ruddy S, Sledge CB (eds) Textbook of rheumatology, 2nd edn, Philadelphia, WB Saunders, pp 182–196
7. Dingle JT (1979) Recent studies in the control of joint damage. Ann Rheum Dis: 38:201–214
8. Dingle JT (1991) Cartilage maintenance in osteoarthritis: interactions of cytokines, NSAID and prostaglandins in articular cartilage damage and repair. J Rheum 18 Suppl. 28:30–37
9. Muir H, Hardingham TE (1986) Cartilage matrix biochemistry. In: Scott JT (ed) Copeman's textbook of the rheumatic diseases 1, Edinburgh, Churchill-Livingston, pp 177–198
10. Hardingham TE, Fosang AJ, Dudhia J (1994) The structure, function and turnover of aggrecan, the large aggregating proteoglycan from cartilage. Aur J Clin Chem Clin Biochem 32:249–257
11. Kempson G (1980) The mechanical properties of articular cartilage. In: Sokoloff L (ed) The joints in synovial fluid 2. Academic, New York: 177–238
12. Dingle JT, Parker M (1997) Chondroprotection and the role of NSAID: a study of human cartilage metabolism. Brazil J Rheum 37:37–46
13. Hamerman D (1989) The biology of osteoarthritis. N Engl J Med 320:1322–1330
14. Dingle JT (1984) The effect of synovial catabolin on cartilage synthetic activity. Connect Tissue Res 12:277–286
15. Dingle JT (1981) Catabolin – a cartilage catabolic factor from synovium. Clin Orthop 156: 219–231
16. Dingle JT, Horner A, Shield M (1991) The sensitivity of synthesis of human cartilage matrix to inhibition by IL-1 suggests a mechanism for the development of osteoarthritis. Cell Biochem Function 9:99–102
17. Pelletier JP and Martel-Pelletier J (1989) Evidence for involvement of IL-1 in OA cartilage degradation: Protective effect of NSAID. J Rheumatol 16 [Suppl 18]:19–27
18. Shield MJ (1992) Misoprostol: new frontiers: benefits beyond the gastrointestinal tract. Scand J Rheumatol Suppl 92:31–52
19. Dingle JT (1990) Cartilage damage and repair: the roles of IL-1, NSAIDs and prostaglandins in osteoarthritis. In: New frontiers in prostaglandin therapeutics. Excerpa Medica, Princetown, USA, pp 1–15
20. Dingle JT (1993) Prostaglandins in human cartilage metabolism. J Lipid Mediators 6: 303–312
21. Tyler JA (1989) Insulin-like growth factor 1 can decrease degradation and promote synthesis of proteoglycan in cartilage exposed to cytokines. Biochem J 260:543–548
22. Brandt KD (1987) Effects of nonsteroidal anti-inflammatory drugs on chondrocyte metabolism, in vitro and in vivo. Am J Med 83 [Supp 5 A]: 29–34
23. Dingle JT (1996) The effect of NSAIDs in human articular cartilage GAG synthesis. Eur J Rheumatol Inflamm 16:47–52
24. Pelletier JP, Cloutier JM, Martel-Pelletier J (1989) In vitro effect of tiaprofenic acid, sodium salicylate and hydrocortisone on the proteoglycan metabolism of human osteoarthritic cartilage. J Rheumatol 165:646–655

25. Dieppe JT (1993) Drug treatment of osteoarthritis. J Bone Joint Surg [Br] 75:673–674
26. Fell MB, Mellanby EM (1952) The effect of hypervitaminosis-A on embryonic limb bones cultured *in vitro*. J Physical 116:320–349
27. Dingle JT (1992) The use of cytokines and NSAIDs in osteoarthritis: the use of human cartilage in drug assessment. Eur J Rheumatol Inflamm 12:3–8
28. Dingle JT, Parker M (1997) NSAID stimulation of human cartilage matrix synthesis. A study of the mechanism of action of aceclofenac. Clin Drug Invest 14 (5):353–362
29. Dingle JT, Parker M (1997) NSAID stimulation of human cartilage matrix synthesis. Clin Drug Insert 14(5):353–362
30. Gonzales E, De La Cruz C, de Nicolas R et al. (1994) Long term effects of NSAID on the production of cytokines and other inflammatory mediators by blood cells of patients with OA. Agents Actions 41:171–178
31. Rashad S, Revell P, Hemingway A et al. (1989) Effect of non-steroid anti-inflammatory drugs on the course of osteoarthritis. Lancet, II: 519–522
32. Huskinsson EC, Berry H, Gishen P et al. (1995) On behalf of the LINK study group. Effects of anti-inflammatory drugs on the progression of osteoarthritis of the knee. J Rheumatol 22:1941–1946

8.1.3
New and Future Therapies for Osteoarthritis

J.P. Pelletier, B. Haraoui and J.C. Fernandes

8.1.3.1
Introduction

Over the last decade, there have been several interesting advances in the treatment of osteoarthritis (OA), resulting in renewed interest in this field of medicine. Recent progress in the understanding of the pathophysiology of OA has facilitated the development of new drugs and treatments specifically aimed at effectively retarding the disease process. This chapter presents several new agents that have been introduced for the symptomatic treatment of OA. These medications have different mechanisms of action, some of which are not yet fully understood. Clinical studies are currently underway for some of those drugs to determine if they can exert structure–modifying effects to counteract the disease process. This chapter also reviews major fields of investigation that we believe hold promise for the near future.

8.1.3.2
Pharmacological Approach

During the past few years, several investigators and task forces under the leadership of the OARS have classified the drugs used in the treatment of OA into two categories – "symptomatic" and "structure–modifying". The first category of drugs is efficacious in alleviating pain, swelling and stiffness, as well as improving the function of the OA joints, while the latter aims at slowing, stopping or even reversing the structural changes of the disease. These structure–modifying drugs may also have some symptom–relieving properties. Several new compounds are currently being tested for either or both properties, while some "older" drugs are under evaluation for their potential to alter the degenerative process.

A better understanding of the mechanisms of joint damage and repair has led to the development of a new class of molecules that inhibits one or several of the soluble mediators of inflammation, or proteolytic enzymes.

8.1.3.2.1
Systemic Treatment

Diacerhein

Diacerhein, or diacethylrhein, is an anthraquinone derivative that displays several *in vitro* and *in vivo* properties. It inhibits *in vitro* the production of IL-1, and reduces that of metalloproteases (MMP) in human OA cartilage [1]. On the other hand, it stimulates the synthesis of proteoglycan, glycosaminoglycan and hyaluronic acid [2]. In an animal model of OA, *in vivo* diacerhein effectively reduced synovial inflammation and cartilage lesions [3]. Interestingly it does not suppress prostaglandin synthesis.

In human hip OA, diacerhein (50 mg oral BID) was tested alone or in combination with tenoxicam (20 mg QD) over eight weeks [4]. In this double-blind randomized trial, diacerhein was as effective as tenoxicam alone and the combination proved superior. Diacerhein had a slower onset of action, starting two weeks after the initiation of therapy. In another study, diacerhein was compared to naproxen (375 mg BID) in patients with knee and hip OA over a two month period [5]. Diacerhein was as effective as naproxen, however it had a statistically significant carryover effect 30 days after discontinuing treatment. Ongoing studies are being conducted to test the structure–modifying properties of diacerhein.

Avocado/Soybean Unsaponifiables

Avocado/soybean unsaponifiables (ASU) are made of the unsaponifiable extracts of avocado and soybean, in a proportion of one third and two thirds, respectively. ASU was shown to have *in vitro* inhibitory properties against IL-1, and can stimulate collagen synthesis by articular chondrocytes in culture [6]. It has been effective at inhibiting IL-1–induced production of stromelysin, IL-6, IL-8, PGE_2 and collagenase [7].

The clinical efficacy of ASU has been demonstrated in two double-blind placebo–controlled studies for the treatment of knee and hip OA [8, 9]. In a six month treatment period, followed by two months of observation for the carryover effect, ASU was statistically superior to the placebo for the VAS for pain, the Lequesne functional index score, the patient satisfaction scale and the consumption of nonsteroidal anti-inflammatory drugs (NSAID) [8].

Glucosamine Sulphate

As a component of the articular cartilage, glucosamine sulphate (GS) was studied as a possible repair molecule more than 20 years ago. *In vitro* experiments have shown that GS added to chondrocyte cultures stimulates proteoglycan synthesis [10]. Earlier clinical observations were either short term, did not involve large numbers of patients, or were open–label trials. Most revealed a trend towards better symptomatic relief. Lately, in a double–blind randomized trial in knee OA, GS at 500 mg TID was as effective as 400 mg TID of ibuprofen over a period of four weeks [11]. In a similarly designed study, GS was marginally superior to the placebo [12]. GS was also given intramuscularly in a six week double-blind placebo-controlled randomized trial to patients with knee OA [13], where it was shown to be superior to the placebo. To date, studies have addressed only the short term relief obtained with GS, and long term studies dealing with sustained symptomatic relief and structure–modifying properties are needed. Due to its short half–life, some investigators suggest the use of a polymeric form of glucosamine to reduce the frequency of administration [14].

Chondroitin Sulphate

Aside from some *in vitro* stimulatory activity on proteoglycan and collagen synthesis by chondrocytes, chondroitin sulphate (CS) is effective in alleviating the symptoms of knee and hip OA, and in improving joint function [15–17]. In a recent three month double-blind randomized trial versus diclofenac (first four weeks, followed by placebo for two months), CS at a dose of 400 mg TID was shown to be slightly less effective than diclofenac due to its slower onset of action, but superior to the placebo and had a carry-over effect that lasted the duration of the six month study [18].

Hydroxychloroquine, Methotrexate

Due to its efficacy in rheumatoid arthritis (RA), hydroxychloroquine has been used anecdotally in inflammatory erosive OA of the hands. In a retrospective clinical observation, 6 out of 8 treated patients improved [19]. Despite being a retrospective chart review study with a small number of patients, this should stimulate further investigation into the role of hydroxychloroquine as a symptom–modifying, as well as structure–modifying therapy for OA regardless of its site. Methotrexate (MTX) has not been clinically tested in OA, however it displayed little efficacy in a lapin partial meniscectomy model [20].

New Nonsteroidal Antiinflammatory Drugs

The discovery that prostaglandin synthetase (cyclooxygenase (COX)) exists in two separate isoforms, COX-1 and COX-2, and the identification of a new generation of new nonsteroidal antiinflammatory drugs (NSAID) preferentially or selectively blocking COX-2 rather than COX-1, has brought new impetus to finding a safer antiinflammatory drug (Fig. 1). Indeed, in the last few years, discussions have raged about the risk/benefit ratio of NSAID in OA, given the cost, financial as well as in human life and morbidity of their gastrointestinal side effects. There is no question that a certain portion of patients cannot function without NSAID therapy, and that certain NSAID bring more than symptomatic relief. Several *in vitro* and animal studies have demonstrated that, for instance tiaprofenic acid or diclofenac, may reduce cartilage degradation or stimulate proteoglycan production; on the other hand, some NSAID may have deleterious effects [21]. Rather than avoiding NSAID or resorting to combination prophy-

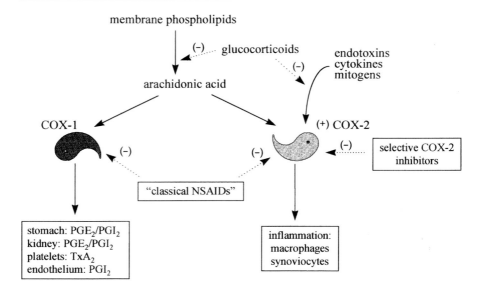

membrane phospholipids

(-) ... glucocorticoids

endotoxins
cytokines
mitogens

(-)

arachidonic acid

COX-1

(-)

(+) COX-2

(-)

(-) ... selective COX-2
inhibitors

"classical NSAIDs"

stomach: PGE$_2$/PGI$_2$
kidney: PGE$_2$/PGI$_2$
platelets: TxA$_2$
endothelium: PGI$_2$

inflammation:
macrophages
synoviocytes

Fig. 1. Prostaglandin synthesis and sites of inhibitory actions by the glucocorticoids, "classical NSAID", and the selective COX-2 inhibitors

lactic therapies with prostaglandin analog or H$_2$-blockers or proton pomp inhibitors, a COX-2 selective NSAID may solve the problem that has plagued the easy handling of this therapy, especially in older, high risk patients. All the new, more selective NSAID have so far faired as well as the old ones in terms of efficacy in OA, but with much less gastrointestinal toxicity [22–24].

8.1.3.2.2
Local Treatment

Corticosteroids

Intraarticular corticosteroid injections have been used for more than four decades in the treatment of OA, mainly of the knee, and to a lesser extent other joints such as the hip or the fingers. Despite extensive clinical experience, certain aspects of this therapy remain controversial: its relative efficacy, the potential deleterious effects and the potential structure–modifying effects. Different chemical formulations have been used with somewhat similar short-term results, all superior to the placebo [25–27]. A retrospective observational study was carried out that evaluated radiographic changes over four to 15 years following repeated intraarticular injections [28]. Despite many flaws in methodology, the authors concluded that such therapy was beneficial, without any evidence to support the suggestion that intraarticular steroids may lead to a more rapid destruction of the joint [28]. This hypothesis is also challenged by animal studies where, on the contrary, corticosteroids were shown to have some beneficial effects retarding cartilage degeneration and osteophyte formation [29].

The long-term role of local corticosteroid injections in the management of OA is still unclear pending well conducted double–blind studies.

Hyaluronic Acid

Hyaluronic acid (HA), a polysaccharide consisting of a long chain of disaccharides (§-D-glucuronyl-§-D-N-acetylglucosamine), is a natural component of cartilage, and plays an essential role in the articular milieu. It is considered not only a lubricant, but also performs a physiological function in the trophic status of cartilage. The clinical use of HA was proposed following studies of OA synovial fluid showing a marked reduction in HA concentration, as well as a shortening in length of the chains. Several studies, sometimes with conflicting results, have been conducted using HA of different molecular weight and obtained from different sources. The term of visco–supplementation was coined by Balazs, who pioneered this form of therapy.

Low molecular weight (500,000 to 750,000 Daltons) HA preparations were compared in well controlled studies to placebos [30–33], or intraarticular corticosteroids [34–36]. Conflicting results were obtained, but in general, pain was reduced for up to six months, and the treatment was well tolerated with the exception of minor transient local discomfort. Recently, a large randomized double-blind placebo controlled trial found no significant differences at 20 weeks between the two groups when compared to their baseline evaluation; however, once stratified according to age and disease severity, HA proved more efficacious than placebo in patients over 60 years of age who had the most severe knee OA [37]. One study demonstrated a certain synergism of action when HA was injected with dexamethasone at one of the five weekly injections [38]. Dougados looked at the structure–modifying potential of HA (Hyalgan) and showed a statistically significant difference in 2 of the 3 evaluated parameters [39]. Further studies are needed to confirm these findings.

High molecular weight HA (Hylan; Synvisc) was evaluated in at least two clinical trials [40, 41]. Scale et al. [40] compared two therapeutic regimens to a placebo; the two and three weekly injections proved superior to the placebo, with a trend towards a more favorable outcome in the group who received three injections. Adams et al. [41] compared the three weekly injections to an NSAID treatment and to the combination of NSAID and Hylan. The results support the hypothesis that treating the pain of knee OA with Hylan is at least as effective as continuous NSAID therapy, and could be used as a replacement or adjunct to NSAID. A retrospective study of 336 patients with 458 treated knees yielded an overall good response in 76 % [42]. In patients who received a second course of treatment, the relief obtained by the first series lasted an average of 8 months. Local side effects were observed in 8 % of patients, and ranged from a transient mild discomfort to an acute synovitis with effusion, requiring drainage and corticosteroid injection or a short course of NSAID treatment.

Treatment of knee OA with HA of low or high molecular weight requires further investigation to better define potential responders, and particularly to evaluate the long–term benefits in retarding or reversing cartilage degradation. For the time being, it is best suited as a symptomatic treatment for patients who do not respond to conventional therapies or who cannot tolerate NSAID.

Glycosaminoglycan Polysulphuric Acid

Glycosaminoglycan polysulphuric acid (GAGPS) has been suggested as a possible intraarticular treatment for OA more than 10 years ago, based on its *in vitro* stimulatory effect on cartilage metabolism [43]. In the past several years, clinical studies have yielded inconclusive results.

Recently, GAGPS was evaluated in one randomized double–blind placebo controlled trial [44]. Pain relief was marginally superior in the GAGPS group at two weeks, with no change documented thereafter. Improvement in the Lequesne's functional index, however, was not statistically significant, and showed a trend favoring GAGPS. Despite the demands of this therapy (two series of five injections at two week intervals), further studies are warranted to demonstrate potential structure modifying properties; only then would it be deemed useful.

Other glycosaminoglycan derivatives have been tried in small uncontrolled studies; therefore, the results were questionable and difficult to interpret. Any new substance should be tested according to the OARS guidelines mentioned earlier.

8.1.3.3
Articular Cartilage Repair

In several tissues such as skin and bone, injury elicits an inflammatory response followed by repair. Lacerations and fractures become filled with a fibrin clot and inflammatory cells. Mesenchymal cells migrate into the clot, proliferate and differentiate, and the lesion becomes plugged with dense scar or native tissue [45]. In early OA, partial thickness defects are common, and no fibrin clot develops within the clefts and fissures or fibrillated cartilage, and neither chondrocytes nor mesenchymal cells migrate into these regions. Consequently, these defects do not become filled with repair tissue. Several approaches have been tested that can possibly induce or help cartilage repair.

8.1.3.3.1
Cellular Grafts

The grafting of cell populations derived from cartilage (chondroblasts, chondrocytes, dedifferentiated chondrocytes) or from bone marrow (mesenchymal cells) into the defect sites is a concept that is being widely tested. This technique is based on the hypothesis that local microenvironmental conditions should then lead to expansion of the cell population and tissue transformation. Cells used for such purposes include chondrocytes [46] and mesenchymal cells [47], but success rates have been extremely varied. Use of cartilage-like matrices as a scaffolding for cell expansion may help enhance cell survival.

8.1.3.3.2
Tissue Grafts

The approach most frequently adopted to induce or improve healing of articular cartilage defects involves the transplantation of biologic material, which includes osteochondral tissue and tissues with chondrogenic potential.

Perichondrial/periosteal grafts can be used as autotransplantation materials for the induction of healing in cartilage defects [48, 49]. There are a variety of protocols designed to improve repair, and although many of the documented findings are encouraging, complete restoration of hyaline articular cartilage tissue or long-term stability has not been achieved. The procedures also involve technical difficulties relating to the mechanical fixation (by suturing or gluing) of transplanted material to the defect surfaces.

Use of cartilage tissue itself as a graft material, or as part of an osteochondral transplant on an autograft or allograft basis in the case of large full-thickness defects, is still the subject of active experimentation [50, 51]. The main problems associated with this approach relate to the attainment of long-term stability and integration of graft-material with the host tissue (at least in the cartilaginous compartment). An additional difficulty is that of tissue storage: subzero temperatures are preferable, but the freezing/thawing steps involve tissue and cell viability problems [51]. Such procedures yield promising intermediate results for severe disabling conditions.

8.1.3.3.3
Combined Grafts

Combined systems can be used, as exemplified by osteochondral grafts for the treatment of full-thickness defects. Transplantation of a single cell type embedded within a biodegradable matrix also represents a combined type of transplantation in that two different materials are placed in the defect space. Such combined systems can be further extended by the introduction of stimulating substances such as growth factors. One example of combined type transplantation is that of dedifferentiated chondrocytes together with a periosteal flap [46] or a single cell type embedded within a biodegradable matrix [52]. There is likely a potential role for this approach in the future treatment of OA cartilage lesions.

8.1.3.3.4
Synthetic Matrices

Synthetic matrices – and preferably biodegradable ones – serve as a scaffolding for transplanted cell expansion into the defect space. Chondrocytes and precursor cells cultured or implanted in a three-dimensional system are less likely to dedifferentiate (chondrocytes) and undergo transformation (precursor cells). For this reason, as well as maximization of cell density and immobilization of transplanted cells *in situ*, the application of matrices is to be recommended.

Natural matrices have been employed: fibrin [53] and denatured collagen-gelatin gels [54]; and a number of biodegradable synthetic materials have been tested: carbohydrate-based polymers such as polylactates [55] and polyglycolic acid [55]. Nonbiodegradable matrices, such as carbon- (2), dacron- [56] and teflon-micromeshes [57] have also been examined. Although reasonable results have been achieved with some of these, foreign body reaction might change the expected life of these implants.

Although the purpose of these techniques is to reestablish normal anatomy to the joint, whether they would effectively reestablish normal joint physiology remains to be determined. Without such re-establishment, the same pathophysiologic process would inevitably degrade these implants and lead again to OA.

The research approach for the next few years will most likely combine cartilage tissue engineering to provide biomechanical stability to the graft and cell recruitment or cell transplantation associated possibly with gene therapy techniques to protect these implants from further degradation [58].

8.1.3.4
Experimental Therapies

8.1.3.4.1
Biologic Agents

Growth Factors

Polypeptide growth factors are areas of potential intervention. They play a major role in the regulation of cell behaviour, including that of articular cartilage. Among the most influential of these factors are insulin-like growth factor 1 (IGF-1), basic fibroblast growth factor (bFGF), and transforming growth factor beta (TGF-β). These and other factors interact to modulate their respective actions, creating effector cascades and feedback loops of intercellular and intracellular events.

Recent data concerning the TGF-β action on OA cartilage has shown that phenotypically altered chondrocytes are more sensitive to TGF-β than normal in the upper layers of cartilage [59]. Contradictory results from experimental models of OA may, however, continue to prevent clinical application of TGF-β [60].

There has been some interest in the experimental treatment of canine OA using intraarticular injections of insulin-like growth factor-1 (IGF-1) [61], both alone and in combination with intramuscular pentosan polysulphate. Combined therapy was successful in blocking proteinase activity and maintaining cartilage structure and biochemistry.

Anticytokines

An interesting approach to reduce proinflammatory cytokine production and/or activity is through the employment of certain cytokines having antiinflammatory properties (Fig. 2). Three such cytokines – IL-4, IL-10, and IL-13 – have been identified as able to modulate various inflammatory processes [62, 63]. Their antiinflammatory potential, however, appears to depend greatly on the target cell [64].

Recombinant human interleukin-4 (rhIL-4) has been tested *in vitro* in OA tissue and has been shown to suppress the synthesis of both TNF-α and IL-1β in the same manner as low-dose dexamethasone [65].

Naturally occurring antiinflammatory cytokines such as IL-10 inhibit the synthesis of IL-1 and TNF-α [66], and can be potential targets for therapy in OA. Augmenting inhibitor production *in situ* by gene therapy or supplementing it

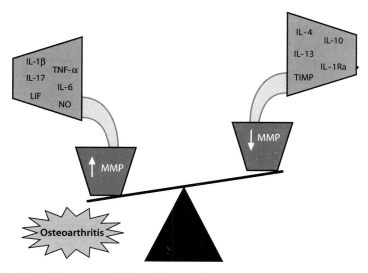

Fig. 2. The balance between cytokines and anticytokines favors cartilage catabolism in osteoarthritis, as well as tissue destruction during the osteoarthritis process

by injecting the recombinant protein is an attractive therapeutic target, although an *in vivo* assay in OA is not available, and its applicability has yet to be proven.

Similarly, IL-13 significantly inhibits lipopolysaccharide (LPS)-induced TNF-α production by mononuclear cells from peripheral blood, but not in cells from inflamed synovial fluid [67]. Although recently discovered, IL-13 has important biological activities: inhibition of the production of a wide range of proinflammatory cytokines in monocytes/macrophages, B cells, natural killer cells and endothelial cells, while increasing IL-1Ra production [68, 69]. In OA synovial membranes treated with LPS, IL-13 inhibited the synthesis of IL-1β, TNF-α and stromelysin, while increasing IL-1Ra production [64]. These results suggest that IL-13 could potentially be useful for the treatment of OA.

8.1.3.4.2
Gene Therapy

Major research efforts over the last few decades have brought forth comprehensive knowledge concerning OA and its etiopathogenesis. Despite this extensive research, the disease remains incurable. A number of biological agents such as proinflammatory cytokine inhibitors, cytokine soluble receptors and antiinflammatory cytokines have demonstrated potentially beneficial therapeutic properties, both *in vitro* and in some *in vivo* models of arthritis [62, 70]. The methods used to deliver these biological agents have often been somewhat difficult to apply to the clinical scenario. Degradation of the protein after oral administration poses a problem, or if injected systematically, the large amount required and the need for frequent injections are often deterrents. This last route of administration can induce adverse effects including an immunological reaction with the appearance of a neutralizing antibody. The necessity of maintaining a sustained level of the agents over time is the major concern with this kind of therapy. In the last few years, much attention has been focused on the use of gene transfer techniques as a method of delivery [71, 72]. Many techniques have been developed using various genes, and a great deal of work is currently devoted to these techniques to facilitate the transfer of genes into joint cells and tissues both *in vitro* and *in vivo* [71, 72]. The attractions of this approach in the treatment of arthritis are multiple, and include the identification of a very specific target, a consistently high local concentration in the joint of the therapeutic protein, and the maintenance of a sustained delivery over time. There is also hope that this type of therapy will reduce the incidence of side effects.

There is at this time no definitive information to indicate the best gene to use for the treatment of arthritis. However, and more specifically with regard to OA, the predominant role of IL-1 in the structural changes of this disease, as well as the relative deficit in the amount of the IL-1Ra, has elicited much attention concerning the use of this gene in OA therapy [73]. This is due in great part to the ability of IL-1Ra *in vitro* to reduce cartilage degradation, and *in vivo* the progression of experimental inflammatory arthritis [62] and OA [74]. Currently, two main systems – viral and non viral – are used for gene transfer to cells [71, 72], with the viral system favoured for the IL-1Ra gene [71]. The reason for this is that they generally allow for a very effective transfer into a large percentage of cells, while maintaining a high sustained level of protein expression which can be extended over a significant period of time. Using the MFG retrovirus, the IL-1Ra gene has been successfully transferred to rabbit and human synovial cells using *ex vivo* techniques [71]. Experiments have demonstrated that these cells can be subsequently transferred successfully *in vivo* into joints, and are able to produce IL-1Ra over an extended period of time [75]. A study done using the experimental dog model of OA has demonstrated that when the IL-1Ra gene is transferred *ex vivo* into synovial cells using the MFG retrovirus, it induces a sustained production *in vivo* of IL-1Ra, which can reduce the progression of the structural changes of OA [76] (Fig. 3). Baragi et al [77] have demonstrated that the *in vitro* human IL-1Ra gene can be successfully transferred into chondrocytes using the Ad.RSV adenovirus, and that the increased production of IL-1Ra can protect the OA cartilage explants from degradation induced by IL-1. Moreover, a recent study has demonstrated that a gene (SVT) can successfully be transferred *in vivo* in rat articular cartilage by a combination of a virus (HUG, Sendai virus) and liposomes [78]. As with any other that allows for a direct *in vivo* transfer of a gene into joint cells, this technology offers interesting advantages.

The treatment of OA using gene therapy is very promising, although still in the very early stage of development. Much work remains to be done, particularly with regard to the development of this technology for *in vivo* use in man. The selection of gene(s) that would offer the best protection against OA also remain to be determined.

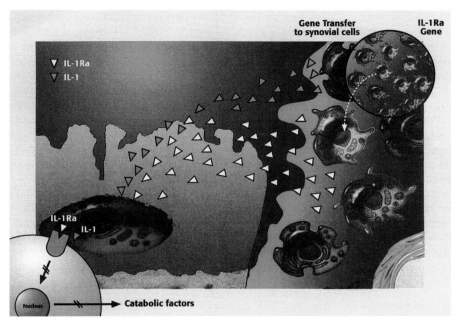

Fig. 3. Schematic representation of the effect of gene therapy using IL-1Ra in osteoarthritic diarthrodial joints. Synoviocytes transfected *ex vivo* with the gene's coding sequence for IL-1Ra using a retroviral vector are injected into the joint, where they graft themselves onto the synovium. They produce enough IL-1Ra protein to displace IL-1 from its membrane receptor and then inhibit the synthesis of catabolic factors. This would lead to a slower rate of cartilage breakdown and reduce OA progression

8.1.3.4.3
Cytokine Inhibitors

Understanding of the role played by cytokines in the pathology of OA is another promising approach. IL-1 seems to be a predominent cytokine implicated in the major events that lead to cartilage destruction [79]. There is some evidence from *in vitro* and *in vivo* experimentation that modulation of IL-1 synthesis may lead to the identification of new targets in therapeutics [80, 81]. A potential role of TNF-α in the disease process cannot, however, be ruled out at this time.

IL-1 Inhibition

Yet another expanding area of OA research is the understanding of cytokine activity in this pathology. There is some evidence that modulation of IL-1 activity could reveal new therapeutic targets [80]. A recent study using the Pond-Nuki dog model has demonstrated that tenidap, a cytokine-modulating drug, can significantly reduce cartilage damage and osteophyte formation while simultaneously inhibiting IL-1 synthesis [81]. New members of this oxyndole family are under experimental assay, and could present a potential area of interest in the future treatment of OA.

The inhibition of cytokine synthesis by a pharmacological approach using p38 kinase inhibitors can reduce availability of IL-1 and TNF-α [82], and MMP [83]. Antisense oligonucleotide therapy using complementary sequence to a non-transduced 5' region of IL-1β RNA has been shown to be effective in reducing IL-1β synthesis [84, 85].

The inhibition of IL-1 activity by modulating the enzymatic conversion of the pro-cytokine (31 kDa) in the active mature cytokine (17 kDa) is an attractive therapeutic target. Intracellular transformation of IL-1 is carried out via a converting enzyme called ICE (IL-1β converting enzyme) [62,86], and can be well be controlled by antisense therapy [87]. A recent *in vivo* study has demonstrated that a new ICE inhibitor effectively reduces the progression of murine type II-collagen induced arthritis (CIA) [88].

Extracellular inhibition of IL-1 can be achieved using either type I (IL-1RsI) or type II (IL-1RsII) soluble receptors. *In vitro* data has recently established some advantages of the latter [89], and some clinical assays are currently underway with rheumatoid arthritis patients. Another option would be the use of anti-IL-1 antibodies to neutralize its activity. Although this technique has been successfully tested in a CIA murine model of inflammatory arthritis [90], no data is yet available for OA.

TNF-α Inhibitors

Soluble TNF-α receptors

The extracellular portion of the two types of TNF-R can be released from the cellular membrane to form soluble receptors (TNF-R55 and TNF-R75) [91, 92]. Both are shed from the OA synovial fibroblasts with a greater amount of release for TNF-R55. Although the exact role of TNF-sR in the control of TNF-α action remains ambivalent, some studies indicate that TNF-sR75 is involved in facilitating the binding of TNF-α to its receptor and/or stabilizing its ligand [92]. Indeed, it was shown that decreasing the shedding of the TNF-R75 may contribute to reducing the response of these cells to stimulation by TNF-α. Moreover, TNF-sR could function as an inhibitor of cytokine activity by rendering the cells less sensitive to the activity of the ligands or by scavenging ligands, not bound to cell surface receptors.

Anti-TNF-α

Anti-TNF-α treatment in murine CIA has been shown to significantly improve the disease [93]. Clinical trials using an anti TNF-α chimeric monoclonal antibody (cA2) in rheumatoid arthritis compared to a placebo group [94] have shown that this approach is very encouraging, for this disease, although TNF-α is not a prominent cytokine in terms of OA.

8.1.3.4.4
Nitric Oxide Synthase Inhibitors

Osteoarthritic lesions are believed to result from an imbalance in the anabolic and catabolic processes that occur during the development of the disease. A decreased synthesis of aggrecan, possibly induced by an excess production of nitric oxide (NO), has been associated with the catabolic events of OA [95]. Nitric oxide is produced in large amounts by chondrocytes, macrophages and inflamed synovium [95, 96] and its synthesis is greatly increased upon stimulation with proinflammatory cytokines [97]. The nitric oxide synthase (NOS) is responsible for the production of NO. The inducible form of NOS (iNOS), which can be upregulated by cytokines, is the main enzyme involved in producing NO in arthritic disorders [95] (Fig. 4).

Recent findings bring attention to the role of NO among identified agents contributing to the imbalance found in the IL-1 system of OA tissue. *In vitro* studies have shown that the cytokine-induced endogenous production of NO by chondrocytes is a potent inhibitor of IL-1Ra synthesis [98]. Moreover, NO can reduce cartilage matrix macromolecular synthesis, and enhance MMP activity, both of which are likely factors contributing to cartilage damage in OA [99, 100]. Recent findings have focused on the potential role of NO in the pathophysiology of OA. A high level of nitrite/nitrate has been found in the synovial fluid and serum of patients [101], and an elevated level of iNOS synthesis/expression detected in OA synovium [102] and cartilage [103]. The increased production of NO may be an additional factor contributing to the excess production of PGE_2 by OA tissues.

These findings with regard to the action of NO on the biological functions of joint tissues leads one to conclude that NO may very well be involved in the pathophysiology of OA and inflammatory arthritis (Fig. 5). Therefore, it is likely that controlling the production of NO in arthritic disease would have a potential therapeutic value. In the experimental models of inflammatory arthritis, treatment with compounds that inhibit iNOS activity either nonselectively, or in a few cases selectively, was shown to reduce the severity of arthritis [95, 104–108]. To date, however, there has been little investigation into the potential of the NOS inhibitor on the progression of OA. One recent study has been con-

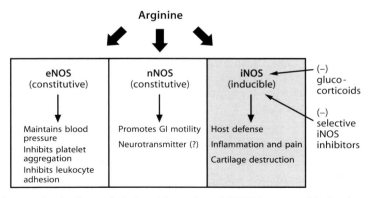

Fig. 4. The constitutive form of nitric oxide synthase (eNOS) is responsible for the maintenance of the biological homeostasis. Under inflammatory conditions, the upregulation of the inducible form of NOS (iNOS) was increased and induced an excessive production of nitric oxide (NO). The activity of iNOS can be blocked by selective inhibitors

Fig. 5. The induction of an increased level of nitric oxide (NO) upregulated the production of prostaglandins, as well as the peroxynitrite, which is responsible for inducing an inflammatory reaction, as well as tissue destruction during the osteoarthritis process

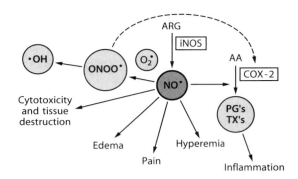

ducted examining the *in vivo* effect of N-iminoethyl-L-lysine (L-NIL), a potent and selective inhibitor of iNOS, on the progression of experimental OA using the anterior cruciate ligament dog model [109]. This study demonstrated that a selective inhibition of iNOS could reduce the progression of early lesions in an experimental OA dog model under prophylactic conditions, and that the inhibition of NO production correlates with a reduction in MMP activity in the cartilage. Treatment with the selective iNOS inhibitor was also associated with a reduction in the level of proinflammatory mediators, IL-1β and PGE_2 and nitrite/nitrate in the synovial fluid, as well as in a marked reduction of the volume of joint effusion. This study provides evidence that *in vivo* cartilage MMP activity can be reduced by inhibiting that of iNOS. Reduction of MMP activity in cartilage is associated with a decreased expression and synthesis of these proteases by chondrocytes, concomitantly with a downregulation of iNOS level and production of nitrite/nitrate. Therefore, the suppression of NO production may aid in the preservation of cartilage by reducing the level of MMP synthesis therein, and inhibiting the formation of peroxinitrite, a toxic, highly reactive oxidant. The reduced degree of synovial inflammation in OA dogs treated with the iNOS inhibitor was associated with a decreased level of IL-1β in OA tissues, and synovial fluid, and may have contributed to the protective effect of L-NIL.

To date, no drugs having disease modifying activity are available for the treatment of OA. This study provides strong evidence that NO produced by iNOS is injurious to the OA joint, and that selective inhibition of this enzyme would provide a novel therapeutic approach treatment. One must keep in mind however that results from the experimental study may or may not translate to the clinical disease in man.

8.1.3.4.5
Metalloprotease Inhibitors

The proteolytic degradation of the extracellular matrix of cartilage in OA has been well documented, and is widely believed to play a major role in the structural changes observed in this disease [73]. Of the different classes of proteases likely involved in this degradative process, the matrix metalloproteases (MMP) are believed to be among the most relevant to OA [73, 110]. These are members of a multigene family that are active at physiological pH, and require heavy metals such as zinc and calcium for activity. MMP are synthesized and secreted as proenzymes, and must be activated by proteolytic cleavage. Some of these proteases are extremely relevant to OA cartilage degradation. The collagenases, particularly MMP-1 (interstitial), MMP-8 (neutrophil), and MMP-13, are believed to be the predominant enzymes involved in native collagen type II degradation [111]. The gelatinases (A and B) and stromelysin-1 are considered the main enzymes involved in the degradation of matrix aggrecans [73, 110]. The increased expression and synthesis of these MMP in OA tissues is likely related to the higher levels of proinflammatory cytokines such as IL-1 and TNF-α found therein [73, 79].

Inhibiting MMP synthesis/activity as a treatment for arthritis has been the focus of very intensive research over the last decade [112]. Although there are natural biological inhibitors of MMP such as the tissue inhibitor of metalloproteases (TIMP), they have very limited possible application as therapeutic agents mainly because of their limitations regarding administration of proteins, as well as mixed results from *in vivo* experiments. Similar limitations are also true with synthetic peptides, therefore, at this time, the most promising inhibitors are chemical agents that can block the activity of MMP.

Antibiotics such as tetracycline and its semisynthetic forms (doxycycline and minocycline) have very significant inhibitory properties that impact MMP activity [112]. Their action is mediated by chelating the zinc which is present in the active site of MMP. Several *in vitro* studies have demonstrated that tetracycline can inhibit collagenases (MMP-1, MMP-13) as well as gelatinases (MMP-2). The IC_{50} towards MMP of semisynthetic drugs is lower, which makes these drugs more attractive. Various tetracyclines have reduced the severity of OA *in vivo* in animal models [112]. Doxycycline was shown to reduce the progression of canine OA, while concurrently reducing MMP (collagenase, gelatinase) activity [113]. A clinical trial is presently underway to explore the therapeutic efficacy of doxycycline in knee OA in men.

The hydroxamate-based compounds are potent inhibitors of MMP [112]. These are believed to work by interacting with the active site of the MMP molecule, binding with the zinc molecule, which inactivates the enzyme. Thiols and carboxylalkyls, also inhibitors of MMP, have a similar mode of action. The hydroxamate compounds are very common as a certain number of them are orally active, and hold interesting potential use in the therapy of arthritic diseases. Several of these compounds are currently under investigation. Among them, CGS27023-A, an orally active stromelysin inhibitor, was shown to block *in vivo* cartilage matrix degradation in rabbits [114]. Another inhibitor, RO-3555 [115], a competitive inhibitor of human collagenases (-1, -2 and -3), inhibits *in vitro* IL-1-induced cartilage degradation. It is also capable *in vivo* of inhibiting articular cartilage degradation in a rat monoarthritic model. Clinical trials are currently being conducted in RA and OA patients. Two hydroxamate inhibitors, BB-1101 and BB-1433, when administered orally, were capable of inhibiting the progression of arthritic lesions in rat adjuvant-induced arthritis [116]. Similarly, another hydroxamic acid derivative named ISC was shown, after oral administration, to reduce swelling and inflammatory parameters [117].

Another means of decreasing MMP levels is to reduce the level of MMP synthesis. There has been very significant progress made in understanding of the complexity of the transcription factors involved in the expression of MMP. Many sequences in the promoter region are responsible for the maximum expression of MMP. Interaction of multiple elements within the promoter appears to govern the regulation of MMP gene expression [112, 118]. Among different factors that can decrease the transcription of MMP are the growth factor TGF-β, the glucocorticoids and the retinoids [112]. The last two factors act on MMP genes via the AP-1 site, however both factors act in a rather nonspecific way as they also interfere with the expression of many other genes making it an nonspecific therapy with several side effects. Nevertheless, novel strategies to specifically inhibit the transcription of posttranscriptional mechanisms of MMP remain an attractive option.

In summary, we believe that, based on our knowledge of the pathophysiology of OA, MMP are intimately involved in the degradation of OA cartilage matrix as well as in the structural changes occurring during the course of the disease. This provides a strong incentive for testing the efficacy of MMP inhibitors as possible structure modifying agents.

References

1. Cruz TF, Tang J, Pronost S, Pujol JP (1996) Molecular mechanisms implicated in the inhibition of collagenase expression by diacerhein. Rev Prat 46:S15–S19
2. Carney SL, Hicks CA, Tree B, Broadmore RJ (1995) An *in vivo* investigation of the effect of anthraquinones on the turnover of aggrecans in spontaneous osteoarthritis in the guinea pig. Inflamm Res 44:182–186
3. Bendele AM, Bendele RA, Hulman JF, Swann BP (1996) Beneficial effects of treatment with diacerhein in guinea pigs with osteoarthritis. Rev Prat Ed Fr 46:S35–S39
4. Nguyen M, Dougados M, Berdah L, Amor B (1994) Diacerhein in the treatment of osteoarthritis of the hip. Arthritis Rheum 37:529–536
5. Marcolongo R, Fioravanti A, Adami S, Tozzi E, Mian M, Zampieri A (1988) Efficacy and tolerability of diacerhein in the treatment of osteoarthritis. Curr Therap Res 43:878–887
6. Mauviel A, Daireaux M, Hartmann DJ, Galera P, Loyau G, Pujol JP (1989) Effects of unsaponifiable extracts of avocado/soy beans (PIAS) on the production of collagen by cultures of synoviocytes, articular chondrocytes and skin fibroblasts. Rev Rhum Mal Osteoartic 56:207–211
7. Henrotin Y, Labasse A, Jaspar JM, De Groote D, Zheng SX, Guillou B, Reginster JY (1998) Effects of three avocado/soybean unsaponifiable mixtures on metalloproteinases, cytokines and prostaglandin E2 production by human articular chondrocytes. Clin Rheumatol (In Press)
8. Maheu E, Mazieres B, Valat JP, Loyau G, Le Loet X, Bourgeois P, Grouin JM, Rozenberg S (1998) Symptomatic efficacy of avocado/soybean unsaponifiables in the treatment of osteoarthritis of the knee and hip: a prospective, randomized, double-blind, placebo-controlled, multicenter clinical trial with a six-month treatment period and a two-month follow-up demonstrating a persistent effect. Arthritis Rheum 41:81–91
9. Blotman F, Maheu E, Wulwik A, Caspar H, Lopez A (1998) Efficacité et tolérance des insaponifiables d'avocat/soja dans le traitement de la gonarthrose et de la coxarthrose symptomatique. Rev Rhum (In Press)
10. Bassleer C, Henrotin Y, Franchimont P (1992) *In vitro* evaluation of drugs proposed as chondroprotective agents. Int J Tissue React 14:231–241

11. Müller-Fasbender H, Bach G, Haase W, Rovati LC, Setnikar I (1994) Glucosamine sulfate compared to ibuprofen in osteoarthritis of the knee. Osteoarthritis Cartilage 2:61–69
12. Noack W, Fischer M, Förster KK, Rovati LC, Setnikar I (1994) Glucosamine sulfate in osteoarthritis of the knee. Osteoarthritis Cartilage 2:51–59
13. Reichelt A, Forster KK, Fischer M, Rovati LC, Setnikar I (1994) Efficacy and safety of intramuscular glucosamine sulfate in osteoarthritis of the knee. A randomised, placebo-controlled, double-blind study. Arzneimittelforschung 44:75–80
14. Talent JM, Gracy RW (1996) Pilot study of oral polymeric N-acetyl-D-glucosamine as a potential treatment for patients with osteoarthritis. Clin Ther 18:1184–1190
15. Mazieres B, Loyou G, Menkes CJ, Valat JP, Dreiser RL, Chorlot J, Masounabe-Puyanne A (1992) La chondroitine sulfate dans le traitement de la gonarthrose et de la coxarthose. Resultats à 5 mois d'une étude aveugle versus placebo. Rev Rhum Mal Osteoartic S9:466–472
16. L'Hirondel J (1992) Klinische doppelblind-studie mit oral verabreichtem chondroitinsulfat gegen placebo bei der tibiofemoralen gonarthrose. Litera Rheumatologica 14:77–84
17. Conrozier T, Vignon E (1992) Die wirkung von chondroitinsulfat bei der behandlug der hüftgelenksarthrose. Litera Rheumatologica 14:69–75
18. Morreale P, Manopulo R, Galati M, Boccanera L, Saponati G, Bocchi L (1996) Comparison of the antiinflammatory efficacy of chondroitin sulfate and diclofenac sodium in patients with knee osteoarthritis. J Rheumatol 23:1385–1391
19. Bryant LR, des Rosier KF, Carpenter MT (1995) Hydroxychloroquine in the treatment of erosive osteoarthritis. J Rheumatol 22:1527–1531
20. Mannoni A, Altman RD, Muniz OE, Serni U, Dean DD (1993) The effects of methotrexate on normal and osteoarthritic lapine articular cartilage. J Rheumatol 20:849–855
21. Huskisson EC, Berry H, Gishen P, Jubb RW, Whitehead J (1995) Effects of antiinflammatory drugs on the progression of osteoarthritis of the knee. LINK Study Group. Longitudinal Investigation of Nonsteroidal Antiinflammatory Drugs in Knee Osteoarthritis. J Rheumatol 22:1941–1946
22. Distel M, Mueller C, Bluhmki E, Fries J (1996) Safety of meloxicam: a global analysis of clinical trials. Br J Rheumatol 35 Suppl 1:68–77
23. Bjarnason I, Macpherson A, Rotman H, Schupp J, Hayllar J (1997) A randomized, double-blind, crossover comparative endoscopy study on the gastroduodenal tolerability of a highly specific cyclooxygenase-2 inhibitor, flosulide, and naproxen. Scand J Gastroenterol 32:126–130
24. Zhao SZ, Hatoum H, Hubbard R, Koepp J, Dedhiya S, Geis S, Bocanegra T, Ware J, Keller S (1997) Effect of celecoxib, a novel COX-2 inhibitor, on health-related quality of life of patients with osteoarthritis of the knee. Arthritis Rheum 40 (Suppl):S88–S88 (Abstract)
25. Dieppe PA, Sathapatayavongs B, Jones HE, Bacon PA, Ring EF (1980) Intra-articular steroids in osteoarthritis. Rheum Rehabil 19:212–217
26. Friedman DM, Moore ME (1980) The efficacy of intraarticular steroids in osteoarthritis: a double-blind study. J Rheumatol 7:850–856
27. Valtonen EJ (1981) Clinical comparison of triamcinolonehexacetonide and betamethasone in the treatment of osteoarthrosis of the knee-joint. Scand J Rheumatol Suppl 41:1–7
28. Balch HW, Gibson JM, El-Ghobarey AF, Bain LS, Lynch MP (1977) Repeated corticosteroid injections into knee joints. Rheum Rehabil 16:137–140
29. Pelletier JP, Mineau F, Raynauld JP, Woessner JF Jr, Gunja-Smith Z, Martel-Pelletier J (1994) Intraarticular injections with methylprednisolone acetate reduce osteoarthritic lesions in parallel with chondrocyte stromelysin synthesis in experimental osteoarthritis. Arthritis Rheum 37(3):414–423
30. Namiki O, Toyoshima H, Morisaki N (1982) Therapeutic effect of intra-articular injection of high molecular weight hyaluronic acid on osteoarthritis of the knee. Int J Clin Pharm Ther Toxicol 20:501–507
31. Bragantini A, Cassini M (1987) Controlled single-blind trial of intra-articulary injected hyaluronic acid in osteo-arthritis of the knee. Clin Trials Journal 24:333–340

32. Dixon AS, Jacoby RK, Berry H, Hamilton EB (1988) Clinical trial of intra-articular injection of sodium hyaluronate in patients with osteoarthritis of the knee. Curr Med Res Opin 11:205–213

33. Dougados M, Nguyen M, Listrat V, Amor B (1993) High molecular weight sodium hyaluronate (hyalectin) in osteoarthritis of the knee: a 1 year placebo-controlled trial. Osteoarthritis Cartilage 1:97–103

34. Leardini G, Mattara L, Franceschini M, Perbellini A (1991) Intra-articular treatment of knee osteoarthritis. A comparative study between hyaluronic acid and 6-methyl prednisolone acetate. Clin Exp Rheumatol 9:375–381

35. Pietrogrande V, Melanotte PL, D'Agnolo B, Ulivi M, Benigni GA, Turchetto L, Pierfederici P, Perbellini A (1991) Hyaluronic acid versus methylprednisolone intra-articularly injected for the treatment of osteoarthritis of the knee. Curr Therap Res 50:691–701

36. Jones AC, Pattrick M, Doherty S, Doherty M (1995) Intra-articular hyaluronic acid compared to intra-articular triamcinolone hexacetonide in inflammatory knee osteoarthritis. Osteoarthritis Cartilage 3:269–273

37. Lohmander LS, Dalen N, Englund G, Hamalainen M, Jensen EM, Karlsson K, Odensten M, Ryd L, Sernbo I, Suomalainen O et al. (1996) Intra-articular hyaluronan injections in the treatment of osteoarthritis of the knee: a randomised, double blind, placebo controlled multicentre trial. Hyaluronan Multicentre Trial Group. Ann Rheum Dis 55: 424–431

38. Grecomoro G, Piccione F, Letizia G (1992) Therapeutic synergism between hyaluronic acid and dexamethasone in the intra-articular treatment of osteoarthritis of the knee: a preliminary open study. Curr Med Res Opin 13:49–55

39. Listrat V, Ayral X, Patarnello F, Bonvarlet JP, Simonnet J, Amor B, Dougados M (1997) Arthroscopic evaluation of potential structure modifying activity of hyaluronan (Hyalgan) in osteoarthritis of the knee. Osteoarthritis Cartilage 5:153–160

40. Scale D, Wobig M, Wolpert W (1994) Viscosupplementation of osteoarthritic knees with hylan: a treatment schedule study. Curr Therap Res 55:220–232

41. Adams ME, Atkinson MH, Lussier AJ, Schulz JI, Siminovitch KA, Wade JP, Zummer M (1995) The role of viscosupplementation with hylan G-F 20 (Synvisc) in the treatment of osteoarthritis of the knee: a Canadian multicenter trial comparing hylan G-F 20 alone, hylan G-F 20 with non-steroidal anti- inflammatory drugs (NSAIDs) and NSAIDs alone. Osteoarthritis Cartilage 3:213–225

42. Lussier A, Cividino AA, McFarlane CA, Olszynski WP, Potashner WJ, De Medicis R (1996) Viscosupplementation with hylan for the treatment of osteoarthritis: findings from clinical practice in Canada. J Rheumatol 23:1579–1585

43. Vacha J, Pesakova V, Krajickova J, Adam M (1984) Effect of glycosaminoglycan polysulphate on the metabolism of cartilage ribonucleic acid. Arzneimittelforschung 34: 607–609

44. Pavelka K Jr, Sedlackova M, Gatterova J, Becvar R, Pavelka K (1995) Glycosaminoglycan polysulfuric acid (GAGPS) in osteoarthritis of the knee. Osteoarthritis Cartilage 3:15–23

45. Grinnell F (1994) Fibroblasts, myofibroblasts, and wound contraction. J Cell Biol 124:401–404

46. Brittberg M, Lindahl A, Nilsson A, Ohlsson C, Isaksson O, Peterson L (1994) Treatment of deep cartilage defects in the knee with autologous chondrocyte transplantation. N Engl J Med 331:889–895

47. Wakitani S, Goto T, Pineda SJ, Young RG, Mansour JM, Caplan AI, Goldberg VM (1994) Mesenchymal cell-based repair of large, full-thickness defects of articular cartilage. J Bone Joint Surg Am 76:579–592

48. Hommings GN, Bulstra SK, Bouwmeester PS, van der Linden AJ (1990) Perichondral grafting for cartilage lesions of the knee. J Bone Joint Surg [Br] 72:1003–1007

49. Kreder HJ, Moran M, Keeley FW, Salter RB (1994) Biologic resurfacing of a major joint defect with cryopreserved allogeneic periosteum under the influence of continuous passive motion in a rabbit model. Clin Orthop 288–296

50. Girdler NM (1993) Repair of articular defects with autologous mandibular condylar cartilage. J Bone Joint Surg [Br] 75:710–714

51. Malinin TI, Mnaymneh W, Lo HK, Hinkle DK (1994) Cryopreservation of articular cartilage. Ultrastructural observations and long-term results of experimental distal femoral transplantation. Clin Orthop 18–32
52. Vacanti CA, Kim W, Schloo B, Upton J, Vacanti JP (1994) Joint resurfacing with cartilage grown *in situ* from cell-polymer structures. Am J Sports Med 22:485–488
53. Hendrickson DA, Nixon AJ, Grande DA, Todhunter RJ, Minor RM, Erb H, Lust G (1994) Chondrocyte-fibrin matrix transplants for resurfacing extensive articular cartilage defects. J Orthop Res
54. Nixon AJ, Sams AE, Lust G, Grande D, Mohammed HO (1993) Temporal matrix synthesis and histologic features of a chondrocyte-laden porous collagen cartilage analogue. Am J Vet Res 54:349–356
55. Freed LE, Marquis JC, Nohria A, Emmanual J, Mikos AG, Langer R (1993) Neocartilage formation *in vitro* and *in vivo* using cells cultured on synthetic biodegradable polymers. J Biomed Mater Res 27:11–23
56. Messner K (1994) Durability of artificial implants for repair of osteochondral defects of the medial femoral condyle in rabbits. Biomaterials 15:657–664
57. Messner K, Gillquist J (1993) Synthetic implants for the repair of osteochondral defects of the medial femoral condyle: a biomechanical and histological evaluation in the rabbit knee. Biomaterials 14:513–521
58. Burmester GR, Perka C, Sittinger M (1997) Tissue engineering: New ways to treat joint destruction in the next millenium. Proceedings of the EULAR Meeting S:288:71
59. Lafeber FPJG, van Roy HL, Van der Kraan PM, van den Berg WB, Bijlsma JW (1997) Transforming growth factor-beta predominantly stimulates phenotypically changed chondrocytes in osteoarthritic human cartilage. J Rheumatol 24:536–542
60. van den Berg WB (1995) Growth factors in experimental osteoarthritis: transforming growth factor beta pathogenic? J Rheum Suppl 43:143–145
61. Rogachefsky RA, Dean DD, Howell DS, Altman RD (1993) Treatment of canine osteoarthritis with insulin-like growth factor-1 (IGF-1) and sodium pentosan polysulfate. Osteoarthritis Cartilage 1:105–114
62. Dinarello CA (1996) Biologic basis for interleukin-1 in disease. Blood 87(6):2095–2147
63. Arend WP (1993) Interleukin-1 receptor antagonist. [Review] Adv Immunol 54:167–227
64. Jovanovic D, Pelletier JP, Alaaeddine N, Mineau F, Geng C, Ranger P, Martel-Pelletier J (1998) Effect of IL-13 on cytokines, cytokine receptors and inhibitors on human osteoarthritic synovium and synovial fibroblasts. Osteoarthritis Cartilage 6:10–18
65. Bendrups A, Hilton A, Meager A, Hamilton JA (1993) Reduction of tumor necrosis factor alpha and interleukin-1 beta levels in human synovial tissue by interleukin-4 and glucocorticoid. Rheumatol Int 12:217–220
66. Katsikis PD, Chu CQ, Brennan FM, Maini RN, Feldmann M (1994) Immunoregulatory role of interleukin-10 in rheumatoid arthritis. J Exp Med 179:1517–1527
67. Hart PH, Ahern MJ, Smith MD, Finlay-Jones JJ (1995) Regulatory effects of IL-13 on synovial fluid macrophages and blood monocytes from patients with inflammatory arthritis. Clin Exp Immunol 99:331–337
68. Defrance T, Carayon P, Billian G, Guillemot J-C, Minty A, Caput D, Ferrara P (1994) Interleukin-13 is a B cell stimulating factor. J Exp Med 179:135–143
69. de Waal Malefyt R, Figdor CG, Huijbens R, Mohan-Peterson S, Bennett B, Culpepper JA, Dang W, Zurawski G, de Vries JE (1993) Effects of IL-13 on phenotype, cytokine production, and cytotoxic function of human monocytes. Comparison with IL-4 and modulation by IFN-gamma or IL-10. J Immunol 151:6370–6381
70. Arend WP, Dayer JM (1995) Inhibition of the production and effects of interleukin-1 and tumor necrosis factor alpha in rheumatoid arthritis. Arthritis Rheum 38:252–160
71. Evans CH, Robbins PD (1994) Gene therapy for arthritis. In: Wolff J A (eds) Gene Therapeutics: Methods and Applications of Direct Gene Transfer. Birkhauser, Boston, pp 320–343
72. Chernajovsky Y, Feldmann M, Maini RN (1995) Gene therapy of rheumatoid arthritis via cytokine regulation: future perspectives. Br Med Bull 51:503–516

73. Pelletier JP, Martel-Pelletier J, Howell DS (1997) Etiopathogenesis of osteoarthritis. In: Koopman W J (eds) Arthritis and Allied Conditions. A Textbook of Rheumatology. 13th edn Williams & Wilkins, Baltimore, pp 1969–1984.

74. Caron JP, Fernandes JC, Martel-Pelletier J, Tardif G, Mineau F, Geng C, Pelletier JP (1996) Chondroprotective effect of intraarticular injections of interleukin-1 receptor antagonist in experimental osteoarthritis: suppression of collagenase-1 expression. Arthritis Rheum 39:1535–1544

75. Müller-Ladner U, Roberts CR, Franklin BN, Gay RE, Robbins PD, Evans CH, Gay S (1997) Human IL-1Ra gene transfer into human synovial fibroblasts is chondroprotective. J Immunol 158:3492–3498

76. Pelletier JP, Caron JP, Evans CH, Robbins PD, Georgescu HI, Jovanovic D, Fernandes JC, Martel-Pelletier J (1997) *In vivo* suppression of early experimental osteoarthritis by IL-Ra using gene therapy. Arthritis Rheum 40:1012–1019

77. Baragi VM, Renkiewicz RR, Jordan H, Bonadio J, Harman JW, Roessler BJ (1995) Transplantation of transduced chondrocytes protects articular cartilage from interleukin-1-induced extracellular matrix degradation. J Clin Invest 96:2454–2460

78. Tomita T, Hashimoto H, Tomita N, Morishita R, Lee SB, Hayashida K, Nakamura N, Yonenobu K, Kaneda Y, Ochi T (1997) *In vivo* direct gene transfer into articular cartilage by intraarticular injection mediated by HVJ (sendai virus) and liposomes. Arthritis Rheum 40(5):901–906

79. Pelletier JP, Di Battista JA, Roughley PJ, McCollum R, Martel-Pelletier J (1993) Cytokines and inflammation in cartilage degradation. In: Moskowitz R W (eds) Osteoarthritis, Edition of Rheumatic Disease Clinics of North America. W.B. Saunders Company, Philadelphia, pp 545–568.

80. Martel-Pelletier J, Mineau F, Tardif G, Fernandes JC, Ranger P, Loose L, Pelletier JP (1996) Tenidap reduces the level of interleukin-1 receptors and collagenase expression in human arthritic synovial fibroblasts. J Rheumatol 23:24–31

81. Fernandes JC, Martel-Pelletier J, Otterness IG, Lopez-Anaya A, Mineau F, Tardif G, Pelletier JP (1995) Effects of tenidap on canine experimental osteoarthritis: I. Morphologic and metalloprotease analysis. Arthritis Rheum 38:1290–1303

82. Lee JC, Laydon JT, McDonnell PC, Gallagher TF, Kumar S, Green D, McNulty D, Blumenthal MJ, Heys RJ, Landvatter SW et al. (1994) A protein kinase involved in the regulation of inflammatory cytokine biosynthesis. Nature 372:739

83. Ridley SH, Sarsfield SJ, Lee JC, Bigg HF, Cawston TE, Taylor DJ, DeWitt DL, Saklatvala J (1997) Actions of IL-1 are selectively controlled by p38 mitogen-activated protein kinease regulation of prostaglandin H synthase-2, metalloproteinases, and IL-6 at different levels. J Immunol 158:3165–3173

84. Fujiwara T, Grimm EA (1992) Specific inhibition of interleukin-1 beta gene expression by an antisense oligonucleotide: obligatory role of interleukin-1 in the generation of lymphokine-activated killer cells. Cancer Res 52(18):4954–4959

85. Manson J, Brown T, Duff G (1990) Modulation of interleukin-1 beta gene expression using antisense phosphorothioate oligonucleotides. Lymphokine Res 9:35–42

86. Cerretti DP, Kozlosky CJ, Mosley B, Nelson N, Van Ness K, Greenstreet TA, March CJ, Kronheim SR, Druck T, Cannizzaro LA (1992) Molecular cloning of the interleukin-1 beta converting enzyme. Science 256:97–100

87. Stosic-Grujicic S, Basara N, Milenkovic P, Dinarello CA (1995) Modulation of acute myeloblastic leukemia (AML) cell proliferation and blast colony formation by antisense oligomer for IL-1 beta converting enzyme (ICE) and IL-1 receptor antagonist (IL-1ra). J Chemother 7:67–70

88. Ku G, Faust T, Lauffer LL, Livingston DJ, Harding MW (1996) Interleukin-1β converting enzyme inhibition blocks progression of the type II collagen-induced arthritis in mice. Cytokine 8:377–386

89. Burger D, Chicheportiche R, Giri JG, Dayer JM (1995) The inhibitory activity of human interleukin-1 receptor antagonist is enhanced by type II interleukin-1 soluble receptor and hindered by type I interleukin-1 soluble receptor. J Clin Invest 96:38–41

90. Joosten LA, Helsen MM, van de Loo FA, van den Berg WB (1996) Anticytokine treatment of established type II collagen-induced arthritis in DBA/1 mice. A comparative study using anti-TNF alpha, anti- IL-1 alpha/beta, and IL-1Ra. Arthritis Rheum 39:797–809

91. Westacott CI, Atkins RM, Dieppe PA, Elson CJ (1994) Tumour necrosis factor-alpha receptor expression on chondrocytes isolated from human articular cartilage. J Rheumatol 21:1710–1715

92. Martel-Pelletier J, Mineau F, Jolicoeur FC, Pelletier JP (1995) Modulation of $TNFsR_{55}$ and $TNFsR_{75}$ by cytokines and growth factors in human synovial fibroblasts. J Rheumatol 22:115–119

93. Williams RO, Ghrayeb J, Feldmann M, Maini RN (1995) Successful therapy of collagen-induced arthritis with TNF receptor-IgG fusion protein and combination with anti-CD4. Immunology 84:433–439

94. Elliott MJ, Maini RN, Feldmann M, Kalden JR, Antoni C, Smolen JS, Leeb B, Breedveld FC, Macfarlane JD, Bijl H (1994) Randomised double-blind comparison of chimeric monoclonal antibody to tumour necrosis factor alpha (cA2) versus placebo in rheumatoid arthritis. Lancet 344:1105–1110

95. Evans CH, Stefanovic-Racic M, Lancaster J (1995) Nitric oxide and its role in orthopaedic disease. Clin Orthop 312:275–294

96. McInnes IB, Leung BP, Field M, Wei XQ, Huang FP, Sturrock RD, Kinninmonth A, Weidner J, Mumford R, Liew FY (1996) Production of nitric oxide in the synovial membrane of rheumatoid and osteoarthritis patients. J Exp Med 184:1519–1524

97. Nathan C (1997) Inducible nitric oxide synthase: what difference does it make? J Clin Invest 100:2417–2423

98. Pelletier JP, Mineau F, Ranger P, Tardif G, Martel-Pelletier J (1996) The increased synthesis of inducible nitric oxide inhibits IL-1Ra synthesis by human articular chondrocytes: possible role in osteoarthritic cartilage degradation. Osteoarthritis Cartilage 4:77–84

99. Järvinen TAH, Moilanen T, Järvinen TLN, Moilanen E (1995) Nitric oxide mediates interleukin-1 induced inhibition of glycosaminoglycan synthesis in rat articular cartilage. Mediators of Inflammation 4:107–111

100. Murrell GAC, Jang D, Williams RJ (1995) Nitric oxide activates metalloprotease enzymes in articular cartilage. Biochem Biophys Res Commun 206:15–21

101. Farrell AJ, Blake DR, Palmer RM, Moncada S (1992) Increased concentrations of nitrite in synovial fluid and serum samples suggest increased nitric oxide synthesis in rheumatic diseases. Ann Rheum Dis 51:1219–1222

102. Grabowski PS, Wright PK, Van't Hof RJ, Helfrich MH, Ohshima H, Ralston SH (1997) Immunolocalization of inducible nitric oxide synthase in synovium and cartilage in rheumatoid arthritis and osteoarthritis. Br J Rheumatol 36:651–655

103. Amin AR, Di Cesare PE, Vyas P, Attur MG, Tzeng E, Billiar TR, Stuchin S, Abramson SB (1995) The expression and regulation of nitric oxide synthase in human osteoarthritis-affected chondrocytes: evidence for an inducible "neuronal-like" nitric oxide synthase. J Exp Med 182:2097–2102

104. Stefanovic-Racic M, Stadler J, Evans CH (1993) Nitric oxide and arthritis. Arthritis Rheum 36:1036–1044

105. Connor JR, Manning PT, Settle SL, Moore WM, Jerome GM, Webber RK, Tjoeng FS, Currie MG (1995) Suppression of adjuvant-induced arthritis by selective inhibition of inducible nitric oxide synthase. Eur J Pharmacol 273:15–24

106. Stefanovic-Racic M, Meyers K, Meschter C, Coffey JW, Hoffman RA, Evans CH (1994) N-monomethyl arginine, an inhibitor of nitric oxide synthase, suppresses the development of adjuvant arthritis in rats. Arthritis Rheum 37:1062–1069

107. Stefanovic-Racic M, Meyers K, Meschter C, Coffey JW, Hoffman RA, Evans CH (1995) Comparison of the nitric oxide synthase inhibitors methylarginine and aminoguanidine as prophylactic and therapeutic agents in rat adjuvant arthritis. J Rheumatol 22:1922–1928

108. McCartney-Francis N, Allen JB, Mizel DE, Albina JE, Xie Q, Nathan DF, Wahl SM (1993) Suppression of arthritis by an inhibitor of nitric oxide synthase. J Exp Med 178:749–754

109. Pelletier JP, Jovanovic D, Fernandes JC, Manning PT, Connor JR, Currie MG, Di Battista JA, Martel-Pelletier J (1998) Selective inhibition of inducible nitric oxide synthase reduces *in vivo* the progression of experimental osteoarthritis. Arthritis Rheum (in press)
110. Dean DD (1991) Proteinase-mediated cartilage degradation in osteoarthritis. Semin Arthritis Rheum 20:2–11
111. Martel-Pelletier J, Pelletier JP (1996) Wanted – the collagenase responsible for the destruction of the collagen network in human cartilage. Br J Rheumatol 35:818–820
112. Vincenti MP, Clark IM, Brinckerhoff CE (1994) Using inhibitors of metalloproteinases to treat arthritis. Easier said than done? [Review]. Arthritis Rheum 37:1115–1126
113. Yu LP Jr, Smith GN Jr, Brandt KD, Myers SL, O'Connor BL, Brandt DA (1992) Reduction of the severity of canine osteoarthritis by prophylactic treatment with oral doxycycline. Arthritis Rheum 35:1150–1159
114. MacPherson LJ, Bayburt EK, Capparelli MP, Carroll BJ, Goldstein R, Justice MR, Zhu L, Hu S, Melton RA, Fryer L et al. (1997) Discovery of CGS 27023 A, a non-peptidic, potent, and orally active stromelysin inhibitor that blocks cartilage degradation in rabbits. J Med Chem 40:2525–2532
115. Lewis EJ, Bishop J, Bottomley KM, Bradshaw D, Brewster M, Broadhurst MJ, Brown PA, Budd JM, Elliott L, Greenham AK et al. (1997) Ro 32–3555, an orally active collagenase inhibitor, prevents cartilage breakdown *in vitro* and *in vivo*. Br J Pharmacol 121:540–546
116. DiMartino M, Wolff C, High W, Stroup G, Hoffman S, Laydon J, Lee JC, Bertolini D, Galloway WA, Crimmin MJ et al. (1997) Anti-arthritic activity of hydroxamic acid-based pseudopeptide inhibitors of matrix metalloproteinases and TNF alpha processing. Inflamm Res 46:211–215
117. Hirayama R, Yamamoto M, Tsukida T, Matsuo K, Obata Y, Sakamoto F, Ikeda S (1997) Synthesis and biological evaluation of orally active matrix metalloproteinase inhibitors. Bioorg Med Chem 5:765–778
118. Vincenti MP, White LA, Schroen DJ, Benbow U, Brinckerhoff CE (1996) Regulating expression of the gene for matrix metalloproteinase-1 (collagenase): mechanisms that control enzyme activity, transcription, and mRNA stability. Crit Rev Eukaryot Gene Exp 6:391–411

8.2
Regulatory Requirements

8.2.1
Preclinical Studies in Osteoarthritis

M. Sisay and R.D. Altman

8.2.1.1
Introduction

We are entering into a new era as a myriad of new approaches to the treatment of osteoarthritis (OA) is under development. While the traditional therapies have been directed at symptoms, many of the new approaches are directed at structure (disease) modification. Indeed, any new agent could conceivably be tested in patients with OA from the time of discovery – as medicines were tested in the past (e.g., foxglove for congestive heart failure). However, because the potential benefits and adverse effects of new medicines are unknown, most new medications are tested in the laboratory first. If there is promise, the medications are then tested for safety, most often in normal volunteers. It is not possible to provide a comprehensive review of all potential preclinical types of trials in a single chapter. We will outline the types of trials that could be performed and emphasize those preclinical trials directed at structure modification.

8.2.1.2
What is to be Studied?

Some potential arenas for basic and laboratory research will be highlighted in a brief summary of the pathogenesis of OA.

OA is a condition of the joint characterized by structural change in the articular cartilage, subchondral bone and surrounding tissue [1], often (but not always) associated with symptoms. Pain is the most common symptom; however, reduced function, deformity, instability and disability are also commonly described. OA is most often slowly progressive, and appears to present as a final common pathway to a variety of different etiologies [2], some of which are known. Either collagen abnormality or physical forces damaging the articular cartilage may be a major pathway to the onset of OA [3].

The diagnosis is mainly based on symptoms and radiological findings. Unfortunately, OA in man is most often diagnosed when the disease is in a late or moderately late stage with advanced destruction of joint cartilage and severe derangement of joint function. Most therapies, to be effective, would probably need to be started in early stage OA.

OA is characterized by a loss of sulfated proteoglycans, abnormal replication of chondrocytes, thinning and erosion of articular cartilage, fibrillation, and osteophyte formation [4, 5]. It mainly affects weight bearing joints (e. g., hip and knee) and some non-weight bearing joints (e. g., hand), but can occur in virtually any diarthroidal joint. The role of OA in the spine is not clear except in relation to the intervertebral disc.

Irrespective of the pathogenesis, ultimately the softening, ulceration, focal disintegration of the articular cartilage and the formation of bone and cartilage excrescences at the joint margins (osteophytes) characterize the disease and are most associated with symptoms [6]. Tissues in and around the joints experience hypertrophy and/or atrophy and limited motion. The cartilage surfaces lose their normal congruity resulting in mechanical instability. Synovial effusions and inflammation may follow. In late stage OA, joint replacement may be necessary.

Significant advances have been made during the past several decades [7, 8] in our understanding of the basic pathologic, biomechanical, biochemical and pathophysiologic process associated with OA. OA is not an inevitable concomitant of aging, but develops as a result of definable alterations in biomechanical and biochemical mechanisms. The advancing knowledge in the etiology, pathogenesis, and complications of OA within the last three decades has helped in the understanding of what abnormalities in OA need to be addressed. In this regard, the study of cells and tissues from cartilage, bone and synovium (from both human and animal), and the use of animals in transitional research provide the basis of new interventions for man. Once developed, these new products need safety studies to determine if they can be used in patients with OA.

8.2.1.3
In Vitro Studies

For symptom modifying agents, *in vitro* studies are mostly directed at safety. Exceptions include those medications that may effect pain and inflammation pathways. Pain pathways that are of particular interest include substance P, calcitonin gene related peptide (CGRP), prostaglandins, opioid receptors, NMDA and other non-narcotic receptors. Inflammatory pathways that have been of particular interest are the cytokines, particularly those that induce the expression of cyclooxygenase 2.

There will be no discussion of safety, since an agent that demonstrates toxicity at the cellular or tissue level is unlikely to be investigated further.

Structure modifying drugs may be partially or entirely directed at a target in the joint, i.e., cartilage, bone, synovium, etc. In order to limit discussion, we will see the kinds of preclinical *in vitro* studies that might be considered in the development of a structure modifying agent with emphasis on cartilage.

8.2.1.3.1
Chondrocyte Cell Culture

The chondrocytes are metabolically active and respond to mechanical, endocrine, biochemical and microenvironmental stimuli with increased rate of synthesis of proteoglycans, type II collagen and degradative enzymes [9–12]. They do not commonly divide but with appropriate stimuli such as a change in the microenvironment the cells divide forming clones [13].

Chondrocytes removed from their matrix (released chondrocytes) are ideally suited to the study of the de novo synthesis and deposition of extracellular matrix. Investigation of the chondrocyte helps identify and perhaps alter pathways of normal development, as well as pathologic metabolism of cartilage. *In vitro* chondrocyte culture reduces the environmental complexity of the *in vivo* tissue. Studies that require separation of cells (clonal analysis) can be performed to investigate matrix deposition as well as factors that influence existing matrix, an ideal setting for examination of the influence of a new agent. An advantage of studying released chondrocytes is that the cells can be cultured at different cell densities to test the influence of cell-cell contacts and cell derived factors. This type of research is important as chondrocytes of different ages and species often have different responses to the same agent or growth factor under the same conditions. OA results from a failure of chondrocytes within the joint to maintain the balance between synthesis and degradation of the extracellular matrix. Study of the chondrocyte may help dissect some of the heterogeneous mechanisms of pathogenesis, i.e., genetic, environmental, and mechanical influences. Extensive studies on the regulation of chondrocyte metabolism by growth factors and cytokines in chondrocyte cultures supports the idea that the relative concentration of such mediators, or an altered response of the cells during degeneration, may determine the rate of progress and final outcome [14] in OA.

Targets of change in chondrocyte metabolism have included collagen type II, production of other cartilage collagens, proteoglycan production (e.g., aggrecan, hyaluronate link and degradation, production of the small proteoglycans and other saccharides), matrix enzyme production (e.g., metalloproteinases), inhibitors of enzyme activity or production, chondrocyte growth and duplication, influence on growth factors and cytokines, etc. These studies may address anatomic, biochemical, and/or physiologic intracellular regulatory mechanisms (e.g., surface receptors, soluble receptors, second messengers, promoters, gene expression).

Characteristically, human articular cartilage has a low ratio of cells to matrix. Differentiated mature chondrocytes, when isolated by enzyme dispersal from the tissue, therefore, have to be taken through several cycles of replication to provide sufficient numbers of cells from transplantation [15]. Traditionally, the most rapid cell growth is achieved by growing chondrocytes as adherent monolayers in the presence of serum. However, during this process the isolated chondrocytes lose their phenotype, become flattened and modulated into a nonspecific fibroblastic like cell capable of producing very little cartilage specific matrix [16]. Therefore, such cells transplanted alone do not produce hyaline cartilage tissue. Modulated chondrocytes, when replanted in suspension as non adherent round cells, or seeded within a gel matrix, slowly regain the chondrocyte phenotype with the ability to express and lay down type II collagen and aggrecan [17], although the efficiency of this reversibility decreases with the number of cell passages. Mixing cells with a gel matrix, such as alginate beads, prior to transplantation is likely to be more successful. Similar benefit may be achieved with specially coated dishes that prevent the chondrocyte from contacting the dish.

Mature chondrocytes modulated to a fibroblastic form in culture are very different from the fibroblastic mesenchymal cells derived from the bone marrow, synovium, or periosteum. Such phenotypic chondrocytes are not multipotential and have a very limited capacity to remodel mesenchymal scar tissue, or to form into calcified cartilage or bone in both *in vitro* and *in vivo* when transplanted into animals.

Some of the studies on chondrocytes have been exciting. Experimental studies placing articular chondrocytes, resuspended in a type I collagen gel, into a cartilage-bone defect, showed a rapid formation of cartilage matrix from the surface to the base of the hole, well below the level of the subchondral bone [18]. However, there was no remodeling of the lower part of the defect to form bone in either the patellar groove or medial femoral condyle of the rabbit knee at 6 months. The repair tissue, therefore, disintegrated and failed, partly because the mechanical loading on the new cartilage plug was different to the surrounding cartilage on a bony base, but also because there was no evidence of integration around the edge of the defect. Other reports [19], describing the use of chondrocytes to fill large osteochondral cavities in the knee of horses, involved also a considerable influx of cells from the subchondral bone, which did give rise to a bony layer within the defect. However, only two third of the newly restored matrix remained at the end of the one year study with a high proportion of fibrocartilage present. Stem cell grafts have demonstrated bony and cartilage repair; however, the repaired tissue inconsistently heals to the surrounding cartilage [20]. The combination of chondrocytes with a growth factor and collagen matrix has shown promise [21].

8.2.1.3.2
Tissue Studies

Since the action of the cartilage as a tissue involves complex interactions, the use of cartilage slices in organ culture allow investigators to study cell-cell, cell-matrix, and matrix-matrix interactions under less synthetic conditions.

The conditions whereby cartilage may repair remains controversial and the subject of continued study [22, 23]. To date, the ability of cartilage to repair is variable and unpredictable [5, 14]. Multiple factors account for this variability as types and magnitude of injuries and the state of the joint as a whole. In addition, these studies have indicated that the structure and integrity of the matrix that was being replaced does not always mimic the macromolecular organization or have the material properties of normal articular cartilage.

The properties of cartilage that dictate the character of selection and collection techniques and sequences in the preparation of cartilage [24] include 1) appropriate clinical documentation of human or animal subjects from whom cartilage has been collected; 2) collection of cartilage under aseptic conditions; 3) avoidance of dehydration by quick collection and temperature and humidity control; 4) after dissection, the prepared blocks or slices are immediately placed in a sterile culture medium or quenched in a low temperature. These concepts also apply to the collection of cells for cell culture.

Animal models have given new insight into the early changes in cartilage associated with OA. However, there is a continuing need to analyze normal and OA human cartilage, especially to correlate these data with the changes seen in the intact animal. Tissue studies allows the investigator to obtain end stage tissue that is frequently not available in animal models. Investigators need to be aware that the ability to interpret the results obtained from such tissues is often limited by inadequate knowledge of the premedication and histology of samples. There is also a need to classify the tissues and their origin adequately so that the results can be compared among laboratories or within the same laboratory over time. Unified cartilage classification would allow comparison of tissues.

Many of the same studies performed on chondrocytes in isolation can be measured in the whole tissue. However, biomechanical testing is more reliable with whole tissues, particularly when testing an intact specimen (i.e., cartilage and bone).

8.2.1.4
Animal Models

Further understanding of OA are aided by the availability of experimental models that simulate human disease [25 – 27]. Animal models provide advantages in the study of the etiopathogenesis of OA and the evaluation of investigative interventions, both for safety and efficacy. Selection of an animal model is dependent upon the object of the study, as different models may better reflect different subsets of OA. Translation of results must take into account that various forms of human OA likely represent subsets. Consideration must be given to the roles played by age, sex, biomechanical alteration, hormones, inflammatory mediators, and immune processes.

One reason for a wide variety of experimental animal models of OA is that no single model is ideal or fully reproduces all aspects of the human disease. However, the models offer distinct advantages over the use of human materials. The onset of the disease is known; the disease can be studied (Table 1) in detail; the progression of the disease can be deduced and many environmental factors that affect the disease can be controlled or modified [28]. Animal models also yield study specimens (e. g., synovial fluid, cartilage, etc) of superior quality and consistency compared with those obtained from humans. With animal models, early OA can be studied.

On the other hand, a number of practical factors must be taken into account when such models are considered for study. Important in such considerations are disease reproducibility, ease of animal handling, time to the development of OA and cost of purchase and maintenance. In some models, pathologic changes occur too infrequently to be of value for statistical purposes.

Experimental models utilizing dogs or pigs involve limitations related to the high cost of animal purchase, the space needed for maintenance, the cost of boarding and the personnel needed to assist in the studies. In contrast, the utility of experimental models developed in small animals such as mice or guinea pigs is limited by the relatively small amount of articular cartilage available to study the parallel evaluations of cartilage pathology and biochemical responses.

Experimental models that induce changes simulating limited components of the OA process are available. Those techniques that only incompletely reproduce selected components of the pathologic and a pathophysiologic process (e. g., degeneration of matrix and cells, regenerative repair characterized by

Table 1. Advantages of animal models in the study of OA

Initiation of disease is known (defined onset)

Progression of disease can be studied in detail and with control of disease progress

Structure modification can be studied

Therapy can be limited to one agent and pharmacokinetics as well as drug interactions can be studied

Disease severity can be monitored by anatomic and radiographic techniques

Tissues from both diseased and normal animals are available in sufficient quantity to study a variety of mechanisms

Environmental and dietary factors can be controlled

Daily physical activity can be controlled

Tissues can be radio-labeled

Modified from Altman [28].

Table 2. Examples of pathological and histopathological changes in cartilage and synovium in models of OA

Model	Species	Cartilage	Synovium
Chemical			
Iodoacetamide	Dog	White; opaque; loss safranin O; chondrocyte loss; fibrillation; osteophytes	Transient focal hypercellularity; no inflammation or fibrosis
Vitamin A	Rabbit	Erosions; osteophytes	Pannus
Papain	Rabbit	Loss PG; fissures; fibrillation; cloning	Hyperplasia
Surgical			
Anterior cruciate ligament transection	Dog	Fibrillation; clefts; cell loss; exposed collagen; osteophytes	Transient inflammation
Posterior cruciate ligament transection	Rabbit	Pitting femur only	No description
Partial medial meniscectomy	Rabbit	ulceration; fissures; loss PG; osteophytes; cloning	Mild inflammation; mild IgG deposition
Total medial meniscectomy	Rabbit	Fissuring; eburnation	No description
Partial lateral meniscectomy	Rabbit	Ulceration; fissures; loss PG; cloning; osteophytes	Mild synovitis
Patellectomy	Rabbit	Chondrocyte degeneration; fibrillation; fissures; cysts; ulceration; limited osteophytes	Inflammation; invasive pannus; granulation/fibrous tissue
Immobilization			
Casting	Dog	Atrophy with intact cartilage surface; loss safranin O	No description
	Rabbit	Loss PG; osteophytes; "loss of tissue integrity"	No description
Compression	Rabbit	Matrix disruption; cloning; loss chondrocytes	No description

PG = proteoglycan.

chondrocyte proliferation and replacement of cartilage matrix components, or secondary synovial proliferative and inflammatory responses) are of value in studying basic cartilage responses to various pathologic stimuli as shown in Table 2 [29]. Other models that simulate the human disease more completely are of greater advantage in studying the total disease process. Both the incomplete and complete models provide opportunity for assessment of therapeutic interventions to possibly prevent, retard, or reverse the disease process. Tissues sampled from animals can be studied for anatomic, biochemical, enzymatic, cellular and subcellular activities with and without an intervention. Few of the studies mentioned above cannot be performed on an animal tissue after *in vivo* or even in *ex vivo* manipulation. Moskowitz [30] has outlined the types of mo-

Table 3. Types of animal models of osteoarthritis[a]

Metabolic and endocrine manipulation
Introduction of various materials intraarticularly into joints
Induction of focal cartilage defects
Primary alterations of joint forces
Limb denervation model
Experimental release of joint contact
Immobilization and compression
Patellectomy and patellar dislocation
Section of cruciate ligaments
Meniscectomy, partial or complete
Extensive surgical manipulation of the joint

[a] Modified from Moskowitz [30].

dels that may help to gain insight into the underlying mechanisms in OA (Table 3). Selected models will be discussed.

8.2.1.4.1
Observational Models

Perhaps the most extensively studied animals are canines. However, many models exist. Involvement may involve the forelegs or hind limbs depending on the animal's feeding habits, e. g., forelegs are most commonly involved in carnivores and hind limbs in herbivores. Vertebral OA including ankylosis of osteophytes is common in quadrupeds; although uncommon in humans, it simulates diffuse idiopathic skeletal hyperostosis. Large canines, such as sheepdogs (the German shepherd in particular), have OA of the hips related to flattened acetabulum and dorsal subluxation. In these animals all pathologic changes seen in human OA are present except pseudocysts. OA is common in race horses involving the carpal bones, which may appear quite early and severe. The hip joint is rarely involved and the stifle (knee) only in work horses pulling carts or plows. The observation of naturally occurring OA in free living colonies of Rhesus monkeys may provide another useful model for comparison with the human disease [23, 24]. OA changes have also been noted in small laboratory animals, different strains of mice or guinea pigs.

8.2.1.4.2
Spontaneously Occurring Animal Models

Spontaneous OA has been described in various strains of small laboratory animals such as mice, hamsters, and guinea pigs. Several strains of mice, particularly the C57BL [22] and STR/IN [25–27] strains have been utilized in studies of the pathogenesis of OA. Lesions occur with variable frequency depending on the mouse strain used, reaching a 50% to 93% incidence in some strains by 15 to 17 months of age allowing for the study of prophylactic intervention. Morphologic differences in histopathologic findings between the cartilage of the medial tibial condyle and cartilage at the patellofemoral articulation in male

STR/IN mice suggest that several pathophysiologic pathways might be involved in induction of lesions in this model [27] allowing the study of interventions for patellofemoral disease (in contrast to tibiofemoral OA). In another study of blotchy mice (BLO stain), which carry a gene causing inadequate crosslinking of collagen, 88 % of the animals studied were shown to develop osteoarthritic lesions [28], an ideal setting for the study of gene therapy. In contrast to mice, rats display an unexplained marked resistance to development of OA [22]. The increased general activity of mice and the greater opportunity to drop from heights within the confined space of the cage may play a role.

OA has also been shown to occur spontaneously in domestic animals, including horses, swine, cattle, and dogs [30].

Joint laxity and OA changes of the hip joint in dogs have been particularly studied as a model for intervention [31–34]. Although these are associated with hip dysplasia in many breeds, German shepherds and Labrador retrievers are most commonly affected. Procollagen accumulation in involved cartilage has been described in the presence of normal total collagen content and a normal rate of collagen synthesis [32]. A partial defect in conversion of procollagen to collagen has been suggested as a target for intervention. Fibronectin, a potential target of intervention, has been shown to be elevated in OA cartilage in the hip dysplasia model, similar to findings in human OA [34]. It is unresolved whether joint laxity appears first in dogs with hip dysplasia or whether cartilage or ligament abnormalities are primary [33]. Joint laxity may be a significant problem in human OA, particularly in those with a hypermobility syndrome. Spontaneous OA has been described in Macaca mulatta monkeys [23, 24]. Osteoarthritic changes were limited and characterized mainly by cartilage fibrillation, chondrocyte clustering and superficial erosions [24].

The use of animals undergoing spontaneous OA for experimental purposes is limited by considerations of disease reproducibility, ease of handling, and cost. In some animals, such as the dog, the disease occurs too infrequently to be of value for statistical purpose. In other species, such as the mouse, large numbers of animals may be required for study to demonstrate statistically significant differences between affected and control groups under analysis; a significant mortality rate compounds the problem. The long time lapse, measured in months and, at times years, between birth and the development of OA, represents an additional disadvantage to the use of any of these spontaneous animal models.

8.2.1.4.3
Interventional Models of OA

There are many models of experimentally induced OA. Lesions of the canine or lapine stifle has been studied as models of posttraumatic OA. Blunt trauma, cruciate deficiency, and abnormal meniscus have received particular attention.

Some of the specific models will be discussed, based on the large numbers of laboratories using these models at this time. However, recent studies with an ovine meniscectomy model have proved it to be a reliable model that closely simulates human OA.

8.2.1.4.4
Anterior (Cranial) Cruciate Ligament Transection Model

Joint instability is induced by anterior cruciate ligament transection of the stifle resulting in a lesions. Both the canine and lapine models have been investigated as models for traumatic OA [28, 30, 42, 43]. In these models the induced joint instability replicates OA seen in humans. The lesion has demonstrated early increases in cartilage hydration, increased proteoglycan synthesis and degradation as well as changes in proteoglycan structure [44]. Canines with ACL deficiency have been extensively studied as a model for OA [45, 46]. As a result of ligament deficiency, an increase in proteoglycan synthesis and hypertrophy of cartilage have been shown at least at the earlier part following the transection [47]. The phenomenon of hypertrophic repair of articular cartilage was also noted in human OA cartilage, from rabbits with partial meniscectomy [48] and rhesus monkey that developed spontaneous OA [31, 32].

8.2.1.4.5
Medial Meniscectomy Model

As described by Moskowitz [49], the medial meniscus of the rabbit is released from the midmedial collateral ligament along with partial excision of the anterior medial aspect of the meniscus. Pathologic changes induced by this procedure in animals resemble certain components of human joint disease, OA secondary to meniscal tear in man [28]. This is because the freed medial meniscus alters the biomechanical force between joint surfaces and may act as a loose body or joint mouse (similar to a foreign body).

8.2.1.4.6
Cartilage Atrophy Induced by Limb Immobilization

Reports have detailed the morphologic features of the degeneration that occurs in articular cartilage with immobilization of a limb [50, 51]. Degenerative changes are marked and appear earlier in areas of mechanical compression, but also occur without contact. The cartilage degeneration due to immobilization may be due to the lack of pumping action, as the nutrition of the cartilage is derived from the synovial fluid. The pumping action during joint is necessary for diffusion of the fluid into the cartilage. Furthermore, synovial fluid production may be reduced by immobilization, which causes degenerative changes in synovial cells and atrophy of the synovial membrane [52].

Of the two models of immobilization reported, immobilization of the leg in extension would result in increased muscle contraction. This method has been reported to cause morphologic changes similar to osteoarthritic cartilage [51]. These include osteophyte formation, fibrillation, pitting and erosion of articular cartilage. In contrast immobilization of the leg in flexion does not lead to morphologic changes of OA [53–55], but may do so upon remobilization with excessive exercise.

The cartilage changes seen with immobilization in flexion are completely reversible if the cast is removed and the dogs are allowed to ambulate freely. Thus limb immobilization in flexion and remobilization can be used as a model of cartilage repair to generate new information concerning the physiologic response of cartilage to loading.

Other frequently used animal models are 'blunt trauma' to the knee of the rabbit or dog [56] or lesion of the meniscus of the rabbit knee which result in the later development of cartilage changes characterized as OA. Prolonged immobilization of the animal knee joint also leads to OA cartilage changes [53, 54].

8.2.1.5
Phase One Clinical Trials

Whereas preclinical cell, tissue culture and animal trials may be directed at both efficacy and safety, the Phase I clinical trial is directed only at safety. Studies are most often conducted on normal male volunteers. Attempts are made to establish the tolerated dose range for single and multiple doses. Even though cell, tissue and animal studies may suggest an effective and safe dose, differences in metabolism, and the clinical setting necessitate dose finding in man. In contrast to some other diseases, Phase I clinical trials in OA are not conducted on severely ill patients (unlike cancer).

Pharmacokinetic trials are usually considered Phase I trials regardless of when they are conducted during the development of a new agent. The types of pharmocokinetic trials that might be considered are listed on Table 4 [58].

Table 4. Types of pharmacokinetic trials

Bioavailability
Peak blood levels
Time to steady-state concentration
Duration of blood concentration
Duration of biological effects
Medication half-life
Accumulation
Time for plasma levels to return to baseline
Microsomal enzyme induction
Distribution characteristics
Plasma protein binding
Metabolism and excretion
Tolerance
Plasma or serum level half-life Vs biological half-life
Drug interaction trials
Comparability trials

Modified from Spilker [58].

References

1. Pelletier JP, Roughley PJ, DiBattista JA et al. (1991) Are cytokines involved in osteoarthritic pathophysiology? Semin Arthritis Rheum, 20 (Suppl 6), 12–25
2. Creamer P, Hochberg MC (1997) Osteoarthritis. Lancet 350:503–509
3. Howell DS, Sapolsky AL, Pita JC, Woessner JF Jr (1976) The Pathogenesis of osteoarthritis. Semin Arthritis Rheum, 5, 365–383
4. Moskowitz RW (1984) Osteoarthritis: a clinical overview. In: Lawrence RC, Shulman LE (eds) Epidemiology of the Rheumatic Disease. Gower Medical Publishing, New York, p 267
5. Peyron JG, Altman RD (1992) The epidemiology of osteoarthritis. In: Moskowitz RW, Howell DS, Goldberg VM, Mankin HJ (eds) Osteoarthritis: Diagnosis and Surgical/Medical Management, 2nd ed. Philadelphia: WB Saunders Inc, pp 15–37
6. Mankin HJ, Mow VC, Buckwalter JA et al. (1994) Form and function of articular cartilage. In: Simon S (ed) Orthopedic Basic science. Chicago, American Academy of Orthopedic Surgons, p 144
7. Dieppe P (1991) Osteoarthritis: clinical and research perspective. Br J Rheumatol 30 (Suppl 1):1–4
8. Davies MA (1988) Epidemiology of osteoarthritis. Clin Geriatr Med 4:241–255
9. Sokoloff L (1974) Cell biology and the repair of articular cartilage. J Rheumatol 1:9–16
10. Mankin HJ (1982) The response of articular cartilage to mechanical injury. J Bone Joint Surg 64 A, 460–466
11. Herman JH, Khosla RC, Mowery CS et al. (1982) Modulation of chondrocyte synthesis by lymphokine rich conditioned media. Arthritis Rheum 25:676–688
12. Rothwell AG, Bentley G (1973) Chondrocyte multiplication in osteoarthritic cartilage. J Bone Joint Surg 55B:558–594
13. Bland JH, Cooper SM (1984) Osteoarthritis: A review of the cell biology involved and evidence for reversibility. Management rationally related to known genesis and pathophysiology. Semin Arthritis Rheum 14:106–133
14. Tyler JA (1991) Cartilage degradation. In cartilage: Molecular aspects (ed. Hall B, Newman S), CRC Press, Boca Raton, FL, pp 213–256
15. Tyler JA, Hunziker EB (1998) Articular cartilage regeneration. In: Brandt KD, Doherty M, Lohmander LS (eds) Osteoarthritis. Oxford University Press, New York, pp 94–108
16. Benya PD, Padilla S, Nimni ME (1978) Independent regulation of collagen types of chondrocytes during the loss of differentiated function in culture. Cell 15:1313–1321
17. Benya PD, Shaffer JD (1982) Dedifferentiated chondrocytes reexpress the differentiated collagen phenotype when cultured in agarose gel. Cell 30:215–225
18. Wakitani S, Kimura T, Hirocka A et al. (1989) Repair of rabbit articular surfaces with allograft chondrocytes embedded in collagen gel. J Bone Joint Surg 71B:74–80
19. Sams AE, Nixon AJ (1995) Chondrocyte laden collagen scaffolds for resurfacing extensive articular cartilage defects. Osteoarthritis Cartilage 3:47–59
20. Caplan AI, Elyaderani M, Mochizuki Y et al. (1997) Principles of cartilage repair and regeneration. Clin Orthop 342:254–269
21. Hunziker EB, Rosenberg LC (1996) Repair of partial-thickness defects in articular cartilage: cell recruitment from the synovial membrane. J Bone Joint Surg 78 A:721–733
22. Buckwalter JA, Mow VC (1990) Articular cartilage repair in osteoarthritis. In: Howell DS, Mankin HJ, Moskowitz RW (eds) Osteoarthritis: Diagnosis and Management. WB Saunders, 2nd edn 1992
23. Buckwalter JA, Rosenberg LC, Hunzer EB (1990) Articular cartilage: composition, structure, response to injury and methods of facilitating repair. In: Ewing JW (ed) Articular Cartilage and Knee Joint Function: Basic Science and arthroscopy. Chap. 2, Raven Press, New York
24. Gardner DL, Mazuryk R, O'Conner P and Orford CR (1987) Anatomical changes and pathogenesis of OA in man, with particular reference to the hip and knee joints. In: Lott DJ, Jasani MK, Birdwood GFB (eds) Studies in Osteoarthrosis, Intervention, Assessment. Wiley, Chichester, pp 21–48

25. Adams ME, Billingham MEJ (1982) Animal models of degenerative joint disease. Curr Topics Pathol 71:265–297
26. Troyer H (1982) Experimental models of osteoarthritis. Semin Arthritis Rheum 11: 362–374
27. Schwartz ER, Greenwald RA (1980) Experimental models of osteoarthritis. Bull Rheum Dis 30:1030–1033
28. Altman RD, Dean DD (1990) Osteoarthritis research: Animal models. Semin Arthritis Rheum 19 [Suppl 1]:21–25
29. Malemud CJ (1988) The biology of cartilage and synovium in animal models of osteoarthritis. In: Greenwald RA, Diamond HS (ed) CRC Handbook of Animal Models for the Rheumatic Diseases. Vol II, CRC Press, Boca Raton, FL, pp 3–18
30. Moskowitz RW (1992) Experimental models of osteoarthritis. In: Moskowitz RW, Howell DS, Goldberg VM et al. (eds) Osteoarthritis: Diagnosis and Medical/Surgical Management. Philadelphia, PA, WB Saunders, pp 213–232
31. Chateauvert JMD, Pritzker KPH, Kessler MJ, Grynpas MD (1989) Spontaneous osteoarthritis in Rhesus Macaques: I. Chemical and biochemical studies. J Rheumatol 16:1098–1104
32. Chateauvert JMD, Grynpas MD, Kessler MJ, Pritzker KPJ (1990) Spontaneous osteoarthritis in Rhesus Macaques: II. Characterization and morphometric studies. J Rheumatol 17:73–83
33. Sokoloff L (1956) Natural history of degenerative joint disease in small animals. I. Pathologic anatomy of degenerative joint disease in mice. Arch Pathol 62:118–128
34. Sokloff L, Gay GE Jr (1956) Natural history of degenerative joint disease in small laboratory animals. II. Epiphyseal maturation and osteoarthritis of the knee of mice of inbred strains. Arch Pathol 62:129–135
35. Schunke M, Tillmann B, Bruck M, Muller-Ruchholtz W (1988) Morphologic characteristics of developing osteoarthritic lesions in the knee cartilage of STR/IN mice. Exp Cell Biol 45:1–8
36. Silberberg R (1977) Epiphyseal growth and osteoarthrosis in blotcy mice. Exp Cell Biol 45:1–8
37. Sokoloff L (1969) The Biology of Degenerative Joint Disease. Chicago, University of Chicago Press, pp 18–21
38. Schnell GB (1959) Canine hip dysplasia. Lab Invest 8:1178–1187
39. Miller DR, Lust G (1979) Accumulation of procollagen in the degenerative articular cartilage of dogs with osteoarthritis. Biochem Biophys Acta 583:218–231
40. Lust G, Bilman WT, Dueland DJ et al. (1980) Intraarticular volume and hip joint instability in dogs with hip dysplasia. J Bone Joint Surg 62 A:576–582
41. Wurster NB, Lust G (1982) Fibronectin in osteoarthritic canine articular cartilage. Biochem Biophys Res Comm 109:1094–1101
42. Pond MJ, Nuki G (1973) Experimentally induced osteoarthritis in the dog. Ann Rheum Dis 32:387–388
43. Hulth A, Lindberg L, Telhg H (1970) Experimental osteoarthritis in rabbits: preliminary report. Acta Orthop Scand 41:522–530
44. Carney SL, Billingham MEJ, Muir H, Sandy JD (1987) Demonstration of increased proteoglycan turnover in cartilage explants from dogs with experimental osteoarthritis. J Orthop Res 2:201–206
45. Adams ME, Brandt KD (1991) Hypertrophic repair of canine articular cartilage in osteoarthritis after anterior cruciate ligament transection. J Rheumatol 18:428–435
46. Brandt KD, Braunstein EM, Visco DM et al. (1991) Anterior (cranial) cruciate ligament transection in the dog: A bona fide model of canine osteoarthritis, not merely of cartilage injury and repair. J Rheumatol 18:436–446
47. McDevitt CA, Muir H, Pond MJ (1973) Canine articular cartilage in natural and experimentally induced osteoarthrosis. Biochem Soc Trans 1:287–289
48. Vignon E, Arlot M, Hartmann D et al. (1983) Hypertrophic repair of articular cartilage in experimental osteoarthrosis. Ann Rheum Dis 42:82–88
49. Moskowitz Rw, Howell DS, Goldberg VM et al (1979) Cartilage proteoglycan alterations in an experimentally induced model of rabbit osteoarthritis. Arthritis Rheum 22:155–163

50. Roy S (1970) Ultrastructure of articular cartilage in experimental immobilization. Ann Rheum Dis 29:634–642
51. Palmoski MJ, Bean JS (1988) Cartilage atrophy induced by limb immobilization. In Greenwald RA, Diamond HS (ed) CRC handbook of Animal Models for the Rheumatic Diseases. CRC Press, Boca Raton, FL, Vol. II, pp 83–87
52. Enneking WF, Horowitz M (1972) The intra-articular effects of immobilization of the human knee. J Bone Jt Surg 54 A:973–985
53. Palmoski MJ, Perricone E, Brandt KD (1979) Development, reversal of a proteoglycan defect in normal canine knee cartilage after immobilization. Arthritis Rheum 22:508–517
54. Polmoski MJ, Brandit KD (1981) Running inhibits the reversal of atrophic changes in canine knee cartilage after removal of a let cast. Arthritis Rheum 24:1329–1337
55. Palmoski M, Brandt K (1982) Immobilization of the knee prevents osteoarthritis after anterior cruciate ligament transection. Arthritis Rheum 25:1201–1208
56. Donohue JM, Buss D, Oegema TR, Thompson RC (1983) The effects of indirect blunt trauma on adult canine articular cartilage. J Bone Joint Surg 65 A:964–957
57. Walton M (1979): Patella displacement, osteoarthrosis of the knee joint in mice. J Pathol 127:165–172
58. Spilker B (1991) Pharmacokinetic principles. In: Guide to Clinical Trials, Raven Press, New York, pp 115–123

8.2.2
Clinical Evaluation of Drug Therapy

J.-Y. REGINSTER, B. AVOUAC and C. GOSSET

8.2.2.1
Introduction

Over the last decades, researchers from all parts of the world have significantly contributed to the better understanding of the pathophysiology of osteoarthritis. Epidemiological surveys and studies provided priceless information regarding the natural history of the disease, its natural course and clinical consequences when untreated [1, 2]. Both the scientific community and the public health authority are now aware of the human, social and economic burden represented by osteoarthritis. Since osteoarthritis mainly but not exclusively, occurs in elderly subjects, the aging process of the population, common to all developed and developing countries, will make this disease an even more dramatic issue in the coming years. Finally, there is now a strong pressure from the patients towards the scientific community to pay attention to medications, devices or practices contributing to the improvement of the quality of life through reduction of impairments or disabilities, rather than dedicated only to the prolongation of life expectancy, neglecting debilitating conditions [3].

Therefore, a large amount of human resources was brought, over the last years, to identify, validate and develop medicines that will be effective in preventing or treating osteoarthritis. This prompted regulatory authorities, scientific organisations and individual experts to re-evaluate the methodology involved in the performance of clinical trials in osteoarthritis [4–11].

The purpose of the present chapter is not to substitute to regulatory agencies in preparing a new set of guidelines neither to chose between the different published documents which one would reflect more accurately the current scientific evidence. It only aims at helping drug developers and clinical investigators to identify the points to consider that have emerged from these previous recommendations [4–11] and that are likely to be taken into account when evaluating the overall risk/benefit ratio of a new medication for osteoarthritis.

8.2.2.2
Classification of Anti-Osteoarthritis Therapy

Medications for osteoarthritis may affect symptoms and/or modify joint structures. Symptomatic treatments decrease pain and reduce functional impairments without necessarily acting on the progression of osteoarthritis. The nomenclature initially proposed recognised fast-acting and slow-acting drugs that induce symptomatic relief [8]. The former are generally prescribed for short periods, except when osteoarthritis is permanently painful and disabling. The drugs most widely used in this class are analgesics or non-steroidal anti-inflammatory drugs (NSAIDs).

Symptomatic treatment with a delayed effect brings a gradual improvement in the symptoms of osteoarthritis with a possible persistent action at the withdrawal of the treatment. These compounds were formerly called Symptomatic Slow-Acting Drugs for Treatment of Osteoarthritis (SYSADOA) [8].

Factors that are considered in trial designs for drugs regulating the symptoms include, not exhaustively, the pharmacokinetics and pharmacodynamics of the compound, time to the onset and peak of clinical response, duration of benefit after dicontinuation, frequency and severity of adverse reactions, effect on pain and other symptoms and signs of the disease [4, 5]. However, the most recent consensual view, shared by a taskforce of the Osteoarthritis Research Society (OARS) [4], the Group for the Respect of Ethics and Excellence in Science (GREES) [5] and the Committee for Proprietary Medicinal Products (CPMP) of the European Agency for the Evaluation of Medicinal Products (EMEA) [10], is that arguments for classifying drugs that induce symptomatic relief into fast and slow subgroups are not compelling. Thus, there is no advantage in creating a separate class for the agents that produce a rapid symptom response from those with a slower benefit [4, 10]. Although drugs that act slowly may have different mechanisms of action from those that act rapidly, there is a range of duration of action of drugs which acts on symptoms. The design of trials should adequately take into account the timing and duration of the action of the drugs on symptoms and these factors may influence the use of any concomitant treatment which is permitted in a trial.

Structure-modifying drugs are aimed at modifying the pathologic process of osteoarthritis. They may either prevent the development of osteoarthritis and/or delay or reverse the worsening of existing osteoarthritic lesions. There were formally called "chondroprotective agents", a concept derived from preclinical studies suggesting that some drugs may reduce the rate of cartilage degradation or increase the rate of cartilage repair. This group of compounds was also labelled as "disease-modifying anti-osteoarthritis drugs" (DMOAD) by analogy to the classification of anti-rheumatoid arthritis drugs [8]. Today, however, no agents have been proved to have structure-modifying properties in human [4].

Based on this consideration, consensual opinion is now emerging that drugs for the treatment of osteoarthritis should be rather classified into two categories, namely symptom-modifying drugs and structure-modifying drugs.

Symptom-modifying drugs are expected to act on symptoms with no detectable effect on the structural changes of the disease. Registration of such drugs would, however, require demonstration of a favourable effect on symptoms with no detectable adverse effect on the structural changes of the disease.

Structure-modifying drugs interfere with the progression of the pathological changes in osteoarthritis. Those drugs may alter the structure with or without independent effect on symptoms. Registration of drugs with structure-modifying, symptom-relieving properties would require demonstration of a beneficial effect on both symptoms and structural indices of the disease.

For structure-modifying drugs with no direct effect on symptoms, some discrepancies are still present between the views expressed in the different sets of guidelines. Experts from the osteoarthritis field appear to be heavily convinced that prevention of further structural joint damage will eventually translate into a significant clinical benefit for the patients and the community, for example, by reducing or postponing the need for prosthetic surgery [5]. Regulatory authorities, however, are more cautious, even if admitting that there is a good indirect evidence that by favourably modifying the natural history of osteoarthritis in terms of structural changes, long-term clinical benefits will occur in a large proportion of patients [10].

8.2.2.3
Study Population

Osteoarthritis is a heterogeneous disorder. Therefore, on a clinical basis, observing an effect of a treatment for osteoarthritis in a major joint does not necessarily mean that it will be effective in every joint. In order to avoid getting registration of a drug for a very specific and/or very limited indication, it is recommended by regulatory authorities that the applicant demonstrates that a proven therapeutic effect in a major joint can be extrapolated to other joints [10].

All sets of guidelines recognise the clinical importance of hip and knee osteoarthritis. Osteoarthritis of the hip is a common and disabling disease. Osteoarthritis of the knee is also both very common and a major cause of functional impairment. For the knee, outcome measures, for both symptoms and structure, are better validated for medial tibio-femoral disease than for lateral or patello-femoral disease. Although osteoarthritis of the hand is a potential target for assessing progression of the disease in trials, it is less important clinically than the hip or knee diseases. If hand osteoarthritis is chosen for evaluating the effect on anti-osteoarthritis drug, trials should better focuse on assessing progression of the disease in proximal and distal interphalangeal joints than in the trapezo-metacarpal joint. In the absence of validated end-points for osteoarthritis of the spine, this structure should not be considered as the primary target for trials evaluating anti-osteoarthritic drugs [5].

Although data may be collected for both right and left joints (e.g. hip and knee) for symptom studies, inclusion criteria for structure studies should limit the target joint to a single site. This will most often be the most symptomatic site. Changes in the contro-lateral joint should be considered as a secondary outcome variable. In the case of hand osteoarthritis, it is recommended to use either both hands or the most symptomatic one [4]. Simultaneous assessment of other joints is always possible and should result in generating supportive evidence of general efficacy.

The OARS taskforce reports that there is a considerable level of controversy, in the scientific community, regarding the use of broad or narrow patients eligibility criterion [4]. As this group mentions, broad patients eligibility allows for generalisation of positive results. However, because of the large amount of variations, broad patients eligibility increases the sample size of the study population required to demonstrate significant differences and may mask the presence of subsets perceiving benefits [4]. Similarly, the CPMP document [10] points out, in accordance with the GREES recommendations [5], that the presentation and natural history of the conditions may be different in younger and older age groups. Therefore, these bodies recommend to preselect and specify the age range of the patients to be entered. However, while a narrow age range will increase group homogeneity, this may be obtained at the expense of the general validity of the data [5, 10].

High-risk groups are special subpopulations of subjects who are more prone to rapidly develop progressive osteoarthritis. They include obese women, with unilateral radiographical osteoarthritis, and men or women who have undergone meniscectomy [12, 13]. This population may be considered in phase II study of structure-modifying drugs but inclusion of a specific high-risk group in phase III studies might decrease the potential for generalisation of the results.

Factors that might affect the rate of evolution of osteoarthritis, include age, gender, obesity, major joints injury, types of use, development abnormalities, familiar osteoarthritis and must be recorded. These variables should be considered for stratification at entry or adjust at data analysis.

All guidelines sets recommend that in studies of patients with idiopathic osteoarthritis, patients should be excluded on the basis of secondary osteoarthritis if they have an history or present evidence of any of the following diseases, in the potential target joints : septic arthritis, inflammatory joint disease, gout, Paget's disease of bone, articular fracture, ochronosis, regular episods of pseudo-gout, acromegaly, haemochromatosis, Wilson's disease, primary osteochondromatosis, major dysplasia or congenital abnormality and heritable disorders (e.g., hypermobility) [4, 5, 10].

To be enrolled in a study, patients should have both symptomatic and structural changes of osteoarthritis in the target joints. Currently, this will mean pain related to use with radiological evidence of joint space narrowing for osteoarthritis of the hip and knee and the diagnosis criteria of the American College of Rheumatism for hand osteoarthritis. Pain and disability at entry need to be recorded and the minimum severity of symptoms at entry will depend on the primary outcome measures being assessed, the potential mode of action of the drugs and the joint site involved [10].

For studies of symptomatic response, the level of symptoms at baseline should be of sufficient severity to permit the detection of changes. For studies of structure-modifying drugs, the patient should present definite radiographic changes of osteoarthritis based on an established score and atlas, e.g., Kellgren and Lawrence radiographic entry criteria : grade 2 or 3 (i.e. sufficient remaining interbone distance to permit detection of worsening/progression) [4, 5, 10].

8.2.2.4
Endpoint

Instruments used to measure outcome in clinical trials of osteoarthritis should be valid, reliable and responsive to changes when such measures exist.

8.2.2.4.1
Symptom-Modifying Drugs

The primary outcome measure should be the pain attributable to the target joint and reported by the patient. Functional disability is considered an important additional endpoint for symptom-modifying drugs. Pain should be measured by self-assessment and use-related and rest pain should be assessed separately. The activity causing pain should be specified. A validated method should be used to grade the degree of joint pain. A 100 mm visual analog scale (VAS) or a five-point Likert scale are accepted tools. The period of assessment should be defined (for example, now, today, this week). Measurements should be serially recorded at appropriate intervals to provide an assessment of the time needed for the onset of pain relief as well as an assessment of the duration of the analgesic effect.

For functional disability, a disease-specific and joint-specific instrument such as the Western Ontario Mac Master University Osteoarthritis index (WO-MAC) [14], the algofunctional index for osteoarthritis (AFI) [15] or the Lequesne's index [16] is recommended to assess disability arising from osteoarthritis of the knee, hip or hand.

Secondary endpoints include the patient's perception of the clinical severity of their osteoarthritis (patient global assessment or global rating), the occurrence and number of flares (even if the concept of flares in osteoarthritis lacks a precise definition hence making it difficult to reliably identify), the physical signs including range of motion, health-related quality of life or utility measures and concomitant medications consumption.

8.2.2.4.2
Structure-Modifying Drugs

The evaluation of efficacy of drugs aimed at modifying the structure of the osteoarthritis joint is the most controversial point between the different sets of published guidelines. Panels of scientists dealing with osteoarthritis consider that measure of joint morphology or direct visualization of the joint should be considered as the primary outcome variable for structure-modifying drugs [4, 5]. This position is not fully agreed on by the recent CPMP guidance set [10]. This regulatory authority questions the robustness of the currently available data showing that a change in the joint structure, without concomitant clinical benefit, can eventually translate into a long-term clinical outcome. They consider that some epidemiological data support the relation between structural changes and a long-term clinical outcome. However, the nature and the magnitude of the structural changes that are likely to be clinically relevant on a long-term basis remain debatable. Therefore, a hard clinical endpoint, as necessity of joint replacement, time to surgery and long-term clinical evolution (pain and disability) would be preferable to assess the efficacy of such drugs. On the other hand, the radiographic measurement of joint space width or osteophytes seems to be a promising tool to assess the progression of osteoarthritis, although it has not yet been fully demonstrated. Consistantly, and provided that the applicant gives some data supporting this surrogate, these changes could be considered, by the CPMP, as alternative primary endpoints. In any case, hard clinically endpoints, as mentioned above, should be assessed during the study [10].

The reproducibility of the radiographic technique is dependent on the control of a number of technical issues. Such standardization is essential in order to reliably assess sequential changes in joint anatomy. The most consistant results will be obtained by carefully adhering to standardized radiographic procedures, based on published, validated data [4, 17, 18].

Films should be read centrally. Material collected during trials (radiographs) should be kept available for re-reading because the techniques for assessing structural changes may be improved or changed during the course of the trial. Other technologies for the evaluation of the severity of osteoarthritis: chondroscopy, magnetic resonance imaging, scintigraphy, ultrasonography or biochemical measurements (serum, urine, joint fluids) may be considered as secondary endpoints. Obtaining reproducible X-rays on successive visits is a prerequisite for reliable assessment of progression of osteoarthritis. The sources of variability in joint space width measurement are numerous (patient positioning, radiographic procedure, measurement process, …). It is essential to standardise radiographic techniques based on published, validated data. The method should define the radio-anatomic position of the joint, beam alignment, and should define the anatomic landmarks for measurements. Positioning of the patient should also be based on validated published methods, but in all cases, weigth bearing (standing) anteroposterior views should be used in studies involving the hip or the knee. Repositioning of the joint can be facilitated by use of foot maps drawn at the time of the initial examination. Correction for radiographic magnification has been shown to improve accuracy and precision of measurements.

Even though a structure-modifying drug may not have an independent effect on symptoms, the CPMP recommends clinical signs and symptoms should be assessed. If both symptom-modifying effect and structure-modifying effect are claimed, the requirements under both categories should be fulfilled [4, 5, 10].

8.2.2.5
Concomitant Interventions

All symptom-oriented studies require discontinuation of prior analgesic and anti-inflammatory medications, including topical agents and steroid injections, prior to initiating treatment with the test drug in order to permit an evaluation of unmodified pain severity. The time of withdrawal should be the time required for the clinical effect to disappear (e.g. five half-lives of drugs).

It is impractical to expect patients to participate in a long-term trial without some potential use of rescue medications for pain.

Many patients with osteoarthritis who are recruited for trials are likely to have exacerbations of symptoms which require treatment during the study, irrespective of the type of study design used. Such concomitant treatment may interfere with outcome measures and should ideally be excluded. However, in long-term studies, it is neither ethical nor practical to exclude all concomitant treatments.

For long-term trials, use of concomitant medications should be permitted on a limited basis. An example may be the use of acetaminophen or paracetamol for escape analgesia. Any escape medication must be discontinued in sufficient time for the clinical effects of the agent to disappear prior to the assessment. For all trials, concomitant treatments (drugs or interventions) that are likely to affect joint structures should be excluded.

Concomitant treatments with physical and/or occupational therapy should be either standardized or adjusted for in the analysis to ensure that the effect of exercise programmes on disease progression do not bias the outcome of the study.

8.2.2.6
Study Design

8.2.2.6.1
Phase II Trials

The goals of phase II trial are to define an ideal effective dose-range and regimen and to provide sufficient patient exposure to demonstrate safety.

Phase II study should provide data over a range of doses. The doses selected for these studies should enable the minimum effective dose and the dose-response profile to be determined. Evaluation of at least three doses is recommended.

Some agents may have both symptom and structure modifying effects, but the optimal dose for modification of symptoms may be different from that which alters structure.

Modification of Symptoms

The duration of phase II studies for symptom-modifying effects will depend on the expected outcome and the mode of action of the drug. Normally, even in the case of a slow acting symptom-modifying drug, its effects would be expected to be apparent in several months.

Modification of Structures

The duration of phase II studies for a drug with structure-modifying effects will also depend on its mode of action, but it is likely to be longer than that required to assess modification of symptoms. Studies over a range of doses and of sufficient duration to show meaningful changes in structure are required. The magnitude of these changes should be predetermined.

8.2.2.6.2
Phase III Trials

Phase III trials are intended to convincingly demonstrate efficacy and safety of the optimal regimen and dose(s) of the test agent. Replication of pivotal studies (studies of primary importance for registration of drugs) for demonstration of efficacy is recommended, even though not specifically requested in the European recommendations [5, 10].

Because of the heterogeneity of osteoarthritis, limiting the number of different joints investigated also can limit the potential for generalisation of the results. In each trial, one joint, preferably the hip or the knee, should be selected as a target joint, although simultaneous assessment of further joints is possible. The primary analysis population should be defined according to the intention to treat principle. The design and duration of this study may differ according to the properties of the drug.

Modification of Symptoms

Studies should have a randomised, double blind, parallel group design. To establish that a symptom-modifying drug does not have deleterious effects on the joint, structural changes should be monitored for at least 1 year.

Modification of Structures

Studies should have a randomised, double blind, parallel group design. Clinical variables, or alternatively structural changes when their surrogacy value is proven, are required as primary endpoints. When structural changes are chosen as primary endpoint, the magnitude of a clinically relevant effect of a drug on such variable should be predetermined based on data solidly established. Due to the expected mechanism of action of these drugs, long-term studies, no shorter than at least 2 years, will be requested both for efficacy and safety assessment.

8.2.2.7
Use of Placebo and Choice of Comparator

8.2.2.7.1
Phase II Trials

Pivotal studies should have a placebo-controlled, randomised, double blind and parallel group design.

8.2.2.7.2
Phase III Trials

For symptom-modifying drugs, active controlled studies are necessary with the most favourable comparator. Three-arm, including placebo and active control studies are recommended. It is possible to show that the beneficial effet is sustained long-term by means of a withdrawal study in which actively treated patients, at the end of the study period, are randomised to continue or discontinue (double-blind) treatment.

For structure-modification, studies should have a randomised, double blind, placebo controlled, parallel group design.

References

1. Altman RD, Hochberg MC (1983) Degenerative joint disease. Clin Rheum Dis 9:681–693
2. Croft P, Cooper C, Wickham C, Coggon D (1990) Defining osteoarthritis of the hip for the epidemiologic studies. Am J Epidemiol 132:514
3. Morales-Torres J, Reginster JY, Hochberg MC (1996) Rheumatic and musculoskeletal diseases and impaired quality of life. A challenge for rheumatologists. J Rheumatology 23:1–3
4. Altman RD, Brandt K, Hochberg MC, Moskowitz R (1996) Design and conduct of clinical trials in patients with osteoarthritis. Osteoarthritis Cartilage 4:217–243
5. Dougados M, Devogelaer JP, Annefeldt M, Avouac B, Bouvenot G, Cooper C, Dieppe P, Ethgen D, Garattini S, Jones EA, Kaufman JM, Lemming M, Lemmel EM, Lohmander S, Menkes CJ, Nuki G, Paolozzi L, Pujol JP, Rovati L, Serni U, Spector TD, Tsouderos Y, Veys EM, Weseloh G, Reginster JY (1996) Recommendations for registrations of drugs used in the treatment of osteoarthritis. Annals of Rheumatic Diseases 55:552–557
6. Avouac B (1991) French recommendations for pharmacological and clinical studies of chondroprotectors. Litera Rheumatologica 13:75–80
7. Avouac B, Dropsy R (1993) Méthodologie des essais cliniques des traitements de fond de l'arthrose. Therapie 48:315–319
8. Lequesne M, Brandt KD, Bellamy N, Moskowitz RW, Menkes CJ, Pelletier JP (1994) Guidelines for testing slow acting drugs in osteoarthritis. J Rheumatology 21 [Suppl 41]:65–73
9. Hochberg MC, Altman RD, Brandt KD, Moskowitz RW (1997) for the Task Force. Design and conduct of clinical trials in osteoarthritis: preliminary recommendations from a task force of the Osteoarthritis Research Society. J Rheumatology 24:792–793
10. European Agency for the Evaluation of Medicinal Products (1998) Points to consider on clinical investigation of medicinal products used in the treament of osteoarthritis. CPMP/EWP/ 784/97
11. Furst D (1995) Guiding principles for the development of drugs for osteoarthritis. Final Draft XVII
12. Spector TD, Hart DJ, Doyle DV (1994) Incidence and progression of osteoarthritis in women with unilateral knee disease in the general population: the effect of obesity. Ann Rheum Dis 53:565–568
13. Roos H, Lindberg H, Gardsell P, Lohmander S, Wingstrand H (1994) The prevalence of gonarthrosis and its relation to meniscectomy in former soccer players. Am J Sports Med 22:219–222
14. Bellamy N, Buchanan WW, Goldsmith CH, Campbell J, Stitt LW (1988) Validation study of WOMAC: a health status instrument for measuring clinically important patient-relevant outcomes to antirheumatic drug therapy in patients with osteoarthritis of the hip or the knee. J Rheumatol 1:95–108
15. Dreiser RL, Maheu E, Guillou GB, Caspard J, Grouin JM (1995) Validation of an algofunctional index for osteoarthritis of the hand. Revue du Rhumatisme (English Edn) S1:43–53

16. Lequesne M. Mery C, Samson M, Gerard P (1987) Indexes of severity for osteoarthritis of the hip and knee: validation-value in comparison with other assessment tests. Scandinavian J Rheumatol S65:85–89

17. Buckland-Wright JC (1995) Protocols for precise radio-anatomical position of the tibiofemoral and patellofemoral compartment of the knee. Osteoarthritis Cartilage 3 SA: 71–80

18. Buckland-Wright JC, Macfarlane DO, Williams SA, Ward RJ (1995) Accuracy and precision of joint space width measurement in standard and macroradiographs of osteoarthritic knees. Ann Rheum Dis 54:872–880

CHAPTER 9

Surgical Treatment of the Cartilage Injuries

M. BRITTBERG

9.1
Introduction

The primary aim of all treatments including the surgical treatment of osteo-arthritis is to give pain-relief and retain and improve joint-function for a pro-longed time. The loss of cartilage function may lead to a painful joint with a decreased mobility. Many factors, i.e. epidemiological, biochemical and mor-phological, are associated with cartilage destruction; however, only trauma is known directly to cause osteoarthritis [1]. To what extent a single lesion of cartilage will progress into osteoarthritis is not known and it is also not known if repairing such a defect with a good quality repair will prevent such a de-velopment. This is important to know when discussing the different treatments for cartilage injuries. The classification when a diseased joint should be called an osteoarthritic joint is also not clear and especially regarding the so-called pre-osteoarthritic joint which could give us difficulties when to evaluate opera-tive techniques and their efficacies. There could be differences in the out-come of treatment of pure local cartilaginous lesions and early osteoarthritic lesions.

This chapter will address the treatments of the local cartilage defects as well as the surgical salvage procedures of the osteoarthritic joint.

There is a direct correlation between the ability of a tissue to repair itself after trauma and the tissue turnover state. Adult articular cartilage has an ex-tremely slow metabolic rate and thereby a very low ability to repair itself after injury. At the edge of a cartilage injury, some mitotic activity can be seen at an early stage after trauma, but it is not powerful enough to repair the defect. Prin-cipally, the initial number of cells that can take part in the repair is of major im-portance. In a mesenchymal tissue, there are primitive prechondrocytes/stem-cells which can differentiate into the cells of the injured tissue in beneficial conditions. The repair of the mesenchymal tissue is thus dependent on the local availability of these chondrogenic cells and the ultimate goal for all types of treatment for a cartilage defect must be to deliver and activate high densities of these stem cells to the injured site.

Some techniques described here are purely meant to be for pain-relief and return of some function while the others could have a place in the prevention and eventually hinder the progress of an early osteoarthritis. The latter ultimately produce and/or deliver different types of repair cells that are thought to appear as mature chondrocytes producing a more or less differentiated hyaline cartilage at the end of differentiation lineage.

9.2
Joint Lavage and Debridement of Fibrillated Cartilage

Burman and associates [2] reported a reduced disability in degenerative arthritic patients following arthroscopic lavage which was attributed to the removal of mechanical irritants in the joint.

The concept of shaving or debriding of fibrillated cartilage, mostly superficially situated, is to remove the irregularities of the lesion to get a smooth stable articular surface. This procedure was first described by Haggart [3] and Magnuson [4]. They removed all intra-articular abnormalities: abnormal synovial membrane, osteophytes, torn menisci and degenerative fibrillated cartilage and performed a so-called "house cleaning" of the joint. The technique has been used in open debridements as well as in transarthroscopic procedures, mainly as a "shaving" technique.

A post-operative temporary relief of pain is often seen but no signs of cartilage repair. The combination of debridement and joint irrigation; lavage could give an effect by eliminating cartilage debris that could cause inflammation; synovitis. However, the value of this treatment is uncertain [5] and as in most studies regarding the treatment of injured cartilage the diagnosis has been osteoarthritis and the studied group consisted of elderly patients in non-randomized studies [6]. It has also been shown that the success of the arthroscopic debridement correlates inversely with the severity of the disease and thus, patients with a mild disease improved the most, particularly when a coexisting meniscal tear was treated [7]. There are a few randomized studies regarding lavage and debridement. Livesley conducted a clinical trial with 37 osteoarthritic patients treated with lavage and physiotherapy and a control group of 24 knees treated with physiotherapy alone. There was better relief of pain in the lavage group and the effect was still present at one year [8]. In another study the effect of arthroscopic lavage and debridement was compared measuring objectively the thigh muscle function before and after the operation. There was some improvement in quadriceps isokinetic torque at six and 12 weeks after joint lavage but not after debridement. Neither method significantly relieved the patient's symptoms [9]. Chang and co-workers [10] compared arthroscopic surgery to closed-needle joint lavage for 32 patients with non-end-stage osteoarthritis. After 1 year, 44% of subjects who underwent arthroscopy reported improvement and 58% of the lavage-group improved. The reasons why in several papers patients benefit from the lavage and debridement of osteoarthritic joints are unclear. To determine if a placebo effect might influence the results of those types of surgery, Moseley and co-workers [11] performed a pilot-study where 5 patients were randomized to a placebo-arthroscopy, three patients randomized to arthroscopic lavage while finally two patients to arthroscopic debridement. The placebo-group reported decreased frequency, intensity and duration of pain and there thus seemed to exist a significant placebo-effect regarding the effect of arthroscopic osteoarthritis treatment. A larger study of this kind is planned by the same authors and will be of great interest.

Arthroscopic lavage success seems to be quite unpredictable and if good results are obtained they often seem to decline rapidly over time. Regarding the extended debridement one can suspect that good results depend to an important part on the lavage effect as part of the procedure as in the randomized studies there were no differences.

9.3
Drilling, Resection or Abrasion of the Subchondral Bone Plate

Pridie [12] introduced drilling of the bare exposed subchondral bone to stimulate fibrocartilaginous ingrowth from the vascular bone marrow. Large areas of bare bone can be repaired by the technique of making several drill holes into the subchondral vascular area (Fig. 1B). Different ways to achieve resurfacing via an opening of the subchondral bone marrow cavity have been tried. Ficat [13] described the spongialization, a resection of the entire subchondral bone plate in chondromalacic patellas, and reported 79% of good to excellent results in their patients. Steadman suggested that an awl should be used instead of a high-speed drill bit and named the technique microfracturing. The awl creates a rough surface around the fractured bone plate which according to Steadman will give a better blood-clot formation [14]. Lanny Johnson [15] introduced the transarthroscopic abrasion arthroplasty where the sclerotic exposed subchondral bone was excised 1–3 mm with a motorized burr to reach intracortical vascularity (Fig. 1A). The resulting fibrin clot formation is protected with non-weight bearing for 2 months.

Evidence exist that the above described techniques will produce a repair mainly consisting of fibrocartilaginous tissue. Despite this, there are reports on an improvement in the patients symptoms [15, 16]. It is to note that the follow-up times in most studies have been short and it has been difficult to compare the treated groups due to lack of common descriptions of the cartilage lesions; single cartilage lesion or generalized OA. Furthermore there is a marked lack of randomized controlled studies.

Buckwalter and Mow [17] claimed that arthroscopic abrasion arthroplasties and debridements may provide temporary relief of symptoms in selected patients when performed by surgeons with considerable experience in cartilage handling. Salisbury and McMahon [18] discussed the role of abrasion arthroplasty in cartilage resurfacing. In a knee with a degenerative meniscal lesion the forces that dislocate the meniscal flap may often create a damage on the adjacent condylar weight bearing cartilage area and the lesion can be debrided after resection of the meniscal flap. This would be a localized area that can be treated by the surgeon in two ways: either accepting the debrided defect now with stable edges or abrade the base of the lesion to get a bleeding bony surface. Salisbury and McMahon [18] state that debridement alone will give reduction in symptoms like locking, catching and effusions for a while but by time the decrease in meniscal load sharing will lead to a gradual cartilage degeneration

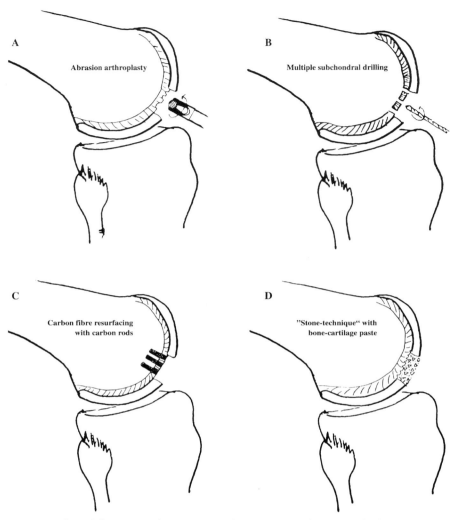

Fig. 1. Cartilage defect repair alternatives. **A** Abrasion arthroplasty. **B** Multiple subchondral drilling. **C** Carbon fiber implantation. **D** "Stone technique" with microfracturing of the subchondral bone + implantation of an osteochondral "paste"

also of the surrounding cartilage. To what extent an abrasion arthroplasty could hinder such a progress is not known. The filling up of the defect might stabilize the edges of the defect but there is doubt that the fibrocartilage tissue repair after abrasion will stand against wear for a prolonged time. The abrasion arthroplasty however is suggested to be used for small chondral defects. The results of an extended abrasion arthroplasty as a treatment for widespread unicompartmental or multicompartmental OA have been more unpredictable and discutable [19].

In older athletes studies have shown that in osteoarthritis debridement alone gave better long-term results than arthroscopic abrasion with debridement and also that arthroscopic abrasion made some patients even worse [20]. Contrary, Friedman et al. [16] in a retrospective study found better results with medial meniscectomies in combination with arthroscopic abrasion arthroplasty in osteoarthritic knees, especially in patients younger than 40 years of age. Even here, we can note the age-dependency of the procedures on the injured articular cartilage.

Interestingly, in a rabbit study a comparison of abrasion burr arthroplasty and subchondral drilling in the treatment of full thickness cartilage lesions was made [21]. The authors reported that both techniques were suboptimal for cartilage defect repair but that at 6 months there was evidence that subchondral drilling may result in a longer-lived repair than abrasion arthroplasty in the treatment of full thickness lesions.

A combined technique for cartilage repair has been described by Stone and Walgenbach [22]. The surgical technique include shaving away loose or fragmented articular cartilage, followed by microfracturing the base of the defect until bleeding occurs. An articular cartilage osteochondral graft is harvested from the inner rim of the intercondylar notch with a trephine. This graft is then morselized in a bone graft crusher, mixing the cartilage with the cancellous bone. The resulting "paste" is finally pushed into the defect and described to be secured by the adhesive proporties of the bleeding bone (Fig. 1D). In 29 patients followed for more than one year, 27 were satisfied with good pain-relief. Sixteen patients had undergone second-look arthroscopies with 7 patients described to have biopsies with an appearance of immature hyaline cartilage, 7 patients with a mixture between hyaline and fibrocartilage repair tissue and 2 with predominantly fibrocartilaginous tissue.

9.4
Osteochondral Allo- and Autografting Techniques

In osteochondral grafting techniques the cartilage defect area and underlying bone is replaced with a matching articular graft that has been harvested either as an allograft from an organ donor (Fig. 2B) or as an autograft. The limited source of autologous grafts has led to an interest in allografts. The chondrocyte has transplantation antigens [23] but the matrix is protective against immunological reactions. Allografts have therefore been tried clinically both in fresh and frozen preparations. A lot of experience has the transplantation unit in Toronto [24]. They have shown that the chondrocytes were found to be viable up to 92 months after transplantation. The use of an osteochondral graft with bone thickness less than 1 cm was of importance prior to or simultaneously with the implantation of the graft as well as it is essential to correct joint malalignment prior to or simultaneously with graft transplantation [25]. In the beginning the indications for allografting was not clearly defined and the early results of the technique consists of a wide variety of patients. By time it has been found that best results are achieved in patients of young age with post-traumatic defects and before the onset of degenerative changes. Long-term

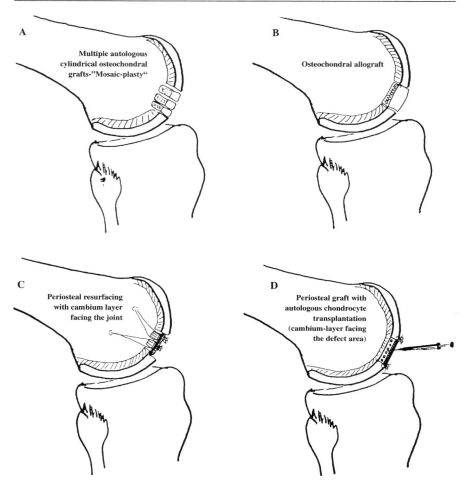

Fig. 2. Cartilage defect repair alternatives. **A** Osteochondral allograft **B** Multiple autologous osteochondral plug implantation; „mosaic-plasty". **C** Periosteal resurfacing with mesenchymal stem cell-cambium-layer facing the joint. **D** Periosteal resurfacing + autologous chondrocyte implantation. Periosteal cambium-layer facing the defect area

results after allografting of posttraumatic defects has been reported by the Toronto group with success rates of 75% at 5 years, 64% at 10 years and 63% at 14 years. Best results were obtained with patients 60 years of age and with traumatically induced defects of the articular surface in the knee joint [26]. New results were presented in 1997 with fresh small-fragment osteochondral allografts that were used to reconstruct post-traumatic osteochondral defects in 126 knees in patients with the mean age of 35 years and followed for mean 7,5 years. Eighty-five % were rated as succesful and the rest as failures. Factors related to failure included here age over 50 years, bipolar defects, malaligned knees and worker's compensation cases [27].

Important to ensure long-term survival of the allografts is that the subchondral bone support must be maintained. However studies have shown that the subchondral bone sometimes is resorbed and that 75% of the failures of cryopreserved grafts were due to subchondral necrosis [28]. Advantages is that a large selection of donors are available and that fresh as well as frozen allografts can be used. The frozen grafts could be more cartilage structural deteriorated and have a lower concentrations of proteoglycans [29]. The frozen grafts make it possible to use it for elective reconstructive surgery while one may have the time to examine the grafts for diseases. The grafts also have the advantage that they have the structure of the normal cartilage and they can be prepared to fit exact the size of the defect to be treated. Disadvantages is a risk for immunologic reactions and disease transmission. The bone component give rise to an immunological response. The surrounding cartilage matrix is protective against immunological reaction while the chondrocytes have transplantation antigenes. Instead autologous osteochondral grafting has advantages; reliability of bony union, a high survival rate of grafted cartilage and no risk for disease transmission. Wagner [30] in Germany used a part of the posterior femoral condyle as an autogeneic graft. Yamashita et al. [31] used an autogeneic graft from the anterior aspect of the medial femoral condyle and Outerbridge et al. [32] used part of the patella to treat osteochondral defect of the knee in ten patients who were followed for 6 and a half years. Function was improved and symptoms were alleviated in all the patients. Matsusue and associates [33] described an interesting alternative technique in which multiple autologous osteochondral grafts were harvested as cylinders from the lateral wall of the patellar groove, non-weight-bearing area. Recently, techniques with small-diameter autologous cylindrical osteochondral grafts have been presented [34, 35]. They are one-stage autogenous osteochondral grafting techniques for the treatment of cartilage defects in different joints. One to several cylindrical osteochondral grafts are harvested from an unloaded area in the knee-joint via arthrotomy or arthroscopy and implanted in a mosaic-fashion in the defect area complemented with an abrasion of the areas between the osteochondral plugs (Fig. 2 A). Bobic [34] presented 12 patients operated on with osteochondral plugs for chondral lesions 10–22 mm in diameter in combination with an anterior cruciate ligament reconstruction. One year MRI control confirmed excellent graft integration and 9/12 patients were examined with arthroscopy and a thin shallow "halo" were noted at the borderzone between graft and normal cartilage. The simplicity of the procedure makes it interesting for the surgeon and we are exspecting future randomized studies with these methods to know their position in the treatment of cartilaginous defects.

9.5
Periosteal and Perichondral Resurfacing (Soft-Tissue Arthroplasty)

Another way to deliver a new cell population to the cartilage defect site is to use periosteal and perichondral implantations. Both these tissues consist of a certain amount of multipotential mesenchymal stem cells with the ability of cartilaginous metaplasia. They have subsequently been used to resurface cartilage defects but with varying success. The results in different studies are difficult to compare since the methods used vary considerably as well as the properties of the experimental grafting materials. In most of the repair studies the periosteal grafting was combined with an opening of the subchondral space permitting cells from the marrow to invade the defects. The number of these pluripotential stem cells seem to decline drastically in the mature periosteum compared to in an immature periosteal graft and O'Driscoll et al. [36] showed that adult periosteum regenerated a repair tissue in adult rabbits that had only 15% type II collagen compared for 93% in the adolescent group. This is important to consider since in most studies of periosteal grafting the animals have been adolescent and the grafting procedures have been combined with an opening into the bone marrow cavity containing pluripotent mesenchymal cells the number of which also decreases steadily with age.

Poussa et al. [37] found that periosteum transplanted as a free graft in the rabbit knee joint formed a cartilaginous body without any bone formation. Rubak et al. [38] used periosteum to treat cartilage defects in the rabbit knee with success and the repair was described as hyaline-like. Similar animal studies regarding the chondrogenic potential of the periosteum have been made by Salter and O'Driscoll and co-workers [36, 39, 40]. They have studied the periosteum as a free graft in the joint and as graft for the repair of rabbit trochlear groove defects as well as for rabbit full thickness patellar chondral defects. They developed the concept of continuous passive motion for resurfacing with periosteal grafts and were able to show that there was a significant higher degree of chondrogenesis in the grafts in continuous passive motion-knees compared to immobilized knees [40]. They also showed that the results were dependent on the orientation of the graft and the age of the animal. Grafting with the cambium layer, rich in mesenchymal multipotential stem cells with osteochondrogenic potential, facing into the joint resulted in the best repair compared to those with the cambium layer facing towards the subchondral bone. The repair quality was also better in adolescent animals compared to in adult animals. The repair could withstand wear up to 1 year post-surgery without any detorioration of the grafted tissue [36].

Vachon et al. [41] used periosteal autografts for repair of large osteochondral defects in 10 horses aged 2 to 3 years old. In each horse, osteochondral defects measuring $1.0 \times 1.0 \text{ cm}^2$ were created bilaterally on the distal articular surface of each radial carpal bone. Control and experimental defects were drilled. Periosteum was harvested from the proximal portion of the tibia and was glued into the defects, using a fibrin adhesive. Control defects were glued, but were not grafted. Sixteen weeks after the grafting procedure, the quality of the repair tissue of control and grafted defects was assessed biochemically. All biochemical variables were compared with those of normal equine articular cartilage taken from the same site in another group of clinically normal horses. The biochemical composition of repair tissue of grafted and nongrafted defects was similar, but clearly differed from that of normal articular cartilage.

In clinical studies Niedermann et al. [42] presented 5 patients with osteochondral defects that were treated with periosteal resurfacing with an excellent result. The defects were drilled subchondrally prior to grafting and the grafts were fixed with fibrin-glue. Hoikka et al. [43] treated 13 patients (mean age 36 years) with patellar chondral defects with free periosteal grafts and followed them for a mean 4 years. The cambium layer faced the subchondral bone and the periosteum was sutured or glued into the defect. 11 patients reached what was called an "acceptable" niveau post-surgery. Korkkala and Hukkanen [44] used free, autogenous periosteal grafts to treat six patients, three with acute traumatic patellar cartilage lesions and three with local sclerotic osteochondritis of the medial femoral condyle. The treatment resulted in satisfactory results with symptomatic amelioration, 14 to 59 months after the procedures. Fourteen patients with osteochondritis dissecans of the femoral condyle (mean size 4 cm^2) treated with periosteal transplantation were reviewed by Angermann and Riegels-Nielsen in 1994. The patients were followed for 1 year and then 43% were free of symptoms. In 29% of the patients defect was reduced in size radiographically while 64% were unchanged. Lorentzen [45] reported from 25 patients with a mean age of 31.4 years that after mean 42 months with periosteal resurfacing and multiple drilling of patellar full cartilage thickness defects 16 patients were graded as excellent and that the remaining 9 patients were graded as good. Five randomly selected cases were biopsied and all were described as showing normal hyaline cartilage. It was pressed that meticulous surgical technique as well as rigorous post-operative continuous passive motion regimen is of outmost importance for a successful outcome of the surgery. The importance of experience to harvest the periosteum has been pointed about often by O'Driscoll who also is currently directing a multi-surgeon randomized, controlled, prospective, partially-blinded clinical trial at the Mayo Clinic of periosteal arthroplasty to treat chondral and osteochondral defects more than 1 cm in size in the knee joint (Fig. 2 C).

Skoog et al. [46] described the potential for the cells in the perichondrium to produce neocartilage with the potential to repair cartilage defects. This evoked an interest for the perichondrium and several animal studies have been done to confirm the chondrogenic potential of the perichondrium [47, 48]. Homminga and al. [49] treated pure chondral lesions in young rabbits with the epiphyses still open with perichondrium and noted hyaline-like repair on the grafted areas. They also found that it might be important to leave the subchondral bone intact while it could play an important role in preventing cartilage degeneration and referred to the studies of Radin and Rose [50].

Amiel et al. [48] reconstructed full thickness cartilage defects in the rabbit knee with rib perichondrium and noted that the differentiation of this basic tissue into a hyaline repair was dependent on extrinsic influences emanating from the environment. They suggested that the presence of motion, low oxygen tension and absence of vascularity could favor hyalinization of the repair. However, despite the initially promising results from periosteal and perichondral graftings, the long-term durability of these grafts still remains uncertain as have shown by Engkvist et al. [51] when they resurfaced patellar cartilage defects in the dogs with perichondrium. Two to eight months post-surgery the repair was of hyaline-character but between 12–17 months post-surgery the graft-tissue degenerated leaving areas of exposed bone bare. However it is important to notice that the results in long-term follow-ups are dependent of the site that has been treated.

Regarding the beneficial results with periosteum and continuous passive motions, few results regarding continuous passive motions and perichondrium have been reported. Kwan et al. [52] reported that continuous passive motions did not improve the quality of the repair tissue when evaluated one year post-surgery compared to free cage activity.

The clinical use of perichondrium to resurface cartilage defects was first described for the wrist and finger joints in human patients [53]. Homminga et al. [54] used autologous costal perichondrium to treat 30 chondral knee defects in patients with mean age of 31. Twenty-five patients were evaluated by arthroscopy 1 year post-surgery, 14 patients were reevaluated at 2 years postoperatively when it was found that 27 of 30 defects had healed with a tissue resembling cartilage. Three biopsies showed a hyaline like morphology. In a later follow-up in a larger study group, 20% of the patients in the Homminga series suffered graft failure and only 40% of the patients had good results after 8 years [55]. Beckers et al. [56] analyzed their result after perichondrial resurfacing for cartilage defects in the knee joint. After a mean follow-up of 32 months, of 80 studied patients, 42 patients were classified as failures and lost grafts. Failure occured at an average of 18 months after the operation, especially in patients with diagnosis of osteoarthritis. In the patella, the results were worse if the defect had previously been drilled. The results were better in young persons; mean age 27 years in the success group compared to 34 years in the failure group. They concluded that the perichondrial grafts should be used for osteochondritis dissecans and early post-traumatic cartilage defects in young persons. Also other authors have found that perichondrial resurfacing seems to be more successful in fairly young patients with posttraumatic defects of the articular cartilage [57]. Graft fixation and graft calcification are major problems in perichondrial grafting and could be responsible for a poor clinical outcome.

Vachon et al. [58] compared the repair effect of perichondral and periosteal grafts on cartilage defects in 6 young horses (2–4 years old). Periosteal autografts were obtained from the medial aspect of the proximal portion of the tibia, and perichondrial autografts were obtained from the sternum. Using arthroscopic visualization, each autograft was placed as a loose body into 1 tarsocrural joint in the horse. The animals were hand-walked daily, starting the day after surgery, for a total of 6 h/wk for 8 weeks. Eight weeks after autograft implantation, radiographs were taken of each tarsocrural joint and were interpreted with regard to mineralization in the transplanted autografts. Grafts were then surgically removed, and examined macroscopically and microscopically for viability, size, and production of chondroid tissue. All autografts appeared viable and most showed evidence of growth. Neochondrogenesis was observed in 5 of 6 periosteal grafts and in 1 of 6 perichondrial grafts. Furthermore, the amount of chondroid tissue produced in periosteal autografts was significantly greater than that produced in the 1 perichondrial graft. The chondroid tissue produced by periosteal autografts had morphologic and matrical staining properties similar to those of hyaline cartilage

A common finding both in animals or in humans is that the grafts produce the best results in young individuals and in traumatic defects. The fact that the number of potential repair cells in any graft declines steadily with age could be one explanation of these effects.

9.6
Cell-Transplantation

It is possible to differentiate between two types of repair with cells: *intrinsic repair* means a replication of chondrocytes from the area adjacent to the defect site while *extrinsic repair* consist of a metaplasia of chondrocytes from other cell types such as connective-tissue stem-cells i.e subchondral marrow cells, synovial cells [59].

Cell transplantation has for a long time been explored as an alternative to other types of repair methods. The cells could be harvested autologously or as allografts from a healthy part of the donor tissue, isolated, expanded *in vitro* and finally implanted into the defect site in high densities. Pure chondrocytes, epiphyseal or mature, allogeneic or autologous as well as other types of mesenchymal cells have been used.

In 1965 Smith [60] perfected the isolation of chondrocytes and chondrocytes were thereafter able to be grown using standard culture methods. Chestermann and Smith [61] isolated chondrocytes from rabbit cartilage and those cells were then transplanted into cartilage defects in the humerus of adult sister rabbits. The defects healed but no hyaline cartilage was found. Bentley and Green [62] transplanted isolated articular cartilage chondrocytes and epiphyseal chondrocytes from young rabbits to cartilage defects on adult rabbits of the same inbreed. A nice repair with hyaline like neocartilage was described in more than 50 % of the defects.

Green [63] reported a significant better repair after heterologous chondrocyte transplantation of chondral lesions of the rabbit knee. Autoradiography confirmed that the implanted isolated chondrocytes were responsible for the repair and three generations of transplanted chondrocytes could be identified by the decrease in intensity in nuclear labelling. Bentley et al. [64] transplanted isolated epiphyseal chondrocytes as allografts into rabbit knee tibial drill holes. Cells were pipetted into the defects with a success rate of 47 % of the defects repaired. Ashton and Bentley [65] compared allografts of intact cartilage, isolated chondrocytes and cultured chondrocytes from the epiphyseal growth-plate and articular surface from immature rabbits inserted into full thickness defects in mature rabbits. Both intact articular cartilage as well as intact epiphyseal growth-plates induced significantly better repair vs controls. Cultured chondrocytes also produced a significantly better repair than when the defects were left ungrafted in arthritic joints.

Yoshihashi [66] studied isolated articular chondrocytes in comparison with normal articular cartilage and used chondrocytes that were released by enzymatic digestion from slices of articular cartilage taken from 8 week old white rabbits. The isolated cells were inoculated in a large number into a 0.28 cm^2 stainless cylinder on a Millipore filter. After 12 hours these chondrocytes were layered by gravity onto the Millipore filter and were cultured in the same medium during 7 days. Subsequently the cell aggregate was transferred to an organ culture system and was fed every other day. Aggregates of cells were sampled at 1, 2, 4, 8, 12 weeks in culture for morphological and biochemical studies. The results obtained were as follows: after one week in culture, deposition of metachromatic matrix was observed under a light microscope only at the periphery of the aggregate of cells. Matrix formation in the whole aggregate occurred after 2 weeks in culture. The tissue reformed in this culture consisted of metachromatic hyaline cartilage like matrix and chondrocytes within lacunae but for cells at the surface arranged in a tangential flattened layer. The collagen in this tissue was of type II mixed with a very small amount of type I. The tissue reconstituted *in vitro* by freshly isolated chondrocytes had characteristics of hyaline cartilage except over the surface. Compared with normal articular cartilage, the cells in this tissue were distributed more randomly and the intercellular hyaline matrix was poor under a light microscope, and collagen fibrils in the matrix observed under an electron microscope were much thinner than those of normal articular cartilage. This method provides a tissue culture model of cartilage organization.

Wakitani and associates [67] implanted osteochondral progenitor cells from the periosteum and bone marrow cells-mesenchymal stem cells into the femoral condyle cartilage defects of rabbit knees. Those cells were preferred opposed to chondrocytes because they were said to be capable of a broader range of chondrogenic expression and that they may recapitulate the embryonic lineage transitions originally involved in the formation of joint tissue. No difference between the bone-marrow cells and the periosteum-derived cells was seen and the best scores were seen at 4 weeks. At twelve weeks the subchondral bone plate was restituted. There was a gap between the host cartilage and the neocartilage but the underlying bone was almost completely united with that of the host.

Goldberg and Caplan [68] compared implantation of mature chondrocytes, so called committed, with mesenchymal stem cells for the repair of full thickness defects in the femoral condyles of adult rabbits. Both cell types repaired the defect with a hyaline-like neocartilage. However the mesenchymal stemcell repair had a more hyaline-like morphology and cartilage zonal characteristics than the repair from the committed chondrocytes. They hypothesized that the open subchondral bone releases host-derived bioactive factors like different growth-factors and cytokines that could influence the biologic properties of the mesenchymal stem cells but not of the already differentiated chondrocytes.

Robinson et al. [69] implanted chondrocytes derived from chick embryos into defects of articular surfaces of young and old adult chickens. The embryonal chondrocytes underwent an accelerated aging process in the old chickens implying that the maturation stages within the implant were shorter in the old animals leading to a shorter healing time.

The above reported cell transplantations have been allografts. The chondrocyte have transplanation antigenes and these cells can theoretically participate in immunological reactions. The cartilage matrix acts as a protective barrier [23]. Kawabe and Yoshinao [70] studied the immune responses to reparative tissue formed by allogeneic growth plate chondrocyte implants. The neocartilage yielded by implantation of these cells into cartilage defects of adult rabbits looked very good in the beginning but began to degenerate two to three weeks after implantation partially because of humoral immune response but also because of cell-mediated cytotoxicity. Host lymphocytes were seen around the allograft at 2–12 weeks.

Lars Peterson and co-workers [71] in 1982 developed a rabbit model to treat cartilage defects in the rabbit patella with autologous *in vitro* expanded chondrocytes and with that model using the knee joints of adult rabbits Grande and co-workers [72] examined the effect of autologous chondrocytes grown *in vitro* on the healing rate of chondral defects not penetrating the subchondral bone plate. To determine whether any of the reconstituted cartilage resulted from the chondrocyte graft an experiment was conducted involving grafts with chondrocytes that had been labeled prior to grafting with a nuclear tracer. Results were evaluated using both qualitative and quantitative light microscopy. Macroscopic results from grafted specimens displayed a marked decrease in synovitis and other degenerative changes. In defects that had received transplants, a significant amount of cartilage was reconstituted (82%) compared to ungrafted controls (18%). Autoradiography on reconstituted cartilage showed that there were labeled cells incorporated into the repair matrix.

The same rabbit model has since then been used and further developed by a group at the Göteborg University. The cultured cells are injected into a premade cartilage defect of the patella of the rabbit and covered with a flap of periosteum, functioning as a biological membrane. This method resulted in a high degree of healed rabbit patellar defects and the repair tissue had a similarity to the original cartilaginous tissue [73]. In october 1987 the technique was first used to treat patients with chronic disabling symptoms of the knee joint with cultured cartilage cells from their own cartilage (Fig. 2 D). The first 23 patients (mean age 27) were presented in the New England Journal of Medicine in 1994 [74].Those patients had local deep cartilage injuries that had been treated with conventional methods without any healing and 16 defects were located on the so called femoral surface and 7 on the patella. In all, 16 patients had "good" or "excellent" knee function at mean three years postoperatively. The best results were found in the femoral group compared with the patella patients that were less successful. The technique appeared to be most successful in patients that had injuries on the femoral surfaces producing a single, localized deep cartilage lesion. This is important to note as opposed to the gradual wear and tear of advancing age. The disappointing outcome of the patella group might have resulted from mechanical misalignements of the patella that were not corrected at the time of transplant surgery.

A new reexamination was done in 1996 on 92 patients with a follow-up between 2–9 years. There was a high percentage of good to excellent results in patients with single femoral condyle lesions (24 patients, 92%) and in patients with osteochondritis dissecans (19 patients, 89%) whereas 75% good to excellent results were obtained in patients with femoral condyle lesions and a concomitant anterior cruciate injury and ligament reconstruction (16 patients). Twenty-one patellar patients with 62% improved and multiple lesions (12 patients) with 75% improved. Twenty-six patients were biopsied and 80% of the biopsies showed a hyaline-like appearance.

In 1995 a randomized controlled multi-center study has started to compare multiple subchondral drilling of the cartilage injury with treatments with a periosteum with or without implantation of the patients own cultured cartilage cells. In August 1997 in the USA the Food and Drug Administration approved the cell technology that uses a patient's own chondrocytes to repair cartilage injuries in the knee. This was the first type of cell technology that have been regulated for the industry of manipulated autologous structure guidance.

9.7
Scaffolds in Cartilage Repair

A scaffold is a material from which the repair cells can receive directions for tissue engineering and the produced tissue will thus have the shape of the original scaffold. Ideally the scaffold should provide a temporary framework until the repair cells have produced its own matrix. Both biologic and synthetic matrices (collagen and fibrin gels, decalcified bone, polyglycolic acids, ceramics and carbon fibers) have been used for the induced repair of cartilage injuries.

The different types of scaffolds can be populated by cells before the introduction into the cartilage defect or the cells may migrate into the scaffold after the implantation. The scaffolds may also function to maintain the cells in the defect after implantation and they could be used together with chondrogenetic factors like TGF-β. Allograft cells or autologous cells can be used. Experimental studies suggest that use of scaffolds may enhance the quality of the repair tissue [75].

A three-dimensional culture system for cultured chondrocytes acts as a template for growth and could hence contribute to phenotypic stability of chondrocytes

The cells that have been used in the scaffolds have varied: allogenic or autologous cells of mesenchymal origin. Muckle and Minns [75] used a meshwork of woven carbon fibers to treat osteochondral defects in rats and rabbits as well as in human osteoarthritic knees (Fig. 1C). Articular cartilage defects were resurfaced with cells from the bone marrow producing a fibrocartilaginous tissue. Seventy-seven percent out of 47 patients had a satisfactory result 3 years after surgery. Similar results with carbon fibre resurfacing was presented by Brittberg et al. [76] with 37 patients classified as having early osteoarthritis of the knee joint. Eighty-three percent of 36 patients followed for 4 years post-surgery had an significant improvement. Recently, Haddad et al. [77] reported on 101 patients (mean age 31 years) with a mean follow-up of 5 years that had been treated with carbon fibre pads in the knee joint. Fifty-three percent of the patellar resurfaced patients were improved while 83% of the femoral condyle lesions had satisfactory results. The long-term outcome with these carbon scaffolds has to be evaluated with randomized studies that are planned as a multi-center international study.

The first to report the use of a matrix for chondrocyte grafting was Itay and collegues [78] that used embryonic chondrocytes in a gel to treat cartilage defects in roosters. They used a resorbable gel with fibrin glue that maintained the transferred chondrocytes within the defects.

Vacanti et al. [79] used biodegradable polyglycolic acid polymers seeded with chondrocytes to resurface joint cartilage defects in the rabbit knee and the treatment resulted in hyaline repair in a high percentage after 7 weeks.

Wakitani and associates [67] used osteochondral progenitor cells to repair large, full-thickness defects of the articular cartilage that had been created in the knees of rabbits. Adherent cells from bone marrow, or cells from the periosteum that had been liberated from connective tissue by collagenase digestion, were grown in culture, dispersed in a type-I collagen gel, and transplanted into three-by-six-millimeter full-thickness defect in the medial femoral condyle. The contralateral knee served as a control. As early as two weeks after transplantation, the autologous osteochondral progenitor cells had uniformly differentiated into chondrocytes throughout the defects and there was no apparent difference between the results obtained with the cells from the bone marrow and those from the periosteum. Twenty-four weeks after transplantation, the reparative tissue of both the bone-marrow and the periosteal cells was stiffer and less compliant than the tissue derived from the empty defects but less stiff and more compliant than normal cartilage. Freed and co-workers [80] used matrices of polyglycolic acids with or without seeded allograft chondrocytes to resurface cartilage defects in the rabbit trochlear groove. The histological score were similar in the experimental groups at 6 months and higher than what has been reported for self-repair in which identical defects were left empty for six months. However, the total contents of glycosaminoglycans and collagen was only one third of that of parent rabbit cartilage.

9.8
Decrease of the Loads of Repair and/or Degenerated Cartilage

One of the theories behind the development of osteoarthritis is that mechanical overload of an articular compartment produces microfractures in the subchondral bone which may lead to an increasing bone stiffness and a subsequent risk for progress of osteoarthritic disease [50]. To achieve an unloading it is possible to do a division of the bone adjacent to the diseased compartment: a so called angular or rotational osteotomy. Most commonly seen for the knee joint. Theories behind the use of osteotomy are:
- there could be a venous congestion subchondrally causing the pain and experimental studies have shown that an osteotomy could changes the intraosseous pressure and eventually give pain relief [81]
- the realignment may take the unfavourable pressure of the diseased area and distribute the pressure more evenly. This may even allow a stimulation to some type of repair of the diseased cartilage [82].

Clinically, Tippett [83] presented the results from a combined operative procedure for treating unicompartmental osteoarthritis with subchondral drilling and a rotational dome osteotomy. Satisfactory results occured in 90% of the patients. However, Akizuki et al. [84] presented a study where patients with osteoarthritic knees were divided into a group of 51 knees treated with abrasion arthroplasty and osteotomy and another group of 37 knees that were treated with osteotomy alone. The first group showed a significantly better local repair of affected area but there was no difference between the groups in the clinical outcome at 2 to 9 years postoperatively.

Nagel et al. [85] found that it seems that the results regarding activity level after tibial osteotomies is generally lower than the preoperative level and than gradually decreases with time. They suggested that tibial osteotomies could be recommanded for patients less than 60 years of age, relatively preoperatively active and with a wish to in future participate in activities with stresses of impact loading across the affected joint, not suitable for a prostheses. Only one randomized study with tibial osteotomies compared with arthroplasties has been found [86]. They found no difference between a group of high tibial osteotomy and unicompartmental knee arthroplasty 1 year post-surgery but both group were improved. Two retrospective, comparative studies between osteotomy and unicompartmental arthroplasty showed results for the unicompartmental replacement as significantly better after 5–17 years [87, 88]. The technical skill of the performing surgeon is a critical factor as well as the surgeon ability to select the most suitable patient for osteotomy.

9.9
Resection and Interpositional-Arthroplasties

A way to eliminate large destroyed articular cartilage areas is to excise the diseased part and let the bare bone ends be kept apart to let the blood clot formation organize into a fibrocartilaginous tissue. These methods can give quite substantial pain relief however to the sacrifice of joint stability. Examples of resection or excision arthroplasties are resection of the acromio-clavicular joint and first metatarsophalangeal joint resection, resection arthroplasty for a failed hip fracture.

To get a better stability the resection arthroplasties may be combined with an interposition of soft tissues like fascia, tendons, muscle and adiposal tissues. An example is the interposition with tendon flexor carpi radialis after basal joint resection of the thumb metacarpal joint for degenerative osteoarthritis [89]. Pain relief is noted but loss of strength in pinch-grip. Fascia lata has been used as an alternative to arthrodesis in young patients with post-infectious destroyed articular cartilage in the knee joint and with good functional results reported 25–35 years post-interpositional surgery [90]. As in most biological articular resurfacing the results seem to be most successful in younger patients.

9.10
Artificial Joint Arthroplasties

The modern ideas of joint-replacement have their origin in the Smith-Peterson cup arthroplasty followed by the Charnley concept [91] of using polymethyl-acrylate as a fixator between the subchondral bone plate and the artificial material. An arthroplasty could be an excisional, partial or total one and the material could be of biological as well as of artificial origin. The total joint arthroplasty must be considered as a definitive treatment, and as the failure of an arthroplasty risk to result in a less than optimal function other types of less definite procedures must carefully be considered first. However, total arthroplasties are nowadays highly reliable and have reported good to excellent results in more than 90% of the cases and survival rates of 90–95% at ten years. The relief of pain and improved joint function seem to be almost very predictable and for elderly people a very safe and secure method when suffering from a moderate to severe osteoarthritis. In younger, active patients wear and loosening of the prosthetic components is a problem and the focus is the interface between the cement and underlying bone. This means that here the alternative techniques described for more local cartilage defects may have a place in the future and that explains the explosion of research for reliable biological articular resurfacing methods.

9.11
Arthrodesis

A final solution to severe cartilage injuries and osteoarthritis is to eliminate the destroyed joint surfaces and induce bony fusion, arthrodesis. Any joint can be fused and the pain relief and stability will be paid by loss of movements. Some joints as the first metatarsophalangeal joint can be fused without great disadvantages while others like the knee and hip-joint will cause significant disadvantages for the patient. The word arthrodesis is for many patients an ugly word and a lot of patients refuse to be operated with such an operation even though they suffer from considerable joint pain.

However, arthrodesis is still a method to consider especially in young active patients with severe cartilaginous surface injuries and especially when there is a concomitant subchondral bone loss.

9.12
Discussion and Future Perspectives

Animal experiments as well as clinical studies have shown that with a variety of operative techniques it is possible to stimulate a repair of chondral and osteochondral defects with a cartilaginous tissue. However, there still are no prospective, randomized studies evaluating the effectiveness of the different treatments and a lot of research is needed to learn the best way of perfecting a cartilage regeneration. It is also difficult to transfer a technique that is primarily developed to treat a local cartilage defect to an organ failure like ostearthritis. It has been said that it is unlikely that any of the different cartilage repair methods will be generally successful; structural and functional abnormalities of the diseased joint as well as the patients expectations and demands of the activity level will decide the surgeons treatment plan [92]. The surgeon is responsible for maintaining his/hers professional skills as well as acquiring new knowledge in clinical work. At the same time, the surgeon is obliged to look upon the new developments in each clinical field critically. To prevent a disease seems more attractive than to cure an already developed disease and therefore it is of great importance to find out if an early surgical treatment of a cartilage injury could prevent a progression into a more widespread disease, osteoarthritis.

The future of treatment could be found in a bioengineering approach, programming cells or tissues to respond and regenerate cartilage and subchondral bone. The increasing knowledge about the use of growth factors and the possibility to use genetic transduction procedures to induce the different musculoskeletal cells to secrete factors stimulating repair or inhibiting destructive cytokines will let us combine pure instrumental orthopaedic surgery with the highest technology of biochemistry; for future treatment of cartilaginous and other types of musculoskeletal injuries *biomedical surgery* will be the new concept.

References

1. O'Connor BL, Brandt KD (1993) Neurogenic factors in the ethiopathogenesis of osteoarthritis. Rheum Dis N Am 19:581–604
2. Burman MS, Finkelstein H, Mayer L (1934) Arthroscopy of the knee joint. J Bone Joint Surg 16: 255–268
3. Haggart GE (1941) Surgical treatment of degenerative arthritis of the knee joint. J Bone Joint Surg 22 (Br):717
4. Magnuson PB (1941) Joint debridement, surgical treatment of degenerative arthritis. Surg Gynecol Obstet 73:1–9
5. Bentley G, Dowd G (1984) Current concepts of etiology and treatment of chondromalacia patellae. Clin Orthrop 189:209–228
6. Buckwalter JA, Lohmander S (1994) Operative treatment of osteoarthritis: Current practice and future development. J Bone Joint Surg 76 (Am):1405–1418
7. Aichroth PM, Patel DV, Moyes ST (1991) A prospective review of arthroscopic debridement for degenerative joint disease of the knee. Int Orthop 15:351–355
8. Livesley PJ, Doherty M, Needoff M, Moulton A (1991) Arthroscopic lavage of osteoarthritic knees. J Bone Joint Surg 73 (Br):922–926
9. Gibson JN, White MD, Chapman VM, Strachan RK (1992) Arthroscopic lavage and debridement for osteoarthritis of the knee. J Bone Joint Surg 74 (Br):534–537
10. Chang RW, Falconer J, Stulberg SD, Arnold WJ, Manheim LM, Dyer AR (1993) A randomized, controlled trial of arthroscopic surgery versus closed-needle joint lavage for patients with osteoarthritis of the knee joint. Arthritis Rheum 36:289–296
11. Moseley JB, Wray NP, Kuykendall D, Willis K, Landon G (1996) Arthroscopic treatment of osteoarthritis of the knee: A prospective, randomized, placebo-controlled trial. Am J Sports Med 24:28–34
12. Pridie KH (1959) A method of resurfacing osteoarthritic knee joints. J Bone Joint Surg 41 (Br):618–619
13. Ficat RP, Ficat C, Gedeon PK, Toussaint JB (1979) Spongialization: A new treatment for diseased patellae. Clin Orthop 144:74–83

14. Steadman PB, Pegg SP (1992) A quantitative assessment of blood loss in burn wound excision and grafting. Burn 18:490–491
15. Johnson LL (1986) Arthroscopic abrasion arthroplasty. Historical and pathologic perspective: Present status. Arthroscopy 2:54–59
16. Friedman MJ, Berasi DO, Fox JM, del Pizzo W, Snyder SJ, Ferkel RD (1984) Preliminary results with abrasion arthroplasty in the osteoarthritic knee. Clin Orthop 182:200–206
17. Buckwalter JA, Mow VC (1994) Cartilage repair in osteoarthritis. In: Moskowitz RW, Howell DS, Goldberg VM, Mankin HJ (eds) Osteoarthritis. Diagnosis and medical/surgical management. WB Saunders, 2 edn, Philadelphia, pp 71–108
18. Salisbury RB, Mc Mahon MR (1994) Joint debridement and abrasion arthroplasty for degenerative joint disease of the knee joint. In: Parisien SJ (ed) Current techniques in arthroscopy. Current Medicine, Philadelphia: pp 147–167
19. Bert JM, Maschka K (1989) The arthroscopic treatment of unicompartmental gonarthrosis: a five-year follow-up study of abrasion arthroplasty plus arthroscopic debridement and arthroscopic debridement alone. Arthroscopy 5:25–32
20. Goldman RT, Scuderi GR, Kelly MA (1997) Arthroscopic treatment of the degenerative knee in older athletes. Clin Sports Med 16:51–68
21. Menche DS, Frenkel SR, Blair B, Watnik NF, Toolan BC, Yaghoubian RS, Pitman MI (1996) A comparison of abrasion arthroplasty and subchondral drilling in the treatment of full thickness cartilage lesions in the rabbit. Arthroscopy 12:280–286
22. Stone KR, Walgenbach AW (1997) Surgical technique and initial results for articular cartilage transplantation to traumatic and arthritic defects in the knee joint. In: Abstracts of the 2nd Fribourg International Symposium on cartilage repair, Fribourg, Switzerland: p 52
23. Elves MW (1974) A study of the transplantation antigenes on chondrocytes from articular cartilage. J Bone Joint Surg 56 (Br):178–185
24. Mc Dermott AG, Langer F, Pritzker KP, Gross AE (1985) Fresh small-fragment osteochondral allografts. Long-term follow-up study on the first 100 cases. Clin Orthop 197:96–102
25. Zukor DJ, Gross AE (1989) Osteochondral allograft reconstruction of the knee. Part 1: A review. Am J Knee Surg 2:139–149
26. Mahomed MN, Beaver RJ, Gross AE (1992) The long-term success of fresh, small-fragment osteochondral allografts used for intra-articular post-traumatic defects in the knee joint. Orthopaedics 15:1191–1199
27. Ghazavi MT, Pritzker KP, Davis AM, Gross AE (1997) Fresh osteochondral allografts for post-traumatic osteochondral defects of the knee. J Bone Joint Surg 79 (Br):1008–1013
28. Mankin HJ, Fogelson FS, Trasher A (1976) Massive resection and allograft transplantation in the treatment of malignant tumours. N Engl J Med 294:1247–1255
29. Stevenson S, Li XQ, Martin B (1991) The fate of cancellous and cortical bone after transplantation of fresh and frozen tissue-antigen-matched osteochondral allografts in dogs. J Bone Joint Surg 73 (Am):1143–1156
30. Wagner H (1964) Operative Behandlung der Osteochondrosis dissecans der Kniegelenke. Zeitschr Orthop 98:333–355
31. Yamashita F, Sakakida K, Suzu F, Takai S (1985) The transplantation of an autogeneic osteochondral fragment for osteochondritis dissecans of the knee. Clin Orthop 201: 43–50
32. Outerbridge HK, Outerbridge AR, Outerbridge RE (1995) The use of lateral patellar autologous graft for the repair of a large osteochondral defect in the knee. J Bone Joint Surg 77 (Am):65–72
33. Matsusue Y, Yamamuro T, Hiromichi H (1993) Case report. Arthroscopic multiple osteochondral transplantation to the chondral defect in the knee associated with anterior cruciate ligament disruption. Arthroscopy 9:318–321
34. Bobic V (1996) Arthroscopic osteochondral autograft transplantation in anterior cruciate ligament reconstruction: a preliminary clinical study. Knee Surg Sports Traumatol Arthrosc 3:262–264
35. Hangody L, Kish G, Karpati Z, Szerb I, Udvarhelyi I (1997) Arthroscopic osteochondral mosaic plasty for the treatment of femoral condylar articular defects. A preliminary report. Knee Surg Sports Traumatol Arthrosc 5:262–267

36. O'Driscoll SW, Keeley FW, Salter RB (1988) Durability of regenerated articular cartilage produced by free autogenous periosteal grafts in major full thickness defects in joint surfaces under the influence of continuous passive motion. J Bone Joint Surg 70 (Am):595–606

37. Poussa M, Rubak J, Ritsilä V (1981) Differentiation of the osteochondrogenic cells of the periosteum in chondrotrophic environment. Acta Orthop Scand 52: 235–239

38. Rubak J, Poussa M, Ritsilä V (1982) Chondrogenesis in repair of articular cartilage defects by free periosteal grafts in rabbits. Acta Orthop Scand 53:181–186

39. Salter RB, Simmonds DF, Malcolm BW, Rumble EJ, McMichael D, Clements NDF (1980) The biological effect of continuous passive motion on the healing of full thickness defects in articular cartilage. An experimental investigation in the rabbits. J Bone Joint Surg 62 (Am): 1232–1251

40. O'Driscoll SW, Salter RB (1984) The induction of neochondrogenesis in free intra-articular periosteal autografts under the influence of continuous passive motion. J Bone Joint Surg 66 (Am):1248–1257

41. Vachon AM, McIlwraight CW, Keeley FW (1991) Biochemical study of repair of induced osteochondral defects of the distal portion of the radial carpal bone in horses by use of periosteal autografts. Am J Vet Res 52:328–332

42. Niedermann B, Boe S, Lauritzen J, Rubak JM (1985) Glued periosteal grafts in the knee. Acta Orthop Scand 56:457–460

43. Hoikka VEJ, Jaroma HJ, Ritsilä VA (1990) Reconstruction of the patellar articulation with periosteal grafts. Acta Orthop Scand 61:36–39

44. Korkkala O, Hukkanen H (1991) Autogenous osteoperiosteal grafts in the reconstruction of full thickness joint surface defects. Int Orthop 15:233–237

45. Lorentzon R (1997) Treatment of deep cartilage defects in the knee with periosteum transplantation. In: Abstracts of the 2nd Fribourg International Symposium on cartilage repair, Fribourg, Switzerland: p 77

46. Skoog T, Ohlsén L, Sohn A (1972) Perichondral potential for cartilaginous regeneration. Scand J Plast Rec Surg 6:123–125

47. Engkvist O, Ohlsén L (1979) Reconstruction of articular cartilage with free autologous perichondrial grafts. An experimental study in rabbits. Scand J Plast Reconstr Surg 13:269–274

48. Amiel D, Coutts RD, Abel M, Stewart W, Harwood F, Akeson WH (1985) Rib perichondrial grafts for the repair of full thickness articular cartilage defects. A morphological and biochemical study in the rabbits. J Bone Joint Surg 67 (Am):911–920

49. Homminga GH, van der Linden TJ, Terwindt-Rouwenhorst WAW, Drukker J (1989) Repair of articular cartilage defects by perichondral grafts. Experiments in the rabbit. Acta Orthop Scand 60:326–329.

50. Radin EL, Rose RM (1986) Role of the subchondral bone in the initiation and progression of cartilage damage. Clin Orthop 213:34–40

51. Engkvist O (1979) Reconstruction of patellar articular cartilage with free autologous perichondrial grafts. Scand J Plast Reconstr Surg 13:361–369

52. Kwan MK, Woo SL-Y, Amiel D, Kleiner JB, Field FP, Coutts RD (1987) Neocartilage generated from rib perichondrium: A long-term multidisciplinary evaluation. Trans Orthop Res Soc 12:277

53. Pascaldi P, Engkvist O (1979) Perichondrial wrist arthroplasty in rheumatoid patients. Hand 11:184–190

54. Homminga G, Bulstra SK, Bouwmeester PSM, van der Linden AJ (1990) Perichondral grafting for cartilage lesions of the knee. J Bone Joint Surg 72 (Br):1003–1007

55. Brittberg M, Lindahl A, Homminga G, Nilsson A, Isakssson O, Peterson L (1997) A critical analysis of cartilage repair. Acta Ortop Scand 68:186–191

56. Beckers JMH, Bulstra SK, Kuijer R, Bouwmeester SJM, van der Linden AJ (1992) Analysis of the clinical results after perichondral transplantation for cartilage defects of the human knee. Abstracts from the 19th symposium of the ESOA-Joint Destruction and osteoarthritis, Nordwijkerhout, Netherlands: p 157

57. Seradge H, Kutz JA, Kleinert HE, Lister GD, Wolff TW, Atasoy E (1984) Perichondral resurfacing arthroplasty in the hand. J Hand Surg 9 A:880–886

58. Vachon AM, McIlwright CW, Trotter GW, Nordin RW, Powers BE (1989) Neochondrogenesis in free intra-articular, periosteal and perichondrial autografts in horses. Am J Vet Res 50: 1787–94

59. Sokoloff L (1974) Cell biology and the repair of articular cartilage. J Rheumatology 1:1–10

60. Smith AV (1965) Survival of frozen chondrocytes isolated from cartilage of adult animals. Nature 205:782–784

61. Chestermann PJ, Smith AU (1968) Homotransplatation of articular cartilage and isolated chondrocytes. J Bone Joint Surg 50 (Br):184–197

62. Bentley G, Greer RB (1971) Homotransplantation of isolated epiphyseal and articular chondrocytes into joint surfaces. Nature 230:385–388

63. Green WT (1977) Articular cartilage repair, behaviour of rabbit chondrocytes during tissue culture and subsequent allografting. Clin Orthop 124:237–250

64. Bentley G, Smith AV, Mukerjhee R (1979) Isolated epiphyseal chondrocyte allografts into joint surfaces. Ann Rheum Dis 37:449–458

65. Ashton JE, Bentley G (1986) Repair of articular surfaces by allografts of articular and growth-plate cartilage. J Bone Joint Surg 68 (Br):29–34

66. Yoshihashi Y (1983) Tissue reconstitution by isolated articular chondrocytes *in vitro*. Nippon-Seikeigeka-Gakkai-Zasshi 57:629–641

67. Wakitani S, Goto T, Pineda SJ, Toung RG, Mansour JM, Caplan AI, Goldberg VM (1994) Mesenchymal cell-based repair of large, full thickness defects of articular cartilage. J Bone Joint Surg 76 (Am):579–592

68. Goldberg VM, Caplan AI (1994) Cellular repair of articular cartilage. In: Kuettner KE, Goldberg VM (eds) Osteoarthritic disorders. Am Acad Orthop Surg, Monterrey: pp 357–364

69. Robinson D, Halperin N, Nevo Z (1989) Fate of allogeneic embryonal chick chondrocytes implanted orthotopically as determined by the host's age. Mechanisms of ageing and development 50:71–80

70. Kawabe N, Yoshinao M (1991) The repair of full thickness articular cartilage defects. Immune responses to reparative tissue formed by allogeneic growth plate chondrocyte implants. Clin Orthop 268:279–293

71. Peterson L, Menche D, Grande D, Pitman M (1984) Chondrocyte transplantation: an experimental model in the rabbit. In: transactions from the 30th Annual Meeting of Orthopaedic Research Society, Atlanta, Palatine III, Orthopaedic Research Society: p 218

72. Grande DA, Pitman MI, Peterson L, Menche D, Klein M (1989) The repair of experimentally produced defects in rabbit articular cartilage by autologous chondrocyte transplantation. J Orthop Res 7:208–218

73. Brittberg M, Nilsson A, Lindahl A, Ohlsson C, Peterson L (1996) Rabbit articular cartilage defects in the knee with autologous cultured chondrocytes. Clin Orthop Rel Res 326: 270–283

74. Brittberg M, Lindahl A, Nilsson A, Ohlsson C, Isaksson O, Peterson L (1994) Treatment of deep cartilage defects in the knee with autologous chondrocyte transplantation. New England Journal of Medicine 331:889–895

75. Muckle DS, Minns RS (1990) Biological response to woven carbon fibre pads in the knee. A clinical and experimental study. J Bone Joint Surg 72 (Br):60–62

76. Brittberg M, Faxèn E, Peterson L (1994) Carbon fiber scaffolds in the treatment of early knee osteoarthritis. A prospective 4-year follow-up of 37 patients. Clin Orthop 307: 155–164

77. Haddad FS, Norman D, Bentley G (1997) Articular cartilage resurfacing with carbon fibre pads. In : Abstracts of the 2nd Fribourg International Symposium on cartilage repair, Fribourg, Switzerland: pp 80

78. Itay S, Abramovici A, Nevo Z (1987) Use of cultured embryonal chick epiphyseal chondrocytes as grafts for defects in chick articular cartilage. Clin Orthop 220:284–303

79. Vacanti CA, WooSeob K, Schloo B, Upton J, Vacanti JP (1994) Joint resurfacing with cartilage grown *in situ* from cell-polymer structures. Am J Sports Med 22:485–488

80. Freed LE, Grande DA, Lingbin Z, Emmanuel J, Marquis JC, Langer R (1994) Joint resurfacing using allograft chondrocytes and synthetic biodegradable polymer scaffolds. J Biomed Mat Res 28:891–899

81. Arnoldi C, Lemperg RK, Linderholm H (1975) Intraosseous hypertension and pain in the knee. J Bone Joint Surg 57 (Br):360–363

82. Odenbring S, Egund N, Lindstrand A, Lohmander LS, Willen H (1992). Cartilage regeneration after proximal tibial osteotomy for medial gonarthrosis. An arthroscopic, roentgenographic and histologic study. Clin Orthop 277:210–216

83. Tippett JW (1991) Articular cartilage drilling and osteotomy in osteoarthritis of the knee. In: Mc Ginty JB, Caspari RB, Jackson RW, Poehling GG (eds) Operative arthroscopy, Raven, New York: pp 325–339

84. Akizuki S, Yasukawa Y, Takizawa T (1997) Does arthroscopic abrasion arthroplasty promote cartilage regeneration in osteoarthritic knees with eburnation? A prospective study of high tibial osteotomy with abrasion arthroplasty versus high tibial osteotomy alone. Arthroscopy 13:9–17

85. Nagel A, Insall JN, Scuderi GR (1996) Proximal tibial osteotomy. A subjective outcome study. J Bone Joint Surg 78 (Am):1353–1358

86. Weidenhielm L, Olson E, Brostrom LA, Börjesson-Hederström M, Mattson E (1993) Improvement in gait one year after surgery for knee osteoarthritis: a comparison between high tibial osteotomy and prosthetic replacement in a prospective, randomized study. Scand J Rehabil Med 25:25–31

87. Broughton NS, Nerwman JH, Baily RA (1986) Unicompartmental replacement and high tibial osteotomy for osteoarthritis of the knee. A comparative study after 5–10 years' follow-up. J Bone Joint Surg 68 (Br):447–452

88. Weale AE, Newman JH (1994) Unicompartmental arthroplasty and high tibial osteotomy for osteoarthritis of the knee. A comparative study with a 12 to 17-year follow-up period. Clin Orthop 302:134–137

89. Eaton RG, Glickel SZ, Littler JW (1985) Tendon interposition arthroplasty for degenerative arthritis of the trapeziometacarpal joint of the thumb. J Hand Surg 10 (Am):645–654

90. Anfinsen OG, Sudmann E (1988) Fascia lata plastikk i kneleddet. Tidsskr Nor Laegeforen 108: 1020–1022 (in Norwegian)

91. Charnley J (1969). Arthroplasty of the hip. A new operation. Lancet 1:1129–1132

Scientific Basis of Physical Therapy and Rehabilitation in the Management of Patients with Osteoarthritis

J.-M. CRIELAARD and Y. HENROTIN

10.1
Introduction

The goals of physical therapy and rehabilitation in the treatment of osteoarthritis (OA) are prevention, relief of pain, restoration or maintenance of movement, offsetting function loss and physical impairment reduction.

Prevention aims to avoid joint dysfunction or to stabilize or delay osteoarthritis progression. Prevention can be achieved by educational programs, weight loss, joint malalignment correction, joint stability improvement, biomechanical stress decrease, joint protection, environmental accommodation and psychosocial problem management.

The second therapeutic aim is to relieve pain. Pain is frequently the first reported symptom and is often associated with reduced joint function. In response to this pain, muscles go into spasm, often creating a deforming force. Muscle spasm can increase joint pressure and alter normal kinematics. Pain relieving is capital to improve the quality of life and to avoid adverse effects such as decreasing muscle activity, muscle atrophy, physical aversion, osteopenia, interruption of sleep and psychosocial stress.

The third goal is to maintain muscle strength and elasticity, and preserve a functional range of motion. Reduction of the range of joint motion disrupts normal occupational, leisure or daily activities and causes overuse of surrounding joints and provokes psychosocial problems. Muscles perform an important protective function for joints by maintaining normal alignment and serve as excellent shock absorbers.

Rehabilitation must also provide supportive measures to compensate for a functional deficit of the patient and protect the damaged joint. Orthoses, adaptive and assistance devices and environmental design contribute toward reaching these objectives.

Finally, rehabilitation aims to reduce impairment. Aerobic exercise programs realised may improve physical capacity and function of patient with lower-limb and spine OA.

There are many modalities that may be therapeutically employed to accomplish both general and more specific goals. In this chapter, we describe the scientific basis of physical therapy and the rehabilitation methods used in the management of patients with OA.

10.2
Physiotherapy Techniques

Physiotherapy techniques are valuable therapeutic adjuvants for the treatment of osteoarthritic (OA) symptoms. These agents are efficient to treat specific joint problems but are inappropriate to treat generalized OA. Analgesia and muscle relaxation methods may also be used to prepare future rehabilitation and improve muscle performance.

10.2.1
Muscle Relaxing Action

Muscle spasm is a source of pain and limitation of joint motion. Moreover, muscle spasm increases intra-articular pressure and stress to which the cartilage is subjected. Moreover, muscle spasm reduces muscular blood flow and provokes local ischaemia. Tendons are also sources of inflammatory process secondary to tensile stress generated by muscle spasm. Intra-articular pressure enhancement and tendon inflammation generate pain resulting in induced or amplified muscle spasm. Muscle spasm inhibition is an important therapeutic target in OA management.

Muscle relaxation may be obtained by massage, deep and superficial heating or low frequency electrical current and hydrotherapy. Heat therapy may be obtained by conduction (heating pad, hubbard tank, parafango, paraffin, etc), radiation (infrared), convection (sauna, steam room) or diathermy (short waves, microwaves). Local application of heat increases blood flow to the area, decreases pain and muscle spasm and causes general relaxation. Increased muscular blood flow promotes cellular metabolite elimination (lactate, CO_2, etc) and energizing source dispatching (O_2, glucose, ...). In addition, superficial heat produces sedation and analgesia by acting on free nerve endings [1]. Heat application also induces muscle relaxation by decreasing spindle neuromuscular excitability [2].

10.2.2
Analgesic Action

The cardinal symptom of the osteoarthritis (OA) is pain. The pathogenesis of pain in osteoarthritis is multifactorial. Cartilage itself is aneural and therefore is not the source of pain. Consequently, the pain in osteoarthrosis originates from non-cartilaginous intra-articular and peri-articular structures. Possible intra-articular sources and causes of pain include intra-articular hyperpressure induced by joint swelling, overloading on exposed subchondral bone, trabecular microfracture, laceration of intra-articular ligament, pinching of synovial villi, shearing and distension of joint capsule and secondary inflammatory synovitis. Reduction of venous drainage with subsequent vascular congestion of bone, muscle spasm and peri-articular tendon inflammation constitute the extra-articular sources of pain in OA. Before starting the analgesic treatment, physician must choose the right target and identify the origin of pain.

Analgesia may be obtained by heat or cold therapy, ultrasound, pulsed electromagnetic field, ionization, electrotherapy, acupuncture or electro-acupuncture or vibrotherapy.

Cold is used to decrease pain and inflammation and may be generated by ice pack, cryogel, local spray, or cold stream gazeous systems [3]. Superficial cooling decreases muscle spasm has been demonstrated to decrease muscle spindle activity and raise the threshold of pain [4, 5]. The use of vapocoolant sprays upon areas of painful muscle trigger points has been highly successful [6].

Deep heat is delivered by short-waves, micro-waves and ultrasound. The methods are also useful in treating painful musculoskeletal disorders. One study has shown that pain in OA of the hip and knee is significantly reduced by short-wave diathermy [7]. Superficial heat delivery by infrared light also improve pain and disability in patients with knee and hand OA.

In a pilot, prospective double-blind randomized study, pulsed electromagnetic fields (PEMF) decreased pain and improved functional performance of patients suffering of OA of the knee, hand or ankle [8]. Treatment consisted of 18 half-hour periods of exposure during approximately 1 month in a specially designed noncontact air-coil device which produced a low frequency (less than 30 Hz), varying, pulsed electromagnetic field averaging 10–20 Gauss of magnetic energy [8]. The pulse phase duration was 67 ms, including 15 micropulses with a pause duration of 0.1 s. Moreover, the benefit appeared to remain for at least one month after completion of treatment. However, the mechanism involved is not yet clearly understood. Morever, short-wave diathermy and PEMF stimulate glycosaminoglycans synthesis by chondrocytes suggesting that electromagnetic fields may favorize cartilage repair [9, 10].

Ultrasound is generally employed in the treatment of a wide range of acute and chronic musculoskeletal disorders but meager evidence from well-designed controlled study has cast doubt upon its effectiveness [11]. Ultrasound waves are sound waves with a frequency greater than audible sound (> 20,000 Hz). The most common therapeutic ultrasound frequencies used in physical therapy are 1 and 3 MHz. Ultrasound generates thermal and non-thermal effects. Two modes of application – continuous or pulsed – may be delivered by an ultrasound generator. Some of the local thermal effects produced are increased blood flow, increased pain threshold, increased metabolic rate and increased extensibility of soft tissues [12–15]. Energy exposures of 0.5–2 watts/cm² for 10 to 15 min is recommended. Non-thermal effects include increase of cell membrane permeability, calcium transport across the cell membrane, nutrient exchange, and phagocytic activity of macrophage. Non-thermal effects may be obtained by pulsed ultrasound emission. When the pulsed mode is applied, the thermal effects are reduced but the non-thermal effects remain unchanged. This mode of ultrasound application can result in non-thermal effects as pain relief without induction of deep-heating. This modality of application is recommended in the presence of tissue inflammation such as synovitis. Currently, pulsed ultrasound is used at a power range of 2 to 3 Watts/cm². Little information is available on the effectiveness of ultrasound in the treatment of OA. One study reported that pain in OA of the hip and knee is significantly reduced by ultrasound. It was also showed that there was significant additional improvement when ultrasound was combined with a nonsteroidal anti-inflammatory agent [7]. On the other hand, Falconer et al. [16] failed to demonstrate in a randomized, double-blind, sham controlled clinical trial that ultrasound therapy with exercise is more effective in reducing pain and increasing joint mobility of OA than exercise without ultrasound.

Electrotherapy is widely used for the treatment of acute and chronic pain. The most generally applied electrotherapeutic modality is Transcutaneous Electrical Nerve Stimulation (TENS). TENS currents are generally characterized by the pulse amplitude, the pulse duration and pulse frequency. The current characteristics normally employed are low frequency mono or biphasic pulses of short duration. TENS is usually delivered in one of three modes: conventional TENS (50–100 Hz), accupuncture-like TENS or strong low rate TENS (SRL) (2–8 Hz), and burst mode TENS or "brief intense" TENS. These modes have different electrical parameters and are thought to use different biological mechanisms to achieve their analgesic effects [17]. A rational basis for the relief of pain by the use of TENS is provided by the gate control theory. Large diameter, cutaneous fibers ($A\alpha\beta$ fibers) are preferentially stimulated by TENS. This stimulation mechanism inhibits the transmisssion of painful stimuli to the spinal cord. Pain relief by acupuncture-like TENS was found to be reversible by naloxone, which suggest that relief is due to the activation of descending endophinergic system. Two recent overview in the literature [18, 19] have analyzed the results of studies using TENS for the treatment of osteoarthritic knee pain. They concluded at the presence of many deficiencies in the design of the reported studies and the description of electrode placement and TENS parameters used was found lacking. The common limitations of the surveyed studies in these reports were small sample sizes, lack of information on the ability and validity of the outcome measures as well as lack of standardization of the TENS protocol. Moreover, a powerful placebo response was often related in the surveys examined. However, the majority of these studies claim that TENS therapy has a superior effect on pain relief than that of the placebo group, irrespective to the TENS parameter used [20–25]. The reviewed studies also suggested that no single mode of TENS delivery is superior in relieving osteoarthritic knee pain. No consensus exists on the duration of treatment with TENS for osteoarthritic pain. In the reviewed trials, TENS application duration varied from 20 to 30 min sessions. Often pain relief was short in duration and only a small percentage of patients appeared to achieve a lasting reduction in pain following TENS therapy. A recent double-blind, randomized, placebo controlled study of 86 patients with OA of the knee reported that monophasic low frequency (100 Hz) pulsed electrical stimulation, delivered at night for 4 weeks, provided significant improvement in knee pain and duration of morning stiffness [25]. Based upon these and other reported findings, the authors concluded that TENS produced clinically relevant reduction of pain and improvement of function and would be an appropriate treatment for patients that cannot tolerate non-steroidal anti-inflammatory drugs, with cardiac, liver or renal disease, that required repeated intra-articular injections or when surgery was not possible.

Galvanic current exerts sedative action (anode effect) and facilitates trans-cutaneous penetration of water soluble drugs (i. e. NSAIDS) and saline solution (i. e. $CaCl_2$ 1%) [7]. Nevertheless, there are no controlled trials in the literature demonstrating the efficacy of this treatment on OA symptoms.

Acupuncture and electro-acupuncture have been applied to manage pain in patient with osteoarthritis. Two studies failed to demonstrate a significant difference between the treatment [26, 27] and placebo group while one showed a long-term effect on painful relief [28]. In the oldest study, forty patients with OA in various joints were randomly treated either by conventional acupuncture or sham acupuncture as control. Pain level in both groups improved significantly, but there was no significant difference between the treatment and placebo groups [26]. A recent randomized placebo-controlled study, involving 40 patients with OA of the knee showed that real and sham acupuncture significantly reduced pain, stiffness and physical disability, but no difference was found between the two groups [27]. The long-term effect of acupuncture treatment was studied in 29 patients with severe OA of the knee. The evaluation during and after the 50-week trial showed a significant reduction in pain and analgesic consumption in the treated group compared with the control group [28].

Finally, literature reports that transcutaneous mechanical vibration (100 Hz) can relieve both acute and chronic pain [29]. As described for TENS, mechanical vibration acts by $A\alpha\beta$ fibers activation.

10.2.3
Antiinflammatory Action

In some patients at some phases of the disease, an inflammatory component may be present in osteoarthritis (OA). Such inflammation is focal, being most pronounced where the synovium is adjacent to cartilage lesion [30 – 32]. Inflammation of synovial membrane may contribute to cartilage loss by production of inflammatory cytokines such as IL-1 or TNFα, which in turn results in release of matrix metalloproteases, such as collagenases and stromelysin, as well as prostaglandins, plasminogen activators and free radicals. Anti-inflammatory action may be conducted by cold application, ionization of non-steroidal anti-inflammatory drugs or ultrasound therapy conducted with a anti-inflammatory gel.

10.2.4
Hot or Cold Application on Osteoarthritic Joint

In active osteoarthritis, destructive enzymes are produced in the inflamed joints. The activity of these cartilage-degrading enzymes, particularly aggre-canase, stromelysin and collagenase, is influenced by joint temperature. Enzymatic activity increases with increasing temperature, resulting in increased breakdown of cartilage and other tissues [33]. In active osteoarthritis, the mean joint temperature is slightly elevated [34]. Therefore, one goal of physical therapy should be to decrease intra-articular temperature. In patients with inflammation of the knee joint, the application of ice chips for 30 min or nitrogen cold air for 6.5 min decreases the intra-articular temperature by 6.1 °C and by 3.3 °C, respectively. Treatment with ligno-paraffin increases the temperature in the joint cavity by 1.7 °C [35]. Others found that 30 min applications of hot pack at 42 °C increased mean intra-articular temperature by 1.2 °C [36]. After 15 min of micro-wave treatment, joint temperature increases by 4.0 °C in one study and 2.9 °C in another. Finally short-wave diathermy increased intra-articular temperature by only 1.4 °C [37]. The depth of penetration of ultrasound is greater than that of short-wave or micro-wave diathermy. Only ultrasound can raise the intra-articular temperature of the hip joint [38]. Therefore, treatments that elevate intraarticular temperature, such as micro-wave diathermy, short-wave diathermy, superficial heat and ultrasound treatment are unsuitable for treating OA with secondary synovitis. At temperatures of 30 °C or below, the activity of destructive enzymes is negligible. This can be achieved with local applications of cold (i.e., ice chips) for 20 to 30 min [37]. Cooled inflamed joints spare the cartilage. If the patient nevertheless prefers heat, as is sometimes the case, superficial heat application should be no more than 5 to 10 min [35].

10.3
Rehabilitation Techniques

Physical disability is one of the major symptoms of OA of a loading joint (spine, knee, hip, ankle). Multiple factors as alteration of the physical capacity, environmental, social, psychological influences interact to cause physical disability. Physicians may improve physical capacity by increasing aerobic power, strength, joint function and gait.

10.3.1
Traction

Traction may be used to relieve pressure on a compressed nerve root, a degenerative intervertebral disc or articular cartilage. Traction force must be applied progressively and can be associated with pumping movement. Superficial heat applied before or during traction may help to reduce muscle spasm and then improve traction effectiveness. Traction force equal to 5–7 kg is recommended for cervical application. Lumbosacral traction has been used to decrease pain in patients with discogenic disease or facet syndrome. Traction is used at a force equal to or greater than one half the body weight. The distance between the vertebral bodies is increased by a few millimetres [39]. Most studies report a low success rate in reducing back pain or radicular pain. However some patients do respond and it is sometimes applied when other modalities or stretching techniques have not resulted in relieving pain.

10.3.2
Massage

The beneficial effects of massage include relaxation of soft tissues, decreased muscle spasm and trigger points, break-up tissue adherence, increased muscle flexibility, improved venous and lymphatic flow with reduction of oedema and increased local blood flow to an area. Different types of massage have been described: gentle gliding over the skin without moving the underlying tissues (effleurage), muscles kneading and rolling manipulation, vigorous cross-fibre friction over tendons or ligaments, neuromuscular massage, myofascial release. Massage with topical NSAIDs on osteoarthritic joint has been widely used for centuries in several countries in the Europe and in the United States. A novel approach to topical treatment of joint pain and inflammation consists of using capsaicin, a substance that results in the depletion of substance P from the nerve. Substance P is active not only as a neurotransmitter important for mediating pain sensation but also as a potent pro-inflammatory cytokine and active mediator of cartilage damage [40, 41].

10.3.3
Hydrotherapy and Spa Treatment

The use of water as a therapeutic mode is termed hydrotherapy. As an exercise medium, water provides many benefits such as the property of buoyancy that helps to suspend the body and allow partial weight bearing during rehabilitation. The deeper the submersion, the less weight is borne. This property is important during exercise program with patient suffering of OA of the loading joints. The temperature of the water also may be beneficial. A warm bath promotes relaxation, increases blood flow to the muscles and decreases pain. As suggested by some previous studies, swimming and water exercises are excellent means of exercising elderly people with generalized OA. Forty-nine patients with OA of the peripheral joint were treated with hydrotherapy in a recent trial. Results showed a decreased pain level and improved mobility [42]. In a randomized, tap-water controlled, double-blind trial, thermal water was tested in 62 patients with OA of the knee, treated in a non-spa environment. By the end of the 3-week treatment, pain decreased significantly more in the thermal water group compared with the control group [43].

Modern spa therapy is a combination of different therapeutic factors including natural specific remedies of the spa (mineral waters, mud, climate, etc), drug treatment, physical therapy, dietary measures, psychological guidance and social measures [44, 45]. The use of spring water in therapy date back in the history of medicine. Traditionally and empirically, the therapeutic value and indication of thermal spring waters are linked to its composition, mineral concentration and temperature of the water. Thermal water containing high concentration of sulphate, bicarbonate, sodium chloride, bicarbonate chloride and other trace elements (zinc, copper, etc) is usually recommended for treating patients with osteoarthritis. Six months after the completion of a two week spa therapy with 12 patients with symptomatic OA of the knee, a measurable decrease of pain and tenderness in the joint resulted which underlines the long lasting effects of this combined therapy [46]. The same prolonged beneficial effects of spa therapy on joint pain, functional impairment and quality of life were observed in a recent randomized, controlled trial of 188 patients with OA of the hip, knee and lumbar spine [47].

10.3.4
Excercise Therapy

The treatment goals of excercise in OA are to (1) reduce impairment and improve function (i.e., decrease pain, increase range of motion (ROM) and strength, normalize gait, and facilitate activities of daily living); (2) protect joints from further damage (i.e., reduce joint stress and improve biomechanics); and (3) prevent disability and improve health status [48].

10.3.4.1
Range of Motion Exercises

Joint stiffness in osteoarthritic patients may result from (1) capsular distension secondary to increased amount of synovial fluid; (2) retraction of the capsule, periarticular ligaments or tendons; (3) loss of articular cartilage with varying amounts of fibrosis osseous ankylosis; (4) joint surface incongruity, mechanical block (osteophytes, loose bodies); (5) muscles spasm and (6) pain (muscular sideration).

Moreover, physician must keep in mind that loss of the range of motion in one joint affects the biomechanics of the adjacent proximal and distal joints. For example, when older persons with knee OA are compared to non-arthritic controls, range of motion (ROM) in both limbs and at all joints (hip, knee, ankle), are reduced [49, 50]. Altered joint biomechanics modifies normal limb motion, increases joint stress, enhances energy consumption during movement, exacerbates pain and instability. Furthermore, limitations in the motion of lower-extremity joints profoundly modify the normal gait kinematics. For example, patient with knee OA have lower knee angular velocity and knee range of motion but a compensatory increase in hip angular velocity than age-, mass- and gender matched control subjects. Moreover, they have an increasing loading rate in unaffected leg after heel strike and exert less peak vertical force during push-off [49, 51]. In addition, it is now accepted that continuous passive motion has a trophic action on cartilage and can promote cartilage repair [52]. For these reasons, recovering functional ranges of motion are an important goal of the rehabilitation of OA patients.

Many types of ROM exercises are usually applied in the treatment of OA patients.

- In passive ROM exercises, joint mobilization is performed by a therapist or splints.
- In assisted ROM exercises, the patient moves the joint through its maximal ROM and the therapist assists with the terminal stretch.

- In active ROM, the patient moves the joint through its full range of motion. Joint mobilization can be facilitated by physiotherapy or massage application. Infrared, short-wave, micro-wave, and ultrasound reduce joint stiffness and improve ROM [53, 54].

10.3.4.2
Strengthening Excercises

Many papers have reported the relationship between knee osteoarthritis and weakness of the quadriceps [55–59]. Some of these studies claim that pain is a secondary consequence of the loss of strength and activity associated with arthritis. Muscle weakness or asymmetric muscular activity may generate an unstable joint. Stress on an unstable joint may then lead to strain on innerved tissues and provoke pain and disability. Other studies postulate that the pain, secondary to decreased strength, may lead to or accentuate the overall functional losses seen in OA. Pain induces reflex muscle activity inhibition, a decrease of the limb function or even immobilization. This creates a vicious cycle of disuse, muscle weakness, pain and disability (Fig. 1) [60, 61].

In persons with symptomatic osteoarthritis of the knee, quadriceps muscle weakness is common and is widely believed to result from disuse atrophy secondary to joint pain and swelling [62]. This phenomenon is commonly called "Arthrogenous Muscle Inhibition" (AMI). Inhibition of muscle function has been reported in both normal and arthritic knee joints when increasing the intra-articular fluid volume and hydrostatic pressure [63]. Another study shows that maximal isometric strength is markedly lower in the presence of an effusion and that an aspiration of joint produced a significant increase in strength [64]. Meanwhile, AMI is also observed in patients without pain and joint effu-

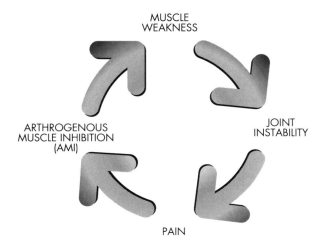

Fig. 1. Vicious cycle of disuse implicating muscle weakness and pain. Muscle weakness induces joint instability and consequently pain. Pain induces reflex muscle activity inhibition that may lead at muscle weakness

MUSCLE WEAKNESS

JOINT INSTABILITY

ARTHROGENOUS MUSCLE INHIBITION (AMI)

PAIN

sion suggesting that AMI involves other mechanisms. A histochemical study has shown a decrease of the relative number of type II fibers in the gluteus medius and tensor fasciae lata of patients with severe hip osteoarthritis (OAH) requiring joint replacement in comparison with age-matched control groups. The diameter of both types of fibers (I and II) is also significantly smaller in OAH than in the non-OA patients [65]. The relative increase in type I fibers may increase the stiffness of the muscle and may render the joint more susceptible to osteoarthritis by altering its shock absorbing potential. Interestingly, quadriceps weakness may be present in patients who have osteoarthritis but do not have muscle atrophy [66]. These observations suggest that muscle weakness is not necessarily bound to muscle atrophy or pain and joint swelling and that weakness may be due to muscle dysfunction [59]. Muscle dysfunction may be secondary to limb deformity, muscle fatigue or impaired proprioception. Electromyographic analysis of quadriceps during isometric contraction at a knee flexion of 30° and 60° shows significantly higher activity for people with genu varum in comparison with people with normal tibial alignment with a preferential activation of rectus femoris [67, 68]. This relative high percentage utilization of the quadriceps femoris may serve to explain the high energy requirement of ambulation and the susceptibility of those with knee OA to fatigue during prolonged activities. In turn, because fatigue is associated with abnormal co-ordination of muscle and impaired muscle shock absorption, this may explain why patients with limb deformity might be especially susceptible to joint damage during walking and standing.

Furthermore, some studies suggest that quadriceps weakness is a primary risk factor for knee disability and progression of joint damage in persons with osteoarthritis of the knee [59, 69]. Madsen et al. demonstrated that a slight increase in strength (+19% of the mean for men and +27% of the mean for women) could result in a decrease of from 20% to 30% in the odds of having osteoarthritis.

Some studies have quantified the loss of quadriceps and knee flexor in gonarthrosis. Both isometric and isotonic torque of knee extensor has been found to be lower in OA than in healthy reference groups [70] but no change of the shape of torque-angle curve was observed. Some studies have also stayed that the knee flexor torque is lower than normal, but that the loss in strength is not as great as in the extensors [71]. Isokinetic study also showed that unlike hamstrings weakness, quadriceps weakness is common [59, 72]. Isokinetic testing of knee musculature in patient with unilateral gonarthrosis revealed that peak torque and work reduction of quadriceps is more marked at low (60°/sec; –23%) than at high (240°/sec; –15%) angular velocity (Figs. 2 and 3). Moreover, flexor knee weakness is more commonly observed at high angular velocity [73].

Strengthening exercises in the treatment of OA have been promoted because muscles serve as shock absorbers around the joint and if stronger would be protective. Moreover, some studies have reported that exercises to strengthen the quadriceps relieve joint pain and improved physical function in persons with osteoarthritis of knee suggesting the role of muscle weakness in the

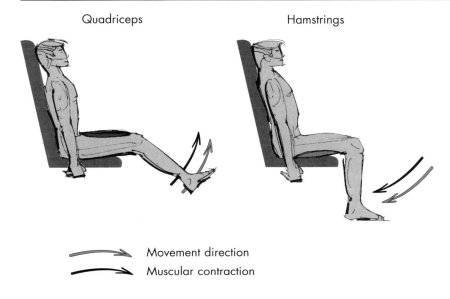

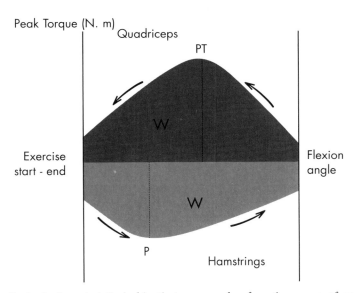

Fig. 2. A characteristic isokinetic torque-angle of motion curve of quadriceps and hamstrings. PT = peak torque corresponding at the highest torque output of the joint produced by muscular contraction as the limb moves through the range of motion ; W = peak work defined as the area under the torque versus angular displacement curve [81, 82]

Quadriceps Peak Torque

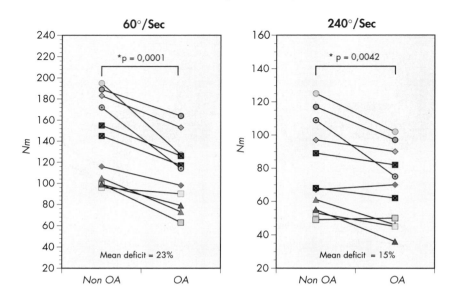

Quadriceps maximal total work

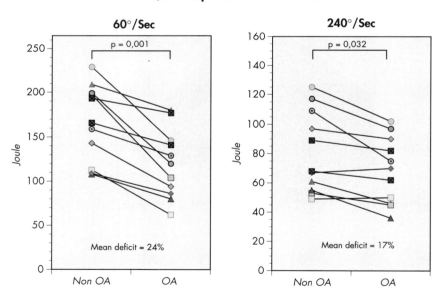

Fig. 3. Quadriceps peak torque and work of eleven patients (5 women and 6 men) suffering unilateral gonarthrosis. The average age of the tested patients was 52 years old (range 41–62). Muscle strength expressed as peak torque (Nm) and maximal work (J) was assessed by iso-kinetic dynamometers as a concentric contraction mode and at angular velocity of 60°/sec and 240°/sec. To obtain comparable data on peak torque and maximal work, range of motion was assessed using a window of 100°. Statistical difference between groups was performed using the paired Student's t-test

pathogenesis of joint pain and disability [55, 74, 75]. Nevertheless, before starting a strengthening program, it is necessary to treat pain, swelling and capsule stiffness to reduce AMI factor that may undermine effective rehabilitation by preventing strength increase of affected muscle groups. Moreover, pressure generated by extensor muscle activation in knee joints with effusion affects the synovial microcirculation by compressing the capillaries [76]. Intermittent ischaemia may be of etiopathogenic significance in the development of joint injury [77, 78]. This element must be considered when elaborating the strengthening program. These findings suggest that exercises that strengthen muscle can prevent the development or progression of pathologic changes of osteoarthritis or decrease the risk for joint pain or disability.

Exercises designed to increase muscle strength can be divided into three types: isometric, isotonic, and isokinetic.

- In isometric exercises, muscles are contracted without changing their length or causing joint movement. The contraction is held for a specified time (6 s), relaxed and repeated five or ten times. Antagonist co-activation is recommended. Indeed, Himeno et al. [79], showed that nearly equal pressure distribution over the complete femoro-tibial articular surface results if forces generated by the agonist is counterbalanced by antagonist activation. Such arrangements reduce the overall articular surface pressure and prevent focal surface damage [80].
- In isokinetic exercises, the joint moves through a range of motion with a constant speed of movement. Resistance is variable so that increased muscular force results in increased resistance rather than increased acceleration. Interfacing of microprocessors with isokinetic dynamometers allows a rapid quantification of a variety of parameters of muscle function including peak torque, angle-specific torque, work, power, endurance indexes and speed of contraction can be measured to evaluate changes in clinical studies. Many of these offered parameters have been overlooked by poor scientific evidence concerning their validity, reproducibility and/or clinical importance decreasing their applicability for routine use [81]. In patient rehabilitation, the major benefit of isokinetic training is that the dynamometer could accommodate to the decrease force applied at a painful arc of motion and reduce the resistance. Nevertheless, it is reported that isokinetic exercise, particularly at low speed, produces heavy loads on the involved joint and may therefore, place risks upon healing tissues, especially in healing cartilage defects where pain control is not always very effective.

Recently, Miltner et al. [83] described the influence of isokinetic exercise on the intra-articular oxygen partial pressure of an osteoarthritic joint. They concluded that a velocity of 60°/sec (slow dynamic tension) leads to a reduction of the intra-articular pO_2 below the resting value whereas a velocity of 180°/sec leads to improvement of the intra-articular metabolic condition [83]. It is known that pathological reduction of the intra-articular oxygen partial pressure has deleterious consequences for the metabolism of chondrocytes. Nevertheless, the most dangerous mechanism for cartilage integrity occurs when hypoxia is followed by a tissue reoxygenation. A panel of studies has shown that exercise of the inflamed human knee (including inflammatory osteoarthritis) induced hypoxic-reperfusion injury mediated by reactive oxygen species [77]. The mechanism of synovial ischaemia-reperfusion is now well understood. In the osteoarthritic knee, the mean resting value of the partial oxygen pressure is significantly decreased. Exercise of the knee with inflammatory synovitis is associated with a large increase in intra-articular pressure, exceeding the capillary perfusion pressure, and in certain cases the systolic blood pressure, and consequently leads to tissue hypoxia [84]. During this period of raised intra-articular pressure, the synovial fluid pO_2 falls. When rest allows, intra-articular pressure decreases, a reperfusion of blood occurs creating a ischaemia-reperfusion phenomenon [77] (Fig. 4). Oxygen tension suddenly increases and active oxygen species are formed, more particularly at the level of altered mitochondria chain. Evidence is presented that the microvascular endothelial cells and chondrocytes are the predominant source of active oxygen species (AOS) in osteoarthritic joint exposed to hypoxia-reoxygenation [78, 85]. Active oxygen species may induce damage in all matrix components and decrease synovial fluid viscosity [86–88]. Moreover, hypoxia induces endothelial cell synthesis

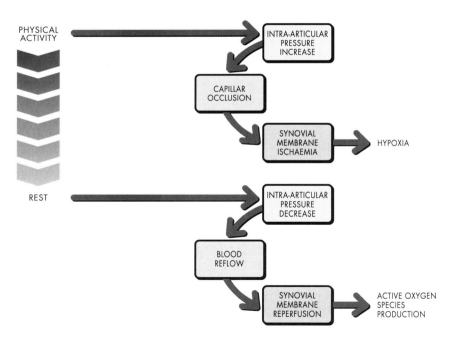

Fig. 4. Ischaemia-reperfusion phenomenon occuring in synovial membrane during repetitive exercises of an inflamed joint

and release of IL-1 [89]. IL-1 is one of the most soluble cytokines responsible for cartilage degradation in OA.

Closed chain exercise could be privileged since qualitative geometrical analysis indicates that the antagonists provide regulated stabilizing functions to distraction forces generated by the agonist muscles, as well as support this evidence of equalizing articular surface pressure distribution meant to preserve and prolong the cartilage integrity [80].

– In isotonic exercises, the joint is moved through an arc of motion, with or without additional resistance with muscle shortening and lengthening. Isotonic exercises can be also included in strengthening programs. Nevertheless, isotonic program must be conducted in undamaging range of motion and with submaximal resistance.

Finally, some studies have described the beneficial effects of a quantitative progressive exercise program (QPE) conducted for muscle strength, endurance and contraction speed over a three month period. The QPE program is composed of isometric, isotonic, isotonic with resistance, endurance and speed contractions prescribed in a progressive sequence [90]. Nevertheless, this program fails to correct the abnormal gait pattern observed for OA patient. An additional gait retraining seems to be necessary to "re-program" the locomotor pattern [91].

10.3.4.3
Stretching Exercises

Stretching exercises aim to increase length of shortened muscle surrounding the OA joint. Muscle shortening may be a consequence of long-term muscle spasm, skeletal deformity or limited joint motion. Thus, muscle shortening induces abnormal joint strain and limitation of joint motion. After 4 weeks of stretching exercises with or without additional ultrasound, active ROM and isometric strengthening exercises, increased ROM and gait velocity was demonstrated [16]. Leivseth et al. [92] studied passive stretch therapy in six patients with OA of the hip. Stretching force was applied perpendicular to the adductor muscles with the hip flexed to 45° and maximally abducted without moving the hip joint. A 30 sec stretch was followed by a 10 sec pause and repeated for 25 min, 5 days a week for 4 weeks. Hip abduction increased a mean of 8.3° and patients reported reduced pain. After therapy, muscle biopsies showed hypertrophy of type I and II fibers with an increase in muscle glycogen content. Stretching is not used for an inflamed joint and care must be taken in the presence of a joint effusion, as forceful stretching can rupture capsule. However, it is most useful in the presence of tight muscles, tendons and joint capsule.

performance and reduced pain in the aerobic exercises group than in the health education groups [105]. Another study showed that subjects who participate in aerobic walking or aquatics programs for 12 weeks, presented significant improvement over control subjects who participated in only non-aerobic ROM exercise, in terms of aerobic capacity, gait velocity, anxiety and depression [95]. On the other hand, no significant differences between groups were observed for duration of morning stiffness or grip strength. To avoid excessive loading stress during aerobic training, Mangione et al. [106] proposed treadmill exercise program at 20% or 40% of body weight support. This method permitted recommended training intensities to be obtained in elderly people with OA, but may not provide pain relief in this group.

10.3.5
Proprioceptive Reeducation

Neuromuscular systems control the mechanical environment of the joint and protect joint structure against excessive shearing, tensile or loading strain. Several studies comparing the ability of healthy volunteers and those with OA of the knee to reproduce knee angles in weight bearing and non-weight bearing circumstances demonstrated that proprioception is altered in OA volunteers [107–110]. Gait velocity, cadence, stride length and gait cycle each negatively correlates with either active angle reproduction test result suggesting that patients used slower locomotion to compensate for poor proprioception [107]. The origin of the proprioceptive deficit is not yet clearly identified and does not appear to exclusively be a local result of disease in knee OA [110]. In animal studies, deafferation (ipsilateral L4-S1 root ganglionectomy or neurectomy) of structurally intact, stable joints does not induce joint degeneration. Neurectomy involved the three primary articular nerves, leaving intact the sensory nerves from muscles, tendons, skin and small accessory joint nerves. This finding suggests a minor role for articular receptors in healthy joints. However, in unstable joints, deafferation greatly accelerates joint degeneration, suggesting that sensory input is important in protecting the unstable joint from rapid breakdown [111, 112]. Moreover, these animal experiments reveal that sensory inputs are temporarily important in protecting the unstable joint suggesting that central nervous system acquires the ability to protect the unstable joint even in the absence of ipsilateral afference. The authors conclude that there exist two sets of protective muscular reflexes (PMR). One set protects normal joints and is independent of ipsilateral sensory input. It could be driven by sensation from the contralateral limb, the forelimbs, the visual system and vestibular system, all of which influence a variety of CNS programs. The other set of PMR apparently protects unstable or injured joints from rapid breakdown and heavily depends on ipsilateral sensation that influences CNS programs. These observations speak for neuromuscular mechanism involvement in the etiopathogenesis of OA and argument for proprioceptive training of OA joint. Some studies have shown that proprioception can be enhanced by wearing orthoses or an elastic bandage [113]. Muscular training, unloading or loading proprioceptive exercises, gait training, biofeedback and electrical stimulation have been proposed as other approaches to enhancing proprioception [114–116].

10.3.6
Orthoses and Assistive Devices

Some orthoses have been developed for the treatment of gonarthrosis. Revel [117] preconised a rest unloading compartmental orthosis inducing valgus or varus depending of the damaged compartment in the treatment of femorotibial arthrosis. He reported that the use of this orthosis during the night or at least 4 h a day during rest periods for 29 months induced a decrease of pain, hydarthrosis and analgesic drugs consumption in most of the cases studied. Valgus knee bracing (Generation II bracing) produces statistically significant pain relief in older patients with medial compartment severe gonarthrosis in comparison of age-matched control groups. In addition, GII knee braces worn on a daily basis for 12 months increase isokinetic quadriceps muscle strength, increase femoro-tibial angle and decrease lateral movement of the center of gravity during gait in OA patients [118, 119]. The decrease in the center of gravity range caused by a reduction in lateral swing might improve joint stability thereby decreasing the load on the medial compartment. A second pain-relieving factor could be the increase in quadriceps muscle strength.

An orthosis (Joint Active Systems, Effingham, Ill.) that utilizes principles of stress relaxation (constant displacement) and static progressive stretching was used to re-establish range of motion. The orthosis is designed to facilitate permanent (plastic) deformation of soft tissue through incremental increases in displacement. A progressive stretching protocol creating an incremental series of stress-relaxation states is also allowed. The orthosis is also designed to displace the fulcrum of the applied force away from the center of rotation of the joint. Shifting the fulcrum away from the joint line reduces compressive bending stresses [120].

Recently, it was demonstrated that tape applied with a force pulling the patella medially provides significant reduction of pain in patients with osteoarthritis affecting the patellofemoral joint. Patella taping is a simple, safe and inexpensive treatment procedure that can be combined with other therapeutic intervention and which patients can learn to use themselves [121, 122].

Keating et al. [123] demonstrated that the use of lateral heel wedges relieved pain in patients with mild or severe medial osteoarthritis of the knee. The wedge prescribed provided lateral heel elevations of 6.35 mm and lateral sole elevation of 4.76 mm. Shock absorbing viscoelastic shoe soles and insoles provide much relief for many people with lower limb and back osteoarthritis [124].

In elderly people with lower limb osteoarthritis, walking sticks and walkers must be prescribed to maintain functional status without exacerbating pain. In hip OA, proper use of a cane on the contralateral side can reduce joint reaction forces at the hip by as much as 50 per cent [125].

Spinal orthosis may also provide significant pain relief for patients with OA in the lumbar, thoracolumbar and cervical areas. Spinal brace can limit motion and reduce loading strain by maintaining the spine in a semi-erect position and supporting weak muscles.

Orthosis technology for the hand has greatly evolved since the development of low temperature, thermoplastic orthotic materials. Low temperature material can be softened in hot water and then molded directly to the contours of the patient. Most therapists consider the use of orthotics for immobilizing or restricting the joints to reduce inflammation. However, orthoses can be designed to stabilize individual joints to improve functional dexterity or strength of the hand or digits. Orthoses can now be selectively designed to correct joint, soft tissue or muscle contracture [126]. Orthotic treatment of the OA hand can be small cylinder orthoses fitted to slip over inflamed DIP joints. They limit motion and prevent trauma, allowing patients to use their hands in activities that otherwise would be painful. The thumb is one of the most frequently observed localization of OA. Orthotic treatment aims to stabilize the carpometacarpal joint in abduction with a web space C-bar that block thumb adduction and allows full interphalangial joint flexion [127]. Nevertheless, if active wrist flexion and extension elicit pain in the base of the hand or thumb, there is a good chance that more than one trapezial surface is affected by OA. Indeed, in one study of 200 candidates for surgery for OA of the CMC joint 86% had involvement of trapezial joints [128]. Pantrapezial arthritis requires a rigid, circumferential wrist orthosis that prevents wrist and thumb CMC joint motion.

10.4
Educational Action

Severals studies have shown that pain or disability in osteoarthritis does not correlate with cartilage loss. In such pain, educational factors seem important. It was reported that severe knee pain in osteoarthritis is associated with low educational attainment, especially with people having fewer than 8 years of education [129]. For this reason, various different educational interventions have been developed and they appear to give equivalent results. Two important works [130, 131] showed that regular contact via monthly telephone calls from health care workers improved pain and function of patients with knee OA. However, the most investigated educational program is unquestionably the back school program. In a review of 16 randomized clinical trials on the efficacy of back school programs, seven studies reported positive results and seven others reported negative results of back school in comparison with control groups [132]. It is interesting to note that the four trials with the best methodology reported beneficial effects of back school [133–136]. These studies indicate that back school may be effective in occupational settings in acute, recurrent or chronic condition. Nevertheless, the reported benefit of back schools are usually of a short duration. The most promising type of interventions seem to be the "Swedish back school" or derived programs and are quite intensive (a 3 to 5-week stay in a specialized center). The original "Swedish back school" consists of four lessons lasting about 45 min [137]. During the lessons, information is given on the anatomy and function of the back. Patients also receive instructions on isometric abdominal muscle exercises and are encouraged to increase their activity level during leisure time. This original Swedish program underwent some modifications. Exercises, relaxation, ergonomics counseling, postural education and psychotherapy were progressively introduced in back school program.

10.5
Concluding Remarks

Osteoarthritis is principally a disease of elderly people characterized by pain, joint stiffness and swelling, muscle weakness and spasm, disability and physical fitness alteration. Improvement of the algo-functional status of OA patients is the principal goal of the physical therapy and rehabilitation. Physicians have some physiotherapy and rehabilitation techniques at their disposal to efficaciously treat OA symptoms (Fig. 5). However, treatment success will depend on the feeling and the discrimination of the physician in the use of these methods. Physician action must be adapted to the stage and the extent of arthritis, the joint involved, the presence or absence of inflammatory process, the alteration of joint biomechanics, the patient's life style, the handicap, the compliance with treatment, the patient's medical problems and how they may affect the rehabilitation process. Osteoarthritis is often interspersed with congestive episodes due to inflammation of synovial membrane and often accompanied by chondrolysis. In osteoarthritis, clinical signs of inflammation are moderate and often difficult to diagnose. Physicians must be attentive to the increase of pain

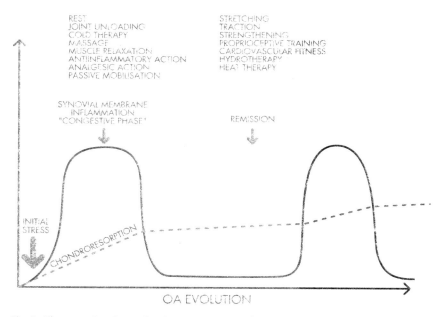

Fig. 5. Therapeutic schema for the management of patients with osteoarthritis

intensity and morning stiffness, the appearance of nocturnal pain and joint swelling and the reduction of walking time for loading limb. In the presence of inflammatory process, the physical therapist must immediately reconsider its therapeutic attitude. Rest, joint unloading (i.e., orthosis, cane, etc), analgesic (i.e., TENS, acupuncture, ultrasound, pulsed electromagnetic field, etc) and anti-inflammatory actions (i.e., cold therapy, ionization), massage, passive joint mobilization in a limited range of motion should be privileged during congestive episodes. When inflammation is relieved, progressive stretching, strenghtening, proprioceptive and aerobic exercises may be prescribed to reduce impairment and improve function. Exercise programs must be accommodated to the functional capacity and need of the patient and reconsidered in the presence of joint pain and swelling.

Prevention is another challenge of rehabilitation in the management of OA. Primary prevention aims to avoid or delay OA appearance. It may be obtained by educational programs, weight control, joint instability and biochemical disorders correction, professional and sports joint stress reduction. Secondary prevention aims to stop or slow OA progression. This aim may be achieved by orthosis, devices, educational programs and environmental adaptation.

We can conclude that physical therapy and rehabilitation play a crucial role in the management of OA. Physical therapy and rehabilitation may not only act on symptoms but also prevent or reduce disability and improve overall health status.

References

1. Lehman J, Brunner G, Stow R (1958) Pain threshold measurement after therapeutic application of ultrasound, micro-waves, and infrared. Arch Phys Med Rehabil 39:560–565
2. Fischer E, Solomon S (1965) Physiological responses to heat and cold. In: Therapeutic heat and cold. Edited by Licht S. New haven, CT, E Licht: pp 126–169
3. Chick H, Carayon A-L, Rogon J-C, Cohpan A (1966) Cryothérapie gazeuse dans le traitement des traumatismes chez le sportif de haut niveau. Sport Med 84:29–33
4. Mennell J (1973) Spray and stretch treatment for myofascial pain. Hosp Phys 12:47–52
5. Benson T, Copp E (1974) The effects of therapeutic forms of heat and ice on pain threshold of the normal shoulder. Rheumatol Rehabil 13:101–104
6. Travell J (1952) Ethylchloride spray for painful muscle spasm. Arch Phys Rehabil Med 33: 291–298
7. Svarcova K, Trnavsky K, Zvarova J (1988) The influence of ultrasound, galvanic currents and short-wave diathermy on pain intensity in patient with osteoarthritis. J Rheum 67:83–85
8. Trock D, Bollet A, Dyer R, Fielding L, Minner W, Markoll R (1993) A double-blind trial of the clinical effects of pulsed electromagnetic field in osteoarthritis. J Rheumatol 20:456–460
9. Vanharanta H, Eronen I (1982) Short-wave diathermy effects on ^{35}S-Sulfate uptake and glycosaminoglycan concentration in rabbit knee tissue. Arch Phys Med Rehabil 63:25–28
10. Liu H, Abbot J, Bee J (1996) Pulsed electromagnetic fields influence hyaline cartilage extracellular matrix composition without affecting molecular structure. Osteoarthritis Cartilage 4:63–76
11. Gam A, Johannsen F (1995) Ultrasound therapy in musculoskeletal disorders: meta-analysis. Pain 63:85–91

12. Gersten J (1955) Effect of ultrasound on tendon extensibility. Am J Phys Med 34:362–369
13. Aleya W, Rose D, Shires E (1956) Effect of ultrasound on threshold of vibration perception in a peripheral nerve. Arch Phys Med 37:265–267
14. Duarte L (1983) The stimulation of bone growth by ultrasound. Arch Orthop Trauma Surg 101:153–159
15. Dyson M, Pond J, Joseph J, Warwick R (1968) The stimulation of tissue regeneration by means of ultrasound. Clin Sci 35:273–285
16. Falconer J, Hayen K, Chang R (1992) Effect of ultrasound on mobility in osteoarthritis of the knee. Arthritis Care and Research 5:29–35
17. Lundeberg T (1995) Pain physiology and principles of treatment. Scand J Rehabil Med Suppl 32:13–42
18. Aubin M, Marks R (1995) The efficacy of short-term treatment with transcutaneous electrical nerve stimulation for osteo-arthritic knee pain. Physiotherapy 81:669–675
19. Robinson J (1996) Transcutaneous electrical nerve stimulation for the control of pain in musculoskeletal disorders. JOSPT 24:208–226
20. Taylor T, Hallett M, Flaherty L (1981) Treatment of osteoarthritis of the knee with transcutaneous electrical stimulation. Pain 11:233–240
21. Smith C, Lewith G, Machin D (1983) TENS and osteoarthritic pain: preliminary study to establish a controlled method of assessing transcutaneous nerve stimulation as a treatment for the pain caused by osteoarthritis of the knee. Physiotherapy 69:266–268
22. Lewis D, Lewis B, Sturrock R (1984) Transcutaneous electrical nerve stimulation in osteoarthritis: A therapeutic alternative. Ann Rheum Dis 43:47–49
23. Fargas-Babjak A, Rooney P, Gerecz E (1989) Randomised trial of Codetron for pain control in osteoarthritis of the hip/knee. Clin J Pain 5:137–141
24. Grimmer K (1992) A controlled double blind study comparing the effects of strong burst mode TENS and high rate TENS on painful osteoarthritic knee. Aust J Physiotherapy 38:49–56
25. Zizic T, Hoffman K, Holt P, Hungerford D, O'Dell J, Jacobs M, Lewis C, Deal C, Caldwell J, Cholewczynski J, Free S (1995) The treatment of osteoarthritis of the knee with pulsed electrical stimulation. J Rheumatol 22:1757–1761
26. Gaw A, Chang L, Shaw L (1975) Efficacy of acupuncture on osteoarthritis pain. N Engl J Med 293:375–378
27. Takeda W, Wessel J (1994) Acupuncture for the treatment of pain and osteoarthritic knees. Arthritis Care and Research 7:119–122
28. Christensen B, Luhl I, Vilbek H (1992) Acupuncture treatment of severe knee osteoarthritis. A long term study. Acta Anaesthesiol Scand 36:519–525
29. Tardy-Gervey M-F, Guieu R, Ribot-Ciscar E, Roll J-P (1993) Les vibrations mécaniques transcutanées: effets antalgiques et mécanismes antinociceptifs. Rev Neurol 3:177–185
30. Lindblad S, Hedfors E (1987) Arthroscopic and immunologic characterization of knee joint synovitis in osteoarthritis. Arthritis Rheum 30:1081–1088
31. Walker E, Boyd R, Wu D, Lukoschek M, Burr D, Radin E (1991) Morphologic and morphometric changes in synovial membrane associated with mechanically induced osteoarthrosis. Arthritis Rheum 34:515–523
32. Haraoui B, Pelletier J-P, Cloutier J-M, Faure M-P, Martel-Pelletier J (1991) Synovial membrane histology and immunopathology in rheumatoid arthritis and osteoarthritis. Arthritis Rheum 34:153–163
33. Hollander J (1974) Collagenase, cartilage and cortisol. N Engl Med 290:50–51
34. Horvath S, Hollander J (1949) Intra-articular temperature as a measure of joint reaction. J Clin Invest 28:469–473
35. Oosterveld F, Rasker J (1994) Treating arthritis with locally applied heat or cold. Semin Arthritis Rheum 24:82–90
36. Weinberger A, Fadilah R, Lev A, Pinkhas J (1989) Intra-articular temperature measurements after superficial heating. Scand J Rehab Med 21:55–57
37. Oosterveld F, Rasker J (1992) Effects of local heat and cold treatment on surface and articular temperature or arthritic knee. Arthritis Rheum 35:146–151

38. Darlas Y, Solassol A, Clouard R, Normand H, Allas T, Perrin J, Fernandez Y (1989) Ultrasonothérapie: calcul de la thermogenèse. Annales de Réadaptation et de Médecine Physique 32: 181–192

39. Cyriax J (1988) Manipulations, massages et infiltrations. In "Manuel de médecine orthopédique". Ed Masson (Paris): pp 43–46

40. Halliday D, McNeil J, Betts W, Scicchitano R (1993) The substance P fragment SP-(7–11) increases prostaglandin E2 intracellular calcium Ca^{2+} and collagenase production in bovine articular chondrocytes. Biochem J 292:57–62

41. Creamer P, Hochberg M (1997) Osteoarthritis. Lancet 350:503–508

42. Ahern M, Mc Farlane A, Leslie A, Eden J, Roberts-Thomson P (1995) Illness behaviour in patient with arthritis. Ann Rheum Dis 54:245–250

43. Szucs L, Ratko I, Lesko T, Szoor I, Genti G, Balin G (1989) Double-blind trial on the effectiveness of puspokledany thermal water on arthrosis of knee-joints. J Royal Soc Health 109:7–9

44. Balint G, Szebenyi B (1995) Research and training at spa resorts in Europe. Rheumatol in Europe 24:149–152

45. Schmidt K (1995) Scientific basis of spa treatment in rheumatic diseases. Rheumatol in Europe 24:136–140

46. Elkayam O, Wigler I, Tishler M, Rosenblum I, Caspi D, Segal R, Fishel B, Yaron M (1991) Effect of spa therapy in Tiberias on patients with rheumatoid arthritis and osteoarthritis. J Rheumatol 18:1799–1803

47. Nguyen M, Revel M, Dougados M (1997) Prolonged effects of 3 week therapy in a spa resort on lumbar spine, knee and hip osteoarthritis: follow-up after 6-months. A randomized control trial. Br J Rheumatol 36:77–81

48. Minor M, Allegrante J (1997) Osteoarthritis and exercise. In: Osteoarthritis. Public health implications for an aging population. Edited by D Hammerman. The Johns Hopkins University Press. pp 150–165

49. Messier S, Loeser R, Hoover J, Semble E, Wise C (1992) Osteoarthritis of the knee: effects on gait, strength and flexibility. Arch Phys Med Rehabil 73:29–36

50. Jesevar D, Riley P, Hodge W, Krebs D (1993) Knee kinematics and kinetics during locomotor activities of daily living in subjects with knee arthroplasty and in healthy controls. Phys Ther 73:229–242

51. Messier S (1994) Osteoarthritis of the knee and associated factors of age and obesity: effects on gait. Med Sci Sports Exerc 26:1446–1452

52. Salter R (1994) The physiologic basis of continuous passive motion for articular cartilage healing and regeneration. Hand Clinics 10:211–219

53. Lehman J, Mc Millan J, Brunner G, Blumberg J (1959) Comparative study of the efficiency of short-wave, micro-wave and ultrasonic diathermy in heating the hip joint. Arch Phys Med Rehabil 40:510–512

54. De Lateur B, Stnebridge J, Lehmann J (1978) Fibrous muscular contractures: treatment with a new direct contact micro-wave applicator operating at 915 MHz. Arch Phys Med Rehabil 59:488–490

55. Fischer N, Pendergast D, Gresham G, Calkins E (1991) Muscle rehabilitation: its effect on muscular and functional performance of patients with knee osteoarthritis. Arch Phys Med Rehabil 72:367–374

56. Hall K, Hayes K, Falconer J (1993) Differential strength decline in patients with osteoarthritis of the knee: revision of the hypothesis. Arthritis Care and Research 6:89–95

57. Madsen O, Bliddal H, Egsmose C, Sylvest J (1995) Isometric and isokinetic quadriceps strength in gonarthrosis; inter-relations between quadriceps strength, walking ability, radiology, subchondral bone density and pain. Clin Rheumatol 14:308–314

58. O'Reilly S, Jones A, Doherty M (1997) Muscle weakness in osteoarthritis. Curr Op Rheumatol 9:259–262

59. Slemenda C, Brandt K, Heilman D, Mazzuca S, Braunstein E, Katz B, Wolinsky F (1997) Quadriceps weakness and osteoarthritis of the knee. Ann Intern Med 127:97–104

Dekker J, Tola P, Aufdemkampe G, Winckers M (1993) Negative affect, pain and disability in osteoarthritis patients: the mediating role of muscle weakness. Behav Res Ther 31: 203–206

Ettinger W, Afable R (1994) Physical disability from knee osteoarthritis: the role of exercise as an intervention. Med Sci Sports Exerc 26:1435–1440

Hurley M, Newham D (1993) The influence of arthrogenous muscle inhibition on quadriceps rehabilitation of patients with early, unilateral osteoarthritic knees. Br J Rheumatol 32:127–131

Lebeck P, Moritz U, Wollheim F (1989) Joint capsular stiffness in knee arthritis. Relationship to intra-articular volume, hydrostatic pressures, and extensor muscle function. J Rheumatol 16:1351–1358

Fahrer H, Rentsch H, Gerber N, Beyeler C, Hess C, Grunig B (1988) Knee effusion and reflex inhibition of the quadriceps. J Bone Joint Surg 70:635–638

Sirca A, Susec-Micheli M (1980) Selective type II fiber muscular atrophy in patient with osteoarthritis of the hip. J Neurol Sci 44:149–159

Madsen O, Brot C, Petersen M, Sorensen O (1997) Body composition and muscle strength in women scheduled for a knee or hip replacement. A comparative study of two groups of osteoarthritis women. Clin Rheumatol 16:39–44

Marks R, Percy S, Semple J, Kumar S (1994c) Comparison between the surface electromyogram of the quadriceps surrounding the knees of healthy women and the knees of women with osteoarthrosis. Clin Exp Rheumatol 12:11–15

Marks R, Percy S, Semple J, Kumar S (1994d) Quadriceps femoris activation changes in genu varum: a possible biomechanical factor in the pathogenesis of osteoarthritis. J Electromyogr 170:283–289

Wu M, Lai I, Tsauo J, Lien I (1990) Isokinetic study of muscle strength in osteoarthritis knees of females. J Formos Med Assoc 89:9773–9779

Wessel J (1996) Isometric strength measurements of knee extensors in women with osteoarthritis of the knee. J Rheumatol 23:328–331

Nordesjö L, Nordgren B, Wigren A, Kolstad K (1983) Isometric strength and endurance in patients with severe rheumatoid arthritis or osteoarthrosis in knee joints. Scand J Rheumatol 12:152–156

Madsen O, Brot C (1996) Assessment of extensor and flexor strength in the individual gonarthrotic patient: interpretation of performance changes. Clin Rheumatol 15:154–160

Henrotin Y, Croisier J-L, Dumont R, Huskin J-P, Dubuc J-E, Leflot J-P, Reginster J-Y, Crielaard J-M (1997) Isokinetic testing of knee musculature in patient with unilateral gonarthrosis. Rev Rhum (Engl Ed) 11:740

Marks R (1993a) The effect of isometric quadriceps strength training in mid-range for osteoarthritis of the knee. Arthritis Care and Research 6:52–56

Schilke D, Johnson G, Housh T, O'Dell J (1996) Effects of muscle-strength training on the functional status of patients with osteoarthritis of the knee joint. Nurs Res 45:68–71

Stevens C, Williams R, Farrell A, Blake D (1991) Hypoxia and inflammatory synovitis: observations and speculation. Ann Rheum Dis 50:124–132

Blake D, Unsworth J, Outhwaite J, Morris C, Merry P, Kidd B, Ballard R, Gray L, Lunec J (1989) Hypoxic-reperfusion injury in the inflamed human joint. Lancet 1:289–293

Henrotin Y, Deby-Dupont G, Deby C, De Bruyn M, Lamy M, Franchimont P (1993) Production of active oxygen species by isolated human chondrocytes. Br J Rheumatol 32:562–567

Himeno S, An A, Tsumura H (1986) Pressure distribution on articular surface. Proc North Am Biomech Congress Montreal, Canada, pp 97–98 (Abstract Book)

Baratta R, Solomonow M, Zhou B, Letson D, Chuinard R, D'Ambrosia R (1988) Muscular coactivation. The role of the antagonist musculature in maintaining knee stability. Am J Sports Med 16:113–122

Kannus P (1994) Isokinetic evaluation of muscular performance: implications for muscle testing and rehabilitation. Int J Sports Med 15:S11–S18

102. Rejeski W, Brawley L, Ettinger W, Morgan T, Thompson C (1997) Compliance to exercise therapy in older participants with knee osteoarthritis: implications for treating disability. Med Sci Sports Excerc 29:977–985

103. Minor M, Hewett J, Webel R, Dreisinger T, Kay D (1988) Exercise tolerance and disease related measures in patients with rheumatoid arthritis and osteoarthritis. J Rheumatol 15: 905–911

104. Beals C, Lampman R, Banwell B, Braunstein E, Albers J, Castor C (1985) Measurement of exercise tolerance in patients with rheumatoid arthritis and osteoarthritis. J Rheumatol 12: 458–461

105. Ettinger W, Burns R, Messier S, Applegate W, Rejeski W, Morgan T, Shumaker S, Berry M, O'Toole M, Monu J, Craven T (1997) A randomized trial comparing aerobic exercise and resistance exercise with a health education program in older adults with knee osteoarthritis. The fitness arthritis and senior trial (FAST). JAMA 277:25–31

106. Magione K, Axen K, Haas F (1996) Mechanical unweighting effects on treadmill exercise and pain in elderly people with osteoarthritis of the knee. Phys Ther 76:387–394

107. Skinner H, Barrack R, Cook S, Haddad R (1984) Joint position sense in total knee arthroplasty. J Orthop Res 1:276–283

108. Marks R, Quinney H, Wessel J (1993b) Proprioceptive sensibility in women with normal and osteoarthritic knee joints. Clin Rheumatol 12:170–175

109. Marks R (1996) Further evidence of impaired position sense in knee osteoarthritis. Physiol Res 1:127–136

110. Sharma L, Pai Y-C, Holtkamp K, Rymer W (1997) Is knee joint proprioception worse in the arthritic knee versus the unaffected knee in unilateral knee osteoarthritis? Arthritis Rheum 40:1518–1525

111. O'Connor B, Visco D, Brandt K, Myers S, Kalasinski L (1992) Neurogenic acceleration of osteoarthrosis. J Bone Joint Surg Am 74:367–376

112. O'Connor B, Visco D, Brandt D, Albrecht M, O'Connor A (1993) Sensory nerves only temporarily protect the unstable canine knee joint from osteoarthritis. Arthritis Rheum 36: 1154–1162

113. McNair P, Stanley S, Strauss G (1996) Knee bracing: effect of proprioception. Arch Phys Med Rehabil 77:287–289

114. Marks R (1994a) Correlation between knee position sense measurements and disease severity in persons with osteoarthritis. Rev Rhum 61:365–372

115. Marks R (1994b) Reliability of knee position sense measurements in healthy women. Physiother Can 46:37–41

116. Barrack R, Skinner H, Cook S (1994) Proprioception of the knee joint, paradoxal effect of the training. Am J Phys Med 63:175–181

117. Revell M, Mayoux-Benhamou M, Mathieu A (1989) Rééducation des arthroses femorotibiales non operables. Utilisation d'une orthèse de décharge compartimentale. Ann Readapt Med Phys 32:167–171

118. Matsuno H, Kadowaki K, Tsuij H (1997) Generation II knee bracing for several medial compartment osteoarthritis of the knee. Arch Phys Med Rehabil 78:745–749

119. Horlick S, Loomer R (1993) Valgus knee bracing for medial gonarthrosis. Clin J Sport Med 3: 251–255

120. Jansen C, Windau J, Bonutti P, Brillhart M (1996) Treatment of a knee contracture using a knee orthosis incorporating stress relaxation techniques. Phys Ther 72:182–186

121. Cushnaghan J, Mc Carthy C, Dieppe P (1994) Taping the patella medially: a new treatment for osteoarthritis of the knee joint? BMJ 308:753–756

122. Kowall M, Kolk G, Nuber G, Cassisi J, Stern S (1996) Patellar taping in the treatment of patellofemoral pain. A prospective randomized study. Am J Sport Med 24:61–66

123. Keating M, Farris P, Ritter M, Kane J (1993) Use of the lateral heel and sole wedges in the treatment of medial osteoarthritis of the knee. Orthopaedic Review 12:921–924

124. Voloshin D, Wosk J (1981) Influence of artificial shock absorbers on human gait. Clin Orthop Rel Res 160:52–56

125. Neumann D (1989) Biomechanical analysis of selected principles of hip joint protection. Arthritis Care Res 2:146–155

126. Melvin J (1995) Orthotic treatment of the hand. What's new? Bull Rheum Dis 44:5–8

127. Melvin J, Carlson-Rioux J (1989) Compliance and effectiveness of a thumb CMC-MCP orthosis for OA of the CMC joint. Arthritis Care and Research 2:510–517

128. Swanson A, de Groot-Swanson G (1976) Osteoarthritis in the hand. J Hand Surg 1:210–216

129. Hannan M, Anderson J, Pincus T (1992) Educational attainment and osteoarthritis. Differential associations with radiographic changes and symptom reporting. J Clin Epidemiol 45:139–147

130. Rene J, Weinberger M, Macuzza S, Brandt K, Katz B (1992) Reduction of joint pain in patients with knee osteoarthritis who have received telephone calls from lay personel whose medical treatment regimes have remained stable. Arthritis Rheum 35:511–515

131. Weinberger M, Tierney W, Cowper P, Katz B, Booher P (1993) Cost-effectiveness of increased telephone contact for patients with osteoarthritis: a randomized controlled trial. Arthritis Rheum 36:243–246

132. Koes B, van Tulder M, van der Windt D, Bouter L (1994) The efficacy of back schools: a review of randomized clinical trials. J Clin Epidemiol 47:851–862

133. Bergquist-Ullman M, Larsson U (1977) Acute low-back pain in industry. Acta Orthop Scand 170:111–117

134. Linton S, Bradley l, Jensen I, Sprangfort A, Sundell L (1989) The secondary prevention of low-back pain. A controlled study with follow-up. Pain 36:197–207

135. Hurri H (1989) The Swedish back school in chronic low back pain. Part I. Benefits. Scand J Rehabil Med 21:33–40

136. Mellin G, Harkapaa K, Hurri H, Jarvikoski A (1990) A controlled study on the outcome of inpatient and outpatient treatment of low back pain. Part IV. Scand J Rehabil Med 22:189–194

137. Zachrisson-Forssell M (1980) The Swedish back school. Physiotherapy 66:112–114

a network. However, the functions of other recently discovered matrix proteins including a 36 kDa protein, a 39 kDa protein (termed GP-39), and a 21 kDa protein still need to be clarified.

Concerning the biochemical basis characterising the functional properties of articular cartilage, recent studies have explained the complex interactions between water content, PGs and collagen fibers under physiological conditions and when cartilage is submitted to loading. These observations will contribute to a better interpretation of the role of obesity, one of the most important risk factors for osteoarthritis (OA).

Chapter 2
Epidemiology and Economic Consequences of Osteoarthritis

2.1
The American Viewpoint
(J.C. Scott, M. Lethbridge-Cejku and M.C. Hochberg)

Arthritis and musculoskeletal diseases are the most common chronic diseases and causes of physical disability in the United States (US). The costs to the US economy are striking. $ 54.6 billion in 1988, $ 64.8 billion in 1992. Although there is very little doubt that OA is responsible for the vast majority of these costs, data concerning its exact prevalence are few and frequently controversial. The authors underline that some important basic aspects necessary to perform reliable epidemiological studies on OA, such as a standard definition of OA, clinical classification and radiological criteria, have been only recently established. Thus, results from old studies should be interpreted with care.

Much of the information in the US is derived from the First National Health and Nutrition Examination Survey (NHANES-I), conducted from 1971 to 1975. A clinical diagnosis of OA, based on symptoms and physical findings by examining physician, was found in 12 percent of 6913 examinees aged 25 to 74. Using estimates for the 1990 US Population, the National Arthritis Data Work Group estimated that over 20 million adults have physician-diagnosed OA. The prevalence of OA increases with age. No data on time trends of the prevalence of OA in US are available.

Concerning the risk factors, overweight may be considered the most important modifiable factor for the development of knee OA in both sexes. The NHANES-I study indicates a significant direct association between body mass index (BMI) and OA of the knee, both its occurrence and its worsening. Similar results were obtained by Hochberg and colleagues, who examined participants in the Baltimore Longitudinal Study of Aging. Furthermore, these authors found no correlation between body fat distribution and the presence of knee OA. Concerning the association of obesity with hip OA, the relationship is to lesser strength than to OA of the knee.

Data from NHANES-I were also utilised to study the relationship between occupation and knee OA. Subjects who worked in jobs with either increased strength demands or higher knee-bending demands had greater odds of radiographic knee OA. These data were confirmed in the Framingham study. Concerning hip OA, in the only US study, Roach and colleagues observed that men with hip OA had 2.5 fold greater odds of having performed heavy workloads than controls. Furthermore, duration of heavy workloads seem an additional important risk factor.

The authors concluded with some important suggestions concerning the prevention of OA: avoiding overweight should be included as the primary prevention. Secondary prevention strategies include weight loss, and regular, low intensity, aerobic physical exercise in knee OA. Since recent data from the Framingham Osteoarthritis Study observed that elderly people with a low dietary intake of antioxidants, especially vitamin C and E, as well as those with low serum levels of vitamin D, have high rates of progression of radiographic changes of knee OA, dietary supplementation with these vitamins may be considered as useful in elderly people with knee OA.

2.2
The European Viewpoint
(X. Badia Llach)

In recent years, studies on OA epidemiology have notably increased in European countries. Some recent studies have introduced new methodologies, such as self-reports of joint pain. Using this technique, the prevalence in Spanish communities was estimated to be 12.7% for rheumatic diseases, of whom 43% have OA. A Swedish study using self-reports found that 30–43% of female and 15–25% of male subjects aged 70–79 reported joint complaints, and that knee joints were the most common sites in both sexes.

Concerning risk factors, among the few studies which have investigated the impact of genetic factors on OA in Europe, Spector et al. recently found significant differences, in term of prevalence, between identical and non-identical twins, with a clear genetic effect concerning hand or knee OA in women, and genetic influences ranging from 39% to 65%. Let us add the results of a recent English survey on genetic predisposition of hip OA (1): the relative risk for hip OA in siblings (n:611, from 398 families) of ascertained hip OA patients were found as high as 5.1 in men and 2.6 in women for moderate OA, and close to twice the rate with severe OA.

The importance of overweight has also been confirmed in Europe not only for the knee but also for hip OA. Interestingly, it was found that although overweight was a risk factor in the development of hip OA, it appeared to be less important than physical work load and sport, with the etiological fraction related to the three factors being 55% for sports, 40% for physical work and 15% for obesity. We recently reviewed the literature on sport practice and OA (2); the relative risk in certain sports such as football, tennis and long distance running are from 2 to 5 (mainly 2–3) according to extensive Scandinavian studies, providing the practice is of high level.

The author underlines the economic implications of OA, with consequent relevant socio-economic costs, most of which being related to arthroplasties and pharmacological treatment. Among drugs, the cost implications of non-steroidal anti-inflammatory drugs (NSAIDs) are greater. As demonstrated by a recent unpublished study performed in Spain, a significant part of these costs are related to the adverse drug reactions frequently associated with NSAIDs. Thus, the "true" cost of a NSAID is not normally reflected in its prescription price.

Xavier Badia Llach offers some useful examples in reducing OA costs. Concerning the above mentioned NSAIDs, a study demonstrated that reducing the prescription of NSAIDs, reducing dosage, switching to less toxic NSAIDs and using targeted prophylactics could lead to a reduction of up to 50% in the cost of these drugs.

Chapter 3
Experimental Models of Osteoarthritis

3.1
In Vitro Models for the Study of Cartilage Damage and Repair
(Y. Henrotin and J-Y. Reginster)

In vitro models have provided important information on normal and pathological chondrocyte functions and activities. In their extensive review, the authors underline the numerous difficulties in obtaining reliable culture models and the possible bias in the interpretation of the results. A major challenge is the reproduction of the complex extracellular environment without modifying the specific phenotype of chondrocyte. Several culture models have been proposed, however, each culture system is particularly suitable for exploration of one particular aspect of chondrocyte metabolism while unable to reproduce the complexity of *in vivo* chondrocyte functions.

Among the several aspects to be considered is the variability of metabolic activity and the responsiveness to exogenous stimuli of chondrocyte through the depth and localisation of the tissue. Other important causes of variability are the age of the donor and the pathological status of the joint from which the cartilage is harvested. Differences in technical models used for chondrocyte isolation, such as enzymatic digestion, may modify some characteristics of chondrocyte response. Thus receptors can be down-regulated or damaged, cell-matrix interactions mediated by integrins can be disrupted, and residual matrix components contaminating isolated cells may deregulate chondrocyte synthesis. These observations are particularly useful in the interpretation of studies concerning cytokine and growth factor effects. Furthermore, when chondrocytes are seeded in a support plastic, they lose their cartilage-specific phenotype and show a fibroblastic-like morphology.

Concerning the type of culture, monolayer is useful to study cell differentiation. Chondrocytes re-express the differentiated phenotype when they are transferred from a monolayer to suspension. Thus, three-dimensional culture models have been developed allowing optimal studies on matrix formation, since chondrocytes conserve their phenotype for several weeks. Moreover, cultures of chondrocytes in a three-dimensional matrix allow tissue engineering for transplantation in cartilage defects.

3.2
Animal Models of Osteoarthritis
(K. D. BRANDT)

Due to the difficulty in obtaining joint tissues from humans with OA with the pathological changes are advanced, animal models are very useful in studying the evolution of OA and the effects of drug administration. Unfortunately, at present, no animal model is flawless; Thus researchers are frequently obliged to verify their observations using different models.

Among the numerous models reviewed in this chapter, Brandt emphasizes the validity of the "canine cruciate-deficiency model", which has frequently been criticised as a model of cartilage injury and repairs, rather than of OA. Brandt clearly validates this as a model of OA, mainly for biochemical and RMI aspects of progressive cartilage changes, as observed in OA. In this model, cartilage degeneration, with fibrillation and thinning, gradually develops failure of the joint, with loss of cartilage down to bone which may take 3–5 years. Furthermore, this model is useful to evaluate the role of additive factors in accelerating OA, such as neurogenic deficiency and subchondral bone changes.

If dorsal root ganglionectomy or articular nerve neurectomy precedes ligament transection, fullthickness ulceration of the cartilage occurs within only weeks, resembling Charcot neuropathic arthropathy in humans. The canine cruciate-deficiency model has also furnished information on the role of subchondral bone in OA. Radiographic studies of dogs that had undergone cruciate ligament transection revealed that typical articular cartilage changes of OA can occur in the presence of osteopenia and that the stiffening of subchondral bone is not a requisite for the initiation of early cartilage changes in this OA model. This finding conflicts with the hypothesis of E. Radin who theorised that the major role of the subchondral bone stiffening is in the initiation and progression of OA (4). On the other hand, this point of view is now supported by the data mentioned by J. Martel-Pelletier et al: there is an enhanced bone remodeling at the subchondral plate "at the onset of or during the OA process" (see chapt. 4.4). Indeed, the two opposite conditions fo the subchondral bone, osteosclerosis/osteopenia, may be detrimental to cartilage: a hard stiffened bone basis enhances loading pressure and impact effects on the overlying cartilage; on the contrary, the loss of subchondral bone density could theorically disturb mechanical strain in the overlying articular cartilage, leading to degeneration. In keeping with these observations, Brandt recently demonstrated that the administration of a biphosphonate inhibits re-absorption and subchondral bone formation, although it had no effect on osteophyte formation.

As for other animal models, the canine cruciate-deficiency model has raised some criticism concerning its value in closely predicting the therapeutic activity of drugs in humans. Despite these limits, the numerous data on the mechanisms of OA obtained from animal models have led to better identification of the targets of therapeutic interventions, which of course should be subsequently verified in humans (see new and future therapies, chapt. 8.1.3).

Chapter 4
Pathophysiology of Osteoarthritis

4.1
Role of Mechanical Factors in the Aetiology, Pathogenesis and Progression of Osteoarthritis
(G. Nuki)

As largely demonstrated by epidemiological studies, mechanical factors play an important role in the development and progression of OA. However, this process may be accelerated by many other concomitant factors, including ageing, hypermobility, trauma, occupational and sports activities, and overweight. In this context, the authors point out the role of the meniscectomy. About 70% of patients develop radiological evidence of knee OA 20 years after meniscectomy. Further, the high prevalence of knee OA in former soccer players and American football players has largely been attributed to the high incidence of meniscectomy and cruciate ligament injuries in these athletes. However, overuse of hip and knee joints in sport practiced at high level involves by itself, without trauma, an increased risk of OA of the lower limb [2].

Concerning the pathogenesis of OA, the biochemical properties of the cortical and subchondral bone are essential for the protection of articular cartilage from damage following impact loading. In turn, the mechanical functions of cartilage and its ability to withstand loading are dependent on the structural integrity of its extracellular matrix proteins. Static loading is associated with depression of matrix synthesis while dynamic, high frequency, cyclical loading is associated with increase of up to 50% in proteoglycan synthesis. Overloading and unloading of articular cartilage are both associated with proteoglycan depletion (as Sokoloff stated many years ago [3]), while proteoglycan synthesis and cartilage thickness are increased by the mechanical stresses associated with physiological exercise. Since chondrocytes are responsible for the synthesis of matrix proteoglycans and collagen, changes in their characteristics may influence the production of these substances. The author and his colleagues have developed an experimental technique to measure membrane potentials and proteoglycan metabolism in human articular chondrocyte culture following cyclical pressure-induced microstrain. The results of these studies showed that cyclical pressure induced strain leads to membrane hyperpolarisation and increases proteoglycan synthesis. These responses could be blocked with gadolinium, a blocker of stretch-activated ion channels. More recently, the same authors have demonstrated that neutralising antibodies to IL-4 and IL-4 recetors, will block mechanically induced membrane hyperpolarisation, suggesting a new regulatory function for this cytokine in articular cartilage.

4.2
Role of Biomechanical Factors
(P. Ghosh)

As demonstrated by numerous epidemiological studies, certain work and sport activities which involve long-term repetitive joint usage, can increase the risk of developing OA, in keeping with the pathogenetic role attributed to mechanical factors. However, it is difficult to distinguish cartilage degeneration directly related to these occupational activities from secondary cartilage changes arising from injury to other joint tissues, such as menisci and ligaments despite experimental and clinical observations of "pure" overuse of joints (in 2). To study these aspects, the author investigated the relative effects of moderate or strenuous exercise on the synthesis and degradation of the large aggregating PGs (aggrecan), on two small dermatan sulphate-containing PGs, DS-PGII (biglycan) and DS-PGI (decorin), in standard bred horses. The results showed that in horse carpal joint regions normally subjected to high contact stress such as the dorsal radial facet, strenuous running activities altered the chondrocyte metabolism of PGs. The synthesis of aggrecan was decreased while the synthesis of decorin was elevated. Due to the important function of decorin in the repair and remodelling of the connective tissues, its enhanced synthesis could be interpreted as a response of traumatised chondrocytes to mechanical overload.

Gosh and collaborators have also studied the role of meniscectomy in increasing stress on the cartilage and inducing OA. In cartilage from meniscectomised ovine joints, the synthesis of DSPGs is elevated in those regions submitted to abnormally high mechanical stresses. The major DSPG found in these regions is decorin, which was up-regulated in the cartilage subjected to high focal stresses. Other concomitant factors contributing to these biochemical changes of cartilage subjected to mechanical stresses include: prostanoids and PGE2 in particular, cytokines interleukin IL-1β and tumor necrosis factor TNF-α, and nitric oxide free-radicals. It has been observed that traumatic injury to cartilage can stimulate the production of arachidonic acid and that PGE2 may interact with chondrocyte receptors and alter gene expression. Mechanical injury to chondrocytes could also generate small amounts of IL-1β, which may in turn lead to the release of mediators of matrix destruction.

In conclusion, chondrocytes can readily adapt to changing mechanical injuries by synthesising an extra-cellular matrix useful in dissipating stress and protecting it from lesions. However, by increasing the level and duration of the loading or changing the normal mechanics of the joint complex though injury or surgery, the ability of the chondrocyte to respond to these additional stresses is diminished. Ageing or chemical injury are additional factors in the acceleration of this process.

4.3
Genetic and Metabolic Aspects
(C. J. WILLIAMS and S. A. JIMENEZ)

In this chapter the authors review the studies which support the importance of genetic factors in the development of OA. This hypothesis was first suggested many years ago following the observation of familial cases of Heberden's and Bouchard's nodes. Since then, a number of rare hereditary forms of OA have been identified, including primary generalised OA, several osteochondrodysplasias (OCD) and multiple epiphyseal dysplasias (MED) and the familial crystal-associated arthropathies.

Progress in molecular biology techniques has focused attention on collagen abnormalities. Many mutations have been described for type II procollagen, encoding the main collagenous component of articular cartilage. In families with early-onset OA, generalised OA and OCD, COL2-A1 mutations with heterozygous base substitutions of either arginine 519 to cysteine or arginine 75 to cysteine were found. Although mutations in the COL2-A1 gene have been also identified in most families with arthro-ophtalmopathy (Stickler syndrome), in some cases linkage with this locus was excluded and the studies were oriented towards other minor collagen types, including IX, X and XI. Abnormalities linked to COL11-A2 locus were observed in members of families with variants of Stickler syndrome. In a family with Marshall syndrome, characterised by early-onset symptomatic OA affecting the knees and lumbosacral spine, the clinical phenotype was associated with a splicing defect in the COL11-A1 gene, causing the deletion of 18 aminoacids from the triple helical domain of the $\alpha 1$ (XI) collagen chain. Mutations in the type X collagen gene, which encodes a major collagen of the growth plate cartilage, have been indentified in the most common of MED, Shmid type. In this syndrome, associated with an autosomal dominant mode of inheritance, at least 17 mutations in the gene for type X collagen have been characterised.

Familial occurrence of primary generalised OA, the only subset with a frequent genetic component, has been supported by many studies. Clinical presentation and HLA typing of these forms suggests a polyenic inheritance, rather than a single gene defect. Concerning the familial crystal-associated arthropathies, large family aggregations, mainly associated with autosomal dominant inheritance, have been demonstrated in patients with articular chondrocalcinosis or calcium pyrophosphate-deposition disease (CPPD). In these subjects, the disease shows an early onset, usually between the second and fifth decades of life, and a rapid progression into a severe form of OA. In a family from Chiloe Islands, affected with a severe, precocious OA, ankylosis, late-onset spondyloepyphyseal dysplasia and CPPD, a heterozygous mutation in the COL2-A1 gene resulting in an arginine 75 to cysteine substitution was identified.

In conclusion, the numerous molecular defects identified in familiar cases of primary generalised OA and CPPD demonstrated that accurate molecular studies may lead to the exact causative gene defects in many individuals with severe and precocious OA. The knowledge of these defects will in turn permit accurate diagnosis, thus improving the possibilities of preventive therapeutic approaches. The availability of easier and cheaper molecular tests is most likely a basic condition for rapid progress in thid field. However, such precise genetic and familial forms of OA represent a minority in the spectrum of OA in a whole.

4.4
Biochemical Factors in Joint Articular Tissue Degradation in Osteoarthritis
(J. Martel-Pelletier, J. Di Battista and D. Lajeunesse)

In recent years, many authors have focused their attention on the role that biochemical factors play in OA, since they are considered essential for the relationships between the different joint areas contributing to cartilage degeneration, in particular synovial membrane and subchondral bone. An increase in protease activity has recently been observed in osteoblasts from the subchondral bone. Moreover, osteoblasts secrete a number of growth factors and cytokines. Transforming growth factor TGF-β levels are elevated in OA subchondral bone explants and insulin growth factors (IGF) are elevated in OA osteoblast-like cell cultures. These findings suggest that subchondral bone sclerosis is more related to the onset or the progression of OA rather than as a consequence of this disease. The authors' hypothesis is that at the onset of or during the OA process, enhanced bone remodelling at the subchondral bone plate, coupled with repetitive impulse loading leading to local micro-fractures and/or an imbalance of the IGFI/IGFBP system due to an abnormal response of subchondral osteoblasts, promotes subchondral bone sclerosis. This, in turn, may also create local micro-fractures of the overlying cartilage and promote cartilage matrix damage.

Among biochemical factors important in OA are the enzymes and their inhibitors. The metalloproteases (MMP) family is composed of three principal groups: collagenases, stromelysins and gelatinases. Three collagenases have been identified in human cartilage and found to be elevated in OA: MMP-1, MMP-8 and MMP-13. There is recent evidence, showing their different topographical distributions, of a selective involvement of each collagenase at preferential sites during the disease process. Moreover, in OA cartilage, MMP-1 seems involved mostly during the inflammatory process, whereas MMP-13 is implicated in the remodelling phase. For the second and third groups of MMPs, only stromelysin-1 (MMP-3) and the gelatinase 92 kD (MMP-9) appear to be involved in OA. Finally, another group of MMPs localised at the cell membrane surface, namely membrane type MMP (MT-MMP), has recently been discovered.

In joint tissue MMP biological activity is controlled by three physiologically-specific tissue inhibitors of metalloproteses (TIMP): TIMP-1, TIMP-2 and TIMP-3. The increased levels of active MMPs found in OA tissues are partially due to a relative deficit of TIMPs, but also to the effects of some physiological activators, such as PA/plasmin system and cathepsin B. In this context, key roles are played by IL-1β and TNF-α. These cytokines are considered to be the major catabolic systems involved in the destruction of joint tissue. In chondrocytes they not only increase the synthesis of proteases, but also decrease the synthesis of collagens type II and IX and PGs. In articular chondrocytes, IL-1β produces an increase of MMP synthesis parallel with a decrease in TIMP-1 synthesis, thus resulting in an imbalance of the system. The high sensitivity of OA chondrocytes to the stimulation of IL-1 and TNF is probably due to the increase of receptors types I IL-1R and TNF-R55. New highlights for pharmacological interventions in OA will probably derive from better knowledge of the mechanisms regulating the specific intra-cellular receptors of IL-1β and TNF-α in the joint cells involved in OA. Therapeutic assays in this area are in progress.

Among cytokines, a new discovered IL-17 is interesting since it may upregulate the production of pro-inflammatory cytokines as well as MMP in target cells and increase the production of NO in chondrocytes. NO is produced in larger amounts in OA cartilage, mainly when stimulated by pro-inflammatory cytokines, which enhances the expression of the inducible NO synthase (iNOS),

in the articular cartilage. Furthermore, repeated local injections of TGF-β may induce marked and prolonged upregulation of chondrocyte PG synthesis and stimulate osteophytes in the murine knee joint. It may thus be hypothesized that cartilage pathology may be induced by both overproduction as well as impaired signaling of TGF-β. Another interesting observation concerning the pathogenic effect of this growth factor is the recent observation that TGF-β, despite its well known general anti-protease activity, may enhance the level of MMP-13 (collagenase-3) in activated chondrocytes.

In conclusion, the authors suggest that the traditional theory attributing beneficial effects in OA to growth factors because they activate the repair processes should be revised. Destructive cytokines and degradative enzymes, as well as an excess of some growth factors, may be responsible for the changes in normal homeostasis associated with the development of OA. Appropriate approaches to the new therapies of OA should carefully consider these aspects. In this context, further progress can be derived from better knowledge of receptor expressions and/or signaling associated with the OA chondrocyte phenotype.

4.6
Role of Crystal Deposition in the Osteoarthritic Joint
(G. M. McCarthy)

Despite frequent findings of crystals in OA tissue, most of the questions concerning their role in OA remain unanswered. In this chapter, G. McCarthy attempts to elucidate the aspects which are thought to be relevant for their clinical or laboratory evidence.

The most intriguing and, at same time, the most difficult to be studied are the basic calcium phosphate (BCP) crystals. These crystals, which are found in 30–60% of OA synovial fluids (SF), may sometimes cause destructive or erosive arthropathy. At present, it is unclear why in some cases BCP crystals are associated with dramatic inflammatory reactions and in most cases are apparently innocuous. Some authors claim that crystals in OA joints are simply an epiphenomenon of cartilage degeneration. However, as suggested by G. McCarthy, in ths case we would expect to see CPPD or BCP crystals in the sites most commonly affected by primary OA. Instead, crystal deposition disease frequently involves the shoulder, wrist and elbow, joints rarely affected by primary OA. Alternative hypotheses are that degeneration and crystal formation may be parallel events of common derivation or, in an intermediate view called "amplification loop", that a primary metabolic abnormality leads to degeneration, but secondary crystal deposits accelerate deterioration.

The basis of cartilage damage by calcium-containing crystals remains unanswered. It is possible that damage may be caused by matrix-degrading enzymes released by synovial lining cells after ingestion of crystals rather than by direct chondrocyte injury. Other than the ability to induce metalloproteases, crystals may have mitogenic properties and may stimulate prostaglandin synthesis. Recent studies have extensively explored the mechanism of crystal-induced mitogenesis. Interestingly, experiments utilising fibroblasts have demonstrated that phagocytosis followed by intracellular crystal dissolution occurs when BCP crystals and fibroblasts come into contact with each other and that this process contributes to BCP crystal-induced mitogenesis. Furthermore, in these cells, the mitogenic response to BCP crystals is associated with PKC (Protein Kinase C) activation, but not with phophatidylinositol 3-kinase or tyrosine – kinase activation, confirming that the cell activation by BCP is selective in mechanism. Other steps in this process involve transcription factor NF-κB (Nuclear Factor-κB) and proto-oncogene induction.

Concerning the matrix degradation induced by calcium containing crystals, the role of inflammatory cytokines is unclear. At present, neither BCP nor CPPD crystals seem able to induce IL-1 *in vitro*. However, currrent data supports direct stimulation of MMP production by fibroblasts and chondrocytes upon contact with calcium-containing crystals.

In the chapter conclusion, the author offers some interesting suggestions concerning the therapy of these forms. Phosphocitrate, a potent inhibitor of hydroxyapatite crystal formation, seems useful in protecting articular tissues from the harmful biologic effects of calcium-containing crystals. The mechanism of this action is most likely related to the inhibition of mitogenic effect of BCP crystals. G. McCarthy also suggests that misoprostol, a PG1 analogue used to prevent gastrointestinal damage induced by NSAIDs, may be proposed in the future due to its ability to interfere with the biological effects of BCP crystals.

Chapter 5
Diagnosis and Monitoring of Osteoarthritis

5.1
Direct Visualization of Cartilage
(X. AYRAL and M. DOUGADOS)

A simplified arthroscopy (ambulatory "chondroscopy" under local anesthesia) aiming at repeated evaluation of the articular cartilage is now available. A 2.7 mm arthroscope (usually 4 mm) is used. It is as well or better tolerated as MRI: 95% of patients accept a second chondroscopy one year later. The beneficial effect of chondroscopy (symptom improvement: 82%) is attributed to joint lavage (about 1 liter). However, we must mention that in a more recent study, the authors found only 40% of patients treated by lavage remained improved at six months [5]. With the SFA score and the global VAS score for quantifying the articular cartilage lesions in continuous variables, the intra-observer reliability coefficient is 0.928 and 0.989 respectively; this allows for valid comparison of lesions one year apart (videotaped arthroscopy). Sensitivity to change (worsening) in 41 patients was highly significant ($p = 0.0002$) in such a time-span. The VAS chondropathy score is correlated to the joint space narrowing on radiographs (r between 0.59 and 0.64). Eventually, chondroscopy could become a new tool for assessing possible structure-modifying drugs versus placebos in the near future.

5.2
Radiographic Imaging of Osteoarthritis
(C. Buckland-Wright)

Taking into account recent advances, radiographic imaging of OA is to be considered from three points of view: the diagnosis of OA, the following up, and the specific needs of the latter in therapeutic trials.

1. Diagnosis of OA should be performed as early as possible. In the three main sites – knee, hip and hands – the subchondral bone reaction to the cartilage lesion seems to be the best indicator of incipient OA, especially osteophytes; most often, it appears earlier than joint space narrowing (JSN). According to certain studies, up to 40% of osteoarthritic knees exhibit oteophytosis and well developed subchondral bone sclerosis, whereas JSN is minimal or absent. However, JSN is more significant and sensitive to change. A slight JSN is more convincing than a tiny osteophyte notably in elderly people. Moreover, a few types of OA, especially the "atrophic" and rapid forms of hip OA and certain cases of knee OA involve JSN without any osteophytosis.

What views are required from the radiologist? With regard to knee OA, at least anteroposterior, mediolateral and skyline views, since OA involves both tibiofemoral and patellofemoral compartments in about 50% of cases (Dieppe 1994, MacAlindon 1992). In patients without JSN on the standard anteroposterior view, the film in semiflexed (BW) or, most often, the schuss position may disclose such a JSN, since cartilage loss is usually predominant at the postero-inferior part of the condyle. We would like to point out that, in reality, the semiflexed position of Buckland-Wright corresponds to a very partial flexion; most often, from 2° to 10° yet, the maximum thinning of the cartilage is usually located more posteriorly, largely beyond the joint space site encompassed by this semi flexed position. It is much closer to the joint space encompassed by the schuss position (30° flexion). Likewise, in incipient OA of the hip, if the anteroposterior radiograph does not show any uniquivocal JSN, do not conclude that it is lacking: the faux profil (partial oblique view) of the hip detects an anterosuperior or a posterior JSN in close to 75% of such cases [6].

2. For the purpose of following up OA with good X-rays reproducibility, the following recommendations are essential: each joint should be radiographied separately; the central X-ray beam must be centered on the targeted JS; fluoroscopy is recommended; a standing position is preferable to assess the JSN both in knee and hip OA patients. In fact, the faux profil view is performed exclusively in a standing position.

3. In therapeutic trials of possible structure-modifying (ex-"chondroprotective") drugs, the primary criterion is the progression of radiographic features of OA, principally the annual rate of JS loss over 2 to 3 years in OA of the hip or knee. To enhance the reproducibility of yearly outcome measures, it was shown that strict position of the patient and correct orientation of the central X-ray beam are the most important parameters, the source of variation larger than the variation from measurement of the radiographic JS itself, at least in regard to OA of the knee. In the near future, relatively new views such as the schuss view of the knee, and the faux profil of the hip ought to be validated in the frame of

such trials: JSN is probably more advanced in such views, and perhaps faster, and more sensitive to change. Future studies should address this issue. Fine "manual"measurement of the JS was performed in the past with a ruler, then with callipers and is now made with a magnifying glass with a graduation in 0.1 mm engraved in the glass [7]. The mean JS loss is 0.20 or 0.35 mm per year in hip OA, and 0.15–0.25 in common knee OA. SD is at least as large as the mean. The coefficient of variation (CV) of the manual measurement at the narrowest point of the JS is 4–5% with the keenest eyes (intraobserver reproducibility).

Other methods of measurement were proposed and have been validated. The radiographs being centred, it is now possible to measure JSN, not only at its thinnest site, but within a relevant area of the JS on machines yielding a digitized image of the radiograph. Indeed, macroradiography can reduce the CV but the device is very scarce. In the knee, size of osteophytes correlates well with JS loss, however is more difficult to quantify. A few authors have proposed a global scoring comprising osteophytes, JSN, sclerosis and even cysts to replace the classical Kelgren-Lawrence grading. Nevertheless, JS loss per year seems easier to measure and is more responsive. These qualities, along with a reduced CV, lead to a smaller patient sample size. Currently, this sample size should be from 150 to 250 patients per group, in randomized double blind trials versus placebo, in the field of possible structure-modifying drugs. Moreover, we recently showed with Dougados et al. that the rapidity of JSN over one year is a good predictive factor of the severity of the OA of the hip [8]. This also seems useful in daily practice.

5.3
Magnetic Resonance Imaging in Osteoarthritis
(Y. Jiang, C. G. Peterfy, J. J. Zhao, D. L. White, J. A. Lynch and H. K. Genant)

This chapter summarizes the principal and main techniques of MRI, especially for bone and joint and result yields in normal cartilage and OA: high T2 signal from the articular cartilage (CA) depends not only on the high rate of water within the CA, but also on the state of the H2 molecule (water bound to collagen in some parts or free) and on the linear direction of collagene fibres which differ from one CA layer to another. On intermediate echo time (TE) images, normal CA shows a trilaminar appearance: a low signal (superficial lamina); an intermediate signal (upper radial zone); a low signal (deep zones). On T2, CA becomes homogenous in signal intensity.

In OA, the first magnetic sign is T2 signal enhancement in areas of matrix damage in deep, intermediate or superficial layers before loss of thickness. When these high signal foci are close to the CA surface, arthroscopic views confirm abnormalities as "blistering" for example. With more sophisticated techniques, it is likely that some chemical compositional changes in OA CA would be detectable by MRI in the future.

The morphologic changes usually occur later. They are best shown (high contrast at the articular surface and CA – bone interface) with a fat supressed T1, 3D gradient echo technique (Peterfy 1996). Focal defects so disclosed were verified by arthroscopy. 3D reconstructed images of the CA may lead to quantifying thinning, volume, geometry and surface topography of CA. Volume MRI measurement was checked for correlation with the true CA volume scraped from the bone in autopsy. This technique could serve for long term trials of possible structure-modifying drugs. However, it is time – and human input – consuming. The ultimate project is to achieve mapping of the OA CA, to register and to compare it over time with the final image, as arthroscopists are able to do now (see chapter 5.1). Today, we are relatively far from this target. Eventually, MRI will not be limited to CA expertise, but could yield images of all the other components of the joint: bone (and its trabecular architecture), and tissues not shown by X-ray: synovium and its grade of inflammation over time, synovial fluid, ligaments, muscles. However, several different and time-consuming techniques of acquisition (including contrast in many cases) are necessary to cover all these structures.

As a comment, we must stress that:

1) early internal alterations of the CA are often far from the painful stages of OA. Its detection could be useful from a prophylactic point of view in high risk subjects (sport, occupation, heredity...)

2) quantitation of magnetic images of CA could be used for assessment of possible structure-modifying drugs. However, such measurements would require several years to be validated by plain or microfocal radiographs [7]. Currently longitudinal studies with MRI have not been validated.

5.4
The Role of Molecular Markers to Monitor Breakdown and Repair
(L. S. LOHMANDER)

A major interest in the study of cartilage derived molecules or fragments concerns their value as OA disease markers. As suggested by the author, these biochemical markers may serve as a window on the pathological processes in the joint and may be useful in elucidating degradation mechanisms, in predicting prognosis and in monitoring response to treatment. However, most studies proposing molecules for this important role have been criticised, mainly due to the presence of many confusing factors in the marker determination and in the difficulty in adequately determining the specific source of the different markers found in the various tissues.

While recent studies have failed to confirm the originally suggested usefulness of keratan sulfate or other molecules as diagnostic tests for generalised OA, these markers may serve to evaluate disease severity or staging in some conditions. Concerning their prognostic value, some interesting reports have pointed out that serum determination of some substances, including hyaluronan, COMP or chondroitin sulfate epitope 846, may predict the progression of knee OA. Another possible role of biochemical markers may be to monitor response to therapy, as sensitive surrogate outcome measures in clinical trials of new disease-modifying treatments. Given that markers may reflect the dynamic state of cartilage metabolism, they may be used as prognostic tools to identify patients at risk of rapid progression, to identify the responders to treatment, and to assess the degree of response. However, to appropriately use these markers, their variability over time, both in the individual and among individuals, should be known. In a recent study, S. Lohmander reported the assay results on samples of synovial fluid, serum, and urine obtained on 8 different occasions during one year from 52 patients with incipient knee OA. Both among-patient and within-patient coefficients of variation varied for markers in different body fluid compartments, with the lowest variability for serum keratan sulfate and the highest for synovial fluid markers. Among these, aggrecan fragments showed the least variability and the matrix MMP the highest. The degree of variability within patients is lower than among patients, thus confirming the need to ascertain the baseline concentrations in clinical trials which propose to use these markers as outcome measures.

In conclusion, the progress in developing sensitive assays has allowed a quantification in body fluids of new molecules which have notably improved our understanding of the OA processes. Despite originally enthusiastic reports, none of these substances may be considered at present capable of satisfying all functions required to be considered as a OA disease marker, such as detecting sub-clinical OA, assessing disease activity, predicting long-term evolution, and evaluating the response to treatment. However, there is increasing evidence that this major goal may be attainable using a combination of different markers, each reflecting a different aspect of the disease process.

Chapter 6
Evolution and Prognosis of Osteoarthritis
(E. VEYS and G. VERBRUGGEN)

It is very difficult, if not impossible, to state an individualised prognosis of OA for a given patient. OA is too much a heterogeneous condition: it is primary or secondary, atrophic or hypertrophic, mono- or polyarticular (generalized OA), etc. The predictive value of the main relevant factors are still either incompletely demonstrated unknown, or unreliable. However, the course of knee and finger OAs – not hip OA – are addressed in this chapter and interesting data are provided. They relate mainly to X-ray changes.

With regard to methodology for assessing the radiological stages of OA, it is pointed out that the qualification of "absent, doubtful, moderate, severe" for every radiographic feature of OA is not sensitive enough and leaves much room for personal bias. Quantitative scoring is preferable. For example, in knee OA, the following scoring system for osteophytes is proposed: at inclusion, each knee osteophyte is scored + 0.2. During follow-up, occurrence of an osteophyte is scored +1 (and disappearance – 1); enlargement or a decrease in size of an existing osteophyte is scored + or – 0.5 respectively. Summing these numbers results in a general joint score. Narrowing of joint space (JSN) is easier to measure more precisely. Subchondral bone sclerosis, cysts and attrition are more difficult to be quantified. Nevertheless, eventually, a summative or global score including the degree of every radiographic sign of OA is obtained.

Summarizing ten cohort studies on the natural course of OA knee, Veys points out that the main predictive factors of subsequent deterioration are as follows: presence of OA in the hands, knee pain at entry, crepitus, joint swelling, instability, chondrocalcinosis. The pejorative predictive value of body mass index as well as of positive bone scan (scintigraphy) are debated; nearly half of the patients with a favorable outcome over years had had a positive bone scan. It is noteworthy that a close correlation exists between the evolution of disease in both knees in individual cases. Last but not least, the weak correlation between clinical outcomes and X-ray changes are once more emphasized. We would recall that, regarding hip OA, the rapidity of the JSN over one year is a valuable predictive factor of severity [8].

The finger joints involved in OA are mainly the distal interphalangeal (DIP), but also the proximal interphalangeal (PIP) joints. Three quarters of the DIP and half of the PIP are affected in patients five years after the onset of symptoms.

The progression of non erosive finger OA is very slow: scoring changes only at 2–3 year intervals (however, quantitative microfocal radiography is more sensitive). Osteophytes and erosion or collapse of the subchondral bone plate are the most reliable variables.

The evolution of erosive OA of the finger joint (mainly the PIP, and also the DIP, but neither the MCPH nor the trapezo-metacarpal joint) is different. It occurs in more than one third of patients with common finger OA at onset followed for 3–5 years. After a phase of stationary OA occurs a phase of joint space disappearance and joint erosion, then finally a stage of joint remodelling (with large osteophytes and clinical Heberden and Bouchard nodes) or fused joints. Such is the natural history of finger OA. Nevertheless, many patients remain steady, without erosive or inflammatory OA, and are most often asymptomatic.

Chapter 7
Impact of Osteoarthritis on Quality of Life
(J. POUCHOT, J. COSTE and F. GUILLEMIN)

Quality of life (QoL) instruments, addressed by J. Pouchot, J. Coste, F. Guillemin are generic or disease specific or even patient specific. Table summarizes the main determining criteria; disease specific are more responsive, though generic-specific could be valuable when scoring only in certain domains. A recent use of the patient-specific scale called MAC TAR seemed to be as responsive as the disease-specific ones in patients with OA treated by total replacement.

Only two instruments are specifically devoted to OA – which are algofunctional indices (AFI) rather than QoL, strictly speaking. The latter are not so responsive to therapeutic changes (i. e. in trials) as the former: QoL strictly speaking are responsive to "massive" treatment such as total joint replacement (confirming obvious good results) and not clearly as responsive to analgesics or NSAIDs, except in some experiences with AIMS, which is rather time-consuming. It is noteworthy that the psychosocial domain of the WOMAC failed to demonstrate enough responsiveness in a 6 week NSAIDs treatment and then was dropped by its author, N. Bellamy [9].

The AFI and some QoL can be performed by telephone interview.

Among the other uses of AFI or QoL, let us mention the following ones: 1) to follow up the natural course of the disease and the impact of the patient's education/rehabilitation; – 2) to aid the surgical decision: scores meaning "time for hip or knee replacement" are published with regard to the Lequesne's indices [10], WOMAC, NHP, AIMS; – 3) OA contrasted to other disease: patients with OA rated better scores than those with RA (and even those with fibromyalgia, lombar pains, and degenerative cervical spine disease concerning pain and psychological outcomes…). Interestingly, domains of energy and sleep measured with NHP are more impairing in OA patients than in several classes of chronically ill patients such as stroke victims; – 4) Medico-economic studies: several techniques such as QUALYs use, utility measures are able to assess the economic benefit of health interventions; they will certainly be more widely used in the near future. As for the practice of trials, the time consuming long questionnaires tend to be avoided.

Table 1. Main Quality of Life (QoL) instruments (in **bold** types, those, easily usable in OA) – (according to data from chapter 7)

		SCORE						
		Number items	Dimen sions	Separat (profil)	Global index	Self-admin	Inter-view	Time spent
GENERICS								
Short Form 36 (SF 36)		36	8	+		+	+	5 – 10'
Nottingham Health Profile (NHP)		38	6	+	–	+	–	5'
Sickness Impact Profile (SIP)		136	12	+	+	+	+	30'
Quality of Life Being (QWB)		3	+	+	+	–		20'
European QoL (Euro QoL)		5	+	+	+	–		
DISEASE SPECIFIC	FOR:							
Lequesne's for hip/knee (1987)	OA	11	3	–	+	–	+	3 – 4'
WOMAC for hip and knee (1988)	OA	24	3	+	+	+	+	8 – 10'
Health Assessment Question. (HAQ)	RA, OA ±	20	8	+	+	+	+	5 – 10'
Arthritis Impact Measur. Scale (AIMS)	Ra, OA ±	45	9	+		+		20'

Chapter 8
Medical Management of Osteoarthritis

8.1
Medical Aspects

8.1.1
Basic Principles in Osteoarthritis Treatment
(D. CHOQUETTE, J-P. RAYNAUD and E. RICH)

Non pharmacological management of OA is important and often underused in some countries. Direct data are rather scarce with regard to weight loss in OA treatment: only one paper points to a strong correlation between weight loss (3–6 kg mean) and a reduction in symptoms, more so for knee than hip OA. Conversely, the harmful role of obesity in knee OA is well established concerning the risk of occurence and the risk of worsening. Unfortunately, with regard to physical therapy in OA of the knee, the distinction between the patellofemoral and the tibiofemoral types are not often made, although the results of some treatments, are probably different according to such types, especially the strengthening of the quadriceps muscle, which seems to us more effective in the patellofemoral type. The latter may also be improved with regard to pain by special medial taping of the patella. Using a cane is likely to be one of the best treatment for both knee and hip OA, but rarely accepted by patients before an advanced stage of the disease. Shock-absorbing shoes are more easily adopted. Kneeling and squatting favor knee OA, and should be avoided.

Pharmacological management. Analgesics are the first treatment to advise, and could improve 30% of patients with knee OA. Some well known studies support that analgesics and NSAIDs are of (almost) the same efficacy in OA. However, we would like to underline that more than 30% of OA patients are improved by NSAIDs and every practitioner knows that NSAIDs are, as a whole, more effective in OA. However, they represent a risk factor by their gastrointestinal toxicity, especially in the elderly. A substantial portion of the latter seems able to stop NSAID therapy and are still off these drugs up to 6 months later. Analgesics themselves are not devoid of possible side effects: liver and kidney functions should be monitored during chronic administration. The use of narcotics is addressed: it is justifiable in certain patients, for short periods, but difficult to overcome side effects are frequent, especially in the elderly. Topical agents such as capsaicin are perhaps underprescribed, particularly in OA of the fingers, toes or knees. A recent review of 86 studies concluded that topical agents are effective and safe.

Intraarticular injections. Repetitive intraarticular injections of corticoids do not seem detrimental to cartilage. A retrospective study of 4 to 15 years of IA steroids injections did not find any severe side effects. However, efficacy itself is still discussed despite an ancient paper of Dieppe et al. showing that steroids are superior to placebos. Improvement seems better if an iffusion exists and is aspirated before the injection of steroids. Triamcinolone hexacetonide seems more effective than Betametazone.

Hyaluronan in various molecular weights (500–700 kD to 4000–5000 kD) seems effective if OA of the knee is of low grade. Duration of the effect, when positive, seems longer than with steroids: 2 to 6 months. However, we know that there are several negative trials and it is likely that such negative studies will never be published.

Among other substances possible to inject by the intraarticular route, Orgotein is mentioned. It seems effective with a coherent effective dose curve from 4 to 16 mg with 2 to 4 weekly injections, and the improvement lasts several months. Other therapies stated are radiation synovectomy, which was not found to be different from triamcinolone: good efficacy at month 3, however, at month 6, improvement disappeared. For knee OA, simple lavage during arthroscopy is perhaps an effective symptomatic treatment. A rate of 40 % of patients remained improved at month 6 in a recent study [5].

8.1.2
Non-steroidal Anti-inflammatory Drugs Administration in the Treatment of Osteoarthritis
(J. T. DINGLE)

The author reminds us of the basic notion: which alterations are repairable, which are not? The depletion of the glycosaminoglycans (GAG) network is to a certain point able to be repaired. The GAG turnover is rapid and, in a 90 year old subject is still 50 % that of the juvenile turnover. On the contrary, the turnover of collagen is close to 20 times slower, and likely not capable of repair. The capillary invasion from the subchondral bone to the overlying cartilage results in calcification and ossification which cannot be eliminated.

IL-1 is not so much a direct agent of catabolism for articular cartilage (AC) as an inhibitor of the activity of the growth factors like IGF-1 on matrix synthesis. This deleterious action begins at low concentrations of IL-1. How is IL-1 released into the joint? Probably as an episodic flow after trauma, overuse, or other precipitating factor.

Dingle reminds us that the tools are currently at our disposal for assessing the effects of different substances (including NSAIDs) on AC vitality: not only on animal, but also on humans organ culture (nevertheless on short term). Moreover, administration of NSAIDs *in vivo* to patients for 10–20 days before a total replacement for knee or hip OA permits *ex vivo* studies on the human AC metabolism. GAG synthesis is mainly measured by the uptake of $^{35}SO_4$ in precise conditions and collagen synthesis by ^3H Proline. For the latter, incorporation time is 16 days as opposed to 20 hours for GAG, because of the much slower turnover of collagen. Moreover, several dozen specimens of a given AC should be analysed because of the large variability of the findings from one site to another, and obviously a sufficient number of patients (interindividual variability is also very large) is necessary to obtain significant means. The main conclusions of Dingle's and others works are as follows: the femoral head AC has a lower GAG synthetic activity than that of the femoral condyles, both in normal and in OA conditions. However, the more severe the OA, the lower the GAG synthetic activity. In patients briefly (10–20 days) given NSAIDs before operating, the variability of GAG synthetic activity was very large, in comparison with those who were not treated by NSAIDs. *In vitro* and *in vivo* studies of different NSAIDs showed the inequality of the latter on the AC metabolism. 3 groups may be distinguished: a) Nimesulide, Ibuprofen, Indomethacin and Naproxen frankly depressed GAG synthesis-b) Diclofenac, Piroxicam, Aspirin, Nabumetone (and paracetamol) seem to be „neutral"-c) Aceclofenac, Tenidap, and Tolmetin are stimulatory. However, this quality decreases in more advanced OA, although it remains significant. The stimulatory action of aceclofenac disappeared in the absence of serum; this action was found again in the presence of growth factor IGF-1 instead of serum. Many of these results on GAG were confirmed by studies on *collagen* synthetic activity.

GAG synthesis studied *ex vivo* after NSAIDs *in vivo* is significantly lower than from untreated patients. This synthesis doubled after *in vitro* NSAID wash out incubation of the *ex vivo* specimens. As a perspective for the future, we would like to conclude as follows: the underlying integrity or repairability power of the joint cartilage should be considered *in vitro* and *in vivo* when treating patients with a given drug, apart from its effect on inflammation and pain. However, let us add that the deleterious effect of NSAIDs on cartilage in a long term *in vivo* study in humans was shown using only indomethacin (the LINK's study). The opposite, i.e., favorable effect of a given NSAID retarding the OA process in the long term is still to be demonstrated with the help of a structure-modifying drug trial design. Moreover, let us not forget that the main side effect limiting the use of NSAIDs in general are other than in the AC itself. More long-term, controlled, randomized trials addressing both the structure-modifying and the gastrointestinal actions of NSAIDs should be carried out.

8.1.3
New and Future Therapies for Osteoarthritis
(J.P. PELLETIER, B. HARAOUI and J.C. FERNANDES)

Three quarters of this extensive and exciting chapter addresses new perspectives and the remainder known therapies.

Pharmacological approaches. Among the relatively new treatments for OA are four slow acting drugs for which we propose the term symptomatic slow acting drugs in OA (SYSADOAs) [11]: diacerhein, avocado/soybean unsaponifiables (ASU), glucosamine sulfate and chondroitine sulfate. They have a moderate efficacy on pain and functional indices, with no clear superiority of one over another. For example, in the latest clinical trial of diacerhein in knee and hip OA, just published [12], responders (patients with a 30% improvement in both pain and in algofunctional indices) were 41% in the diacerhein group and 25% in the placebo group (p = 0.018). SYSADOAs have a delayed onset of action (about 6–8 weeks) and a certain carryover effect (about one month). Therefore, it is not recommended to prescribe such drugs beyond 2 months if they cannot be either reducted or withdrawn. That must be systematically checked. SYSADOAs did not exhibit severe adverse reactions.

In the field of NSAIDs, new compounds which selectively inhibit the cyclo-oxygenase-2 (cox-2) would be as efficacious as the classical NSAIDs but with much less gastrointestinal toxicity.

Among the *local treatments*, other then intra-articular corticosteroid injections, hyaluronan (hyaluronic acid) seems to be of interest, despite some conflicting results (two negative trials out of about ten, and to our knowledge, three negative studies not published). The high molecular weight hyaluronan (Hylan, Synvisc) was shown to be at least as effective as continuous NSAID therapy in knee OA, with no or minor (local) side effects. A current study argues that responders are 70% with an improvement averaging 8 months. However, let us recall that the placebo effect in intra-articular therapy is high (25–50%) and high on functional indices [10].

Grafts of cells, tissue, or synthetic matrices are justified as a possible cartilage repair process, since neither fibrin clot, nor mesenchymal cells appear in the fissures of articular cartilage (AC). However, despite the encouraging success of combined grafts in localized and limited AC defects in rather young patients, this treatment currently remains irrelevant to the widespread OA cartilage lesions (see chap. 9).

Experimental therapies. This is presently an exciting topic in OA. A large spectrum of potential treatments have been explored or proposed in the last decade. Anticytokines or antiinflamatory cytokines IL-4, IL-10 and IL-13 potentialities greatly depend on the target cell.

Gene therapy is a logical approach to introduce biological agent organisms active in OA but which degrade as a protein after oral administration. The gene transfer is achieved with the help of certain retrovirus. Transfer of the IL-1 antagonist receptor (IL-1Ra) to cells subsequently introduced into joints induces sustained production of IL-1 Ra over a long time span. That reduces the progression of structural changes in experimental OA by blocking the action of IL-1 on targeted cells, i.e. chondrocytes or synoviocytes. Its use in man *in vivo* still requires many studies.

IL-1 inhibition. Modulation of IL-1 activity was found to be experimentally successful using tenidap, p 38 kinase inhibitor and either IL-1 soluble receptors (notable IL-1RsII) or anti IL-1 antibodies. Currently, the target is rheumatoid arthritis (RA), OA being a possible perspective.

TNF-α inhibitors. TNF-α soluble receptors (TNF-α sR) seem to facilitate stimulation of cells by TNF-α; this stimulation could be reduced by decreasing TNF-α-sR shed from the OA synovial fibroblasts.

Nitric oxide synthase inhibitors. The inducible form of nitric oxyde synthase (iNOS) is the main source of NO in arthritic disorders; its excess likely decreases synthesis of aggregan. NO is produced in large amounts by chondrocytes, macrophages and inflamed synovium; its synthesis is greatly increased by inflammatory cytokines. NO is a potent inhibitor of IL-1 Ra synthesis; it can reduce matrix synthesis and enhance metalloproteases activity. iNOS is injurious to the OA joint in animals. The iNOS inhibitor reduces synovial inflammation and the level of IL-1α in OA in dogs. Is this a novel therapeutic approach in human OA?

Metalloprotease inhibitors. In this field, a few chemical or biological agents discovered to be active *in vitro* or in animal OA are already in trial in humans. Matrix metalloproteases MMP (collagenases, gelatinases A and B, stromelysin-1...) are known to be among the most active in the OA process, at physiological pH, provided heavy metal such a zinc and calcium are available for their active sites. Natural inhibitors of MMP, Tissue Inhibitor of MP (TIMP), are proteins and therefore unusable as a drug. Chemical agents able to block MMP activity are the most promising. Tetracycline and its semi synthetic forms (doxycycline, minocycline) act by chelating the zinc necessary for MMP activity. They can inhibit collagenases as well as gelatinases. Doxycycline reduces canine OA and is now in a phase II–III trial in human knee OA. Additional trials are in progress with RA and OA patients using other inhibitors, hydroxamate-based compounds which bind with zinc such as RO35 55, and are active on human collagenases. It also seems possible to alter the molecular transcription of MMP gene expression by TGF-β, glucocorticoïds and retinoïds.

Indeed, the road from *in vitro* data and animal experiments to human OA is a long and hard one, often disappointing. However, with so many novel strategies in view, we can reasonably hope that at least one of them will yield a true new treatment of human OA in the near future.

8.2
Regulatory Requirements

8.2.1
Preclinical Studies in Osteoarthritis
(M. Sisay and R.D. Altman)

Outlined by M Sisay and RD Altman, the preclinical studies in OA constitute a very useful basis to cautiously interpret the results from laboratory work, according to certain limitations of technique and pitfalls. For example, in certain *in vitro* studies, the reader should be aware of the cell density of the released chondrocytes in culture, their age and phenotype, as their responses to the same agent (cytokine, enzyme, growth factor) may vary considerably according to such parameters. Likewise, monolayer cultures (the most rapid technique) in which cells adhere to the dish, cause chondrocytes to lose their phenotype; they become non-specific, fibroblastic-like cells unable to produce a significant amount of matrix, especially hyaline cartilage tissue. They are not multipotential like fibroblastic mesenchymal cells of the bone marrow, synovium, or periostum; they have very little capacity to remodel mesenchymal scar tissue. On the contrary, modulated chondrocytes replanted in suspension as non-adherent round cells, notably within a gel matrix such as alginate beads, retrieve their phenotype and are able to express type II collagen and aggregan. Experimental grafts yield variable results. Often, after a promising onset phase, the repair tissue disintegrated and failed, mainly because integration with the surrounding cartilage around the edge of the receiver defect was not achieved. However, a combination of chondrocytes with a growth factor and collagen matrix seems more promising. In another example, the large cavities of horses'-knees, cells from the subchondral bone give rise to matrix surrounding new formed bone; however, after one year, a large amount of fibrocartilage of poor quality is found, reminding us of poor fibrocartilage rising up from the Pridie's holes performed through the subchondral bone, an old surgical process attempted in the 1960's in human OA. Even when cartilage tissue slices or blocks are used instead of chondrocytes in suspension to fill in the defect, the result is not always a macromolecular organisation in the replaced matrix able to mimic articular cartilage.

Some spontaneous OA, occuring frequently enough in certain animal strains, are an exciting tool for researchers. For example, the C57BL and the STR/IN strains of mice present a 50 to 93% incidence of OA lesions, appearing progressively at 15–17 months of age. The blotchy mice, a strain which carries a gene causing an inadequate cross-link of collagen, is close to the ideal model: 88% of the animals develop OA lesions. However, in many cases, animals showing spontaneous OA are costly, very irregularly affected and require a long time between birth and OA observation. Consequently, interventional models are most often used. The anterior cruciate ligament transection in dogs and rabbits, resulting in instability, replicates human OA well (see chapt. 3.2). Medial meniscectomy in rabbits generates some aspects of human OA. A hopeful perspective could be an ovine meniscectomy, a model that closely simulates human OA, as shown recently.

Let us be reminded by the judicious remark by Sokoloff "Cartilage can survive in a large range of sollicitations, but below and beyond, it will suffer" [3]. Indeed, a few models of experimental OA use limb immobilization to induce OA: in extension of the limb, immobilisation creates muscle contraction and lesions like OA; in flexion, it does not lead to OA, unless followed by excessive exercise. However, followed by normal exercise, it could serve to study cartilage repair and the substances able either to enhance or to inhibit this process.

In summary, animal models of OA, especially the interventional ones, permit the study of the true onset of the disease, its progression and the impact of different agents (drugs, mechanical factors, etc…) analysed sequentially, the severity of the lesions monitored and precisely measured by anatomic and radiographic techniques, including radio-labelling. The main methods and targets in the field are very carefully listed in Tables I to IV of this chapter.

8.2.2
Clinical Evaluation of Drug Therapy
(J-Y. REGINSTER, B. AVOUAC and C. GOSSET)

Denominations and definitions of the different classes of drugs are opportunely recalled by J-Y. Reginster, B. Avouac and C. Gosset in this chapter: the old designation of fast-acting and symptomatic slow-acting drugs in OA (SYSADOAs) [11] are now gathered under the general heading of *Symptom-modifying drugs.* The old appellation "chondroprotective drugs", replaced in 1994 by the term of "disease-modifying anti osteoarthritis drugs" (DMOADs) [11] have been called *"structure-modifying drugs"* for 2 years. By definition, the latter are aimed at either preventing or slowing down, or even reversing the structure (anatomical) OA lesions. No such drug exists today. The design of trials should be different for each class so defined: the primary outcome must be chosen among symptoms (i.e. pain, functional index) in the first class and chosen to reflect the possible structure alteration (i.e. narrowing of joint space, osteophytosis variations) in the second class of drugs mentioned above.

Which topographic type of OA is to be chosen? Osteoarthritis of the spine is excluded as a "bad model" for trials. The best models are hip and knee OA. Methodologies for these target joints are well known. As an example of perspective for the coming years, let us consider OA of the hand. Studies of hand OA as a model for trials are now in progress, with the introduction of functional indices such as Dreiser's index (15 in chapt. 8.2.2) or the AUSCAN index, in the process of validation [13], and of a pain interval timing index, a self-recording of the painful days over time proposed by E. Maheu, taking into account that pain is very irregular in hand OA [14]. In that model, a possible structure-modifying drug may now be assessed with the help of the sequence of degradation described by Veys and Verbruggen (see chapt. 6) or with the macroradiography advocated by Buckland-Wright (chapt. 5.2).

The target of the trial is usually the most painful joint: for example, the tibiofemoral compartment (the patellofemoral one is not a "good model") [15]. The contralateral joint could belong to the secondary assessment criteria. Moreover, if a given OA joint is proven to be improved in a trial, the applicant must also bring evidence of a similar favourable action on other OA joints before obtaining right to present his drug as an "antiosteoarthritic" drug in general. Similar, when reading the report of a trial, the practitioner should consider whether the positive results can be extrapolated to a large population of OA patients or remain limited to a rather narrow subset of the disease.

With regard to the diagnostic criteria for hip and knee OA, allowing for homogenous groups of patients, discrepancy remain between the American College of Rheumatology (ACR) criteria, according to which osteophytosis could be the only radiological sign, and the European Agency: Reginster et al. who specify joint space narrowing (JSN) as a necessary sign in hip and knee OA. This requirement, and the list of diseases to be excluded according to these authors, is close to the European diagnostic criteria for hip and knee OA [15] while far from the ACR criteria. With regard to the X-ray criteria for diagnosis, we personally believe that, in the near future, with the help of the schuss position for the knee, the faux profil (partial oblique view) for the hip [6] JSN will be easier and more frequently elicited and will give a more consistant basis to the diagnosis, especially for the possible structure-modifying drug trials. For entry in the latter, reference to the atlas of Altman et al. [16] could allow more precision in the diagnosis and the stage at which OA patients are recruited.

With regard to assessment criteria (or outcome measures, or end points), the four following were proposed as sufficiently validated to constitute a "core set" in trials for hip and knee OA: *pain – functional index – global assessment of the patient – imaging if the trial duration is ≥1 year* [17]. With regard to possible structure-modifying drug trials, imaging (currently the X-ray) should be the primary criterion: measurement of the JSN over 2 to 3 years by manual or automatic process on digitized film is now admitted as reliable (see chapt. 5.2 and [7]). As recently shown with a large group of 436 hip OA patients, the rate of JSN per year is a good marker of OA severity. It yields a predictive clue for the future necessity of total hip replacement (THR) – the more rapid the JSN, the greater the risk of undergoing a THR [8]. However, two important remarks on the JSN as criteria pointed out be Reginster et al. should be highlighted: 1) multiple recommendations must be followed with regard to the strict reproducibility of positioning of the patient (see references "Ravaud" in chapt. 5.2), the direction and centering of the X-ray beam, and the measurement itself on films which must be centralized (only one selected measurer), 2) However, a drug slowing down the structural lesions may be more or less devoid of effect on symptoms, at lest in the mid-term. Then, the European Agency recommends assessing carefully symptoms in such a trial; it is reasonable to require that an improvement of pain and function must accompany the positive structure modification, if any at least, over 1 or 2 years.

Chapter 9
Surgical Treatment of the Cartilage Injuries
(M. BRITTBERG)

In recent years, the introduction of new techniques to stimulate repair of chondral and osteochondral defects has notably modified the surgical approaches to the treatment of cartilage injuries. Unfortunately, the exact value of some of these techniques is still uncertain and needs to be further established by long-term and accurate studies.

Among the more exciting innovation proposed in the field of cartilage repair are the osteochondral allo- and autografting techniques, used to replace cartilage defects and underlying bone with a matching articular graft that has been harvested either as an allograft from an organ donor or as an autograft. The best results of allografts are achieved in young patients with post-traumatic defects and before the onset of degenerative changes. Recently, Ghazawi et al. reported their experience with fresh small-fragment osteochondral allografts reconstructing post-traumatic knee defects of 126 patients followed for a mean of 7.5 years, 85% have had good results. The failure factors included age over 50 years, bipolar defects, misaligned knees and worker compensation cases. However, allografts have some important disadvantages, such a risk for immunologic reactions and disease transmission, thus increasing attention has been focused on autologous osteochondral grafting. Among the different recently proposed techniques, of interest are those which utilise small-diameter autologous cylindrical osteochondral grafts, harvested from an unloaded area in the knee via arthrotomy or arthroscopy and implanted in a mosaic-fashion in the defect area, complemented with an abrasion of the areas between the osteochondral plugs. Excellent results of this relatively simple technique were observed by MRI after one year.

The effectiveness of periostal and perichondral implantations in delivering new cell populations to the cartilage defect needs to be further evaluated, due to the variability of the results in the different studies. Better results are obtained in patients with osteochondritis dissecans and early post-traumatic cartilage defects in young persons.

Young age is a prerequisite necessary to obtain the best results in graft techniques, probably due to the fact that the number of potential repair cells in grafts declines steadily with age.

Another interesting area is that of cell-transplantation. Among the different techniques used, that introduced by Brittberg in 1987 is interesting. The cultured cells from knees of patients with chronic disabling symptoms are injected into a cartilage defect and covered with a flap of periosteum. Of 23 patients (mean age 27), 16 had defects in the femoral surface and 7 in the patella. After a mean of three years, all patients with femoral defects had good or excellent knee function. The restored cartilage is hyaline cartilage. The best results were observed in patients with injuries of the femoral surfaces producing a single, localised deep cartilage lesion. In a recent re-examination with follow-up between 2–9 years, the best results were observed in patients with single femoral condyle lesion and with osteochondritis dissecans. The importance of this technique was confirmed in 1997 by the approval of the USA Food and Drug Administration of the cell technology that uses a patient's own chondrocytes to repair cartilage injuries in the knee.

These new approaches have changed the role of the surgeons, who are increasingly attracted by prevention of the disease rather than the cure of an already developed one. Therefore, to obtain optimal results, it is necessary that the surgeon should be able to combine the more advanced surgical techniques with the highest knowledge obtained by researchers in the field of cartilage injuries, in a new exciting working area which Brittberg propose to call "biomedical surgery". Would it be daring to hope for a technique derived from this one and suitable for incipient osteoarthritis cartilage lesions in the future? The issue seems very different from the repair of a localised traumatic lesion in young patients.

Chapter 10
Scientific Basis of Physical Therapy and Rehabilitation in the Management of Patients with Osteoarthritis
(J-M. CRIELAARD and Y. HENROTIN)

The scientific basis mentioned in the title is largely and carefully stressed by the authors. One of the pivotal facts recalled is that a relevant (i. e. sufficient, exactly adusted) contraction of adequate muscles during movement – especially in charge – is the major protective and shock absorbing agent for the joint. Muscular weakness and impaired proprioception are detrimental to OA joints in action. In turn, painful and even some painless OAs tend to inhibit full muscle contraction (Arthrogenous Muscle Inhibition: AMI) resulting in muscular disuse and weakness, a truly vicious circle. Synovial membrane behaviour under dynamic conditions is also well explained, notably the *ischaemia-reperfusion phenomenon*: hypoxia followed by tissue reoxygenation is deleterious for chondrocyte metabolism and cartilage integrity. Effort and exercise, particularly in certain (excessive) rehabilitation bouts, result in increasing intraarticular pressure (especially in OA joint with effusion or flare of inflammation), which provokes tissue ischaemia by capillar occlusion. Hypoxia favours synthesis and release of IL-1. Subsequent rest decreases intraarticular pressure and consequently provokes blood reflow and synovial membrane reperfusion, which generates active oxygen species. The latter may induce damage in all matrix components. This is one example. Many other interesting physiopathological mechanisms having favorable or detrimental effects on OA joints during exercise or efforts in daily life were studied and were often discarded within the past decades.

A number of physical therapy techniques are stated by the authors. However, they clearly point out the randomized controlled trials (RCT). The RCT are difficult to carry off and relatively rare on the matter, but they exist, and deserve to be emphasized.

With regard to the analgesic action, an interesting double blind versus placebo RCT showed that pulsed electromagnetic fields (18 sessions of 30 min for 1 month) are able to decrease pain and to improve functional status in knee, hand and ankle OA patients. Another RCT of this therapy addressed to painful knee OA recently confirmed this beneficial effect [18]; with 9 daily sessions of 60 min, improvement of pain and Lequesne's index were significant at month 3, testifying a delayed but long carry over effect.

Transcutaneous electrical nerve stimulation (TENS) was appraised in two recent overviews of the literature. Many methodological flaws in the design of most of the studies prevent positive conclusions. Acupuncture and electro-acupuncture comprise three negative and one positive significant result (RCTs).

A word about local applications of cold or heat: although double blind RCT design is not possible, it is concluded that, on the whole, cold application (ice chips, cold packs) seem preferable; cooling inflamed joints tends to spare the cartilage, as enzymatic activity decreases.

And lastly, let us mention local massages with capsaïcin: this P substance antagonist benefits from a renewal of interest.

Rehabilitation techniques are numerous.

Spa therapy, despite obvious difficulties, was tested according to a like RCT design with a significantly positive result in two studies in knee, hip and lumbar OA patients.

Aimed at fighting arthrogenous muscle inhibition and muscle hypotrophy, a quantitative progressive exercise program has been shown to yield beneficial effects when performed for a three month period. The programm is comprised of isometric (no joint movement) and isotonic (an arc of motion with or without resistance) exercices, followed by endurance and speed contraction training sessions. Likewiese, in a controlled trial, aerobic exercises improved mobility and physical performance and reduced pain significantly in comparison with a simple educational program.

Before prescribing exercise aimed at gaining an incremental range of motion and/or strengthening muscles, the practitioner must ensure that there is neither effusion, nor inflammatory flare in the targeted joint, nor a threatening of a chondrolysis episode. The target should be chosen with proper judgment: for example, strengthening of the quadriceps, particularly the vastus mediatis, is especially useful in patients with patellofemoral OA.

Devices, orthesis and educational actions. Pain and discomfort resulting from patellofemoral OA were also reduced by a simple device: a tape pulling the patella medially (statistically significant result). Other devices were tested successfully: in patients with medial tibiofemoral knee OA, valgus knee bracing produced significant pain relief. Shock absorbing viscoelastic shoe soles and insoles provide relief in many patients with lower limb OA and are likely to be a preventive treatment of OA worsening. Use of a walking stick (probably the best "second line" treatment for hip or knee OA) may reduce forces over the joint up to 50 % as far as the hip is concerned. Unfortunately, patients often do not obey us concerning the walking stick, ulesss they are obliged to adopt it at an advanced stage of their OA, when it is too late.

Last but not least, educational actions – among which back schools are the best known, have beneficial effect; even simple regular contact via monthly telephone calls from health care medical auxiliaries have been shown in two reliable works to provide improvement in pain and function in knee OA patients. This procedure probably acts as a recall of the patient's duties concerning exercise, prevention of pain, and other instructions as well as psychotherapeutic support.

Is it useful to add a conclusion to a chapter entitled "Conclusions"? Let us say only that we remember that, fifty years ago, osteoarthritis was treated like a poor relation in the family of rheumatic diseases. Now, and increasingly over the last few decades, OA is more and more studied on a scientific basis by researchers, clinicians (new tools for measuring OA and its development), epidemiologists, radiologists, physiotherapists and – last but not least – orthopaedic surgeons, who have given our patients an invaluable present: the hip and knee prosthesis. We have to find "as soon as possible" (next decade? next century?) a "second line" treatment slowing down or – who knows? – stopping the disease. Thus, we would be able to validate the second part of the beautiful motto adopted formerly by the French League against Rheumatism "more years to life and more life within those years".

References

1. Lanyon P, Doherty S, Muir K, Doherty M (1998) Strong genetic predisposition to hip osteoarthritis. Arthritis Rheum 41–9 (suppl): S 351
2. Lequesne M, Dang N, Lane N (1997) Sport practice and osteoarthritis of the limbs. Osteoarthritis Cartilage 5:75–86

3. Sokoloff L (1969) The biology of degenerative joint disease. Chicago. Chicago Press
4. Radin EL, Rose RM (1986) Role of subchondral bone in the initiation and progression of cartilage damage. Clin Orthop 213:34–40
5. Ayral X, Mézières M, Dougados M (1998) Are there predictive factors of symptomatic efficacy of joint lavage in knee osteoarthritis? Rev Rhum (Engl Ed) 65:674
6. Lesquesne M, Larédo JD (1998) The faux profil (oblique view) of the hip in the standing position. Contribution to the evaluation of osteoarthritis of the adult hip. Ann Rheum Dis 57:676–681
7. Lequesne M (1995) Quantitative measurements of joint space during progression of osteoarthritis: "chondrometry" in: Kuettner K, Goldberg V (Eds) Osteoarthritis disorders. Rosemont Am Acad of Orthopaedic Surg 30:427–444
8. Dougados M, Gueguen A, Nguyen M, Berdah L, Lequesne M, Mazières B, Vignon E (1999) Requirement for total hip replacement: an outcome measure of hip osteoarthritis? J Rheumatol 26: in press
9. Bellamy N, Buchanan WW, Goldshith H et al. (1998) Validation study of WOMAC, a health status instrument for measuring clinically important patient relevant outcomes to anti-rheumatic drug therapy in patients with osteoarthritis of the hip or knee. J Rheumatol 15:1833–1840
10. Lequesne MG (1997) The algofunctional indices for hip and knee osteoarthritis. J Rheumatol 24:779–781
11. Lequesne M, Brandt K, Bellamy N, Moskowitz R, Menkes CJ, Pelletier JP, Altman R (1994) Guidelines for testing slow acting drugs in osteoarthritis. J Rheumatol 21:65–73
12. Lequesne M, Berdah L, Gerentes I (1998) Efficacité et tolérance de la diacerhéine dans le traitement de la gonarthrose et de la coxarthrose. Rev Prat 48:S31–S35
13. Bellamy N, Haraoui B, Buchbinder R, Hall S, Muirden K, Roth J, Hobby K, MacDermid J, Campbell J (1996) Development of a disease specific health status measure for hand osteoarthritis clinical trials. Assessment of symptom dimensionality. Scand J Rheumatol, Suppl 106, 5 (abstract)
14. Mahue E, Dewailly J (1997) Weekly self-assessment of painful joints in hand osteoarthritis (HOA): a new assessment tool. Preliminary validation study. Arthritis Rheum, Suppl 9, S236 (abstract)
15. Lequesne M, Méry C (1980) European guidelines for clinical trials of new antirheumatic drugs. EULA Bulletin 9:171–175
16. Altman RD, Hochberg M, Murphy WA, Wolfe F, Lequesne M (1995) Atlas of individual radiographic features in osteoarthritis. Osteoarthritis Cartilage 3 (Suppl A): 3–70
17. Bellamy N, Kirwan J, Altman R, Boers M, Brandt K, Brooks P, Dougados M, Lequesne M, Strand V, Tugwell P (1997) Recommendations for a core set of outcome measures for future phase III clinical trials in knee, hip and hand osteoarthritis. Results of consensus development at OMERACT III. J Rheumatol 24:799–804
18. Perrot S, Marty M, Kahan A, Menkes CJ (1998) Efficacy of pulsed electromagnetic therapy in painful knee osteoarthritis. Rev Rhum (Engl Ed) 65:715

Subject Index

abrasion or resection, subchondral bone plate 433–435
aceclofenac 378–384
– compared with indomethacin 381
– GAG and collagen synthesis 384
– in vivo and in vitro studies 383
acetabular dysplasia 108
ACL (anterior cruciate ligament) 115
ACR (American College of Rheumatology) system 240, 241
acromegaly 102
activator protein-1 (AP-1) 220
activity, physical 27, 31, 32
acupuncture 455
aerobic power, increasing 458
aetiology, pathogenesis and progression of OA, mechanical factors 101–133
age/ageing 42, 43, 103, 104, 127, 128
aggrecan (PGs) 7, 117, 118, 122, 127, 299, 301, 304, 305
– catabolism 122
– fragments 304
– synthesis 127
aggrecanase 122, 127
– cleavage site in G_1-G_2 122
AHSG (α_2-HS glycoprotein) 221
AIMS (arthritis impact measurement scales) 336
allo- and autografting techniques 435–437
American viewpoint, epidemiology 20–38
ammonium 215
AMP, cyclic 221
analgesics/analgesic action 342, 454–457
anatomy/anatomical
– joints 248
– progression 323
anchorin 10
anesthesia 229
– general 229

– local 229
animal models of OA 81–100, 412–418
– biomechanic factors 116–120
– interventional models 416
– observational 415
– pitfalls, DMOADs 82–94
– spontaneous OA 83–85, 415
– surgical models 85
ankle, MRI 274
ankylosis 146
anterior (cranial) cruciate ligament trasection model 417
anticytokines 394
antiflammatory action 457
antiosteoarthritis therapy, classification 422
antisense oligonucleotide therapy 398
anti-TNF-α 398
α_1 antitrypsin 143
apoptosis 128
arachidonic acid 127
arthritis
– AIMS (arthritis impact measurement scales) 336
– apatite associated destructive 210
– *Charcot* (neuropathic) 108
– gouty arthritis 144, 145
– MACTAR (*McMaster* Toronto arthritis patient preference disability questionaire) 337
– nodal 143
– periarthritis (*see there*) 211
– reactive 304
– rheumatoid 102
arthrodesis 447
arthrography, MR 289
arthro-ophthalmopathy, hereditary 137
arthropathies
– chronic pyrophosphate 211
– cuff tear 210
– crystal-associated 143, 144

arthroplasty
- abrasion 434
- artificial joint arthroplasties 447
- periosteal and perichondral resurfacing
  (soft-tissue arthroplasty) 438–441
- resection or excision arthroplasties 446
arthroscope
- needlescopes 230
- small glass lens 230
arthroscopy 228
- French Society of Arthroscopy (see SFA)
  238, 239
- scoring systems for chondropathy, validation 241–244
articular
- cartilage 1–19, 101, 136, 246, 252, 260,
  277–286
- - destruction 260
- - function 12–19
- - laoding 109, 110
- - MRI 277–286
- - structure 1–12
- chondrocytes 109, 220
- explants 118, 119
aspirin 378, 382, 383
assistive devices 470
atrophy induced by limb immobilization
  417
autoantigens 189
autocrine pathways 128
autologous
- chondrocytes 443
- cylindrical osteochondral grafts 437
autosomal
- dominant 136, 137, 140, 141, 145, 148
- recessive 136
avocado/soybean unsaponifiables (ASU)
  388

back school programs 471
bafilomycin A 215
ballet dancing 115
basic principles in OA treatment 356–370
BCP (basic calcium phosphate) 144, 148,
  210
Beguin system 236
biglycan (DS-PGI) 10, 117, 118
biochemical
- factors
- - joint articular tissue degradation in OA
  156–187
- - normal articular cartilage 277
- markers 296
biomechanical factors and OA 115–133
- articular cartilage 15

- cartilage and exercise: long distance
  running 115–120
- cartilage and injury: meniscectomy
  120–126
biopsy, guided 228
bone
- BMP (bone morphogenetic proteins)
  190, 196
- - BMP-2 196
- BSP (sialoprotein) 302
- dysplasias 102
- marrow (see there) 286, 287
- mineral density 101, 106
- subchondral bone (see there) 106, 107,
  115, 157–163, 246, 257, 297
- viscoelasticity 107
Bouchard's nodes 134, 142, 325
bursitis 148

calcific periarthritis 211
calcified zone, MRI 278
calcium 141
- basic calcium phosphate (BCP) 144, 148,
  210
- calcium-containing crystals (see crystal
  deposition) 143, 210–227
- calcium urate 215
- chondrocalcinosis 145–147, 149
- hypercalcemia 142
- pyrophosphate dihydrate (CPPD) 144,
  210, 212, 213
- - deposition disease (CPPDD) 102, 134,
  145–147
- soft tissue calcification 148
candidate genes 135, 138, 146
canine synovial fibroblasts 215
capsaicin 361
carbon fibers 444
carbon-micromeshes 393
carboxylalkyls 401
cardiovascular fitness 468, 469
carpal joints 118
carpometacarpal (CMC) joints
- first 104, 258, 320
- of the thumbs 104, 258
cartilage
- articular (see there) 1–19, 101, 136, 246,
  252, 277–286
- atrophy induced by limb immobilization
  417
- biomechanical factors (see there)
  115–133
- CDMP (cartilage-derived morphogenetic
  proteins) 190, 193
- degeneration 291, 371

– diagnosis, direct visualization 228–246
– effect of loading 13
– extracellular matrix proteins 146, 148
– fibrillation 107
– growth
– – factors and cartilage repair 188–209
– – plate cartilages 136, 140–142
– human 374
– hypertrophy 128, 188
– impacted 127
– link protein 141
– loss 246, 373
– – matrix synthesis 373
– oligomeric matrix protein (COMP) 11,
  149, 299, 302, 304
– preservation 259
– proteolytic enzymes capable of cartilage
  destruction 371
– remodeling, subchondral bone 162,
  163
– repair (see there) 370–372, 392–394
– signal, abnormal cartilage 282
– structure and function 370
– superficial zones 127
– and synovial membrane (see there)
  163–169
– thickness 253, 282, 285
– in vitro models, study of damage and
  repair 53–81
– volume 284
CDMP (cartilage-derived morphogenetic
  proteins) 190, 193
cell-transplantation 441–444
cellular grafts, repair 392
cervical spine 40, 41
c-fos 216, 217
Charcot (neuropathic) arthritis 108
chondrocalcinosis 145–147, 149
chondrocyte(s) 2, 53, 119, 126, 142, 203, 204,
  214
– adaptive phase 126
– anabolic and catabolic activities 127
– articular 109, 220
– cell culture 410
– cultures (see there) 58–67
– deshielded 129
– hypertrophic phase 126, 142
– immortalized 65, 66
– metabolism (see there) 53, 67–69
– oxygen tension 67
– receptors 127
chondrodysplasias/osteochondrodysplasias
  (CD/OCD) 108, 135–141, 149
– Jansen type metaphyseal chondrodysplasia 141, 142

– metabolic joint diseases, etiology
  (see there) 143–149
– MCD (methyphyseal chondrodysplasias)
  141, 142, 149
– MED (multiple epiphyseal dysplasias)
  135, 140, 141
– OCD (other ostesochondrodysplasias)
  139, 140
– PGOA (primary generalized OA) 142, 143
– rheumatism, chondrodysplastic 136
– Schmid type metaphyseal chondrodysplasia 141
– SED (spondyloepiphyseal dysplasia) 136,
  137, 146
– Stickler syndrome 137–139
chondroitin sulfate 5
– proteoglycan core protein 141
chondroitin sulphate (CS) 389
– 4-sulphate 117
– 6-sulphate 117
– sulphate
– – epitopes 301
– – ratio 301
chondropathy, scoring system 229, 241
– arthroscopic scoring systems for
  chondropathy, validation 241–244
chondrophyte 197
chondroprotection 372, 385
chondroscopy 228
c-jun mRNA 220
classification 22–26
– anti-osteoarthritis therapy 422
– Beguin system 236
– clinical criteria 24–26
– Locker system 236
– newer classifications 234
– Noyes system 234, 235
– previous 231–233
– radiographic criteria 23, 24
– Stabler system 234, 235
– subsets 101, 102
cleft palate 137, 139
clinical trials/clinical evaluation 418, 421,
  425
– evaluation of drug therapy 421–429
– outcome 425
– research 228
cloning, positional 149
cloroquine 215
c-myc 216, 217
COL$_2$A$_1$ 137, 138, 146
COL$_9$A$_2$ 141
COL$_{11}$A$_1$ 139
COL$_{11}$A$_2$ 138, 139
cold or heat therapy 455

collagen(s) 3, 118, 277, 371
- collagen-gelatin gels 393
- fibers 13, 149, 290
- fibrils/fibrous collagen 277
- fibrous 277
- synthesis 374, 384
- - aceclofenac 384
- tensile strength providing 371
- type II-collagen 5, 137, 140, 141, 149, 219, 299, 300, 302
- - α chain fragments 302
- - C-propeptide 299, 302
- type III-collagen N-propeptide 302
- type VI-collagen 141
- type IX-collagen 6, 141, 149
- type X-collagen 141, 142, 149
- type XI-collagen 6, 138, 149
collagenase-1 (MMP-1) 219, 302
collagenase-3 (MMP-13) 202, 219
COMP (cartilage oligomeric matrix protein) 11, 149, 299, 302, 304
- fragments 304
comparator 428
compartment
- knee
- - medial 252, 259
- - patellofemoral and tibiofemoral 250, 251, 261, 263
- matrix (see matrix compartment) 4
computerized measurement, joint space 261, 264
congenital
- congenital/developmental classification 102
- hip dislocation 102
contraceptive pills 44
contrast agents, MRI 272, 283
corticosteroids, intraarticular injections 342, 361, 390
costs 39, 45, 46, 47
- containment strategies 48
- iatrogenic factor 46, 47
- pharmacological treatment 46
- shadow price 46
- surgical treatment 48
COX-1 (cyclooxygenase 1) 389
COX-2 170, 172, 389
- phospholipase A₂/cyclooxygenase 220
coxa vara 141
CPPD (calcium pyrophosphate dihydrate) 144, 210, 212, 213
CPPDD (calcium pyrophosphate dihydrate deposition disease) 134, 145–147
C-reactive protein 304
cross-cultural issues/differences, QoL 350

crystal-associated arthropathies, deposition disease 143, 144, 148, 210–227
- calcium-containing crystals 222
- clinical associations 210–212
- cytokines 222
- inflammation 221, 222
- location and identification 212, 213
- mixed crystal 212
- treatment, implications for 222, 223
- in vitro studies 214–221
cuff
- arthropathy, cuff tear 210
- rotator cuff (see there) 148, 289, 290
culture of chondrocytes 58–67
- chondron culture 64, 65
- co-culture system 66
- culture medium composition 71
- culture system 53
- environment 67
- explant culture 64
- immortalized chondrocytes 65, 66
- in monolayer 58, 59
- in suspension 59–64
cyclic loading 119
cycloheximide 220
cyclooxygenase pathway 127
cysts, subchondral 145, 257, 286, 316
cytokines 127, 165–169, 222, 372, 384, 397
- anti-cytokines 394
- anti-inflammatory 169
- calcium-containing crystals 222
- and growth factors 372, 384
- inhibitors 168, 169, 397
- - of pro-inflammatory cytokines 168, 169
- interaction with growth factors 384
- production 127
- pro-inflammatory and nitric oxide (NO) 165–168

3D (three dimensional) images 268, 284
- 3D MRI 284
dacron-micromeshes 393
DAG (diacylglycerol) 216
damage and repair of cartilage, in vitro studies 53–81
debridement 432
decorin (DS-PGII) 10, 117, 118
- in connective tissues 118
dedifferentiation 192
definition 26, 101
deshielded chondrocytes 129
development of OA lesion 372
- abnormalities, developmental 107, 108
- IL-1 activity 385

diabetic neuropathy 108
diacerhein/diacethylrhein 388
diacylglycerol (DAG) 216
diagnosis and monitoring 228 – 311
– direct visualization of the cartilage
  228 – 246
– molecular markers to monitor breakdown and repair 296 – 311
– MRI (magnetic resoance imaging) 228,
  268 – 295
– radiographic imaging 228, 246 – 268
diamond dust 215
diclofenac 378, 382, 383
disability 20, 21, 27
diseases (see syndromes)
dissolution, intracellular 215
DMDs (disease-modifying drugs) 343
DMOADs 228, 231
dogs
– exercised 116
– meniscectomy 120
doxycycline 401
drilling, resection or abrasion, subchondral
  bone plate 433 – 435
drugs
– aceclofenac (see there) 378 – 384
– adverse drug reactions 46
– analgesics 342
– aspirin 378, 382, 383
– avocado/soybean unsaponifiables (ASU)
  388
– capsaicin 361
– clinical evaluation of drug therapy
  421 – 429
– corticosteroids, intraarticular injections
  342, 361, 390
– cytokines (see there) 127, 165 – 169, 222,
  372, 384
– diacerhein/diacethylrhein 388
– diclofenac 378, 382, 383
– DMDs (disease-modifying drugs) 343
– doxycycline 401
– ibuprofen 378, 382, 383
– indomethacin (see there) 378, 381 – 383
– ketoprofen 382
– minocycline 401
– nabumetone 378
– naproxen 378, 381, 383
– narcotics 360
– nimezulide 378
– NSAIDs (nonsteroidal antinflammatory
  drug administration) 46, 47, 248, 342,
  360, 370 – 387
– piroxicam 378
– orgotein 364

– SSADs (smptomatic slow acting drugs)
  343
– structure modifying drugs 410
– tenidap 378
– tetracycline 401
– tolmetin 378
– tramadol hydrochloride 360
DS-PGI (biglycan) 117, 118
DS-PGII (decorin) 117, 118
dwarfism 140

economic
– burden 421
– impact 34
educational action/patients education 343,
  357, 471
– QoL 343
efficacy 428
EHDP (binding of (^{14}C) ethane-1-
  hydroxyl-1, 1-diphosphonate) 213
eicosanoids 127
electrical therapy, low frequency 454
electro-acupucture 455
electrotherapy 455
endochondral ossification 142
endocytosis 215
environment
– chondrocyte culture environment
  67 – 73
– – ionic and osmotic environment
  68, 69
– extracellular 53
enzymes/enzyme inhibitors 163 – 165
epidemiology and economic consequences
  20 – 52
– American viewpoint 20 – 38
– European viewpoint 38 – 52
– regional variation 41
– studies and surveys, epidemiological 38,
  421
epinephrine 229
epiphyseal dysplasia 138
– MCD (methyphyseal chondrodysplasias)
  141, 142, 149
– MED (multiple epiphyseal dysplasias)
  135, 140, 141
– SED (spondyloepiphyseal dysplasia) 136,
  137, 146
epitope 299
ethnicity 44
etiology of metabolic joint diseases
  143 – 149
– calcium pyrophosphate dihydrate deposition disease (CPPDD) 134, 145 – 147
– crystal-associated arthropathies 143, 144

etiology of metabolic joint diseases
- gout 144, 145
- hydroxyapatite deposition disease
  (HADD) 144, 148, 149
European
- quality of life scale (EuroQoL) 335
- viewpoint
- - epidemiology 38-52
- - incidence 41
evolution and prognosis of OA 312-330
- heterogeneity of OA 312-314
- population studies 315-327
exercise therapy 460-467
experimental models of OA 53-100
extracellular
- environment 53
- matrix (ECM) 3

Fairbanks 140
fat suppression, MRI 275, 276
femoral head 137, 140, 143, 374
- ex-vivo femoral head GAG synthesis
  376
- human condyles 374
FGFs 191, 193, 195
fibril organization and function, articular
  cartilage 5
fibroblasts
- canine synovial fibroblasts 215
- growth factor (bFGF) 394
- human foreskin fibroblasts (HFF)
  217
fibromodulin 10
fibronectin 10
fibrous collagen 277
finger joint OA (see also hand joints)
  320-327
- erosive OA 320
fracture stress 104
free radicals 127, 128
French Society of Arthroscopy (see SFA)
  238, 239
function loss 453
functional status 332
fura-2 215

gadolinium 288
GAG (glycosaminoglycan) synthesis 371,
  374, 376-378, 384
- aceclofenac 384
- ex-vivo femoral head 376
- in-vitro NSAID treatment on 377, 378
- measurement of 374
GAGPS (glycosaminoglycan polysulphuric
  acid) 392

gelatinase
- gelatinase A and B 401
- 92 kD gelatinase (gelatinase B/MMP-9)
  219
gender 43
gene(s)
- candidate genes 135, 138, 146
- expressions 127
- therapy 395-397
genetic(s)
- anticipation 143
- defects 128
- factors 41
- linkage analysis 146-149
- and metabolic aspects 134-156
- - chondrodysplasias/osteochondro-
    dysplasias (CD/OCD) 135-140
- - hereditary OA 134, 135
- molecular genetics 149
- reverse genetics 149
glenohumeral joints 148
global assessment 236
glucosamide sulphate (GS) 388
glycoproteins 221, 277
- AHSG (α_2-HS glycoprotein) 221
glycosaminoglycan 7, 117
- polysulphuric acid (GAGPS) 392
gout 143-145
- gouty arthritis 144, 145
- HPRT-related 144
- pseudogout 211
gradient echo 271, 275
grading systems 239, 256
- SFA (French Society of Arthroscopy)
  238, 239
growth
- factors 149, 372, 394-402
- - anti-cytokines 394
- - and cartilage repair 188-209
- - basic fibroblast growth factor (bFGF)
    394
- - fibroblast growth factor (FGFs) 191,
    193, 195
- - gene therapy 395-397
- - IGFs (see there) 158, 190, 194, 203, 216,
    372, 394
- - Ils (see there) 372, 397, 398
- - interaction of cytocines and growth
    factors on cartilage metabolism 384
- - PDGF (platelet-derived growth factor)
    191, 196, 216
- - TGFs (see there) 190-203, 222, 394
- - TNFs (see there) 398-402
- plate cartilages 136, 140-142
guidelines 234, 423

- Osteoarthritis Research Society Clinical Trials guidelines 251
- videotaping 244

HADD (hydroxyapatite deposition disease) 144, 148, 149
hand joints
- radiography 248, 249, 256, 257
- - finger joint OA 320–327
- - joint space narrowing 256
- small hand joints 39
Harris hip score 346
health (*see also* quality of life)
- HAQ (health assessment questionnaire) 335
- health care access 347
- HRQL (health related quality of life) 332
- index 333
- profiles 333, 334
- - Nottingham health profile (NHP) 334
- public health authority 421
- status 332
hearing loss, sensorineural 137, 139
heat or cold therapy 455
heating therapy, deep or superficial 454
Heberden's nodes 134, 142, 325
hemochromatosis 102, 146
heritable OAs 134
heterogeneity of OA 312–314
HFF (human foreskin fibroblasts) 217
hip
- congenital dislocation 102, 107
- injury 33
- OA 40, 261
- QoL
- - *Harris* hip score 346
- - *Lequesne's* knee and hip index 336
- - *Merle d'Aubigné* hip score 346
- radiographic imaging 254–256, 260, 261
- - joint space width 255
- - position of joint space 254
- - X-ray beam 255
- subchondral sclerosis 261
histological composition 277
HLA A_1B_8 143
hormonal factors 115
horses, standard bred horses 117
hospital admission 45
HPRT (hypoxanthine guanine phosphoribosyl transferase) 143, 144
- gout, HPRT-related 144
- $HPRT_1$ 143–145
hyalgan 391
hyaluronan (hyaluronic acid) 301, 302, 362–364, 371, 391

hyaluronate 3, 104
hydrotherapy 454, 459
hydroxyapatite
- deposition disease (HADD) 144, 148, 149
- pseudopodagra 211
hydroxychloroquine 389
3-hydroxypyridinium cross links[g] 303
hylan (HA) 391
- GF-20 363, 364
hypercalcemia 142
hypermobility 102, 104
hyperparathyroidism 146
hyperuricemia 144
hypomagnesemia 146
hypophosphatasia 146
hypoxanthine guanine phosphoribosyl transferase (HPRT) 143, 144

iatrogenic cost factor 46, 47
ibuprofen 378, 382, 383
IGFs (insulin-like growth factor) 158, 190, 194, 203, 216, 372, 394
- IGF-1 194, 195, 216, 372, 394
- IGF-binding proteins 190
- receptor 190
IKK (IκB kinase) 217, 218
- activation 218
incidence, Europe 41
indomethacin 378, 381–383
- compared with aceclofenac 381
- LINK study 381
- in vivo and in vitro studies 383
inflammation/inflammatory 127, 165–169, 221, 222, 320, 325, 326
- calcium-containing crystals 221, 222
- cytokines (*see there*) 165–169, 372
- inhibitors of pro-inflammatory cytokines 168, 169
- mediators 189
- NSAIDs (nonsteroidal antinflammatory drugs) 46, 47, 248, 342, 360, 377
- OA 320, 326
- - erosive OA 325
- repair 197
injury, joints 32, 33
- hip 33
- knee 33
iNOS (inducible NO synthase) 194, 196, 203
- knockout 203
inosital triphosphate (IP_3) 216
interleukin (IL)
- IL-1 194, 196, 203, 217, 220, 372, 384, 385, 397
- - cytokine IL-1 384
- - inhibition 397

interleukin (IL)
- - knockout 203
- - OA development due to episodes of
  IL-1 activity 385
- IL-1β 127, 128, 166, 167, 169–172, 203,
  398
- - converting enzyme (ICE) 398
- - signaling pathways 170–172
- IL-1Ra 168, 194, 396, 399
- IL-1RsI 398
- IL-1RsII soluble receptors 398
- IL-1sR 168
- IL-4 194, 394
- IL-10 194, 394
- IL-13 394
- IL-17 195
interphalangeal (IP) joints 320
- distal (DIP) 320
- proximal (PIP) 320
interventional animal models 416
isokinetic exercises 465
isometric exercises 465
isotonic exercises 467

Jansen type MCD (metaphyseal chondrodysplasia) 141, 142, 149
jogging 115
joints
- anatomy 248
- articular tissue degradation in OA
  156–187
- - subchondral bone (see there) 157–163,
  246
- artificial joint arthroplasties 447
- carpal 118
- carpometacarpal (CMC) 104, 258, 320
- effusion 287
- finger (see also hand joints) 320–327
- fluid 148, 287, 288, 298
- - MRI 287
- force attenuation 107
- function and gait 458
- glenohumeral 148
- hand, small joints 39
- hip 254, 255
- injury 32
- interphalangeal (IP) (see there) 320
- lavage 230, 363, 432
- metacarpophalangeal (MCP) 320
- neuropathic joint disease 108, 109
- patellofemoral, radiography 250
- space
- - computerized measurement 261, 264
- - radiographic margins 247–256
- - narrowing 246, 247, 249, 256, 263

- - width 247, 249, 255, 257
- synovial 1, 247

κB 217, 218
- IκB 217
- IκB kinase (IKK) 217
- NF-κB (nuclear factor kB) 217
- - NF-κB-inducing kinase (NIK) 218
Kellgren's system 38, 40
keratan sulfate 7, 301, 303
- epitopes 301
ketoprofen 382
knee
- compartment, medial 252, 259, 263
- - tibio-femoral 263
- fully extended, radiography 247
- injury 33
- OA 40
- primary outcome measure 261
- QoL, Lequesne's knee and hip index 336
- radiography 250–254, 259–262, 315–320
- - cartilage thickness 253
- - cysts, attrition and desaxation 316
- - joint space measuring 251, 253
- - joint space narrowing 259, 316
- - joint space width 259
- - micro-/microfocal radiography 261,
  315
- - osteophytes 256–260, 316
- - precision of joint space width 262, 263
- - radiographic progression 315–320
- - reproducibility 262
- - schuss position 259
- - scores, summative, global or overall
  317
- - semi-flexed position 252
- - skyline view 253
- - standing semi-flexed view 251, 253
- - subchondral bone sclerosis 246, 260,
  261, 263, 316
- - therapeutic trials 253
- - X-ray beam 251
- tidal knee irrigation 365
Kniest dysplasia 139
kyphoscoliosis 137

LAP (latency associated peptide) 191
lapine model of OA 214
latex beads 215
lavage
- joint lavage 230, 363
- saline 365
Lawrence's system 38, 40
Lequesne's knee and hip index 336
Lesch-Nyhan syndrome 144

leukemia inhibitory factor (LIF) 195
leukocytosis 221
LIF (leukemia inhibitory factor) 195
ligaments
- ACL (anterior cruciate ligament) 115,
  417
- MRI 289
limb immobilization, cartilage atrophy
  induced by 417
link protein 9
L-NIL (N-iminoethyl L-lysine) 400
Locker system 236
lumbar spine 40, 41, 137
lumbosacral spine 139
lysosomotrophic agents 215

MACTAR (*McMaster* Toronto arthritis
  patient preference disability questionaire)
  337
magnetization (*see also* MRI) 270
- longitudinal 270
- transfer 276, 277, 284
- - subtraction 284
- transverse 270
MAPK (mitogen activated protein kinases)
  217
- p42/p44 217
markers
- biochemical 296
- molecular, to monitor breakdown and
  repair 296 – 311
- - uses of 303 – 307
marrow/bone marrow
- edema 286, 287
- MRI 287
Marshall syndrome 139
massage 459
matrix
- cartilage loss matrix synthesis 373
- compartment 4
- - interterritorial 4
- - pericellular 4
- - territorial 4
- extracellular (ECM) 3
- metalloproteinases (*see* MMPs) 122, 127,
  159, 163, 164, 202, 214, 219, 302, 304, 400,
  401
- proteins 10, 11
- - COMP (cartilage oligomeric matrix
  protein) 11, 149, 299, 302, 304
MCD (methyphyseal chondrodysplasias)
  141, 142, 149
- *Jansen*-type 149
McKusick type 141
McMaster University OA index 336

mechanical
- factors 101 – 114
- - biomechanical factors (*see there*)
  115 – 133
- overload 119
- stress on chondrocyte metabolism 69,
  126
MED (multiple epiphyseal dysplasias) 135,
  140, 141
medical
- management of OA 356 – 430
- - medical aspects 356 – 408
- - regulatory requirements 408 – 429
- treatment of OA, QoL 342 – 344
- - nonsteroidal antiinflammatory drug
  administration 46, 47, 248, 342, 343,
  360, 370 – 387
- - rehabilitation and education 343
medicoeconomic studies 346, 347
membrane hyperpolarisation 109
meniscal tears 290
meniscectomy 105, 120 – 126, 289, 417
- animal models 120, 417
- - in dogs 120
- - in sheeps 120
- lateral 120
menisci 115
- MRI 289, 290
Merle d'Aubigné hip score 346
metabolic aspects/diseases/metabolism
  102, 134 – 156, 374
- chondrocytes, metabolism 53, 67 – 69
- - mechanical stress 69, 126
- - oxygen tension 67
- - pH effect 70
- etiology of metabolic joint diseases
  (*see there*) 143 – 149
- interaction of cytocines and growth factors on cartilage metabolism 384
- measurement of human cartilage
  metabolism 374
- non-arthritic and osteoarthritic
  cartilages, relative metabolism 375
metacarpophalangeal (MCP) joints 320
methodology 421
methotrexate (MTX) 389
metaphyseal chondrodysplasias (*see* MCD)
  141, 142, 149
microscopy, electronic 212
- SEM (scanning electron microscope) 212
- TEM (transmission electron microscopy)
  212
Milwaukee shoulder syndrome (MSS) 148,
  210
mineral density 101, 106

minocycline 401
misoprostol 221
mitogen activated protein kinases (MAPK)
  217
mitogenesis 218
mitogenic properties 214
MMPs (matrix metalloproteinases) 122, 127,
  159, 163, 164, 202, 214, 219, 304, 400, 401
- B/MMP-9 gelatinase (92 kD gelatinase)
  219
- and inhibitors 302
- membrane type 164
- MMP-1 (collagenase-1) 219, 302, 401
- MMP-3 (stromelysin) 219, 300, 302, 305,
  401
- MMP-8 401
- MMP-13 (collagenase-3) 202, 219, 401
- TIMPs (tissue inhibitor of metalloproteinases) 128, 164, 210, 302, 401
monitoring 296-311
- molecular markers to monitor
  breakdown and repair 296-311
monosodium urate 143, 144
- monohydrate (MSU) 143, 215
morphological parameters 284
motion exercises 460
mouse ₃T₃ cells 215
movement 453
- loading 101
MRI (magnetic resonance imaging) 228,
  268-295
- ankle 274
- arthrography, MR- 289
- articular cartilage 277-286
- basic principles 269
- calcified zone 278
- cartilage
- - thickness 282, 285
- - volume 284
- contrast agents 272, 283
- 3D MRI 284
- fast spin echo 275
- fat suppression 275, 276
- gadolinium 288
- gradient echo 271, 275
- joint fluid 287
- ligaments 289
- magnetic susceptibility effects 271
- magnetization (see there) 270, 276, 277,
  284
- menisci 289
- serial measurements 284
- spin echo 271, 272
- subchondral bone 279
- superficial tangential zone 278

- synovium and joint fluid 287
- technical considerations 269-277
- tendons 289
- three dimensional (3-D) images 268
- T₁ relaxation 270
- T₂ relaxation 271
- trilaminar appearance 282
- upper radial zone 281
MSS (Milwaukee shoulder syndrome) 148,
  210
MSU (monosodium urate monohydrate)
  143, 215
multiple epiphyseal dysplasias (MED) 135,
  140, 141
muscle
- relaxation 454
- weakness 105
mutations 134, 137, 139-142, 145, 147, 149
- recessive 139
myopia 137, 139

nabumetone 378
naproxen 378, 381, 383
narcotics 360
necrosis
- avascular 102
- cellular 128
needlescopes 230
neoepitopes 301
neuropathy/neuropathic joint disease 108,
  109
- Charcot (neuropathic) arthritis 108
- diabetic 108
NIK (NF-kB-inducing kinase) 218
nimezulide 378
N-iminoethyl L-lysine (L-NIL) 400
nitric oxide (NO) 127, 128, 165-168, 194,
  196, 398, 399
- free radical generation 127, 128
- iNOS (inducible NO synthase) 194, 196,
  203
- synthase (NOS) 398, 399
- - inhibitors 398, 399
nodal arthritis 143, 325, 326
- Bouchard's nodes 134, 142, 325
- Heberden's nodes 134, 142, 325
nomenclature 422
non-strenuous exercise 117
Nottingham health profile (NHP) 334
Noyes and Stabler system 234, 235
NSAIDs (nonsteroidal antiinflammatory
  drugs) 46, 47, 248, 342, 343, 360, 370-387
- group classification 377
- cost implications 46
- effect on GAG synthesis 377, 378

- human cartilage 380–383
- topical 360
NTPPPH (nucleoside triphosphate pyrophosphohydrolase) 146
nuclear factor κB (NF-κB) 217

OA (osteoarthritis)
obesity 102
observational animal models 415
occupation 27, 31–33, 42
- risks, occupational 105, 106
- therapy, occupational 358
OCD (other osteochondrodysplasias) 139,
  140
onset 41
orgotein 364
orthoses 470
OSMED (oto-spondylomegaepiphyseal
  dysplasia) 136, 139
Osteoarthritis Research Society Clinical
  Trials guidelines 251
osteoarthritis (see OA)
osteoblasts 160–162
osteocalcin 303
osteochondral
- allo- and autografting techniques
  435–437
- autologous cylindrical grafts 437
- progenitor cells 442
osteochondrodysplasia (see chondrodysplasias) 108, 135–140
osteophytes 116, 198, 203, 256–260, 283,
  286, 316
- central 283
- formation 246
- size 260
osteophytosis 253, 257, 263, 286
oto-spondylomegaepiphyseal dysplasia
  (OSMED) 136, 139
overweight 20, 21, 28–30, 33, 42, 105
oxygen tension, chondrocyte metabolism
  67

PA/plasmin system 159
Paget's disease 102
pain, prevention of 453
paracrine factors 128
parathyroid hormone (PTH) 142, 158
patellofemoral
- compartment 250
- joint, radiography 250, 253
- OA 253
pathophysiology 101–227
- aetiology, pathogenesis and progression
  of OA, mechanical factors 101–114

- biochemical factors, joint articular tissue
  degradation in OA 156–187
- biomechanical factors (see there)
  115–133
- crystal deposition in the OA joint
  210–227
- genetic and metabolic aspects 134–156
- growth factors and cartilage repair
  188–209
patient management 49
PDGF (platelet-derived growth factor) 191,
  196, 216
periarthritis, calcific 211
perichondrial/periosteal grafts
- repair 393
- resurfacing 438–441
Perthes disease 102, 107
PGE 220, 221, 399
- PGE$_1$ 399
- PGE$_2$ 220
PGOA (primary generalized OA) 142, 143
PGs 117, 118
- aggrecan (see there) 7, 117, 118, 122, 127,
  299, 301, 304, 305
- DS-PGI (biglycan) 117, 118
- DS-PGII (decorin) 117, 118
phagocytosis 215
pharmacological treatment of OA 46,
  342–344
- costs 46
- drugs (see there) 342, 343
phenotype 144, 146
phosphatidylinositol 3-kinase 217
phosphatidylinositol 4,5-biphosphate (PIP$_2$)
  216
phosphocitrate 222
phosphodiesterase 216
phospholipase A$_2$/cyclooxygenase 220
phospholipase C 216
phosphoribosyl pyrophosphate synthetase
  (PRPS) 143–145
physical
- activity 27, 31, 32
- impairment 453
- therapy 358, 453–458
physician visits 45
PIP$_2$ (phosphatidylinositol 4,5-biphosphate)
  216
piroxicam 378
PKA (protein kinase A) 170
PKC (protein kinase C) 170, 216
placebo use 428
platyspondyly 137, 138, 140
polyglycolic acid 393
polylactates 393

population 33
- rural 44
- studies 315–327
- urban 44
positioning, radio-anatomical 248, 250, 326
- finger joints 326
- knee 250
- wrist and hand 248
PPi (inorganic pyrophosphatase) 146, 222
preclinical studies in OA 408–422
- in vitro studies (see there) 53–81, 377,
  378, 383, 410, 412
precocious OA 137, 141
prevalence 20, 21, 26, 27, 38, 39
prevention 33, 34
- of pain 453
primary OA 313
- PGOA (primary generalized OA) 142,
  143, 326
probenecid 222
prognosis 43
proprioceptive reeducation 469
prostaglandin 127, 214, 220, 221
- synthesis 214
protein kinase A (PKA) 170
protein kinase C (PKC) 170, 216
proteoglycan(s) 7, 9, 10, 277
- aggregates 9, 109
- chondroitin sulfate, proteoglycan core
  protein 141
- non-aggregating 10
- synthesis 109
proteolytic enzymes capable of cartilage
  destruction 371
protons 269
proto-oncogenes 216, 217
- c-fos 216, 217
- c-myc 216, 217
PRPS (phosphoribosyl pyrophosphate
  synthetase) 143–145
- PRPS$_1$ 144
pseudoachondroplasia 140
pseudogout 211
pseudopodagra, hydroxyapatite 211
psychometric properties in the QoL
  instruments 348–350
- acceptability 350
- interpretability 349
- reliability 349
- responsiveness 349
- validity 349
PTH (parathyroid hormone) 142, 158
- PTH-receptor gene 142
- PTH-related peptide 142
public health authority 421

pulsed electromagnetic field 455
pyrophosphate
- arthropathy, chronic pyrophosphate 211
- CPPD (calcium pyrophosphate dihydrate)
  144, 210, 212, 213
- CPPDD (calcium pyrophosphate dihydrate deposition disease) 102, 134,
  145–147
- PPi (inorganic pyrophosphatase) 146,
  222
- PRPS (phosphoribosyl pyrophosphate
  synthetase) 143–145

quality of life (QoL) (see also health) 39,
  331–355
- applications of instruments 338–347
- - cross sectional and short term
    longitudinal studies in OA 338–340
- - medical treatment of OA (see there)
    342–344
- - OA contrasted to other diseases
    340–342
- definition and conceptual issues 332
- disease-specific instruments 335–337
- - arthritis impact measurement scales
    (AIMS) 336
- - health assessment questionnaire (HAQ)
    335
- - Lequesne's knee and hip index 336
- - Western Ontario and McMaster
    University OA index 336
- generic instruments 333–335
- - European quality of life scale
    (EuroQoL) 335
- - Nottingham health profile (NHP) 334
- - quality of well being (QWB) 334
- - short form-36 items (SF-36) 334
- - sickness impact profile (SIP) 333,
    334
- HRQL (health related quality of life)
  332
- impact of OA 331–355
- medical treatment of OA (see there)
  342–344
- medicoeconomic studies 346, 347
- - health care access 347
- - QALYs (quality adjusted life years)
    347
- methodological problems 348–351
- - cross-cultural issues 350
- - psychometric properties in the QoL
    instruments (see there) 348–350
- - selection of QoL instruments in OA
    348
- patient-specific instruments 337, 338

– – *McMaster* Toronto arthritis patient preference disability questionnaire (MACTAR) 337
– – schedule for the evaluation of individual QoL (SEIQoL) 337
– surgical treatment of OA (*see there*) 344–347

racquet sports 115
radiographic imaging 228, 246–268
– carpometacarpal joints 258
– diagnostic 228, 246–268
– direct measurement 256
– features 248, 249, 256
– – measurements of 248
– hand/wrist and hand (*see hand*) 249, 256, 261, 320–327
– hip (*see there*) 254–256, 260, 261
– knee (*see there*) 250–254, 261, 262, 315–320
– macroradiographs 257, 262
– magnification 248, 253, 261
– measurement reproducibility 256
– methods 247
– microfocal 248, 263, 315
– positioning, radio-anatomical 248, 250
– progression 248
– protocols 249, 261
– – for standard radiography 249
– quantitative methods 256
– radiation synovectomy 365
– reproducibility 262
– standard radiography 264
– technician 248
– therapeutic trials 247, 248
– X-ray beam alignment 248
– X-ray diffraction 212
recommendations 422
recource implications 4
reeducation, proprioceptive 469
regional variation, epidemiology 41
regulatory authorities 421
rehabilitation 343, 453
– and education 343
repair 370–372, 392–294
– cellular grafts 392
– mechanisms 372
– natural matrices 393
– perichondrial/periosteal grafts 393
– scaffolds in cartilage repair 444, 445
– synthetic matrices 393
– tissue grafts 392
resection or abrasion, subchondral bone plate 433–435
rheumatology/rheumatism/rheumatoid

– ACR (American College of Rheumatology) system 240, 241
– arthritis, rheumatoid 102
– chondrodysplastic rheumatism 136
Ribbing 140
risk
– factors 38, 41, 103
– risk/benefit ratio 422
rotator cuff tears 148, 289
– rupture 290
running, long distances 115
rural populations 44

safety 427
saline 231
– lavage 365
scaffolds in cartilage repair 444, 445
scanning electron microscope (SEM) 212
Schmid type metaphyseal chondrodysplasia 141
scoring system 239
– chondropathy 229, 241
– SFA (French Society of Arthroscopy) 238, 239
secondary OA 313
SED (spondyloepiphyseal dysplasia) 136, 137, 146
– OSMED (oto-spondylomegaepiphyseal dysplasia) 136, 139
SEIQoL (schedule for the evaluation of individual QoL) 337
SEM (scanning electron microscope) 212
sensorineural hearing loss 137, 139
serine/threonine kinase receptor 192
SFA (French Society of Arthroscopy) systems 236–239
– grading system 239
– scoring system 239
shadow price (*see also* costs) 46
sheep joints, meniscectomy 120
short form-36 items, QoL (SF-36) 334
sickness impact profile (SIP) 333, 334
signal transduction 142
signaling pathways 169–174
– IL-1β activated 170
– intracellular signaling cascades 169
– TNF-α activated signaling pathways 172–174
skiing 115
smads 192
smokers 44
social
– impact 45
– support 357
soft tissue calcification 148

spa treatment 459
spin echo 271, 272
- fast spin echo 275
- T₁-weighted 272 → T_1-weighted 272
spine
- cervial 40, 41
- lumbar 40, 41, 137
- lumbosacral 139
spondyloepiphyseal dysplasia (SED) 136, 137, 146
spontaneous OA, animal models 83 – 85, 415
sports and exercise 32, 43
- sporting injury 105
SSADs (symptomatic slow acting drugs) 343
Stabler system 234, 235
staurosporine 218
steroids 204
Stickler syndrome 137 – 139
- Wagner syndrome 138
stop codon 138
strain 101
strengthening exercises 461
strength 458
stretching exercises 467
stromelysin (MMP-3) 219, 300, 302, 305, 401
- stromelysin-1 300, 401
studies
- Framingham study 106
study
- design 427
- population 423
subchondral bone 106, 107, 115, 157 – 163, 246, 257, 260
- bone cell physiology 158, 159
- cartilage remodeling 162, 163
- cysts/cyst formation 257, 286
- erosions 257
- marker, molecular 297
- MRI 279
- osteoblasts 160 – 162
- radiography 257, 260, 261, 263
- sclerosis 115, 159, 160, 246, 260, 261, 263, 286, 316
supraspinatus tendon 148
surgical treatment of OA 48, 344 – 347, 431 – 452
- arthrodesis 447
- artificial joint arthroplasties 447
- biomedical surgery 448
- cell-transplantation 441 – 444
- cost factors 48
- debridement 432
- decrease of the loads of repair and/or degenerated cartilage 445, 446

- drilling, resection or abrasion, subchondral bone plate 433 – 435
- joint lavage 432
- osteochondral allo- and autografting techniques 435 – 437
- periosteal and perichondral resurfacing 438 – 441
- QoL 344 – 347
- resection and interpositional arthroplasties 446
syndromes/diseases (names only)
- Jansen 141, 142
- Lesch-Nyhan 144
- Marshall 139
- McKusick 141
- Milwaukee shoulder syndrome (MSS) 148, 210
- Paget's disease 102
- Perthes disease 102, 107
- Schmid 141
- Stickler 137 – 139
- Wagner 138
synovectomy 290, 365
- radiation 365
- tenosynovectomy 290
synovial/synovium
- canine synovial fibroblasts 215
- cells 127
- fluids 148, 287
- joints 1, 247
- lining proliferation 214
- markers, molecular 297
- membrane 163 – 169
- - enzymes/enzyme inhibitors 163 – 165
- - inhibitors of pro-inflammatory cytokines 168, 169
- - pro-inflammatory cytokines and nitric oxide (NO) 165 – 168
- - signaling pathways 169 – 174
- MRI of synovium 287, 288
synovitis 287, 289, 304
synthesis, articular cartilage 8
systemic treatment 359

$_3T_3$ cells, mouse 215
T_1
- relaxation 270
- T_1-weighted spin echo 272
T_2
- quantify T_2 changes 283
- relaxation 270, 271
- T_2-weighted spin echo 275
teflon-micromeshes 393
TEM (transmission electron microscopy) 212

tendinitis 148
– calcific 148
tendonitis 290
tendons
– MRI 289
– rupture 290
– supraspinatus 148
tenidap 378
tenosynovectomy 290
tenosynovitis 290
TENS /transcutaneous electrical nerve
   stimulation) 456
tetracycline 401
TGF-β (transforming growth factor) 190,
   191, 193, 194, 196, 200 – 203, 222, 394
therapy (*see* treatment)
thiols 401
(^{3}H)-thymidine incorporation 215
tibiofemoral compartment 250, 251, 261, 263
TIMPs (tissue inhibitor of metalloproteinases) 128, 164, 210, 302, 401
tissue grafts, repair 392
TNF (tumor necrosis factor)
– anti-TNF-α 398
– TNF-α 127, 128, 166, 167, 169, 172 – 174, 195,
   218, 220
– – activated signaling pathways 172 – 174
– – soluble TNF-α receptors 398
– TNF-R 167
– TNF-sR 168
tolmetin 378
TPA (tumor promoting phorbol diester)
   216, 220
– TRE (TPA response element) 220
trabecular microarchitecture 287
track and field activities 115
traction 458
tramadol hydrochloride 360
transin 219
transmission electron microscopy (TEM)
   212
trauma 44, 105
TRE (TPA response element) 220
treatment/therapy 46, 48, 149
– antisense oligonucleotide therapy 398
– basic principles in OA treatment
   356 – 370
– – goals and categories 356
– cost factor 46, 48
– gene therapy 395 – 397
– new and future therapies 387 – 402
– occupational therapy 358

– QoL 342 – 347
– – medical treatment of OA (*see there*)
   342 – 344
– – surgical treatment of OA (*see there*)
   344 – 347, 431 – 452
– physical therapy 358
– radiographic 247
– systemic treatment 359
trinucleotide repeats 143
tumor
– necrosis factor (*see* TNF)
– promoting phorbol diester (TPA) 216,
   220
twin study 143
– identical twins 143
tyrosine kinase 217

ultrasound 455
urban populations 44
uric acid 143

vibrotherapy 455
videotaping guidelines 241
viscosupplementation 362
visits, physician 45
vitreous
– of the eye 138
– tissue 138
in vitro studies 53 – 81, 377, 378, 383, 410, 412
– aceclofenac 383
– cartilage damage and repair 53 – 81
– chondrocyte cell culture 410
– cristal deposition in the OA joint
   214 – 221
– GAG synthesis 377, 378
– indomethacin 383
– tissue studies 412

water 16
weight/overweight 20, 21, 28 – 30, 33, 42, 105,
   357
Western Ontario and *McMaster* University
   OA index 336
WOMAC Osteoarthritis Index 297
wrist, radiography 249

X-linked traits 144
X-ray
– beam alignment 248
– – hip 255
– – knee 248
– diffraction 212